Editor

JOHN MARQUIS CONVERSE, M.D.

Lawrence D. Bell Professor of Plastic Surgery,
New York University School of Medicine

Assistant Editor

JOSEPH G. McCARTHY, M.D.

Associate Professor of Surgery (Plastic Surgery),
New York University School of Medicine

Editor, section on The Hand

J. WILLIAM LITTLER, M.D.

Chief of Plastic and Reconstructive Surgery,
The Roosevelt Hospital, New York City

SECOND EDITION

RECONSTRUCTIVE PLASTIC SURGERY

Principles and Procedures
in Correction, Reconstruction
and Transplantation

VOLUME TWO
FACIAL INJURIES
THE ORBIT
THE NOSE
THE CRANIUM

W. B. SAUNDERS COMPANY
Philadelphia • London • Toronto • Mexico City • Rio de Janeiro • Sydney • Tokyo

W. B. Saunders Company: West Washington Square
Philadelphia, PA 19105

1 St. Anne's Road
Eastbourne, East Sussex BN21 3UN, England

1 Goldthorne Avenue
Toronto, Ontario M8Z 5T9, Canada

Apartado 26370 — Cedro 512
Mexico 4, D.F., Mexico

Rua Coronel Cabrita, 8
Sao Cristovao Caixa Postal 21176
Rio de Janeiro, Brazil

9 Waltham Street
Artarmon, N.S.W. 2064, Australia

Ichibancho, Central Bldg., 22-1 Ichibancho
Chiyoda-Ku, Tokyo 102, Japan

Reconstructive Plastic Surgery

Complete Set	0-7216-2691-2
Volume 1	0-7216-2680-7
Volume 2	0-7216-2681-5
Volume 3	0-7216-2682-3
Volume 4	0-7216-2683-1
Volume 5	0-7216-2684-X
Volume 6	0-7216-2685-8
Volume 7	0-7216-2686-6

Last digit is the print number: 9   8

CONTRIBUTORS

TO VOLUME TWO

PHILLIP R. CASSON, M.B., F.R.C.S.

Associate Professor of Surgery (Plastic Surgery), New York University School of Medicine. Attending Surgeon, Institute of Reconstructive Plastic Surgery, New York University Medical Center; Bellevue Hospital; Manhattan Eye, Ear and Throat Hospital, and Veterans Administration Hospital, New York.

JOHN MARQUIS CONVERSE, M.D.

Lawrence D. Bell Professor of Plastic Surgery, New York University School of Medicine; Director, Institute of Reconstructive Plastic Surgery, New York University Medical Center; Director of Plastic Surgery Service, Bellevue Hospital; Consultant in Plastic Surgery, Manhattan Eye, Ear and Throat Hospital and Veterans Administration Hospital, New York.

REED O. DINGMAN, M.D., D.D.S., D.Sc.

Professor Emeritus of Surgery (Plastic Surgery), University of Michigan School of Medicine. Active Staff, University of Michigan Medical Center and St. Joseph Mercy Hospital, Ann Arbor, Michigan.

RAY E. ELLIOTT, JR., M.D.

Associate Clinical Professor of Plastic Surgery and Orthopedic Surgery (Hand), Albany Medical College. Attending Plastic Surgeon, Albany Medical Center Hospital, Albany Memorial Hospital, Albany Veterans Administration Hospital, Cohoes Memorial Hospital, and Child's Hospital, Albany, New York.

BROMLEY S. FREEMAN, M.D.

Clinical Professor of Plastic Surgery, Baylor University College of Medicine; Clinical Associate in Plastic Surgery, The University of Texas Medical School at Houston. Attending Plastic Surgeon, Methodist Hospital, St. Luke's Hospital, Heights Hospital, St. Joseph's Hospital, Memorial Baptist Hospital, Veterans Administration Hospital, Ben Taub General Hospital, and Hermann Hospital; Consultant in Plastic Surgery, Texas Children's Hospital and Diagnostic Center Hospital, Houston, Texas.

NICHOLAS G. GEORGIADE, M.D.

Chairman and Professor, Department of Surgery, Duke University Medical Center, Durham, North Carolina.

SERGE KRUPP, M.D.

Surgeon in Chief, Division of Plastic Surgery, Clinic for Plastic and Reconstructive Surgery, University of Basel, Switzerland.

v

J. J. LONGACRE, M.D., Ph.D.†

Late Associate Clinical Professor of Surgery (Plastic Surgery), University of Cincinnati College of Medicine. Attending Plastic Surgeon, Cincinnati General Hospital and Children's Hospital; Director of Plastic Surgery Department, Christ Hospital; Director of Cleft Palate and Craniofacial Clinics, Children's Hospital, Cincinnati, Ohio.

W. BRANDON MACOMBER, M.D.

Professor of Plastic and Reconstructive Surgery, Albany Medical College. Chief of Plastic Surgery, Albany Medical Center Hospital, St. Peter's Hospital, Child's Hospital, Memorial Hospital, and Veterans Administration Hospital, Albany, New York.

JOHN CLARKE MUSTARDÉ, M.B., Ch.B., D.O.M.S., F.R.C.S., F.R.C.S.(Glasg.)

Clinical Lecturer in Plastic Surgery, University of Glasgow. Consultant Plastic Surgeon, West of Scotland Plastic Surgery Unit, Canniesburn Hospital, Glasgow; Royal Hospital

BURGOS T. SAYOC, M.D.

Doctor of Medicine and Surgery, University of the Philippines. Surgeon-Director, Sayoc Eye, Ear, Nose and Throat Clinic and Hospital, Quezon City, Philippines.

WILLIAM W. SHAW, M.D.

Instructor in Surgery (Plastic Surgery), New York University School of Medicine. Assistant Attending Surgeon, Institute of Reconstructive Plastic Surgery, New York University Medical Center. Chief, Plastic Surgery, Bellevue Hospital, New York.

BYRON SMITH, M.D.

Clinical Professor of Ophthalmology, New York Medical College. Consultant in Oculoplastic Surgery, Manhattan Eye, Ear and Throat Hospital and The New York Eye-Ear Infirmary, New York.

AUGUSTUS J. VALAURI, D.D.S.

Professor of Surgery (Maxillofacial Prosthetics), New York University School of Medicine; Clinical Associate Professor of Removable Prosthodontics, New York University College of Dentistry. Chief of the Maxillofacial Prosthetics Service, Institute of Reconstructive Plastic Surgery, New York University Medical Center; Acting Chief of Dental Service, Manhattan Eye, Ear and Throat Hospital; Attending Staff, Bellevue Hospital; Consultant, Veterans Administration Hospital, New York.

DONALD WOOD-SMITH, M.B., F.R.C.S.E.

Associate Professor of Surgery (Plastic Surgery), New York University School of Medicine. Surgeon Director, Department of Plastic Surgery, Manhattan Eye, Ear and Throat Hospital; Attending Surgeon, Institute of Reconstructive Plastic Surgery, New York University Medical Center; Visiting Surgeon in Plastic Surgery, Bellevue Hospital; Attending Surgeon, Veterans Administration Hospital; Consultant, New York Eye and Ear Infirmary, New York.

†Deceased.

CONTENTS

Part Two

THE HEAD AND NECK

CHAPTER 24

THE CLINICAL MANAGEMENT OF FACIAL INJURIES AND FRACTURES OF THE FACIAL BONES

Reed O. Dingman, M.D., and John Marquis Converse, M.D.

Fractures of the Condyle
Nicholas G. Georgiade, M.D.

In the clinical management of facial injuries, it is the responsibility of the physician to restore appearance and function to the best of his ability. In some cases, however, the problems are entirely those of restoration of function, while in others the restoration of appearance is the chief indication for treatment.

Economic, sociologic, and psychologic factors operating in a competitive society make it imperative that an aggressive, expedient, and well-planned program be outlined and maintained in order to return the patient to an active productive life as soon as possible with minimal cosmetic or functional disability.

The incidence of facial injuries is high compared to injuries in other areas because the face is in an exposed position without protective covering. Although there are many etiologic agents, the automobile is responsible for a high percentage of facial injuries and deformities in the United States. In automobile accidents, injuries to the head and facial area occur in 72.1 per cent of all victims (Braunstein (1957) (Fig. 24–1). Approximately 50,000 traffic fatalities occur each year in the United States, and for every person killed, 39 require hospitalization (National Safety Council, 1975). This means over 4,000,000 persons are injured in automobile accidents in the United States each year.

Statistics on the number of injuries due to various etiologic factors are not significant. Although statistics are available in a number of series, there is wide variation in different samples due to social, economic, and geographic factors. In one series (Hagan and Huelke, 1961), the automobile was responsible for 38 per cent of all facial fractures in a highly industrial, motorized area of the Midwest, whereas in another series in Great Britain (Rowe and Killey, 1955), automobile accidents accounted for only 8 per cent of facial fractures in a

599

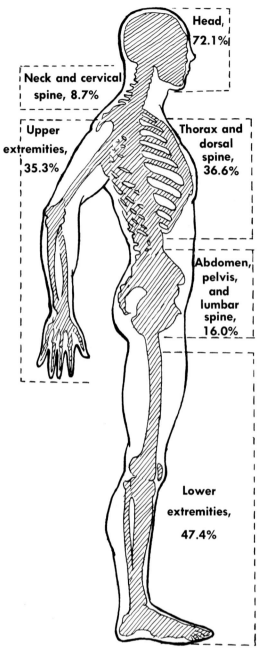

FIGURE 24–1.   Of all persons injured in automobile accidents, 72.1 per cent suffer injury to the head and facial area. All other areas are less frequently involved. (From Patterns of Disease, a publication of Parke, Davis & Co.)

crowded urban area where the social and economic conditions were such that few people used automobiles.

Although protective shoulder slings, head rests, increased padding, "packaging" of the passenger, and decreased speed limits have recently been emphasized, the automobile is here to stay, and "crash" or "crush" injuries of the face involving soft and hard tissues will continue to be a challenge to the plastic surgeon's skill.

Injuries Other Than Automotive

Industrial accidents involve over 2,000,000 persons annually. Most accidents occur in the home, involving over 4,000,000 disabling injuries a year. Dog bites, which often involve the face, are frequent, particularly in children, as a result of the increasing canine population. Athletic injuries of various types involve the face. Military conflicts are the source of the most severe injuries, ballistic missiles disrupting the soft and hard tissues of the face. The popularity of the motorcycle has added another etiologic factor in the causation of facial injuries.

TIMING OF TREATMENT

Timing is especially important in the optimum management of facial injuries. It is axiomatic that soft tissue and bone injuries in the facial area be taken care of as soon as is consistent with the patient's general condition. Early skillful management decreases the possibility of permanent facial disfigurement and serious functional disturbances. It should be kept in mind, however, that facial soft tissue and bone injuries are rarely acute surgical emergencies as far as closure of the wounds or reduction of fractures is concerned. In patients who obviously are losing significant amounts of blood or are in a state of impending shock, bleeding should be controlled and other measures should be instituted to prevent or treat shock and to establish a satisfactory airway.

Facial injuries may be associated with life-threatening lesions; treatment of multiple systemic injuries should take precedence over management of facial wounds. After the airway is cleared, hemorrhage controlled, and measures instituted to control shock, a careful neurologic evaluation is made to rule out intracranial hemorrhage or traumatic lesions of the central nervous system. Damaged or ruptured viscera in the thoracic or abdominal cavity or in the pelvis may endanger life, and every effort should be made to detect and manage these problems before spending valuable time suturing facial lacerations or reducing fractures of the facial bones.

In emergencies, facial lacerations may be quickly sutured by tacking the margins together with a few well-placed sutures. If such a procedure is contraindicated because of the patient's general condition, simply covering the wounds with sterile dressings and applying light pressure will control the bleeding and protect them until it is feasible to achieve definitive closure.

Facial fractures, if they are seen early and if the patient's general condition warrants, may be reduced immediately. When a patient is seen several hours after an accident, the exact condition may be obscured by extensive edema and hematoma in the soft tissue, and delay of treatment is indicated. In these cases, it is best to wait a few days until most of the edema subsides before undertaking reduction and fixation of facial fractures. If it is necessary to defer reduction because of the patient's poor general condition, fractures may be reduced one to three or more weeks later. Fractures treated late may require open reduction, removal of organized tissue from the fracture site, or an osteotomy; nevertheless, fractures can be successfully treated after periods of considerable delay.

EMERGENCY TREATMENT

Establishment and control of the airway is the primary and most important consideration in the clinical management of the acutely injured patient. Asphyxia is a real danger in patients with injuries to the lower jaw or laryngeal region. The mouth should be cleared of broken teeth, clots, dentures, or foreign bodies that might be causing obstruction. Traction on the mandible will pull the tongue and floor of the mouth forward in displaced fractures of the anterior portion of the body of the mandible, in which the tongue falls back into the pharynx. Protraction of the tongue with a suture (Fig. 24–2), towel clip, or forceps may avert asphyxia. Placing the patient in a prone or a sitting position with the head down and forward is helpful in keeping the airway free of mucus and blood. The tongue is displaced forward by gravity, and secretions flow readily from the mouth.

Airway

Emergency Tracheotomy. When tongue protraction and clearing of the oral and pharyngeal airway do not relieve restlessness, air hunger, cyanosis, tracheal tug, retraction of the supraclavicular fossa, or retraction of the intercostal spaces and epigastrium, emergency tracheal intubation or tracheotomy is indicated.

In extremely urgent cases, when nasal or oral tracheal intubation is not feasible, the patient is

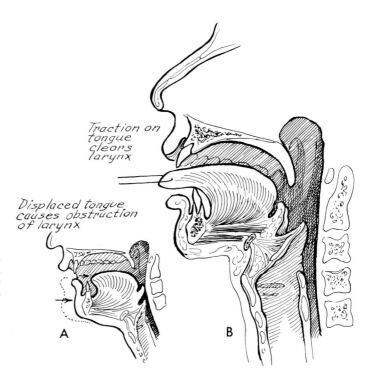

FIGURE 24–2. Relief of respiratory obstruction by protraction of the tongue. *A,* Backward displacement of the tongue causes obstruction of the larynx. *B,* Protraction of the tongue clears the larynx.

placed on the floor or a table with the shoulders supported and the head extended and fixed. A coniotomy is done by incising transversely through the skin and the cricothyroid ligament (conic ligament) between the thyroid and cricoid cartilages (Fig. 24–3).

An emergency low tracheotomy may be done in the following manner: The trachea is grasped between the fingers and the thumb; an incision is made quickly through the skin in the midline between thyroid cartilage and the sternal notch' into the trachea, preferably below the cricoid cartilage; and a cannula, catheter, endotracheal tube, or tracheostomy tube is inserted to keep the opening patent.

Elective Tracheotomy. Early tracheotomy may be a life-saving measure in patients in whom the floor of the mouth, tongue, and hypopharynx become increasingly edematous and interfere with the airway. It should be performed routinely in patients with severe facial fractures associated with intracranial injuries. In some instances, the patient seems to have an adequate airway but maintains it only by sheer effort; he will be more comfortable and recover more quickly if an airway is established by means of a tracheotomy. The tracheal opening, in addition, provides a route by which general anesthesia may be administered. In cases in which it is necessary to pack the nose and to wire the teeth in occlusion to maintain the reduced position of the facial bones, tracheotomy is invaluable in maintaining an adequate airway postoperatively. The tracheostomy tube may usually be removed in

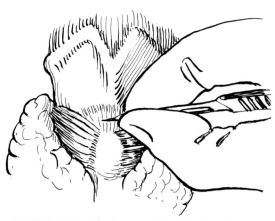

FIGURE 24–3. Coniotomy. The cricothyroid membrane is cut transversely. The direction of the fibers favors opening of the wound to provide an airway. A short protective grip on the knife blade will prevent cutting too deeply and avoid the complication of acute tracheoesophageal fistula.

three to five days as the airway improves with subsidence of the edema.

Every surgeon who treats patients with severely injured facial structures should be well versed in the indications, technique, care, and complications of tracheotomy. Tracheotomy should preferably be an elective procedure, and as soon as any member of the surgical team feels that a tracheotomy is indicated, it should be done without delay. It is difficult to perform a tracheotomy as an emergency procedure at the patient's bedside. Delay of tracheotomy may result in death; on the other hand, if it is done hurriedly as an emergency measure, it may result in surgical complications.

Indications for Tracheotomy

1. Unrelievable obstruction of the airway in the region of the larynx or hypopharynx.

2. The probability of edema that might result in serious decrease of the airway above the larynx.

3. Intracranial injuries with difficulty in maintaining adequate ventilation by normal reflex activity or tracheal intubation.

4. Chest or high spinal cord injuries with loss of normal cough reflexes to clear the bronchial tree of fluids, blood, or secretions.

5. The possibility of prolonged postoperative airway problems.

Techniques of Tracheotomy

CONIOTOMY. This procedure is useful in extreme emergencies when time is of the essence. Coniotomy is performed by making a stab wound or passing a large-bore needle through the cricothyroid membranes (conus elasticus); although not recommended as a routine procedure, the coniotomy may be employed as a life-saving measure (Fig. 24–3). The cricothyroid membrane lies superficially, and the overlying tissues are relatively avascular. When there is sufficient time to do an elective procedure, or when it is a semi-urgent situation under satisfactory conditions, the low tracheotomy is the operation of choice.

LOW TRACHEOTOMY. The low tracheotomy is made below the thyroid isthmus. The opening is generally made between the second and third or between the third and fourth tracheal rings. (See Technique of Elective Tracheotomy).

POSITIONING OF THE PATIENT. The patient should be placed in the dorsal recumbent position with the shoulders elevated (Fig. 24–4). The neck is extended as much as possible so as to bring the trachea into proper relationship

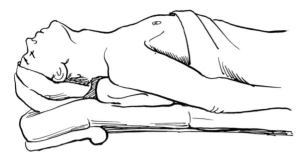

FIGURE 24–4. Tracheotomy is most easily done with the patient in the dorsal recumbent position with his shoulders elevated and head extended.

for entry. This is especially important in the short, fat, bull neck type of patient with heavy musculature. In these patients it is difficult, at best, to penetrate the surrounding soft tissue to enter the trachea.

ANESTHESIA. In the average patient, tracheotomy is relatively easy. The procedure can be done successfully under local anesthesia by infiltrating the skin and deep structures down to the tracheal level. Infiltration of the tissues with local anesthetic solution containing epinephrine (1:100,000) will permit operation with comfort to the patient. A minimum amount of bleeding from small vessels occurs if the operation is deferred for a few minutes after injection of the anesthetic solution.

The operation may be done under general anesthesia when indicated. Endotracheal intubation is desirable. When the tracheal opening is complete, the endotracheal tube is retracted to the level of the tracheal opening, the tracheostomy tube is immediately inserted and the inner trochar removed. The anesthetic agent can then be administered through the tracheostomy opening if indicated.

Technique of Elective Tracheotomy. The elective operation is performed through a 5-cm transverse incision about 2 cm above the suprasternal notch (Fig. 24–5, *A*). The incision should be planned to be directly over the tracheal opening. If possible, the incision line should be planned and marked with ink in the semireclining or sitting patient. This will assure one of making the skin incision directly over the tracheal opening and avoid irritation of the skin, dislodgment of the tube, or tension of the skin against the tube.

The incision is extended through the skin and subcutaneous tissues to the superficial fascia of the neck. Veins that may bleed should be clamped and ligated. The dissection in the

midline should be made either by blunt dissection with scissors or by sharp dissection (Fig. 24–5, *B*). The isthmus of the thyroid may be encountered after separation of the strap muscles of the neck; if it cannot be conveniently retracted, the isthmus is incised in a vertical direction. Large veins crossing the midline at the level of the tracheostomy may be retracted or divided and ligated. The deep fascia overlying

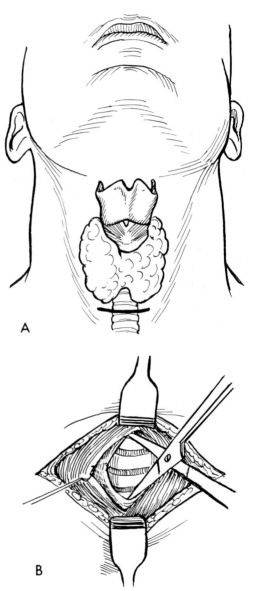

A

B

FIGURE 24–5. Exposure of the trachea for tracheotomy. *A,* A 5-cm transverse incision about 2 cm above the sternal notch provides excellent exposure and results in minimal postoperative scar. The incision is extended to the superficial fascia of the neck. *B,* Dissection through the superficial fascia to the trachea is accomplished by blunt dissection with scissors.

the trachea comes into view, and the glistening cartilages are easily identified. The lower-most portion of the larynx is palpated, and the cricoid cartilage immediately below is identified. A sharp hook on each side of the trachea raises it into position for incision. The hooks securely engaged in the tissues stabilize the trachea for incision. Care in placing the hooks avoids rotation of the trachea. The opening may inadvertently be made off the midline unless care is exercised. The tracheal incision (Fig. 24–6, *A*) is made in the midline through the third and fourth tracheal rings, cutting upward with the knife so as to avoid cutting the transverse communicating veins. Guiding the depth of the incision with the finger will prevent tracheoesophageal fistula, especially in children.

Opinion varies regarding the need for removal of portions of tracheal rings. Many surgeons make a cruciate incision involving two rings in a vertical direction and a transverse limb between the tracheal rings. The cruciate incision offers exposure for the tracheostomy tube, which is anticipated to remain in place two to five days. When the tracheostomy must be maintained for a longer period, a section of the tracheal rings may be excised to provide a more easily maintained opening.

Some surgeons favor a vertical skin incision, feeling that under emergency circumstances quicker access can be obtained through a vertical incision than through a horizontal incision. We mention the vertical incision only to condemn it. The resultant scar is often objectionable and difficult to correct secondarily. Even under emergency circumstances, a transverse incision will give excellent exposure and in most cases will heal spontaneously without leaving an objectionable scar. Revision, if necessary, is accomplished successfully if the original incision has been made transversely.

A tracheostomy tube of adequate diameter and length with the trochar in place must be carefully inserted under direct vision (Fig. 24–6, *B*). Tracheostomy tubes have been inadvertently placed in the fascial space of the neck alongside or in front of the trachea (Fig. 24–7). If the tracheostomy tube is too long, it may irritate the carina or penetrate into one of the main stem bronchi (Fig. 24–8). If the tube is curved too acutely, it may erode the anterior surface of the trachea or cause necrosis of the "party wall" and result in a tracheoesophageal fistula. Semiflexible silicone tracheostomy tubes cause less irritation and are less liable to result in complications than metal tubes.

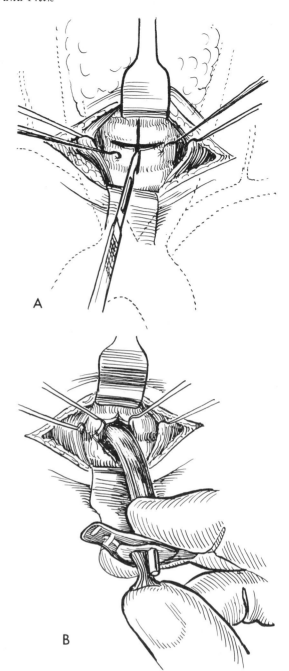

A

B

FIGURE 24–6. Opening the trachea and inserting the tracheostomy tube. *A*, The trachea is stabilized by tissue hooks to prevent rotation. A cruciate incision is made through two tracheal rings and is extended laterally for an equal distance between the cut tracheal rings. *B*, Retraction of incised cartilage edges and insertion of the tracheostomy tube.

After the tube has been inserted, it can be secured to the cervical skin by means of sutures, especially if the anesthesiologist's tube is to be attached (Fig. 24–9). It can be secured at the end of the operation by means of fabric

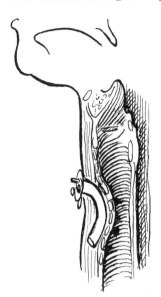

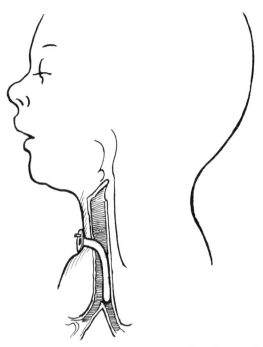

FIGURE 24–7. Blind intubation may result in failure to place the tracheostomy tube inside the trachea. The tube should be inserted under direct vision to avoid this complication.

FIGURE 24–8. A tracheostomy tube of excessive length or curvature may irritate the carina or cause erosion of the wall between the trachea and esophagus. This complication is most likely to occur in children.

tape tied around the neck (Fig. 24–10). The fixation must be secure so that the tube cannot be dislodged from the trachea when the patient coughs or moves the neck. Blood and secretions are carefully aspirated from the trachea.

After insertion of the tracheostomy tube, the wound should not be allowed to close so tightly that air will have difficulty in escaping around the tube proper. If the skin is closed tightly, trapped air may pass along the fascial planes of the face and neck, resulting in troublesome subcutaneous emphysema. The wound is sutured loosely, leaving it funnel-shaped outwardly (Fig. 24–10, *A*), so that air cannot be trapped in the subcutaneous tissues and fascial spaces.

POSTOPERATIVE CARE. Postoperative care of tracheostomy patients requires diligence, imagination, and enthusiasm. It is distressing to see a patient unable to make his wants known, with a tracheostomy tube partially plugged by mucus and crust and a dirty, infected wound and macerated skin about the area of tracheostomy.

The tracheostomy tube should be aspirated frequently with a sterile, disposable catheter to remove mucus, blood, and secretions (Fig. 24–11). The wound should be well protected with gauze dressings changed as frequently as necessary to keep it dry and clean.

The tracheotomized patient is unable to speak. A pad of paper and a pencil at the bed-side for adults are helpful in maintaining communication and give the patient a sense of security.

Humidified oxygen administered through a cuff over the tracheostomy stoma is routinely ordered. Humidification prevents drying of the respiratory mucosa, moistens the gases passing into the bronchi, and facilitates the removal of secretions.

Particular attention should also be paid to in-

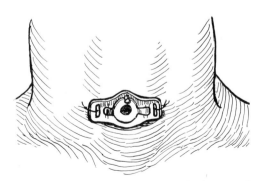

FIGURE 24–9. The tracheostomy tube is secured to the skin of the neck with sutures if general anesthesia is to be administered through the tube; this will prevent dislodgment of the tube during the course of the anesthesia.

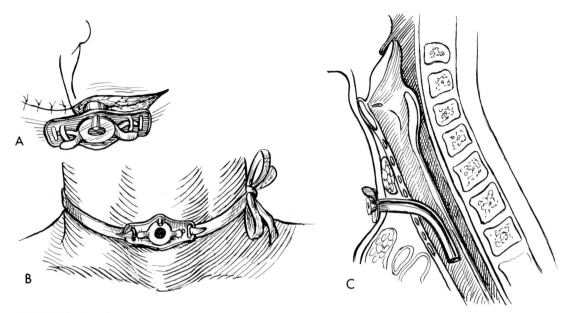

FIGURE 24–10. Closure of the tracheostomy wound and securing of the tube to the neck. *A,* The wound is closed loosely in layers in a conical fashion from below upward to the skin. A tight closure may result in subcutaneous emphysema of the neck. *B,* Fabric tape tied loosely at the side of the neck prevents the dislodgment of the tube and is easily changed when soiled. *C,* The tracheostomy tube lies freely in the trachea without tension and occupies approximately one-half the diameter of the trachea.

termittently deflating the balloon of the cuffed tracheostomy tubes. If the tube has double balloons, they should be alternately inflated. Such care will prevent continuous mucosal pressure and the development of tracheal erosion and tracheoesophageal fistulas.

Complications of Tracheotomy. This seemingly simple, safe operative procedure is not without certain avoidable hazards and complications.

OPERATIVE COMPLICATIONS
1. Severe hemorrhage from vessels of the

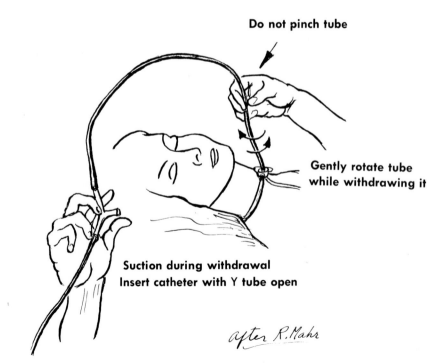

FIGURE 24–11. Care in use of the aspiration tube gives the best results with minimal irritation.

neck. This may be difficult to control if exposure is inadequate.

2. Inadvertent damage of the cricoid cartilage.

3. Acute tracheoesophageal fistula caused by cutting through the tracheoesophageal wall because of inadequate exposure and vision. This happens most often in children.

4. Pneumothorax due to damage of the apex of the pleura of one or both lungs.

5. Hemorrhage from the innominate artery or anomalous median thyroid artery.

POSTOPERATIVE COMPLICATIONS

1. Secondary hemorrhage.
2. Subcutaneous emphysema.
3. Dislodging of the tracheostomy tube.
4. Reinsertion of tube outside the trachea.
5. Wound infection.
6. Erosion of the trachea.
7. Tracheoesophageal fistula.
8. Aerophagia. This may result in distressing abdominal distention, gastrointestinal atony, paralytic ileus, and death.
9. Recurrent obstruction from blood, mucus, and purulent materials in the tube.
10. Ulcerative tracheobronchitis.
11. Lung abscess.

DELAYED SECONDARY COMPLICATIONS

1. Unsightly scar formation.
2. Adherence of the skin to the trachea.
3. Sloughing of tracheal cartilage with tracheal atresia.
4. Persistent tracheocutaneous fistula following long-standing tracheostomy.

The Control of Severe Hemorrhage in Facial Wounds

Lacerations and crush injuries of the facial region may result in near exsanguinating hemorrhage. Methods of control include local pressure with dressings, clamping and ligating large vessels, packing wounds with gauze or hemostatic materials, posterior nasal tamponade, and packing the nasal cavity, sinuses, and palate lacerations (Fig. 24–12). The packs may be removed gradually in two or three days or as soon as the patient's general condition improves sufficiently to permit delayed repair. Approximation of the wound edges with a few well-placed sutures will often control bleeding. Careful final suturing can be accomplished

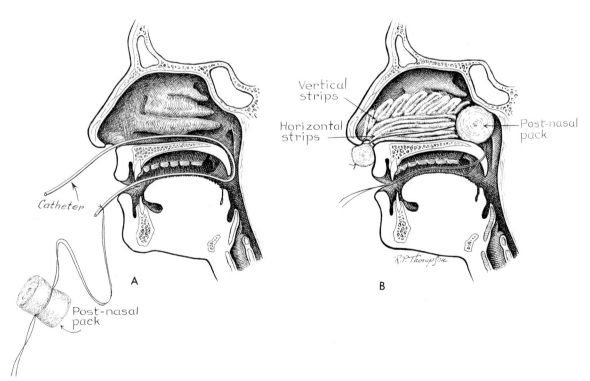

FIGURE 24–12. Technique of packing for the arrest of severe nasal hemorrhage. *A,* The nasal pack is guided into the nasopharynx by a suture attached to a rubber catheter. *B,* With the postnasal pack in place, the lower part of the nasal cavity is packed with horizontal strips, the upper part with vertical strips of gauze. Packs placed in this manner are easiest to remove. (From Kazanjian and Converse.)

later. External carotid ligation is rarely necessary to control bleeding from facial wounds.

Secondary bleeding is not frequently a problem in facial wound management but will respond to the methods mentioned for acute traumatic bleeding. Evaluation of circulating blood volume with replacement therapy if indicated should be done if blood loss has been significant. The patient may swallow several hundred milliliters of blood from severe nasal, oral, or pharyngeal bleeding. Frequent swallowing motions and epigastric distention may give a clue to this type of bleeding. Near exsanguinating hemorrhage may go unrecognized in patients who have persistently swallowed blood.

Prevention and Control of Shock

Impending shock or its presence is frequently noted in association with severe facial trauma. Pallor and clamminess of the skin, depressed blood pressure, feeble rapid pulse, shallow respiration, restlessness, anxiety, and disorientation or unconsciousness are signs of acute peripheral circulatory failure due to derangement of circulatory control or loss of circulating fluid secondary to injury.

Intravenous blood, colloids, electrolytes, and fluid replacement are given as indicated. Positioning of the patient with head down and feet up, sedation, pain relief, and control of hemorrhage is indicated in impending shock or in shock.

PLANNING OF TREATMENT

Because of the complexity of facial injuries in patients with multisystem injuries, the team approach to the management of severe facial injuries has become popular in centers in which specialists in various disciplines are available. The overall plan should be coordinated by the surgeon in charge but should be devised with the cooperation of the neurosurgeon, ophthalmologist, otolaryngologist, and dental, orthopedic, and oral surgeons when their services contribute to the achievement of a satisfactory result. When all of the information and suggestions are available, the surgeon in charge should make the final decisions regarding treatment and see that the plan is executed with skill and expediency.

Clinical Examination

Careful clinical examination is indicated, even if the patient has only minor superficial wounds. These may be abrasions, contusions, or lacerations without evidence of any underlying bone damage. Lesions that appear to be inconsequential may result in a disfiguring scar or dysfunction if not adequately managed. Careful cleansing of the wound, debridement when necessary, and meticulous suturing may prevent conspicuous permanent deformity. Facial lacerations may extend into the eyes, nose, ears, or cranial cavity and may be associated with severe chest, spinal, abdominal, or extremity injuries. Concomitant injuries may require immediate, life-saving treatment, but when the patient is in reasonably good condition, the treatment of facial injuries can be undertaken concurrently with management of injuries in other parts of the body, without the need for an additional operative session and anesthesia.

Classification of the Injury. Wounds of the face and cranium may be classified into three categories: (1) wounds of soft tissue alone; (2) wounds of soft tissue associated with fractures; and (3) fractures without a soft tissue wound.

The soft tissue injury may be a clean, sharp laceration, a laceration with contusion, an abraded wound, a contused wound, an avulsed wound, a puncture wound, a gunshot wound, or a burn wound.

Bone injury is suggested by ecchymosis, edema, or superficial contusion or abrasion over a bony prominence. Subconjunctival hemorrhage with ecchymosis and edema in the region of the orbit suggests fracture of the nasal bones, zygoma, or frontal bone. Ecchymotic and contused tissues over the anterolateral surface of the mandible suggest fracture of the mandible.

Fractures of the facial bones may be diagnosed on the basis of malocclusion of the teeth or open bite deformity due to displacement of the maxilla or mandible. Functional disability suggests fracture of the mandibular condyle, and trismus may be caused by fracture of the zygoma or angle of the mandible. Unequal pupil levels and diplopia are indicative of zygomatic or maxillary fractures.

Bimanual palpation (Fig. 24–13) of the supraorbital, lateral, and infraorbital margins may reveal asymmetry indicating fracture of the maxilla. Fractured nasal bones are diagnosed by tenderness, irregularity, mobility, and crepi-

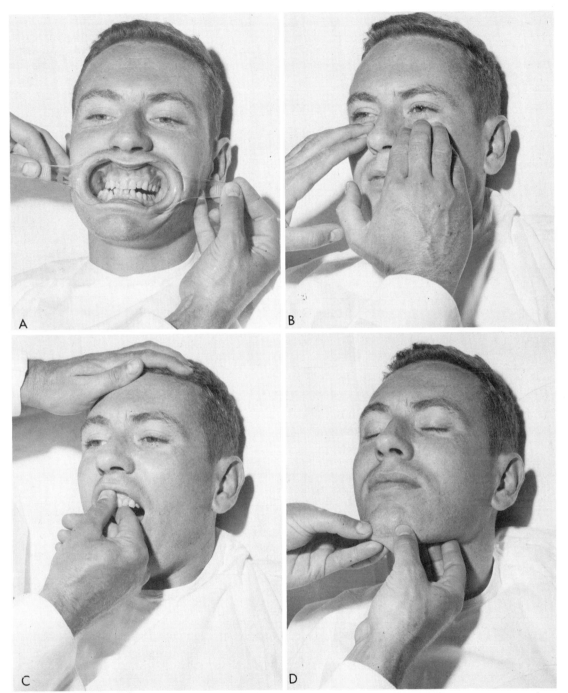

FIGURE 24–13. Clinical signs are helpful in the diagnosis of jaw fractures. *A*, Deviations from normal occlusion and open bite deformity are strongly presumptive of fracture of the mandible. *B*, Comparative bimanual palpation of the bony prominences of the facial skeleton may reveal irregularities which suggest fracture. *C*, In maxillary fracture, movement of the parts usually can be produced by manipulation of the anterior maxillary structures. *D*, Fractures of the body of the mandible with displacement may be detected by palpation of the inferior border of the mandible or by passing the finger intraorally over the mucosa covering the alveolar bone.

tation on digital palpation. Mobility of the middle third of the face when the maxillary anterior teeth are grasped between the fingers and pressure is applied indicates pyramidal fractures (Le Fort II) of the maxilla and middle third of the face or craniofacial disjunction (Le Fort III). Bleeding from the nose may indicate nasal or septal injuries. Fractures of the body of the mandible can be detected by supporting the angle of the mandible and applying up and down manual pressure on the anterior portion of the mandible. Instability and crepitation may be noted when performing this maneuver.

When seen several hours following the injury, fractures may be difficult to diagnose clinically because of facial asymmetry from extensive edema or subcutaneous hematoma. In crushing injuries, associated basilar skull fractures and cribriform plate fractures should be suspected in the presence of cerebrospinal rhinorrhea, bleeding from the ears, paralysis of one or more of the cranial nerves, unconsciousness, unequal pupils, paralysis of one or more extremities, abnormal neurologic reflexes, convulsions, delirium, and irrational behavior.

Roentgenographic Evaluation

Roentgenograms are indispensable in the evaluation of a patient with head and face injuries. Complete cranial and facial bone roentgenograms should be obtained when indicated. Stereoscopic views are desirable, and tomograms may be useful in demonstrating fractures in the region of the mandibular condyle, blowout fractures in the orbital floor, orbital walls, deep orbital region, or cranial base (Fig. 24–14).

Roentgenographic evaluation may be the most important single diagnostic aid. Even though the clinical evaluation may demonstrate obvious fractures and suggest a standard type of management, thorough roentgenographic examination should be made. It may be quite obvious, for example, that a patient has a fracture through the premolar region of the mandible on one side with mild malocclusion. It would be reasonable to apply rubber band traction or intermaxillary fixation to bring the teeth into occlusion.

Roentgenographic examination, however, may demonstrate a fracture of the condyle of the mandible on the opposite side. Even though the plan of treatment would be the

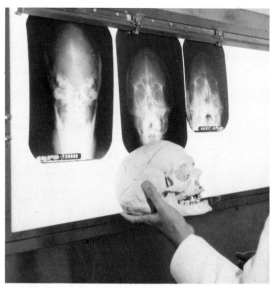

FIGURE 24–14. Examination of a skull is helpful in the interpretation of facial bone roentgenograms.

same, the presence of the fracture should be known to the surgeon and to the patient.

Because of the high incidence of litigation arising from injuries, it is of prime importance to have thorough roentgenographic evaluation of all facial bone injuries. The legal position of the physician who treats injuries of this type without adequate roentgenographic examination may be in jeopardy.

In most instances, roentgenographic evaluation is only one of the means of establishing a diagnosis of fracture. In many cases, however, the roentgenogram provides the only evidence of a fracture. Clinically inherent limitations for demonstrating facial bone fractures by radiography are recognized. The extent and amount of displacement of the fragments is difficult to determine by roentgenography alone. In many views the fracture is partially or totally obscured by overlying or superimposed bone structures of the face, skull, or spine. The total clinical picture, in most cases, is more serious than might be suspected from cursory evaluation of the roentgenographic evidence alone.

Facial bone fractures are not infrequently associated with fractures of the skull or fracture-dislocation of the cervical spine. These structures should be included as part of the total evaluation. If the cervical spine is not demonstrated adequately by the routine views, separate roentgenograms of the cervical spine should be taken, inasmuch as fractures or dislocations of the cervical spine occur in association with severe facial injuries.

The standard routine views of the spine, mandible, and skull are generally adequate. The most valuable and most often employed views are the anteroposterior and lateral views of the mandible, detailed tomograms of the temporomandibular joints, and the facial bone studies, including the Caldwell and Waters views, which are the best to show fractures of the orbit, zygoma, and nasal bones. Fractures of the alveolar structures of the maxilla and mandible, including the teeth, are shown by detailed dental or occlusal views. Soft tissue profile views show edema accompanying the fractures. Occlusal views may be helpful in delineating fractures of the anterior maxillary and mandibular areas. Tomographic roentgenograms of the temporomandibular joints are useful in determining injury to the condyle and joint structures. Blowout fractures of the floor of the orbit and fractures in the region of the cribriform plate and base of the skull are best demonstrated by tomographic techniques.

ROENTGENOGRAPHIC POSITIONS

It is unnecessary for the surgeon to possess a detailed knowledge of roentgenographic techniques, but an understanding of the commonly employed roentgenographic projections will aid in the evaluation and interpretation of the roentgenograms. The roentgenographic views most helpful and informative in the diagnosis and management of fractures of the facial bones are demonstrated and briefly discussed in the following paragraphs.

The Waters Position. The posteroanterior projection is employed for an oblique anterior view of the upper facial bones; the orbits, the malar bones, and the zygomatic arches are well shown. This view is helpful in the diagnosis of fractures of the maxilla and maxillary sinuses, the orbital floor and infraorbital rim, the zygomatic bone and zygomatic arches, and to a lesser extent the nasal bones and nasal process of the maxilla (Fig. 24–15, *A, B*).

The Caldwell Position. The posteroanterior projection is primarily used for demonstration of the frontal sinuses and the anterior ethmoidal cells. The orbital margin, zygomaticofrontal suture, lateral walls of the maxillary sinuses, the petrous ridges, and the mandibular rami are also demonstrated in this projection (Fig. 24–16, *A, B*).

The Fronto-Occipital Anteroposterior Projection. This view is used when injuries prevent examination of the facial bones with the patient in a prone or seated position. This projection gives a satisfactory view of the orbits, lesser and greater wings of the sphenoid, frontal bone, frontal and ethmoidal sinuses, nasal septum, floor of the nose, hard palate, man-

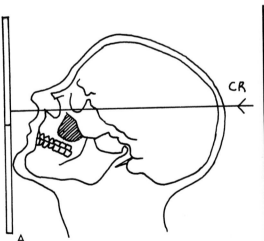
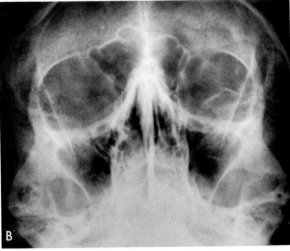

FIGURE 24–15. Waters position. Posterior-anterior view for visualization of maxillary sinuses, maxilla, orbits, and zygomatic arches. This projection may also be helpful in demonstrating fractures of the nasal bones and nasal processes of the maxilla. In this view the petrous ridges are projected just below the floors of the maxillary sinuses. *A*, Position of the patient in relation to the film and the central ray. *B*, Waters view showing internal wire suspension for fixation in fractures of the middle third of the face. (The drawings in Figures 24–15 to 24–38 are reproduced with modifications from the chapter by J. Zizmor in Kazanjian and Converse.)

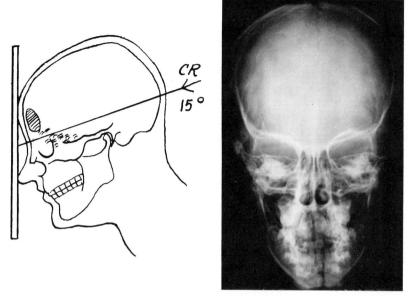

FIGURE 24-16.   Caldwell position. Posterior-anterior view of the skull. This position is used to study fractures of the frontal bone, orbital margins, zygomaticofrontal sutures, and lateral walls of the maxillary sinuses. The paranasal sinuses are shown in this projection. The petrous ridges are shown at a level between the lower and middle thirds of the orbits.

dibule, and upper and lower dental arches (Fig. 24-17, *A*, *B*).

The Reverse Waters Position. The mento-occipital position is also used to demonstrate the facial bones when the patient cannot be placed in a prone position. This projection is used to demonstrate fractures of the orbits, maxillary sinuses, zygomatic bones, and zygomatic arches. The increased part-film distance magnifies the upper facial structures, but otherwise the film is similar to that obtained with the Waters position (Fig. 24-18, *A*, *B*, *C*).

The Optic Foramen—Oblique Orbital Position. This view is best demonstrated with

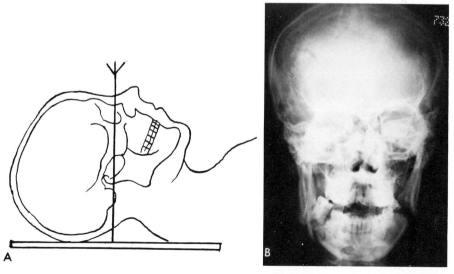

FIGURE 24-17.   The fronto-occipital anterior-posterior projection. When injuries prevent positioning the patient in the prone or seated posterior-anterior position, this position or the reverse Waters projection may be used. *A*, The examination is made with the patient in the dorsal recumbent position. *B*, Bilateral mandibular fractures demonstrated with the fronto-occipital anterior-posterior projection.

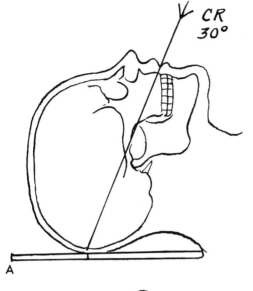

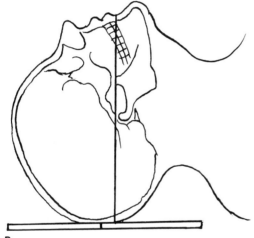

FIGURE 24–18. The reverse Waters position. *A, B,* The mento-occipital position or reverse Waters projection is a view of the facial bones similar to the Waters view except for greater magnification of the facial bones due to the increased distance between the face and the film. *C,* Fractures of the orbits, maxillary sinuses, zygomatic bones, and zygomatic arches are well shown.

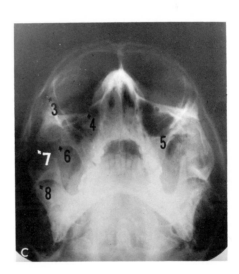

stereoscopic projections and shows the optic foramen and its relationship to the posterior ethmoidal and sphenoidal sinuses. It also shows the lateral wall of the frontal sinuses, the vertical plate of the frontal bone, and the roof and lateral wall of the dependent orbit. Under a bright spotlight the lateral wall of the opposite orbit may be clearly defined (Fig. 24–19).

The Semi-axial (Superoinferior) Projection (Titterington Position). The zygomatic arches, the facial bones, and orbits are well shown in this projection (Fig. 24–20).

The Lateral Anterior Projection (Fuchs Position). This projection gives an oblique view of the zygomatic arch projected free of superimposed structures. The lateral wall of the

maxillary sinus is also well shown in this view (Fig. 24–21).

Lateral and Profile View of the Face. Stereoscopic projections are usually made of this view because of the complexity of the superimposed shadows of the face. This projection demonstrates the lateral profile of the facial bones and soft tissues of the face. This study is important in evaluation of maxillary-mandibular relationships and fractures of the vertical plate of the frontal bone (Fig. 24–22, *A, B*).

Nasal Bones, Lateral Views. This projection gives a detailed view of the nasal bones of the side nearest the film and of the soft structures of the nose. Both sides should be examined

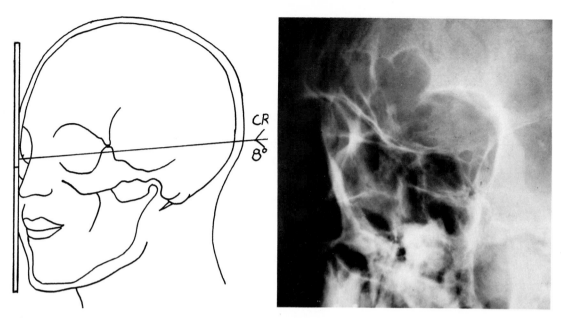

FIGURE 24–19. Optic foramen—oblique orbital position. The oblique posterior-anterior view of the facial bones shows the optic foramen in the lower inferior quadrant of the orbit in relation to the posterior ethmoid and sphenoid sinuses. Fractures, malformations, and tumors of the orbit or optic foramen are best studied in this view.

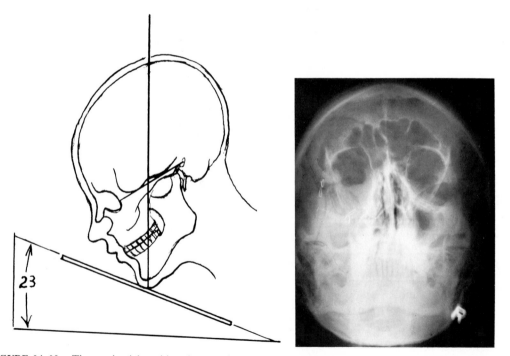

FIGURE 24–20. The semi-axial position, known also as the Titterington position. This projection is helpful in the study of fractures of the zygomatic arches, lateral walls of the maxilla, orbital floors, and orbital margins. The maxillary sinuses, ethmoid and frontal sinuses, and inferior border of the mandible are well shown in this projection.

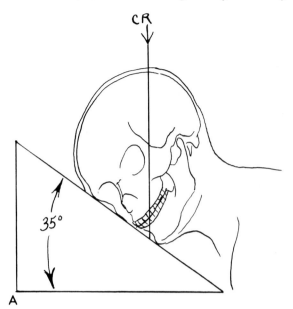

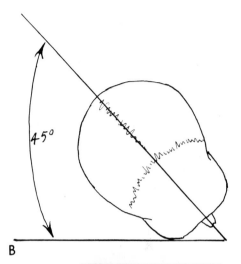

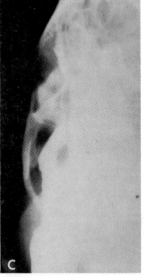

FIGURE 24–21. *A, B,* The lateral anterior projection gives an excellent view of the zygomatic arch projected free of superimposed structures. Fractures of the lateral wall of the maxillary sinus may also be studied in this view. *C,* Fractures of the zygomatic arch are demonstrated by the lateral anterior projection.

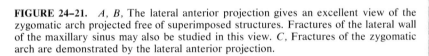

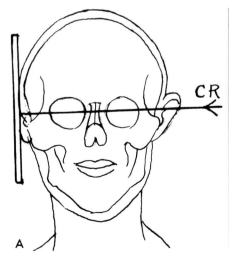

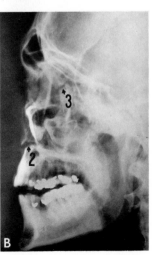

FIGURE 24–22. Lateral and profile view of the face. This view is helpful in the study of fractures of the frontal sinuses, the lateral walls of the orbit, the maxilla, and the mandible. *A,* Position of part to film. *B,* Lateral profile view of the face demonstrating fractures of the zygomaticofrontal suture (3) and the maxilla at the level of the nasal floor (2).

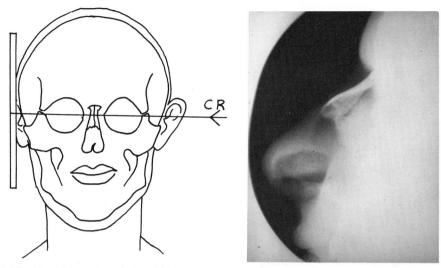

FIGURE 24-23. Nasal bones, lateral view. This projection provides a detailed view of the nasal bone nearest the side of the film. Views from both sides are helpful in the study of fractures of the nasal bones, anterior nasal spine, and nasal processes of the maxilla.

radiographically. One view with this projection should be made with intensifying screens to show the frontal sinuses. Fractures of the nasal bones, the anterior nasal spine and the nasal processes of the maxilla are demonstrated in this view (Fig. 24–23).

Nasal Bones, Axial Projection. The axial superoinferior view of the nasal bones is used to demonstrate medial or lateral displacement of the bony fragments which are not demonstrated on lateral views. The thin nasal bones do not have sufficient body to cast a shadow through the superimposed frontal bone or the anterior maxillary structures. This view demonstrates only those portions of the nasal bones which project beyond a line anterior to the glabella and upper incisor teeth. The view

is not helpful in children or adults who have short nasal bones, concave face, or protruding maxillary teeth (Fig. 24–24).

Superoinferior Occlusal Views of the Hard Palate. Fractures of the hard palate area may be demonstrated by occlusal views with superoinferior projections with the X-ray tube focused and angled to demonstrate the area of interest.

Superoinferior Central Occlusal View of the Hard Palate. This demonstrates the palatine processes of the maxilla and the horizontal plates of the palatine bones and the entire dental arch (Fig. 24–15, *A* to *C*).

Superoinferior Anterior Occlusal View of the Hard Palate. This projection

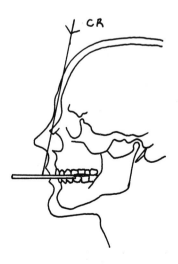

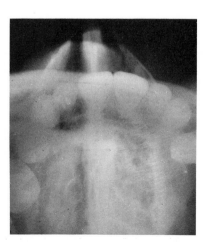

FIGURE 24-24. Nasal bones, axial projection. Superoinferior projection of the nasal bones. This axial view of the nasal bones may reveal fractures with medial or lateral displacement which are not demonstrated on lateral views. Only those portions of the nasal bones that project anteriorly to the line between the glabella and the upper incisor teeth can be demonstrated in this projection. This view is not helpful in the examination of children or adults having relatively small or depressed nasal bones and projecting upper teeth or forehead.

gives a view of the anterior part of the hard palate, the alveolar process, and the upper incisor teeth in greater bony detail than the previous view because the obliquely focused central ray does not penetrate any superimposed bony structures (Fig. 24–26).

OBLIQUE SUPEROINFERIOR POSTERIOR OCCLUSAL VIEW OF THE HARD PALATE. This projection gives an oblique occlusal view of the posterior part of the hard palate unilaterally and the alveolar process and all of the teeth on the upper quandrant of the maxilla.

Fractures of the teeth or alveolar process may be demonstrated by this view (Fig. 24–27).

Submentovertex and Verticosubmental Positions for the Base of the Skull (Fig. 24–28). These views give an axial projection of the mandible, the coronoid and condyloid processes of the rami of the mandible, the zygomatic arches, the base of the skull and its foramina, the petrous pyramid, the sphenoidal, posterior ethmoid, and maxillary sinuses, and the bony nasal septum.

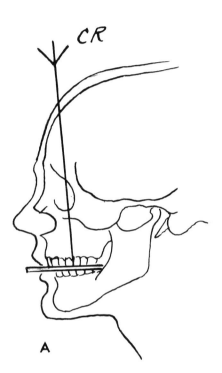

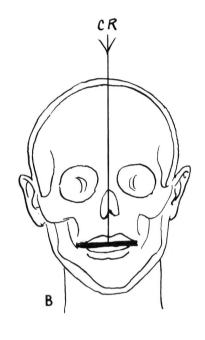

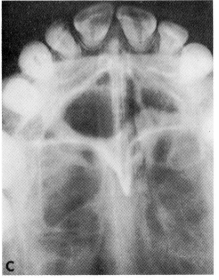

FIGURE 24–25. Superoinferior central occlusal view of the hard palate. This is helpful in the demonstration of fractures of the alveolar process or hard palate. Cysts and bony malformations or defects of the upper dental arch may be demonstrated by this view.

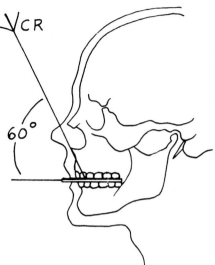

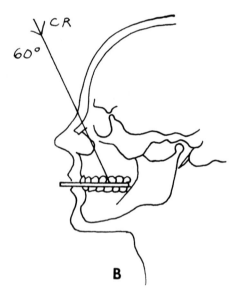

FIGURE 24–26. Superoinferior anterior occlusal view of the hard palate. This view gives details of the maxillary anterior teeth, alveolar process, and the anterior portion of the hard palate. The incisive canal is well demonstrated in this view. This view along with the preceding one is often used to demonstrate bony defects in the cleft palate patient.

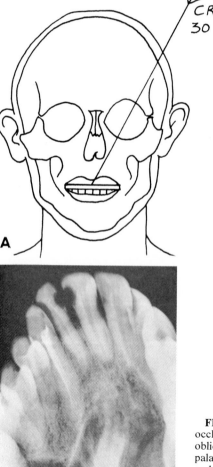

FIGURE 24–27. The oblique superoinferior posterior occlusal view of the hard palate. This projection gives an oblique occlusal view of the posterior part of the hard palate unilaterally. The alveolar process and the teeth and the upper quadrant of the maxilla are demonstrated in detail. Fractures of the alveolar process or teeth may be demonstrated by this view.

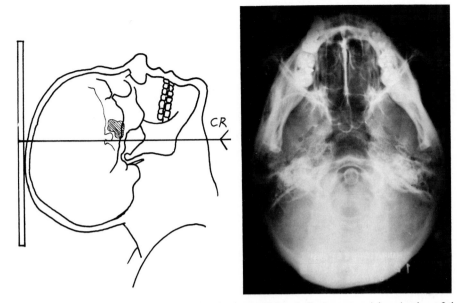

FIGURE 24–28. The verticosubmental position for the base of the skull gives an axial projection of the mandible, including the coronoid and condyloid processes of the rami, the zygomatic arches, the base of the skull and its foramina, the petrous pyramids, the sphenoidal, posterior ethmoid, and maxillary sinuses, and the nasal septum.

Occlusal Inferosuperior Views of the Mandible. Medial or lateral bony displacement in anterior mandibular fractures is well shown by occlusal inferior-superior views of the mandible. This view affords good bony detail of the entire lower dental arch, the mandibular body, the symphysis, the lower alveolar process, and the teeth.

OCCLUSAL INFEROSUPERIOR PROJECTION. This projection is used to demonstrate mesial or lateral displacement of fragments in fractures of the anterior portion of the mandible (Fig. 24–29).

OBLIQUE INFEROSUPERIOR PROJECTION. This projection gives an oblique occlusal view of the anterior mandibular area showing the symphysis, the alveolar process, and the incisor teeth. The bone detail is excellent, and fractures of the symphysis region, alveolar process, or teeth can be well demonstrated (Fig. 24–30).

OBLIQUE SUPEROINFERIOR-SUBMENTAL PROJECTION OF THE MANDIBULAR SYMPHYSIS. This view gives an oblique anteroposterior projection of the mandibular symphysis (Fig. 24–31).

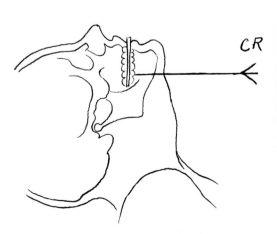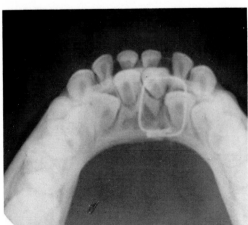

FIGURE 24–29. Inferosuperior occlusal projection of the mandible.

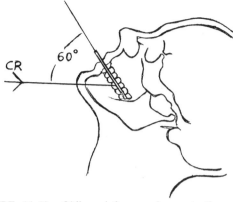
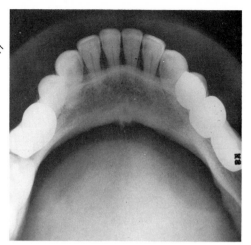

FIGURE 24–30. Oblique inferosuperior projection. This projection shows the mental symphysis, the incisor and canine teeth, and the alveolar processes with excellent bone detail.

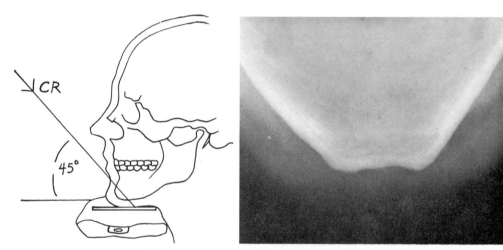

FIGURE 24–31. Oblique superoinferior submental projection of the mental symphysis.

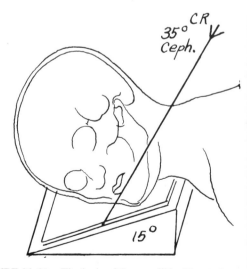
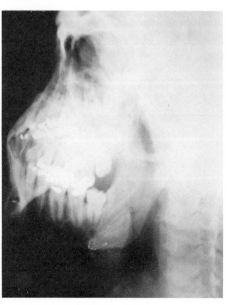
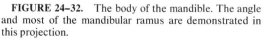

FIGURE 24–32. The body of the mandible. The angle and most of the mandibular ramus are demonstrated in this projection.

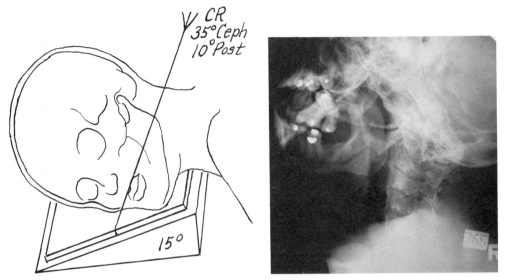

FIGURE 24–33. The ramus of the mandible, in a posteriorly directed oblique lateral view.

Oblique Lateral Views of the Mandible. These positions are used to demonstrate fractures of the mandibular ramus, the body of the mandible, and the symphysis region.

THE BODY OF THE MANDIBLE. This projection provides a lateral view of the mandible posterior to the cuspid tooth and including a portion of the ramus of the mandible (Fig. 24–32).

THE RAMUS OF THE MANDIBLE. This posteriorly directed oblique lateral view shows fractures of the ramus, the mandibular condyle, the condylar and condyloid processes, and the posterior body of the mandible (Fig. 24–33).

THE SYMPHYSIS OF THE MANDIBLE. The anteriorly directed oblique lateral projection of the symphysis of the mandible demonstrates fractures of the symphysis of the mandible, the region of the mental foramen, and the body of the mandible (Fig. 24–34).

POSTEROANTERIOR VIEW OF THE MANDIBLE. Medial and lateral displacement of fractured segments of the mandible may be demonstrated by this view. It demonstrates the symphysis, the body and rami of the mandible, the condyloid and coronoid processes, and the temporomandibular joints (Fig. 24–35).

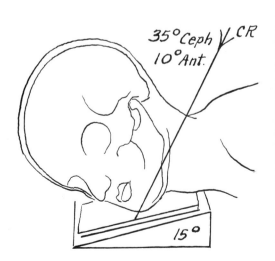
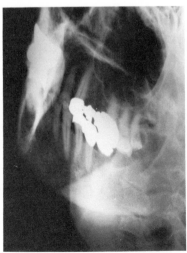

FIGURE 24–34. The symphysis of the mandible is shown by an anteriorly directed oblique lateral view. The regions of the mental foramen and body of the mandible are also shown in detail.

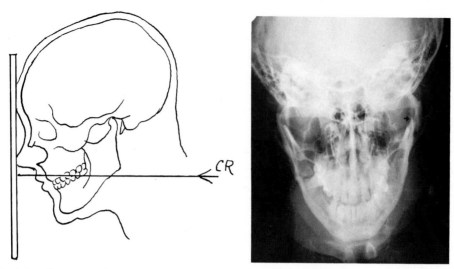

FIGURE 24–35. Posteroanterior view of the mandible. This view demonstrates the symphysis, the body and rami of the mandible, including the coronoid and condyloid processes, and the articular surfaces of the temporomandibular joints.

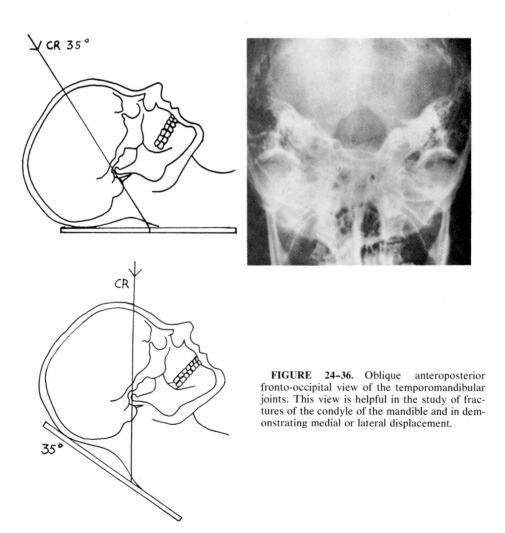

FIGURE 24–36. Oblique anteroposterior fronto-occipital view of the temporomandibular joints. This view is helpful in the study of fractures of the condyle of the mandible and in demonstrating medial or lateral displacement.

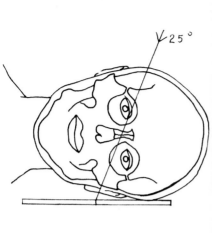

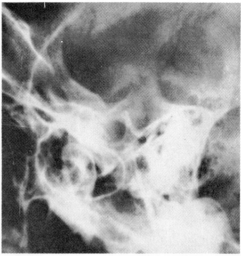

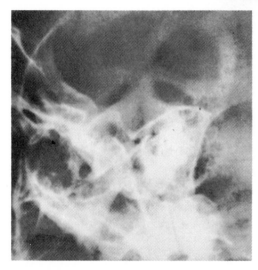

FIGURE 24–37. Lateral transcranial projections of the temporomandibular joints taken in the open and closed position are useful in demonstrating fractures of the mandibular condyle and condylar processes.

The Temporomandibular Joints

OBLIQUE ANTEROPOSTERIOR, FRONTO-OC-CIPITAL VIEW OF THE TEMPOROMANDIBULAR JOINTS. This projection provides an oblique posterior view of the condyloid processes of the mandible and the mandibular fossae of the temporal bones, the petrous bones, the internal auditory canals, the occipital bone, the posterior cranial fossa, and the foramen magnum. Fractures in the region of the temporomandibular joints with displacement medially or laterally can be detected in these views (Fig. 24–36).

LATERAL TRANSCRANIAL PROJECTION. OB-LIQUE LATERAL VIEWS OF THE TEMPOROMAN-DIBULAR JOINTS. The views are taken by the lateral transcranial projection and demonstrate the temporomandibular joints in open and closed mouth positions. The closed mouth view demonstrates the temporomandibular joint, the relation of the mandibular condyle to the fossa, and the width of the joint cartilage. The open mouth view demonstrates the excursion of the head of the condyle, downward and forward, in relation to the glenoid fossa and tubercle. This projection is useful in demonstrating fractures and dislocations of the mandibular condyle and the condylar process. The external auditory meatus and mastoid processes are also demonstrated (Fig. 24–37).

THE MAYER VIEW. The temporomandibular joint, external auditory canal, mastoid process, and petrous pyramid are shown in the unilateral superoinferior view. Medial or lateral displacement of the bony fragments of the mandibular condyle can be shown by this pro-

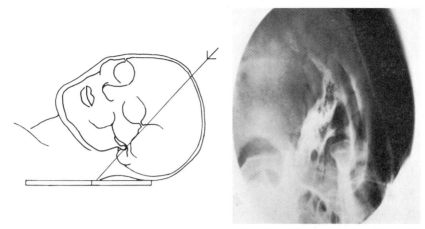

FIGURE 24–38. The Mayer view gives a unilateral superoinferior view of the temporomandibular joint, external auditory canal, mastoid, and petrous processes. This view is helpful in the demonstration of fractures and malformations of the temporomandibular joint and in the study of bony atresia of the external auditory canal.

jection. Fracture-dislocation of the bony portion of the external auditory canal can also be demonstrated by this technique (Fig. 24–38).

The panoramic roentgenogram is a helpful aid in defining the location and displacement of mandibular fractures (Fig. 24–39).

Tomographic evaluation of the temporomandibular joint is discussed in Chapter 31 and that of the orbit in Chapter 25.

GENERAL CONSIDERATIONS IN THE DEFINITIVE TREATMENT OF FACIAL INJURIES

Prophylaxis Against Tetanus. All facial wounds are potentially contaminated, and even though they occur under what might seem to be clean conditions, it is advisable to take ac-

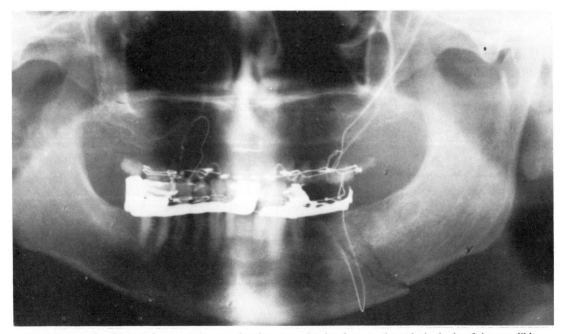

FIGURE 24–39. Panoramic roentgenogram showing postreduction fracture through the body of the mandible.

tive measures against the possibility of the development of tetanus. The efficacy of immunization with toxoid was well demonstrated by the low incidence of tetanus reported by the U.S. Army in World War II; only one case developed in the European Theater by February, 1945 (Graham and Scott, 1946). In the civilian population, most individuals have been actively immunized by their family physician or while in the military service. They should have their serum antibody levels raised by administration of a toxoid booster. If a patient has not been immunized, simultaneous intramuscular injection of 250 units of Hypertet (tetanus antitoxin human) and 1/2 ml tetanus toxoid is recommended. Two additional tetanus toxoid boosters should be given at monthly intervals to complete the immunization.

Treatment of Soft Tissue Wounds. Contusions, abrasions, and lacerations are not life-threatening, but many facial wounds are complex and compound. The more serious ones not only may involve the superficial structures but also may extend into the cranium, orbit, nose, sinuses, or mouth; may affect the seventh cranial nerve, the salivary ducts, or salivary glands; and may be associated with or extend into fractures of the mandible, maxilla, zygoma, nasal bones, orbit, frontal bone, or cranium.

Most civilian wounds occur under relatively clean circumstances, and, with modern techniques under antibiotic coverage they can be treated primarily up to 24 hours following injury. Because of the excellent blood supply of the face, the period from injury to surgery can be extended in clean-cut lacerations. The timing depends upon the judgment of the surgeon, however, and when there is obviously marked contamination with crushing and contusion, delayed primary repair is indicated. The probability of contamination increases rapidly and is directly proportional to the length of time that has elapsed since the time of injury.

Careful examination and evaluation of the wound should be made before any treatment is undertaken. Fractures of the underlying bone should be detected and in many cases treated prior to the soft tissue management. If the fractures are exposed through soft tissue lacerations, it is advisable to ensure fixation of the fractures through the open wound before closing the soft tissues. Injuries to important nerves, ducts, glands, and sinuses require consideration prior to soft tissue closure.

Delayed Primary Wound Closure. When the patient is seen late with extensive edema and subcutaneous hematoma, and when the wound edges are badly contused and some of the tissue devitalized, it is preferable to delay wound closure until conditions for primary healing are more favorable. Limited debridement to remove devitalized tissue, wet dressings, and antibiotic therapy should be the program of treatment until the resolution of edema and acute inflammation and a cleaner appearance of the wound indicate that delayed primary closure will be successful.

The large canine population has resulted in a number of dog bites, particularly in children. An essential precaution, prior to primary suture, is irrigation of the wound with large amounts of saline. Canine saliva contains necrotizing enzymes; the enzyme will produce continuing necrosis of the tissue in the wound if it is not evacuated.

Cleaning of the Wound. All wounds should be carefully inspected for foreign material, and removal of substances such as metal, wood, gravel, dirt, coal, dust, cinders, and powder is imperative to prevent suppuration, delayed healing, and subsequent pigmentation. The wound can be cleansed with detergent soaps and water. In some cases ether, benzene, and alcohol may be necessary to remove materials not soluble in water. Scrubbing with a brush under anesthesia may be required to remove deeply imbedded foreign bodies and to prevent the development of a traumatic tattoo.

Photography. Modern simplified methods of photography make it possible to obtain an accurate photographic record of the patient throughout the course of treatment. Good photographic records are important for insurance and legal purposes. Photographs supplement the written word and enhance the value of medical records. Photographs help the surgeon assess the effectiveness of his therapy by providing a means of review of each case at its termination. The adage that a good photograph is worth a thousand words is in no instance more true than in facial injury cases. Photographs may be worthless unless taken with care and consideration as to lighting, positioning, and composition. In order to adequately show facial lacerations, contusions, and abrasions, the patient should be thoroughly cleansed of dirt, blood, and debris, and overlying clothing and dressings should be removed before the photograph is taken.

For effective use, photographs should be identified with the patient's name, age, and diagnosis, and the date and filed with the patient's record or cross-filed as to diagnosis so that they are readily available for coordinated evaluation and summary of the total treatment.

Instrumentation for the Treatment of Facial Injuries. To facilitate the care of facial injuries, a carefully selected high quality armamentarium is essential. A tray of instruments selected and reserved for the care of facial injuries is recommended. It is distressing at the operating table to find that one or more essential instruments are missing from the set-up. To avoid delay and frustration, a kit of instruments including the materials usually employed in the management of facial soft tissue and bone injuries should be available for ready sterilization at all times. The instruments should be kept in good repair so that the procedures can be performed without annoyance by mechanical problems.

General surgical instruments are available in all operating rooms and consist of basic instruments used in all operations, such as knife handles, hemostats, and suture scissors. A loose-leaf book containing lists of instruments and photographs of instrument table arrangements for various operations done by each surgeon should be available for use by the operating room nurses. Selection and inclusion of all necessary instruments in the set-up before the operation is started will save time at the operating table. Each surgeon has favorite instruments or specially designed instruments for various operations. These should be included in the armamentarium.

Preoperative Considerations. The patient should be in the optimum condition for operative procedures on facial structures. Correction of shock, hypovolemia, dehydration, and electrolyte imbalance should precede all procedures except emergency care. Diabetes should be under control or well covered by the use of insulin and the patient covered with steroids if indicated. Patients with rheumatic or valvular heart disease should be protected by preoperative and postoperative antibiotic therapy. It is advisable to share the responsibility of the patient's general welfare with an internist who may have valuable suggestions in general management.

Anesthesia

General Anesthesia. The use of local or general anesthesia or a combination of the two depends upon the desires and ability of the surgeon, the general condition of the patient, and the facilities available. The extent of the injuries, the general condition of the patient, and the psychologic reaction to surgery in most cases dictate the use of general anesthesia. General anesthesia is usually indicated because the tissues are hypersensitive, and prolonged operative procedures or manipulation of the facial structures may be distressing to the patient under local anesthesia.

Although general anesthesia is preferable for the management of extensive facial trauma, there may be competition for working space owing to the presence of anesthetic equipment in the operative field. A skilled anesthesiologist is needed for the administration of the general anesthesia under these difficult circumstances, and frequently when local anesthesia is utilized, he can offer assistance by the judicious use of intravenous sedative drugs as a supplement to local anesthesia.

Endotracheal transnasal anesthesia is usually satisfactory for the reduction and fixation of fractures of the maxilla and mandible in which the nasal passages are not involved. Endotracheal anesthesia with oral intubation is indicated for fractures of the upper facial area in which it is not necessary to establish intermaxillary fixation. When there is involvement of the mandible, maxilla, and nasal and other facial bones, preoperative tracheotomy under local anesthesia and the administration of an anesthetic agent through the tracheostomy tube are the methods of choice. Anesthesia by this method permits reduction and fixation of the facial fractures, wiring of the teeth, packing of the nose, and application of splints, head frames, and other appliances without concern for airway obstruction during the course of the operation. Postoperative edema of the mouth, neck, and hypopharyngeal area may also present problems if a tracheostomy has not been performed.

Local Anesthesia. An attitude of reassurance, understanding, and sympathy, together with adequate premedication, will permit extensive operations under local anesthesia. Less complicated wounds such as small cuts, bruises, lacerations, and uncomplicated fractures of the facial bones can often be treated

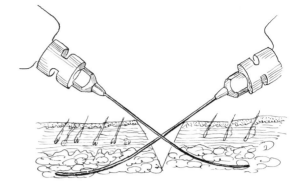

FIGURE 24–40. Pain can be minimized by injecting the subcutaneous tissue through the open wound without passing the needle through the skin. (Redrawn from Straith.)

under local anesthesia in the operating room or an outpatient treatment room.

Adequate premedication is imperative with the use of local anesthesia. The dosage of the selected drug varies with the patient's age and weight. The elderly patient usually requires less premedication. If excitement occurs during surgery, additional sedative medication may be given intravenously.

Local anesthesia is the method of choice in the repair of most soft tissue lacerations. This can be given skillfully without discomfort to the patient if a small, sharp needle is used. The first insertion can be made with minimal discomfort with a 30-gauge needle. Subsequent insertions are made only into already anesthetized areas. In open wounds, pain can be minimized by injection through the wound (Fig. 24–40).

The most effective anesthetic solution at present is lidocaine (Xylocaine), 1 per cent, with 1:100,000 epinephrine. If over 60 ml will be required, the solution may be diluted with equal amounts of balanced saline solution, which will result in a 0.5 per cent solution with 1:200,000 epinephrine. If injected properly this will give anesthesia and satisfactory vasoconstriction if a waiting period of 10 to 15 minutes is permitted before commencing the operation. Infiltration or block anesthesia containing vasoconstrictive drugs is satisfactory and effective for most operative procedures. If the patient's condition contraindicates the use of a general anesthesia, even extensive facial fractures can be operated upon under moderate sedation with gasserian ganglion block or fifth nerve division blocks along with cervical block. In cases in which distortion of the soft tissues due to local injection of anesthetic solutions may be a disturbing factor, local nerve block may be effective. Block anesthesia can be employed in the region of the mandible where the inferior alveolar nerve or the mental nerve may be injected, or into the greater palatine foramen where infraorbital and zygomaticofacial nerve blocks will provide regional anesthesia without distortion. Injection of the supraorbital and frontal nerves suffices for forehead and anterior scalp repairs.

REPAIR OF SOFT TISSUE WOUNDS OF THE FACIAL AREA

Debridement and Care of Soft Tissue Wounds. Thorough, careful cleansing of all soft tissue wounds is imperative before attempting any definitive treatment. All blood and debris should be carefully washed from the tissues by utilizing copious amounts of water and mild detergents. Foreign materials such as glass, hair, clothing, tooth structures, pieces of artificial dentures, paint, grease, gravel, and dirt should be removed. Usually detergent solutions and water will clean the wound adequately. However, in some cases, dirt, carbon, tar, grease, asphalt, etc., may be ground deep into the soft tissues. If permitted to remain, a pigmented scar will result or infection will ensue

(Fig. 24–41). Careful scrubbing of the wounds with handbrush or toothbrush under anesthesia may be necessary to remove foreign material (Fig. 24–42). Dermabrasion over the area will facilitate the removal of intradermal foreign bodies. The use of ether or benzene as a solvent for grease and tar may be necessary.

Careful preoperative attention to these details will avoid infection, faulty healing, scarring, and the need for secondary repair.

In blast injury, minute particles of debris may be forced into the face (Fig. 24–43). These particles should be carefully and individually removed with small curettes. This is a time-consuming procedure, but it assures better end results.

Except for the removal of obviously devitalized portions of tissue, debridement has no place in the management of facial injuries. All tissues that may participate in a satisfactory repair should be retained if there is any possibility of residual vitality in the structures (Fig. 24–44). It is preferable to err on the side of retaining tissues that may not survive than to debride or destroy any tissues that might be important in the final reconstruction. The excellent blood supply of the face makes extensive debridement unnecessary and will permit the survival of tissues retained by only a small pedicle. Wounds of the same magnitude in other areas would necessitate a more radical debridement program.

Pieces of tissue almost completely detached and some small structures that have been avulsed can be sutured back into position as grafts. Many of them will survive. This is useful and practical only in places where reconstructive procedures are unusually difficult, such as the eyelid margin, the ala and tip of the nose, or a segment of the ear. Cooling of the reapplied part may be employed in the postoperative period.

Abrasions. Care should be exercised in the management of abrasions, even though the injury may be superficial, since many of these contain dirt. When first seen, a child with superficial abrasions may not appear to have an injury of consequence. Upon healing, it may be discovered, however, that there is a pigmented residual defect (Fig. 24–45). Dirt, grease, carbon, and other pigments should be carefully scrubbed out of the wound and a light grease dressing applied. This will avoid accidental or traumatic tattoos which result in considerable cosmetic disability (Fig. 24–46).

The Contused Wound. Contusions usually result in extensive edema, ecchymosis, and hematomas which generally subside without active treatment. Subcutaneous hematomas, even though large, will usually absorb gradually, leaving no residual deformity. Contusions may be associated with lacerations and may retard healing. The final results may be inadequate, and secondary repair may be required.

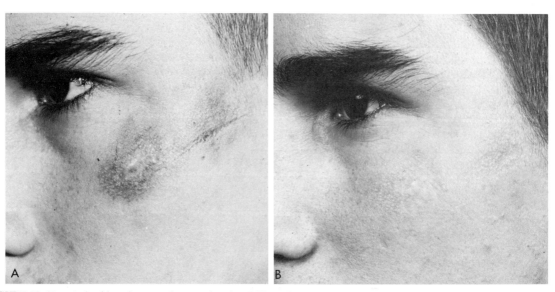

FIGURE 24–41. *A,* Accidental tattoo nine months after falling off a motorcycle on a cinder road. *B,* Two months after removal of intradermal pigment by means of dermabrasion.

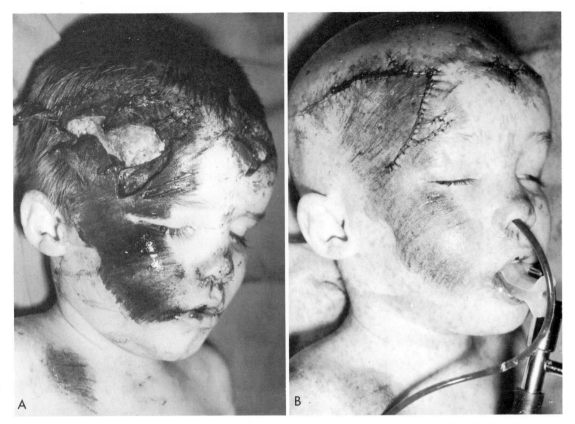

FIGURE 24–42. *A,* Abrasion, contusion, and laceration of the face in a 3 year old child who was knocked down and dragged on the pavement by an automobile. *B,* The wounds were thoroughly scrubbed with a brush and detergent solution, copiously irrigated with normal saline solution, debrided, and sutured. Healing took place with a nonpigmented inconspicuous scar.

The Lacerated Contused Wound. The contused margins of the lacerated wound should be excised. This will lead to earlier, less complicated healing with a superior end result. If the contused marginal tissues are of anatomical importance, it is best to avoid debridement and perform secondary definitive surgery as necessary. This is especially important in eyelid, ear, and nasal alar wounds in which sacrifice of any of the tissues might jeopardize the result (Fig. 24–47).

Deep Lacerations. Lacerations caused by sharp, clean objects, such as a knife, windshield, flying glass, or sharp metal, may extend through all the layers of the soft tissues and may involve important muscles, nerves, glands, and ducts (Fig. 24–48). The muscles of facial expression are so closely associated with the skin that careful closure of the wound in layers will give adequate approximation. Muscle layers should be identified, if possible, and

accurately approximated with fine sutures. Lacerations of the muscles of mastication occur, but complete severance is uncommon. Closure of the muscles in layers, including the overlying fascia, restores adequate function.

It is impractical and unnecessary to identify and suture the terminal branches of the facial nerve. Usually, with reasonably accurate approximation of the tissues, the nerves will regenerate and function will return within 12 to 18 months, if not earlier. If the seventh nerve is severed in the parotid gland, care should be taken to identify and suture the major branches. The branches distal to the laceration can be identified with the help of a faradic nerve stimulator during the first three days after severance of the nerves; no response can be elicited after three days, and the nerves must be located by careful dissection with the aid of binocular magnifying loupes. Dissection of the proximal portion of the nerve is also necessary in order to identify it and to permit

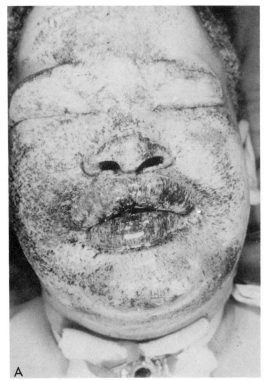

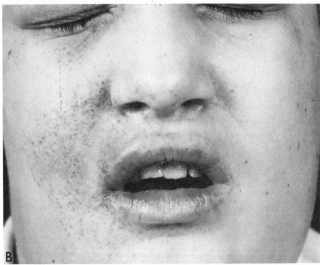

FIGURE 24–43. *A*, Injury in a 14 year old boy two hours after an explosion of a homemade bomb. Inhalation of flame and hot gases resulted in severe edema and obstruction of the upper airway requiring emergency tracheotomy. The wounds were treated by curetting powder particles and thorough scrubbing with a brush and detergents. *B*, Three months post injury. Much of the pigment was subsequently removed by dermabrasion.

approximation with fine sutures under microscopic aid. Every effort should be made to approximate the large segments of the seventh nerve.

The sensory branches of the fifth nerve in the region of the skin are small, and approximation is impractical and unnecessary. Recovery of sensation usually occurs within a few months to a year.

Parotid Duct Lacerations.   Laceration of the parotid duct should be repaired at the time of the wound closure to prevent parotid fistula to the skin surface or to the mucous membrane of the mouth. The latter is not significant, but a parotid fistula to the skin is an annoying lesion (Fig. 24–49). To identify the course of the parotid duct, a line is drawn from the tragus of the ear to the midportion of the upper lip. The

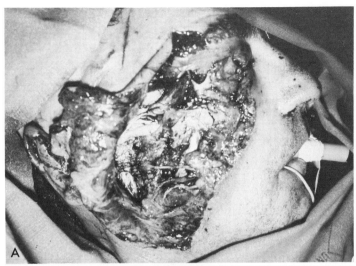

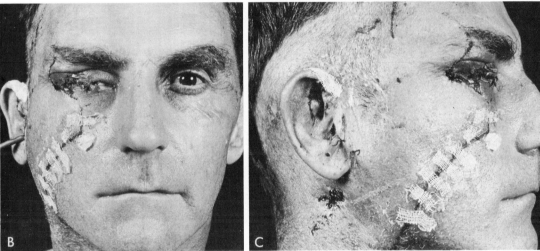

FIGURE 24-44. *A,* Severe laceration from an automobile windshield accident with fracture of the zygoma and orbital margin, exposure of the seventh nerve branches, and laceration of the parotid duct. Treatment consisted of direct wiring of bone fragments, repair of seventh nerve branches, and suture of the parotid duct followed by careful debridement and closure of all soft tissue wounds in layers. *B, C,* Five days postoperatively.

duct traverses the middle third of the line (line AB in Fig. 24–50). Any laceration extending deeply through this area should be suspected of having damaged the parotid duct. Injury can be identified readily by passing a small Silastic tube or silver probe into the opening of Stensen's duct, which is opposite the upper second molar tooth. A tube or probe can be passed through the duct, and if it appears in the wound, it indicates severance of the duct. The proximal end of the duct is then identified by expressing saliva, and the tube is passed into it as far as possible and left in the duct as a splint. An adequate number of sutures are

placed in the substance of the duct to approximate the severed ends around the Silastic catheter (Fig. 24–51). The tubing is cut with the end protruding into the mouth and sutured securely to the mucous membrane so that it cannot be accidently dislodged. The catheter is removed in five to seven days with reasonable assurance that the duct will remain patent.

If Silastic tubing is not available, a 2–0 nylon suture on a large needle can be passed through the substance of the cheek into the duct near the point of laceration, out through the lacerated area into the duct on the proximal side, and brought to the surface of the

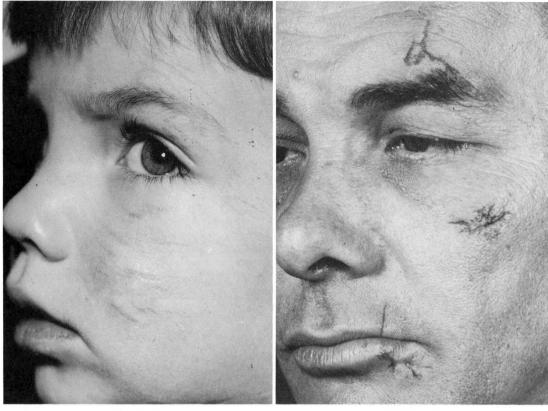

FIG. 24–45.   FIG. 24–46.

FIGURE 24–45. Accidental tatto from a fall. The original wound was considered inconsequential and no treatment was given. The defect required dermabrasion for correction.

FIGURE 24–46. Traumatic tattoo in a garage mechanic. Dirt and grease were forced in the wound at the time of injury and were not removed.

skin. The suture will act as a splint, and the duct can be repaired by suturing. The wound is then closed in layers, and the 2–0 nylon suture is tied loosely over the skin area.

The buccal branch of the seventh nerve traverses the face along the course of Stensen's duct and is usually severed if the duct has been lacerated. If the facial laceration is closed without repair of the parotid duct, the parotid duct syndrome may be evident after a few hours. This is indicated by the presence of paralysis of the muscles of expression to the upper lip, swelling at the site of the wound closure due to pooling of saliva under the skin surface, or draining of saliva between the sutures.

Lacrimal System Lacerations. Lacerations near the medial canthus may sever the canaliculi or damage the sac or other parts of the lacrimal system. If a canaliculus is severed, the severed ends are sutured over Silastic tubing using visual magnification with loupes or a microscope (see Chapter 28).

Submaxillary Duct Injuries. The submaxillary duct is not often injured in fractures or soft tissue injuries unless there is a comminuted type of fracture or gunshot wound to the floor of the mouth. Repair of the submaxillary duct is unnecessary. If unrepaired, a fistula into the floor of the mouth usually results. Scar with obstruction of the duct may require reestablishment of the duct opening or excision of the submaxillary gland.

Injuries to the Soft Tissues of the Orbit. The eye should be carefully inspected for abrasions or lacerations of the cornea or puncture of the globe (Fig. 24–52). In all severe injuries in the orbital area, consultation with an ophthalmologist is desirable in order to detect intraocular injury. An ophthalmologist may not always be immediately available. Visual function should always be checked prior to treatment of a deep laceration or fracture of the orbit region, because decrease or loss of visual function should be verified preoperatively in order to avoid litigation after the treatment is com-

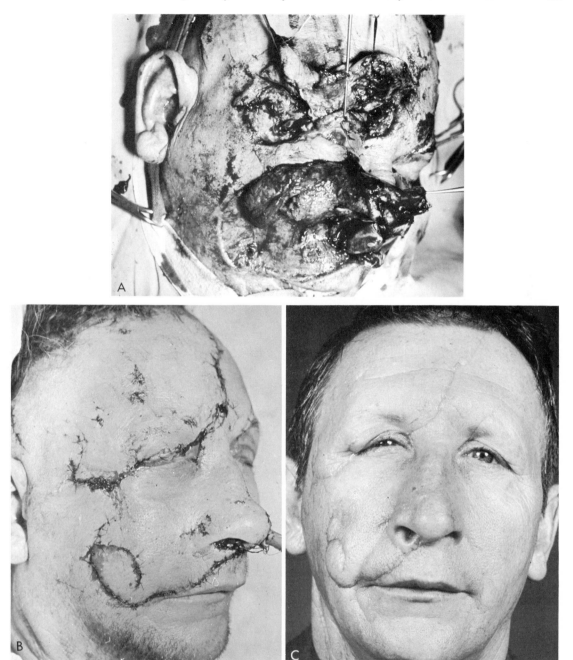

FIGURE 24–47. *A*, Severe soft tissue lacerations and facial bone fractures. Treatment consisted of reduction of fractures through the open wound, cleansing of the soft tissues, minimal debridement, and careful suturing of the soft tissues in layers. *B*, Note that in the right cheek even flaps of tissue based on a very small pedicle survived. Photograph four days postoperatively. *C*, Two months after injury. No tissue was lost and the patient is ready for consideration of definitive repair.

pleted. Miller and Tenzel (1967) have reported a number of simple tests that can be done in the emergency room. Reading a newspaper (the elderly patient wearing his presbyopic correction glasses), the finger counting test (in four quadrants), and the Marcus Gunn pupillary sign are practical means of determining visual function. In the Marcus Gunn test, each pupillary response to a hand-light is sought. If the response is normal on both sides, the light

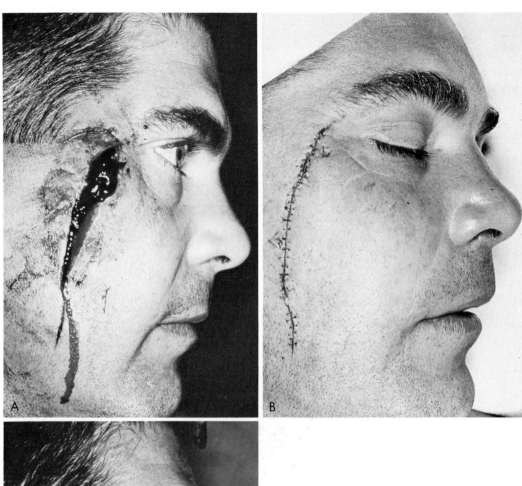

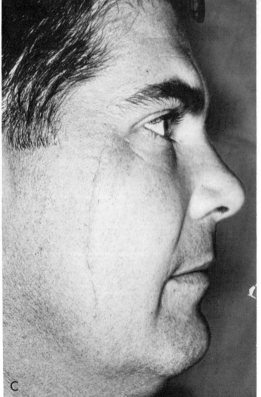

FIGURE 24–48.   *A,* Sharp laceration from a windshield glass cut. Branches of the seventh nerve to the lower lid and lateral nasal area were severed. *B,* The wound was thoroughly cleansed and carefully sutured. No attempt was made to identify or suture the branches of the seventh nerve. *C,* Three weeks following wound closure. The subsequent result was excellent, with complete regeneration of the branches of the seventh nerve within one year. However, with the recent development of microsurgical nerve repair, efforts should be made to identify and anastomose the nerve ends if possible.

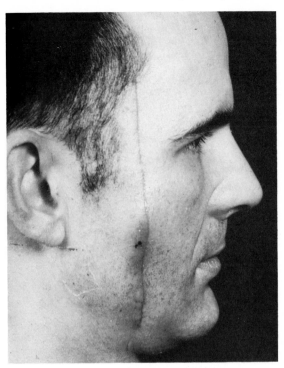

FIGURE 24-49. Subcutaneous swelling with drainage of saliva from a fistula in the right cheek one month following laceration by a knife. Treatment consisted of opening the wound, identifying the parotid duct, and reconstructing the duct over a Silastic catheter.

is moved rapidly from one side to the other. If conduction of the optic nerve is lesser on one side, the pupil will appear to dilate as the light is moved from the sound eye to the involved eye. These simple tests are helpful but should not preclude a careful ophthalmologic examination. Eyelid and associated injuries deserve priority in the scale of the patient's wounds, including those away from the facial area. Lacerations through the eyelid margins require a special technique for repair if a serious cosmetic and functional disability is to be avoided (see Chapter 28).

Lacerations of the Nose. Lacerations of the nose may involve the skin, the lining in the vestibule of the nose, or the mucous membrane of the nasal cavity, most commonly at the junction of the bone and the cartilages. The blow may produce sudden telescopic movements of the soft tissues which are sheared off at their attachments at the bony nasal margin. A thick, boggy, edematous septum may indicate a hematoma, and a septal cartilage laceration may be seen through a tear in the mucoperichondrium. Intranasal suturing following

reduction of the soft and bony structures approximates the lacerated margins. Intranasal lacerations usually need no suturing, as intranasal packing will hold the soft tissues in their proper relationships. The skin of the nose heals well, and even in cases involving extensive lacerations, the final scars are minimal (Fig. 24-53).

Avulsions of the section of the nose near the tip and ala may be repaired by means of the original piece of skin and cartilage if it is available. If the severed tissue is recovered and thoroughly cleansed with saline, it may be sutured into position. In many cases, healing occurs uneventfully, and an important anatomical structure that otherwise might be difficult or impossible to reconstruct can be saved.

Avulsed Wounds of the Facial Area. If the wounds cannot be closed because of avulsion and loss of soft tissue, dressing of the area with a split-thickness skin graft provides immediate closure and avoids infection and prolonged dressing care (Fig. 24-54). Full thickness losses of nasal alar tissue can be repaired by

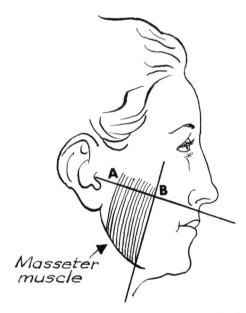

Masseter muscle

FIGURE 24-50. The course of Stensen's duct is deep to the middle third of a line drawn from the tragus of the ear to the mid-portion of the upper lip. This corresponds roughly to the anterior-posterior limits of the masseter muscle. The hilus of the gland is at approximately point A, and the opening of the duct into the mouth is opposite the second maxillary molar tooth deep to point B. The buccal branch of the facial nerve crosses Stensen's duct near point B. Lacerations involving Stensen's duct usually result in severance of the buccal branch of the seventh nerve.

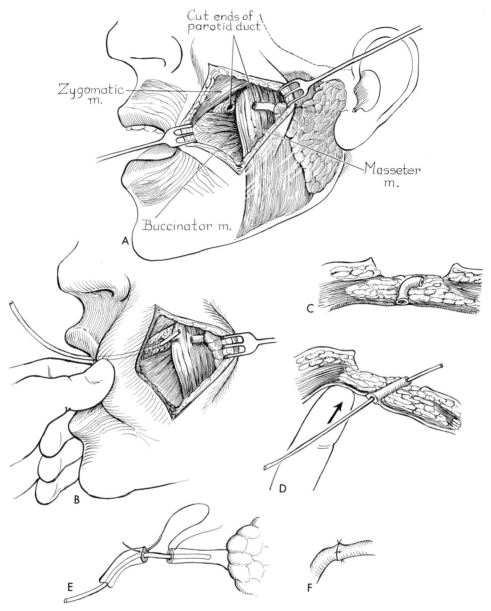

FIGURE 24–51.   Repair of a severed parotid duct. *A*, Severed duct at anterior border of masseter muscle. *B*, A fine-calibered Silastic catheter is threaded through the buccal opening of Stensen's duct. *C*, Angulation of Stensen's duct as it penetrates through the cheek wall. This angulation renders difficult the penetration of the catheter into duct. *D*, Outward stretching of cheek wall tends to straighten duct and facilitate threading of catheter through it. *E*, Direct anastomosis of cut ends of duct using the catheter as a splint. *F*, After suture of the cut ends of the duct. (From Kazanjian and Converse.)

the use of composite grafts from the ear margin as a primary procedure (Fig. 24–55). These grafts will survive if no part of the graft is more than 1.0 to 1.5 cm. away from the nutrient bed (see also Chapter 29).

Lacerations of the Lips.   Lacerations of the lips may involve only the superficial skin and subcutaneous tissues or may extend into the muscle and, not infrequently, involve the mucosa. Bleeding may be profuse if the labial arteries are severed. Pressure or clamping and tying the vessels will control hemorrhage without difficulty. Repair consists of suturing the structures in layers utilizing absorbable sutures for the deep mucosal structures. Accurate ap-

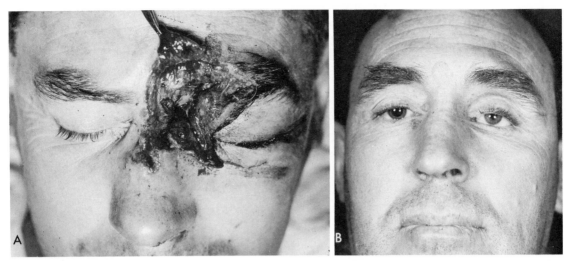

FIGURE 24–52. *A*, Fracture of the nasal bones with detachment of the medial canthal tendon and puncture laceration of the globe. *B*, Result after wiring of the nasal bones through the open wound and reattachment of the medial canthal tendon, suture of the lacerations, and enucleation of the left eye. The left eye has been replaced by a prosthesis.

proximation of the muscle, the vermilion-cutaneous margin, the vermilion-mucosal margin, and the skin is necessary to assure adequate function and appearance of the lip. After careful and thorough cleansing, the lip structures should be closed in layers beginning at the deepest layer and working outward to the skin. Every effort should be made to approximate the musculature in its normal position. The vermilion-cutaneous margin and the mucosal margins are landmarks from which to begin suturing (Fig. 24–56). Inadequate or inaccurate approximation of the vermilion-cutaneous margin leaves a noticeable defect (Fig. 24–57*A*).

Injuries of the Auricle. The ear may be involved in abrasions, contusions, and lacerations. Usually the abrasions heal, and application of a light dressing with moderate pressure will usually control the hemorrhage and prevent subsequent perichondritis and deformity.

Lacerations of the auricle are usually associated with lacerations of the cartilage. The ear may be totally or incompletely avulsed. Even with small pedicle attachments, the ear will usually survive if it is carefully sutured into place and adequately supported with dressings. A few fine catgut sutures to approximate the cartilage will give stability to the ear. Accurate placement of nylon sutures in the skin margins produces excellent results with minimal postoperative deformity (Fig. 24–58).

Avulsion of small or moderate-sized segments of the auricle can be adequately repaired by replacement with composite grafts. Subtotal and total avulsion of the auricle is discussed in Chapter 35.

Care of Extensive Soft Tissue Wounds with Loss of Structure and Tissue. Loss of tissue may preclude wound closure. If an extensive wound, such as one that is produced by gunshot injury, cannot be treated by means of a skin graft or by rotation of tissue from the immediate area, the mucous membrane of the mouth or nasal cavity should be advanced to the skin margin and secured with sutures. By primary closure, infection, delayed healing, and scar contracture will be prevented. Early healing will facilitate the definitive repair and minimize the postoperative dressing problem. Every effort should be made to cover the bone ends with adjacent tissues to prevent infection and necrosis.

The most satisfactory results from repair of facial lacerations are seen in those cases in which the laceration parallels the lines of minimal tension, which are parallel to the expressive skin folds of the face. Fortunate is the patient who has lacerations running in the right direction (Fig. 24–59). The final results may be less than optimal when the lacerations run at right angles or at variance with the lines of minimal tension.

In clean lacerations vertical to the skin surface, it may only be necessary to approximate the tissues to obtain a satisfactory result. When the laceration runs tangential to the skin

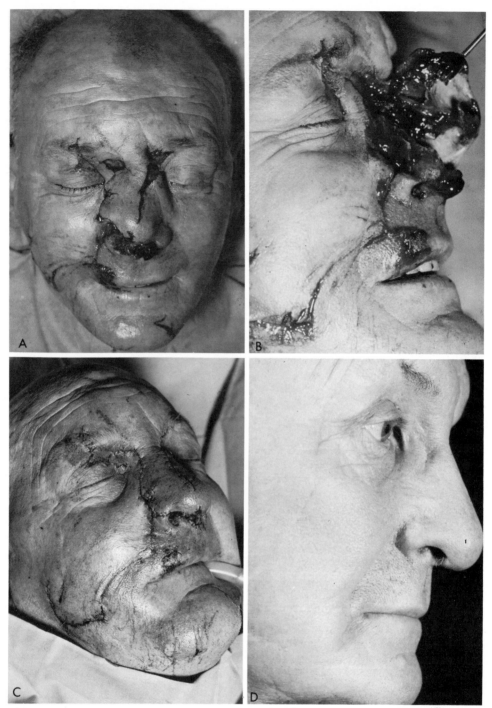

FIGURE 24–53. *A,* Facial injuries sustained in an automobile accident in which the patient was thrown against the windshield. Facial wounds may be much more extensive than they appear on initial examination. The lacerated tissues should be retracted and the wound thoroughly irrigated and cleansed of clots and debris to permit careful inspection. *B,* Retraction of the flaps demonstrated extensive injury to the nasal bones and cartilages. *C,* The fractured nasal bones were reduced and held by direct wiring. The cartilaginous structures were approximated by suturing. The mucous membrane lining of the nose was sutured, and the soft tissues were closed after minimal debridement. *D,* Six months after operation the patient has a patent nasal airway with minimal scarring.

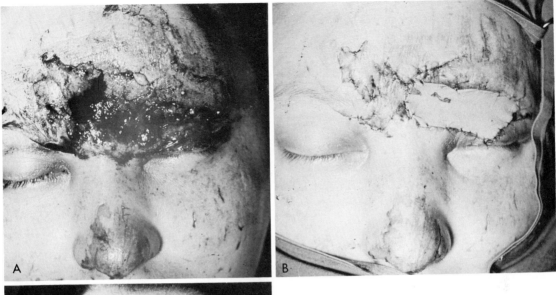

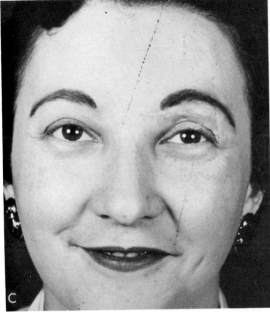

FIGURE 24–54. *A*, Contusions and lacerations suffered in an automobile accident. The patient was thrown into the windshild and sustained extensive multiple lacerations of the forehead and loss of the skin of the upper lid and brow. *B*, Treatment consisted of careful cleansing of the wound, suture of all viable structures into position, and repair of the avulsed area of the lid and brow with a split-thickness skin graft dressing. Whenever possible, primary closure of the wound should be done to avoid infection and minimize subsequent scarring. *C*, Late result after replacement of the split-thickness skin graft with full-thickness postauricular skin and an eyebrow graft.

surface, it is necessary to excise the wound margins at right angles, or slightly less, to the skin surface (Straith, Lawson and Hipps, 1961). Careful debridement (Fig. 24–60) of the contused margins will hasten healing and minimize chances of a conspicuous scar developing. Excision should be conservative, usually not more than 1 or 2 mm into the unaffected skin. The wound must be changed from one of traumatized, uneven margins to one with clean, sharp edges. The margins of the wound must be undermined or undercut sufficiently to prevent undue tension on the wound margins and

to permit closure of the wound in layers with subcutaneous sutures.

The undermining should not produce distortion of adjacent features, such as the angle of the mouth or the ala of the nose. Undermining may be more extensive on one side of the wound than on the other to avoid damage to vessels, nerves, or other important structures. Excision of excess fat and subcutaneous tissues will relieve tension of the wound margins and permit eversion of the skin edges.

Buried fine, clear, nylon or catgut sutures provide subcutaneous fixation with minimal re-

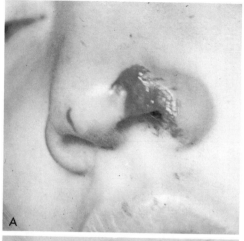

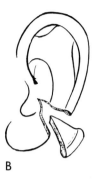

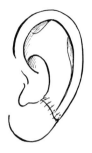

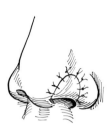

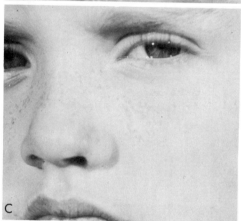

FIGURE 24–55. *A,* Six hours after full-thickness avulsion of the lateral nasal area caused by a dog bite. *B,* Immediate repair with a composite graft from the left ear. The graft contained skin for covering, cartilage for support, and skin for the lining. The auricle provides excellent graft material for repair of nasal tip defects. The thin ear cartilage cover with skin on both sides offers ideal material for repair. The resultant auricular defects are minimal. *C,* One year after repair.

action. Sutures should be placed close enough to relieve all surface wound tension. Interrupted sutures, if used, must be carefully placed and tied without undue tension to avoid suture marks. Interrupted surface sutures should not be used in patients who are subject to the formation of scars.

The subcuticular suture (Fig. 24–61) is excellent for skin closure, as it provides adequate approximation of the tissue margin and can be left in place for three to four weeks without fear of a reaction or leaving suture marks.

Use of fine caliber suture material and atraumatic needles is desirable in facial wounds. Catgut sutures should not be used on the skin surface for the repair of skin wounds, as the cosmetic result is important. These materials cause a foreign body reaction which results in increased inflammation and scar tissue formation.

Sutures placed through the skin surface should be tied at the proper tension so that edema will not cause them to cut through and leave suture scars. Suture marks (Fig. 24–62)

are caused by thin sutures tied too tightly or by sutures left in the tissue too long. Surface sutures should be removed on the third or fourth day and the wound supported with adhesive strips fixed across the wound (Fig. 24–63).

If the wound is long and has been sutured with interrupted sutures, a few sutures should be removed and the wound supported with transverse strips. A few more sutures are removed and another strip applied, and so forth, until all of the sutures have been removed. The supporting strips are maintained for a period of two to three weeks until the tensile strength of the wound will better withstand the adjacent skin tensions.

The Nonsuture Technique of Wound Closure. Gillman, Penn, Bronks, and Roux (1955) proposed that simple approximation of wound margins by use of adhesive tape would be an atraumatic, biologically sound method of wound closure. The nonsuture technique would eliminate the usual disadvantages of surface sutures. This technique has been applica-

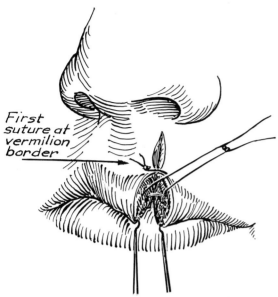

FIGURE 24–56. Repair of vertical lacerations of the vermilion-cutaneous margin. The first suture should be used for approximation of the vermilion-cutaneous border. This will avoid conspicuous irregularity of this portion of the lip following healing.

ble to the treatment of small superficial wounds for many years, but lack of suitable material for firmly approximating large wounds has prevented its adaptation to large wounds. Superficial wounds, especially in children, respond very well to approximation with commercially available sterile adhesive strips.

Dunphy and Jackson (1962) advocated the use of a plastic tape* which has the qualities

---

*Steri-strips. Minnesota Mining & Manufacturing Company, St. Paul, Minnesota.

of porosity and semitransparency; it is nonirritating and can easily be lifted off the skin. The material provides strong resistance to traction in the lateral direction. The authors reported that this tape has practical value for wound closure in a wide variety of operations (Fig. 24–64). Adhesive strapping gives uniform approximation of the tissue margins and eliminates the trauma from sutures. Tapes can be left in place for two to three weeks if indicated, and scar formation is avoided by the lack of lateral pull on the incision.

Dunphy and Jackson stated that there are two phases in gaining tensile strength of the wound: an initial phase of approximately two weeks' duration during which no more than 10 to 30 per cent of the ultimate strength of the wound is obtained, and a second phase, dependent upon function, which may last six weeks, three months, or indefinitely. The first phase in the gain of tensile strength is related to the laying down of collagen, while the second is related to an alteration of the physical state of the collagen fiber (see Chapter 3).

Dressings. Dressings are applied to the wound to relieve tension, to prevent dead space and hematoma formation, to apply pressure for control of oozing or postoperative bleeding, or to provide splinting action for the wound. Dressings vary with the problem and may be individualized to meet the needs. Adhesive strips stuck to the skin will provide support at the wound edges. Light pressure may be applied by the use of elastoplast or an Ace-type bandage. If hematoma or unusual edema is a possibility, elastic pressure bandages must be placed with care and frequently observed to prevent undue pressure and possible necrosis.

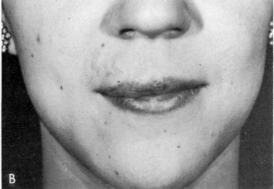
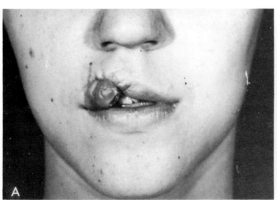

FIGURE 24–57. *A,* Fracture of the maxilla and laceration of the upper lip three months following an automobile accident. *B,* Three months after secondary revision of the upper lip.

A

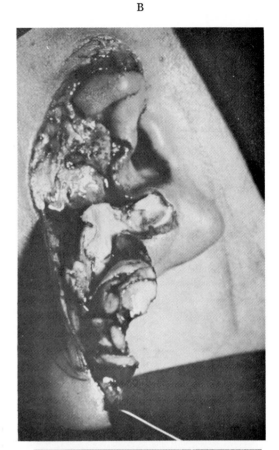

B

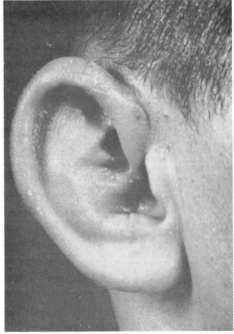

C

FIGURE 24–58. *A*, Sketch to orient the tissues in a severe laceration of the soft tissue and cartilaginous structures of the right ear shown in *B*. *B*, Extensive lacerations of the soft tissues and cartilaginous structures of the ear sustained in an automobile accident. The ear has an excellent blood supply and will often survive, even if attached by only a small pedicle. Every effort should be made to preserve the ear tissue. *C*, Six weeks after injury. Treatment consisted of careful cleansing of tissues and accurate reapproximation of the cartilage and skin.

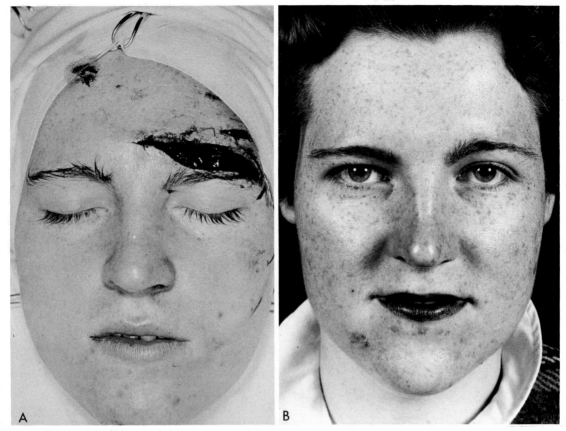

FIGURE 24–59. *A*, Forehead laceration caused by a rear view mirror in an automobile accident. The laceration is favorable for repair because it runs parallel to the skin lines of the forehead. It was closed in layers with fine subcutaneous sutures and a running subcuticular suture. *B*, Six months following repair of the forehead laceration.

Gauze lightly impregnated with petrolatum or xeroform and placed over the wound for the first 24 hours will prevent blood clots and serum from crusting about the sutures. At the end of 24 hours the wound should be carefully inspected, and any tight sutures which seem to

be cutting the skin should be cut at the knot but not necessarily removed.

Most wounds in the facial area can be left exposed without danger of contamination. This permits aeration of the wound and an opportunity for frequent inspection.

With meticulous care, the primary procedure in most instances will be the definitive procedure.

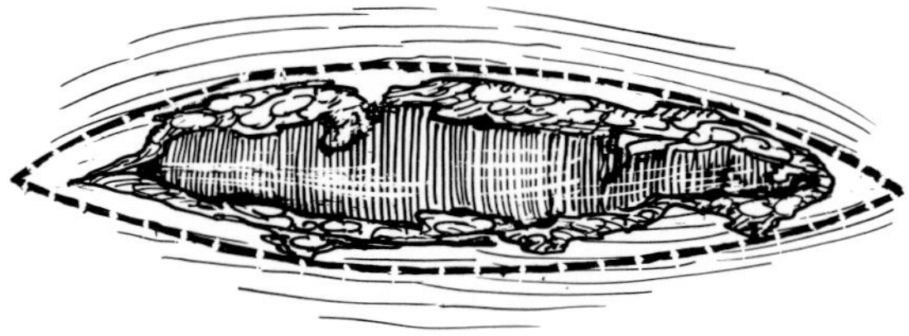

Multiple Small Glass Cuts. A patient who has been injured by multiple pieces of flying glass or whose face has struck a shattered automobile windshield may have hundreds of small, tangential, slicing lacerations. It is obvious that all of these cannot be debrided and sutured, and this is unnecessary. The debris and foreign material should be carefully scrubbed out of the wounds. Those wounds that are significant should be sutured. Surface irregularities, if present after a few months, usually respond to surgical abrasion treatment, as first described by Iverson (1947) (see Chapter 17).

FIGURE 24–60. Careful excision of the contused margins of the wound result in earlier healing with less liability of a conspicuous scar. The excision should be conservative. The two sides of the excised ellipse should be equal in length; thus, a pucker (or dog-ear) will be avoided at one end of the sutured wound.

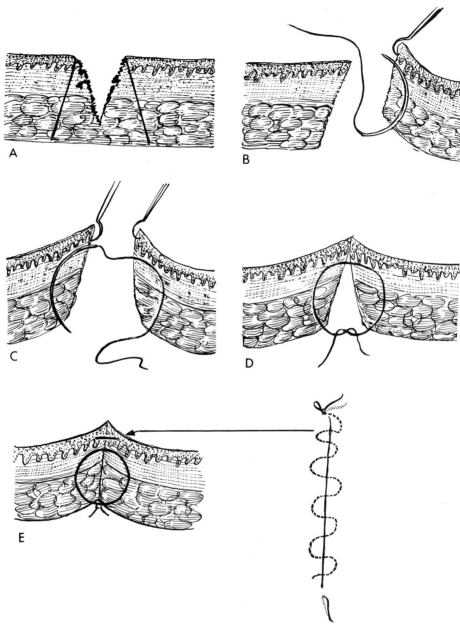

FIGURE 24–61. Method of debriding and suturing a surface laceration. *A,* Slight undercutting of the skin edges provides optimal surfaces for repair. *B,* After undermining the wound margins, the deep structures are closed in layers utilizing fine synthetic or catgut sutures with buried knots to provide subcutaneous fixation and elimination of dead space. *C,* A method of passing the needle to permit tying the knot in the deep portion of the wound. *D,* When the knot is tied, there is some eversion of the tissues at the line of closure. *E,* Eversion of the skin edges along the line of closure obtained by use of subcutaneous sutures and final skin coaptation by means of a subcuticular monofilament nylon suture. The subcuticular suture provides accurate skin closure and may be left in place for three to four weeks.

FIGURE 24–62. Correct and incorrect wound closure. *A,* Usual method of wound closure by interrupted suture. *B,* Following removal of the suture shown in *A,* scar tissue contracture in all directions results in a stretched depressed scar. *C, D,* Correct wound closure. *C* shows the eversion of the skin edges along the line of closure produced by adequate subcutaneous closure and subcuticular approximation of the skin edges with a running suture. *D,* After the suture is removed and scar tissue contracture has progressed, a flat surface with minimal scar and no indentation is the final result.

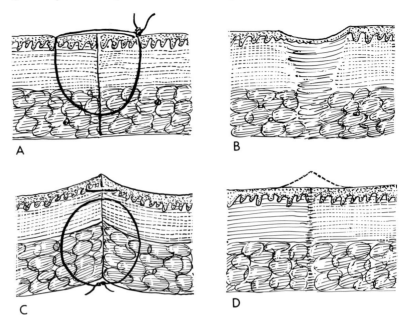

A

B

C

D

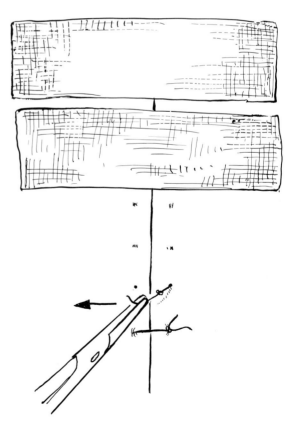

FIGURE 24–63. To avoid suture marks, interrupted surface sutures should be removed on the third or fourth day and the wound supported with butterfly tapes or paper tape strips fixed to the skin with collodion. Sterile adhesive strips for wound support are commercially available. These provide adequate ventilation, remain in position for long periods of time, and provide excellent support to the wound margins.

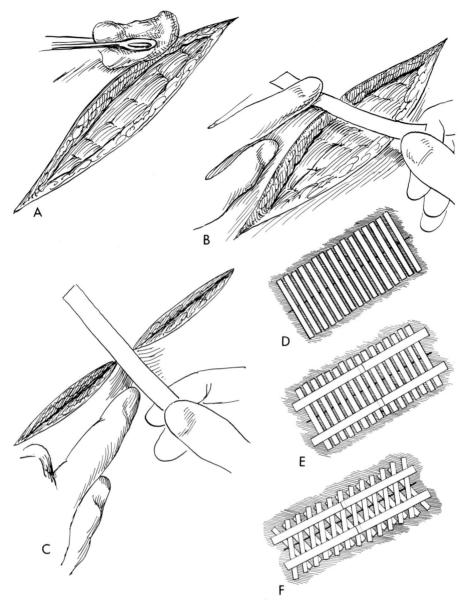

FIGURE 24–64. Use of plastic tape for wound closure. *A,* Clean and dry the skin of the wound area with an ether sponge. *B,* Apply one half of the adhesive strip to one side of the skin at the midportion of the wound, at right angles to the wound, and press firmly into place. *C,* Hold the other end of the strip for traction and appose the skin edges exactly, using fingers or forceps. Compress the free half of the strip into place. *D,* Close the entire wound with additional strips 3 mm apart. *E,* Parallel strips are used as additional reinforcement where unusual tensions are expected. *F,* If more security is desired, crisscross application of the strips is effective.

FRACTURES OF THE JAWS

The Importance of Teeth in the Management of Fractures of the Jaws

The Dentition. The deciduous teeth begin to erupt at five or six months of age. The lower central incisors are generally the first to be noted. By the age of 20 to 24 months, the child has a total of 20 teeth: 10 upper and 10 lower. This is known as the deciduous or temporary dentition. At the age of six, in addition to the temporary dentition, the first permanent or six year molars erupt behind the second deciduous molars. At the age of seven, the maxillary and mandibular central incisor teeth are replaced by the permanent teeth. At the age of nine, the permanent lateral incisors have erupted. At the ages of 10 to 11, the deciduous molar teeth are replaced by the permanent premolar teeth. At ages 12 and 13, the second permanent molar teeth come into position and the deciduous canine teeth are lost and replaced by the permanent canine teeth. At the age of 14, usually all of the deciduous teeth have been exfoliated and replaced by the permanent teeth and the first and second permanent molars in all quadrants are present. The third molars are missing, impacted, or unerupted in some but erupt in most persons after 16 years of age.

If all of the permanent teeth have erupted, the adult has 32 permanent teeth, 8 in each quadrant.

Dental Occlusion. The grinding or incising surfaces of the teeth fit or mesh together into what is known as the occlusion. In normal occlusion the lower arch is smaller than the upper arch and the lower teeth fit just inside the outer surface of the upper teeth. A knowledge of dental occlusion is helpful in the management of facial fractures. A brief study of the mouth of the normal patient will orient the surgeon to the average occlusal relationships. Examination of a nurse or colleague or resident assitant will suffice to remind the examining physician of gross occlusal relationships (Fig. 24–65).

The examiner must be on the alert for abnormalities or deviations from the accepted normal, which for the patient may be his preinjury physiologic occlusion. The preexisting occlusion is easily recognized. Obviously, if the patient had a protruding lower jaw—Class III malocclusion—before injury, it would be impossible to obtain adequate reduction of fragments by attempting to force his teeth into neutrocclusion.

Class I occlusion or neutrocclusion is that in which the mesiobuccal cusp of the upper first molar occludes with the mesiobuccal groove of the lower first molar. The protruding or jutting type of jaw is known as Class III malocclusion (mesioclusion), and the retrusive jaw or the underdeveloped jaw is Class II malocclusion (distocclusion). In addition, there are abnormalities in a lateral direction generally referred to as crossbite or laterognathism.

In the injured patient in whom teeth or segments of bone are missing, it may be difficult to determine what the normal occlusal relationships should be. Usually the patient is not helpful in advising the physician about the preexisting occlusion. Information may be ob-

tained from the patient's dentist, who may have taken X-ray films or casts of the dentition (often referred to as "models") prior to the patient's injury. In older patients, abrasion marks on the teeth may give a clue to the preexisting occlusion. The patient who has had neutrocclusion shows worn surfaces on the outer edge of the lower anterior teeth and on the undersurface of the maxillary anterior teeth. The pa-

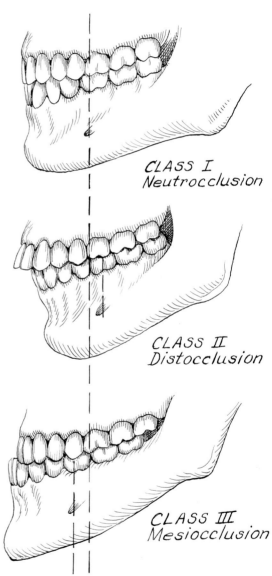

FIGURE 24–65. The classification of occlusion includes three main types. The classification is based upon the position of the mesobuccal cusp of the maxillary first molar in relationship to the mesiobuccal groove of the mandibular first molar tooth. Subdivisions of the three main classes are identified by differences in mesial or lateral positioning of the teeth in the dental arches.

tient with a severely retruded jaw usually will have no wearing of the incisal edges of the lower anterior teeth. The patient who has a protruding lower jaw may have worn surfaces on the outer anterior edge of the maxillary teeth. If the patient has premolar and molar teeth in large segments of the upper and lower jaw, these teeth usually fit into the contours of the opposing teeth. Dental consultation may be helpful in determining the preexisting occlusion.

Inasmuch as the restoration of function is important in the rehabilitation of the patient, it is necessary that the teeth be brought into the best possible occlusal relationship, so that an adequate chewing surface will be restored following reduction, fixation, and consolidation of jaw fractures.

The Dentoalveolar Process. The teeth are intimately associated with the main body of the mandible and maxilla and are held in place by supporting alveolar bone. The alveolar bone is dense on its cortical surface, with a medullary portion supporting the teeth which is highly vascular and spongy in character. Following loss of all of the permanent teeth by extraction or disease, the alveolar portion of the bone usually undergoes atrophy of disuse, with final reduction in size of the mandible to pencil-size thinness and recession of the maxillary alveolar process to the nasal and maxillary sinus cavities (Fig. 24–66).

The Dentition as a Guide in the Reduction and Fixation of Jaw Fractures. The normal teeth are so intimately associated with the mandible and the maxilla that restoration of the occlusion in fractured jaws is tantamount

to anatomical reduction of the fractured segments. In many cases of fracture, simple wiring of the teeth in occlusion provides satisfactory reduction and fixation. The restoration of occlusion is a guide to proper positioning of the maxilla and upper facial bone structures. When the mandible and maxilla are involved, ligation of the teeth in occlusion maintains fixation of the fractured segments.

Surgeons who treat patients with fractures of the facial bones should be acquainted with the normal anatomy of the teeth and tissues of the mouth.

Dental Wiring and Intermaxillary Fixation Techniques

THE GILMER TECHNIQUE. The simplest method of establishing intermaxillary fixation is by the Gilmer method (1887). It was not until 1887 that the importance of the teeth in the fixation of fractures was recognized and described in the American literature. The technique is simple and effective but has the disadvantage that the mouth cannot be opened for inspection of the fracture site without the removal of the wire fixation. This method consists of passing a wire ligature around the neck of all of the available teeth and twisting in a clockwise direction until the wire is tightened around each tooth. After an adequate number of wires have been placed on both the upper and lower teeth, the teeth are brought into occlusion and the wires twisted, one upper to one lower wire. To be consistent and avoid difficulty in removal, it is always advisable to twist wires in one direction, for example, clockwise. The twisted wires are cut short and the ends turned in against the necks of the teeth (Fig. 24–67). Stainless steel wire is most

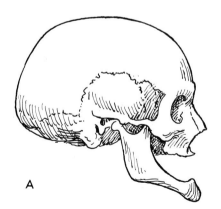
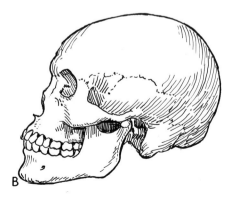

FIGURE 24–66. An edentulous skull *(A)* and a skull containing natural dentition *(B)*. Note the structural changes in *(A)* due to loss of teeth and atrophy of the alveolar process.

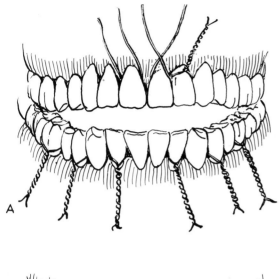

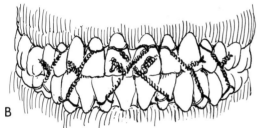

FIGURE 24–67. The Gilmer method of intermaxillary fixation of the teeth in occlusion by intermaxillary wiring.

satisfactory because of its tensile strength and malleability, but brass ligature wire may be used. Gauge 22 to 28 wire is most satisfactory. The size used depends upon the amount of force and stress anticipated. With the Gilmer-

method, the wires are twisted in a vertical direction or crisscrossed to prevent slipping in an anterior-posterior direction.

THE EYELET METHOD. The eyelet method (Eby, 1920; Ivy, 1922) of intermaxillary fixation is useful and has the advantage that the jaws may be opened for inspection by removal of only the intermaxillary ligatures. This method consists of twisting a 20-cm length of 22- or 24-gauge wire around an instrument to establish a loop. Both ends of the wire are passed through the interproximal space from the outer surface. One end of the wire is passed around the anterior tooth and the other around the posterior tooth. One end of the wire may be passed through the loop. In the upper jaw the eyelet should project above and in the lower jaw below the horizontal twist (Fig. 24–68) to prevent the ends from impinging upon each other. After the establishment of a sufficient number of eyelets, the teeth are brought into occlusion and ligatures are passed loop-fashion between one upper and one lower eyelet. The wires are twisted tightly to provide intermaxillary fixation. If it is necessary to open the mouth for inspection, the ligature loop wires may be cut and if necessary replaced without difficulty. If heavy wire is used to form the eyelets, they may be turned to form hooklike projections to which intermaxillary orthodontic rubber bands are attached for traction.

THE ARCH BAR METHOD. Prefabricated arch bars are commercially available. These can be ligated to the external surface of the dental arch by passing 22- or 24-gauge steel wires around the arch bar and around the

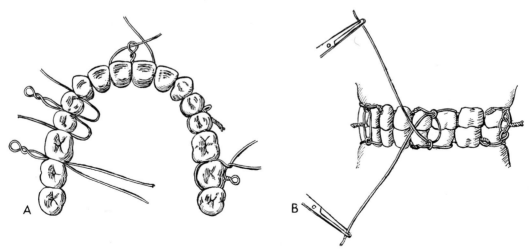

FIGURE 24–68. The eyelet method of intermaxillary fixation popularized by Ivy.

necks of the available teeth. The wires are twisted tightly to hold the arch bars in the form of an arc completely around the dental arch. The arch bars have hooklike projections which are placed in a downward direction on the lower jaw and in an upward direction in the upper jaw (Figs. 24–69 and 24–70).

If an inadequate number of teeth are present owing to trauma or previous extractions, supplementary wiring may be necessary for stabilization of the arch bars. This is sometimes done even if there is a full complement of teeth when traction is expected to be applied with great and prolonged force. Such traction may result in loosening of the teeth if additional support is not provided. Greater stability may be obtained by suspension of the maxillary arch bar from the margin of the pyriform aperture or the anterior nasal spine of the maxilla (Fig. 24–71, *A, B*); greater stability can be attained by drilling through the nasal spine to

and through the floor of the nose on the contralateral side (Fig. 24–72). The mandibular arch bar can be stabilized by one or more circumferential wires around the mandible (see Fig. 24–71, *C, D*).

After the arch bars are secured, orthodontic rubber bands are used between the two arches to bring the teeth into occlusion. The rubber bands pull the teeth into their proper relationship and provide secure fixation. Fractures of several days' duration usually cannot be completely reduced manually because of the presence of organized tissue in the line of fracture. Strong rubber band traction within a period of 24 hours usually brings the teeth into their proper relationship. The use of rubber bands is highly advantageous because they are easily removed. In seven to ten days when the occlusion has settled, the rubber bands are replaced, a few at a time, by 26- or 28-gauge stainless steel wires. The wires are less bulky and easier

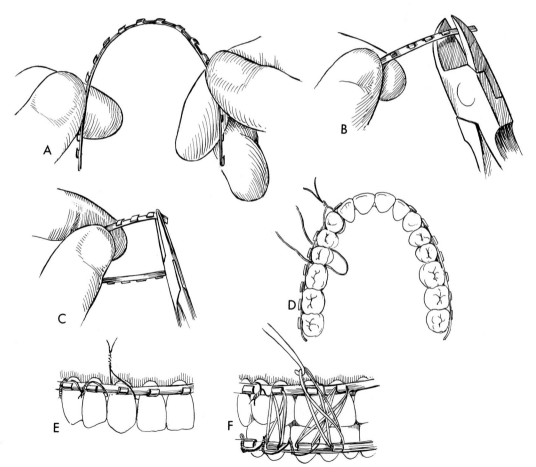

FIGURE 24–69.   Method of adapting and ligating a prefabricated arch bar to the upper teeth and applying rubber bands for intermaxillary fixation.

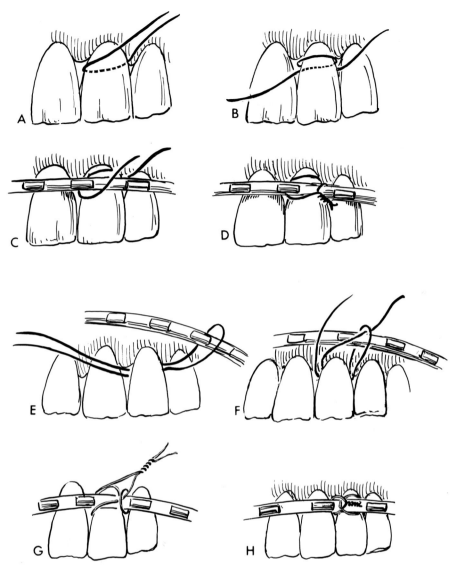

FIGURE 24–70. The conical shape of the maxillary anterior teeth requires special wiring technique to keep the wire and arch bar from slipping. The method of Rowe and Killey provides secure fixation of the arch bar in the maxillary incisor and cuspid area.

to clean with a small toothbrush or Water Pic. At the end of the usual course of treatment, if there is springiness at the site of fracture, fixation is easily reestablished (Fig. 24–73).

THE STOUT METHOD. This method (Stout, 1942) consists of the formation of small wire loops around the upper and lower dental arches to which rubber band traction is supplied (Figs. 24–74 and 24–75).

OTHER METHODS. There are other ways to use wire appliances with rubber bands. An effective method on isolated teeth is that of Kazanjian (1933): a heavy gauge wire is twisted

around the neck of the tooth in a very firm fashion, leaving a button of wire at the neck of the tooth for the attachment of a rubber band (Fig. 24–76).

The arch bar may be attached to the teeth by means of orthodontic bands. This is a precise and accurate method of securely holding the bar (Fig. 24–77). The appliance is time-consuming to construct and is expensive to use in fractures and requires the presence of an orthodontist as a member of the team.

Adaptations of the use of wire ligatures are many. A fracture in which there are stable

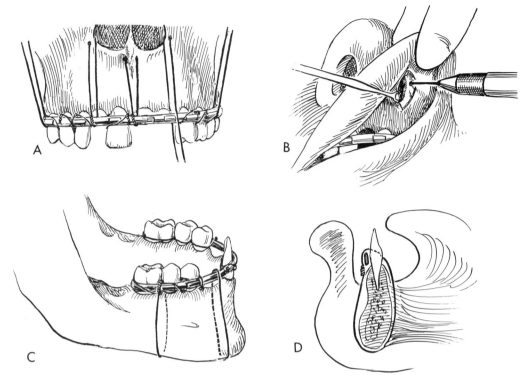

FIGURE 24–71. Supplementary fixation of arch bars is necessary in partially edentulous jaws. Teeth may be missing owing to previous extraction or injury and may be insufficient in number for adequately securing the arch bar. *A,* Support in the maxillary anterior region can be obtained by passing wires through small drill holes at the pyriform aperture of the nasal cavity or through the anterior nasal spine. Additional wires may be suspended from the zygomatic arches. *B,* The approach to the pyriform margin is through a small vertical incision in the labial vestibule of the upper lip. *C, D,* Circumferential wires may be used to give stability to the lower arch bar when an insufficient number of teeth are available for attachment of the bar.

teeth on each side can be secured with a single wire encircling the teeth across the line of fracture or with several wires twisted around adjacent teeth and twisted together (Fig. 24–78).

Splints in Maintenance of Intermaxillary Fixation. Dental splints cast from metal or acrylic resin are useful in maintaining intermaxillary fixation and the continuity of the maxillary or mandibular arch. Appliances of this type are effective but require detailed dental knowledge for construction (Fig. 24–79). The prosthodontist may be able to fabricate acrylic splints to maintain the fragments in alignment during healing (see Fig. 24–96).

Monomaxillary Versus Bimaxillary Fixation. When teeth are present on each side of the fracture line, the use of a splint or prefabricated arch bar obviates the need for intermaxillary bimaxillary fixation to the considerable increase of the patient's comfort. A wiring technique for monomaxillary fixation is illustrated in Figure 24–78.

Fractures of the Mandible

The position and anatomy of the mandible is such that it is frequently subjected to injury and is the facial bone most likely to be fractured. The mandible is a movable U-shaped bone, consisting of a body and two rami and articulating with the skull bilaterally at the temporomandibular joints; it is attached to other facial bones by muscles and ligaments. It also articulates with the maxilla by way of the teeth.

The mandible is a strong bone but has certain areas of weakness. The body of the bone is composed principally of dense cortical bone with a small substantia spongiosa through which blood and lymphatic vessels, and nerves pass. The mandible is thin at the angles where the body joins with the ramus and at the neck of the condyle. The mental foramen through which the mental nerve and vessels extend to the tissues of the lateral aspect of the face and lower lip is large in some individuals and is an

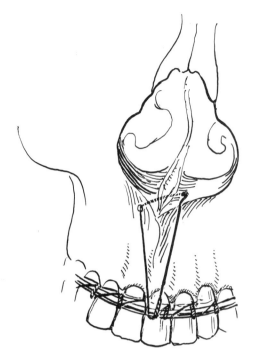

FIGURE 24–72. Alternative technique of passing the wire through the nasal spine and the margin of the pyriform aperture.

area of weakness through which fractures frequently occur. With loss of the teeth from the mandible, atrophic changes in the alveolar portion weaken the bone. Fractures are more frequent through edentulous areas than through areas well supported by adequate tooth structures.

Mandibular movements are determined by the action of muscles attached to the bone. When fracture occurs, displacement of the segments is influenced by the pull of the muscles.

The mandible may be fractured by any external force, the most common causes being automobile accidents, falls, kicks, missiles, blows from fists, trauma from animals, and sports accidents. Fractures may occur in the course of a difficult extraction of teeth or electroshock therapy. Transportation accidents, such as motorcycle, train, and airplane accidents, account for many mandibular fractures.

CLASSIFICATION

Classifications of fractures of the mandible are many and varied. Factors according to which they may be classified are:

THE ETIOLOGY OF THE FRACTURE
Civilian
Military
Crash-type
Gunshot
THE DIRECTION OF THE FRACTURE AND FAVORABILITY FOR TREATMENT
Horizontal
  Favorable
  Unfavorable
Vertical
  Favorable
  Unfavorable
THE SEVERITY OF THE FRACTURE

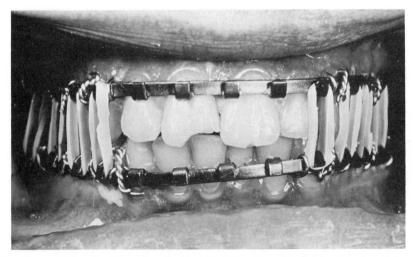

FIGURE 24–73. Intermaxillary fixation with rubber band traction. If a sufficient number of posterior teeth are present to give stability to the arch bars, the anterior teeth are not ligated. Heavy traction on the anterior teeth may loosen the teeth from the alveolar bone. This method provides a quick, easy, and effective means of intermaxillary fixation.

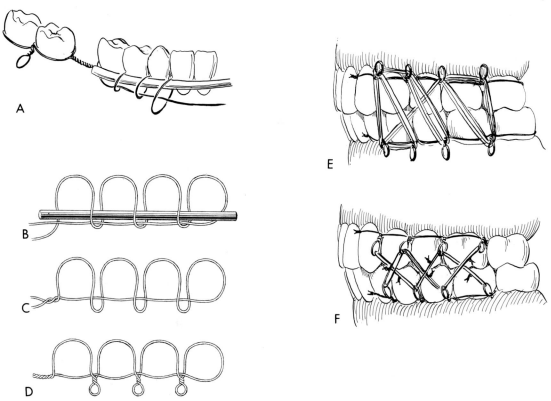

FIGURE 24–74.   Stout's modification of the eyelet technique of intermaxillary fixation. The eyelets are formed by a continuous wire threaded around the teeth and over a soft metal bar which is removed before the eyelets are twisted. *A* to *D*, Method of application of the Stout wire. *E*, The eyelets may be used as hooks over which rubber bands are applied or, *F*, may be used for maxillary wire fixation. (From Kazanjian and Converse.)

Simple fracture—the type in which there is no contact of the fracture site with the outside environment. There is no discontinuity of the overlying soft tissue structures.

Compound fractures—these are fractures in which there is a break through the skin or mucosa and overlying structures with direct communication of the fracture site with the

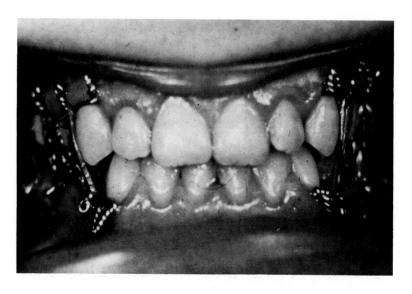

FIGURE 24–75. Fixation of the occlusion by means of intermaxillary multiple loop wiring.

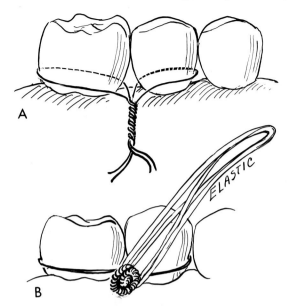

FIGURE 24-76. The Kazanjian button. This method is useful in providing an attachment for rubber band traction in cases where single or insufficient teeth are present in the fragment to permit the application of an arch bar.

outside environment through tears in the soft tissue.

THE VARIETY OF THE FRACTURE

"Greenstick" fracture—in which there is incomplete discontinuity of the bone. The bone structure is bent or partially fractured to resemble a green stick which has been forcibly bent or partially broken.

Simple fracture—in which there is no communication with the outside environment.

Compound fractures—in which there is a communication with the outside environment.

Complex fractures—those in which fractures occur in multiple directions; sometimes into a joint with severe injury to surrounding tissues.

Comminuted fractures—in which there are many small fragments. These may be simple or compound.

Impacted fractures—in which the bone ends are driven firmly together out of position. Force is required to disengage the fragments.

Depressed fractures—those with depression and dislocation of the segments.

THE PREDISPOSING CAUSES TO FRACTURE

Generalized bone disease, such as rickets, osteomalacia, fragilitas osseum.

Localized bone diseases, such as benign and malignant neoplasms, cysts, osteomyelitis or hemangioma of the bone.

Certain anatomical considerations:
Thin areas—the region of the angle of the mandible and the neck of the condyle.

Edentulous areas—in which there is atrophy of the alveolar bone and loss of supporting structures.

The region of a foramen of the mandible or of the maxilla.

THE CAUSES OF FRACTURES

Trauma

Direct—a blow at the site of the fracture which results in discontinuity of the bone.

Indirect—a blow on the opposite side of the jaw or a blow at a distance from the fracture site. This is seen in fractures of the condyle, which may occur from a blow on the chin on the contralateral side. A blow on the symphysis may result in fracture of both mandibular condyles.

THE PRESENCE OR ABSENCE OF SERVICEABLE TEETH IN THE SEGMENTS OF THE MANDIBLE. Kazanjian and Converse (1949) emphasized this classification because it has a practical relationship to the management of the fracture (Fig. 24–80).

Class I—Teeth present on both sides of the fracture line. The teeth can be used as a guide to anatomic reduction and can be utilized for the attachment of wires or appliances to mantain the fragments in position during the healing period. One or more teeth on each side of the fracture may be sufficient even though the upper teeth are not present to permit intermaxillary fixation.

Class II—Teeth present on only one side of the fracture line. The teeth are used for fixation of the mandibular to the maxillary teeth or to hold an appliance to stabilize an edentulous segment.

Class III—The fragments contain no teeth. The teeth may have been dislodged or fractured at the time of injury or may have previously been removed.

MANDIBULAR FRACTURES CLASSIFIED AS TO LOCATION (Dingman and Natvig, 1964)

Parasymphyseal—those that occur in the symphysis area between the lower canine teeth. Fractures vertically through the true symphysis are rare.

Canine—through the cuspid teeth.

Body of the mandible—from the cuspid teeth to the angle of the mandible.

Angle—through the angle of the mandible behind the second molar tooth.

Ramus of the mandible—those fractures between the angle of the mandible and the sigmoid notch.

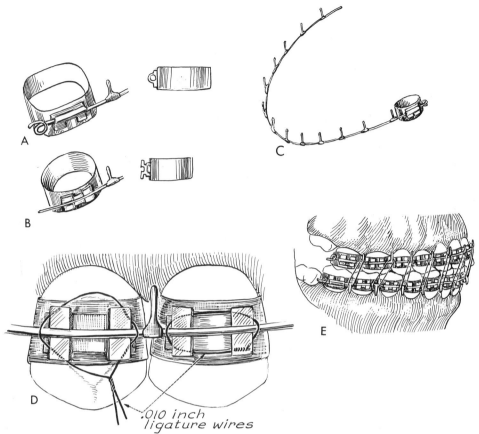

FIGURE 24–77. Edge-wise orthodontic and fixation appliance. *A*, Edge-wise appliance consists of molar bands with rectangular sheath (internal dimensions 0.022 × 0.028 inch) through which edge-wise arch wire is inserted at each end. *B*, Remaining teeth, in each dental arch, carry bands with "twin brackets" (with slot dimensions 0.022 × 0.028 inch) to permit insertion of edge-wise wire (0.021 × 0.025 inch) and secure it in position with ligature ties (0.010 inch). *C*, Arch wire with spurs soldered to gingival side is as it appears prior to final insertion and planned surgery. *D*, Arch wire in position and maintained in position with wire ligatures placed around brackets. *E*, Appliance as it appears at time of surgery with intermaxillary wires (0.028 inch) placed between arches to fix one jaw to the other.

The edge-wise appliance affords the orthodontist the opportunity to make the necessary corrections in tooth position intradentally and interdentally. Obtaining optimum dental alignment and dental arch form in maxillary and mandibular dentition is an essential prerequisite to corrective jaw surgery. It can minimize the maxillary-mandibular disparity and contribute significantly to enhancing surgical results by good interdigitation of the cusps of the teeth, thus securing position and fixation. (From Kazanjian and Converse.)

Coronoid process—in which the coronoid is broken off on a level above the mandibular notch.

Condyle—all fractures of the condyle above the level of the sigmoid notch of the mandible.

Alveolar fractures—segments of alveolar bone with or without attached teeth may be fractured separately or in association with other fractures of the mandible.

THE PRESENCE OF TEETH OR ABSENCE OF TEETH IN THE JAW
    Dentulous
    Partially edentulous
    Edentulous

MUSCULAR CONTRACTION

Seen in some cases of severe destruction of bone due to disease. Muscular contraction in eating may break the weakened bone. This also occurs in electroshock therapy if the jaws are not adequately protected.

CLINICAL EXAMINATION

The common symptoms of fractures of the jaw are the following:

Pain. Pain is usually present on motion and may be noted immediately after the fracture as

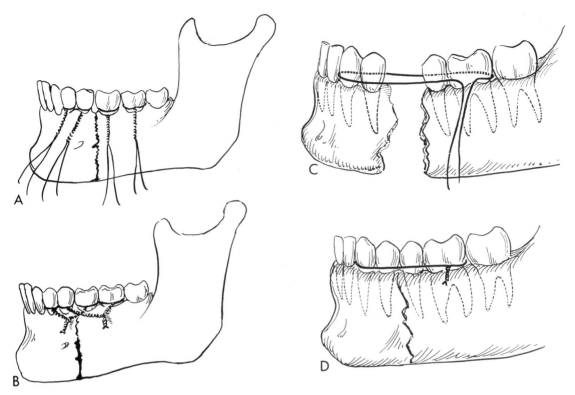

FIGURE 24–78. Method of application of wires for monomaxillary fixation of a fracture of the mandible. *A, B,* Multiple wire technique. *C, D,* Single wire technique.

a result of injury to the inferior alveolar nerve and to adjacent soft tissues.

Tenderness. There is exquisite tenderness over the site of the fracture. This is helpful in localizing the fracture site.

Disability. The patient is unable to open his mouth and refuses to eat usual foods because of discomfort.

Edema. Enlargement of soft tissues at the fracture site is the result of hemorrhage and

FIGURE 24–79. Cast cap splint used for fixation of a mandibular fracture. This type of splint may result in malocclusion as it does not permit accurate evaluation of the occlusal relationship at the time of reduction.

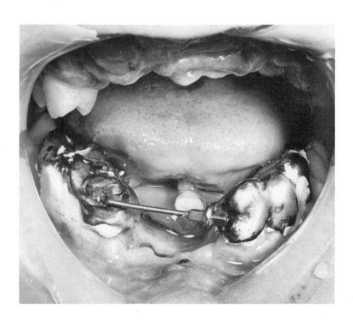

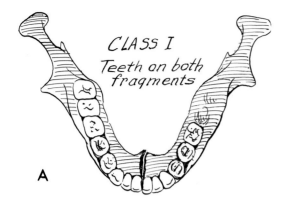

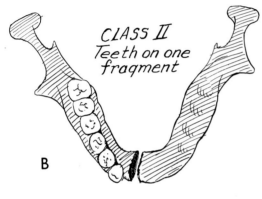

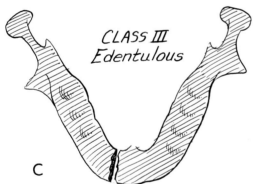

FIGURE 24–80. Classification of mandibular fractures according to the presence or absence of teeth on the fragments. *A*, Class I. *B*, Class II. *C*, Class III. (After Kazanjian and Converse.)

edema. Immediately after the injury there is usually distortion and enlargement of the overlying soft tissues.

Ecchymosis. Hemorrhage may appear as ecchymosis or as hematoma in the soft tissue near the site of the fracture.

Deformity. Owing to fracture-dislocation of the segments, the patient may be unable to open his mouth or may be unable to close it.

Open bite deformity may be present, or the mandible may be shifted to one side or posteriorly, giving a bizarre appearance to the lower facial area.

Abnormal mobility. In fractures of the condyle with displacement, the mandible may shift toward the involved side as the patient attempts to open his mouth. This is caused by nonfunction of the lateral pterygoid muscle on the side of the fracture. On protrusive motion the jaw shifts to the side of the fracture.

Crepitation. The patient may notice a grating sound on movement of the mandible. This is caused by movement of the fracture segments against one another.

Salivation. Pain and tenderness stimulate overactivity of the salivary glands.

Fetor oris. Because of the absence of the normal cleansing activity of mastication, after a day or two debris accumulates around the teeth. Food, blood clots, devitalized tissue, and mucus undergo bacterial putrefaction, resulting in a very offensive breath.

DIAGNOSIS

The diagnosis of mandibular fracture is made on one or more of the following findings:

Clinical Findings

Mobility at the site of the fracture. Bimanual manipulation causes springiness at the site of the fracture, especially in the body of the mandible. One hand stabilizes the ramus of the mandible, while the other manipulates the symphysis of the mandible. Fracture will be demonstrated by movement and discomfort.

Malocclusion. Probably the most reliable finding in fractures of the mandible in dentulous patients is malocclusion. Even the most minute dislocation caused by the fracture will be obvious to the patient inasmuch as the teeth do not mesh or come together in the usual manner.

Dysfunction. The patient is unable to use his jaw and will request soft foods which require minimal movement of the jaw on mastication. Speech is difficult because of pain on motion of the mandible.

Crepitation. This may be noticeable by manipulation at the fracture site, but it is not a frequently used sign because of discomfort to the patient.

Swelling at the fracture site. Swelling is usually quite obvious and may be associated with ecchymosis and subcutaneous hematoma.

Abnormal mobility of the mandible on function with deviation to one side or the other may lead to the diagnosis of fracture.

Tenderness over the fracture site, especially in the region of the temporomandibular joint, is highly suggestive of the presence of a fracture.

Roentgenologic Findings. Roentgenographic examination is imperative. Careful single, stereoscopic views, tomograms, and panoramic roentgenograms should be taken of all fractures, as indicated, with particular attention to the condyles. Occlusal films and dental roentgenograms are helpful in detecting fractures of the symphysis and the alveolar structures of the mandible. (See section on Roentgenographic Positions.)

Muscles Influencing Movement of the Mandible. Muscle action is an important factor influencing the degree and direction of displacement of fractured segments of the mandible. Overcoming the forces of displacement is important in reduction and fixation of the mandibular fragments.

THE POSTERIOR GROUP OF MANDIBULAR MUSCLES. The posterior group of muscles is commonly referred to as the "muscles of mastication." The muscles are short and thick and

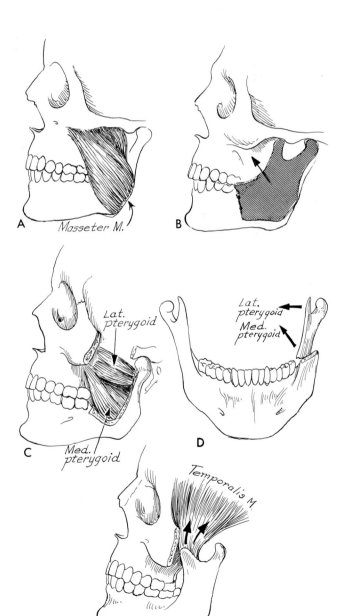

FIGURE 24–81. The posterior group of muscles attached to the mandible. The overall force from the activity of this group of muscles is movement of the mandible upwards, forwards, and medially.

A, The masseter muscle. *B*, Upward displacement in a fracture of the mandible produced by a pull of the masseter muscle on the edentulous proximal fragment. *C*, The medial and lateral pterygoid muscles. *D*, Directional pull of the medial and lateral pterygoid muscles. *E*, The temporalis muscle and its direction of pull. (From Kazanjian and Converse.)

are capable of exerting extremely strong forces on the mandible. The muscles of mastication are the temporalis, masseter, and medial (internal) and lateral (external) pterygoid muscles. The overall activity of this group is to pull the mandible upward, forward, and medially (Fig. 24–81).

Masseter muscle. This is a thick, short, powerful, heavy muscle attached to the zygoma and zygomatic arch. It arises from tendinous fibers in the anterior two-thirds of the lower border of the zygomatic bone and from the medial surface of the zygomatic arch and inserts into the lateral surface of the ramus and into the bone at the angle of the mandible. The masseter muscle is an elevator of the jaw and functions to pull the mandible upward and forward.

Temporalis muscle. This muscle arises from the limits of the temporal fossa. It is broad and fan-shaped. Its fibers converge as it descends to pass under the zygomatic arch and insert into the tip of the coronoid, the lateral and medial surface of the coronoid, and the anterior surface of the ramus as far down as the occlusal plane of the third molar tooth. The anterior fibers are elevators, and the posterior fibers are retractors of the mandible.

Medial pterygoid muscle. This muscle originates in the pterygoid fossa, mainly from the medial surface of the lateral pterygoid process and from the pyramidal process of the palatine bone and maxillary tuberosity. It inserts into the medial surface of the ramus and angle of the mandible. The fibers of the medial pterygoid muscle pass in a downward posterior and lateral direction to the angle of the mandible. Its function is to pull the mandible upward, medially, and forward.

Lateral pterygoid muscle. This muscle has two heads of origin. The upper head arises from the infratemporal crest, the infratemporal surface of the greater wing of the sphenoid bone, and a small area of the squamous part of the temporal bone. The lower head arises from the lateral surface of the lateral pterygoid plate. The upper head inserts into the capsule of the joint and into the articular disc of the temporomandibular joint. The lower head inserts into the anterior surface of the neck of the condyle. The innermost or upper portion pulls the mandible upward, medially, and forward; the external portion pulls the condyle downward and medially and forward. Contraction of the muscle on one side pulls the mandible to the opposite side. Contraction of both muscles simultaneously protrudes the mandible.

THE ANTERIOR OR DEPRESSOR GROUP OF MANDIBULAR MUSCLES. These muscles are considered the opening muscles of the mandible (Fig. 24–82). With the hyoid bone fixed, they depress the mandible. When the mandible is fractured, they displace the fractured segments downward, posteriorly, and medially. This group is made up of the geniohyoid, genioglossus, mylohyoid, and digastric muscles.

Geniohyoid muscle. This muscle arises from the inferior medial spine of the mandible and passes downward and posteriorly to insert into the body of the hyoid bone. Its function is to elevate the hyoid and to depress the mandible.

Genioglossus muscle. This is the main muscle of the tongue and is attached to the genial tubercles on the inner anterior inferior surface of the mandible. Its fibers pass primarily into the substance of the tongue and into the upper surface of the hyoid bone. Its function is to protrude the tongue, elevate the hyoid, and depress the mandible.

Mylohyoid muscle. This fan-shaped muscle acts as a diaphragm for support of the floor of the mouth. It arises from the mylohyoid line on the inner surface of the body of the mandible. Its fibers pass medially to insert into a median raphe and posteriorly to insert into the hyoid bone. Its function is to elevate the hyoid bone and to depress the mandible. Its fibers pull medially, posteriorly, and downward.

Digastric muscle. The digastric muscle arises from the digastric fossa at the inferior medial portion of the mandible bilaterally and extends posteriorly to pass beneath a fibrous sling attached near the lesser cornu of the hyoid bone. Its tendon is continuous with that of the posterior portion which originates from the digastric fossa of the temporal bone. The function of this muscle is to elevate the hyoid and depress the anterior portion of the mandible.

The Temporomandibular Joint. The function and anatomy of this joint is important in consideration of injuries to the mandible condyle (Fig. 24–83). The temporomandibular joint is known as a ginglymodiarthrodial joint; it is capable of a hingelike action as well as a gliding and rotating action. The joint is composed of the articular head of the condyle of the mandible and the mandibular fossa of the squamous portion of the temporal bone (glenoid fossa). The articular surface of each bone is covered by a thin, smooth layer of cartilage surrounded by connective tissue which dif-

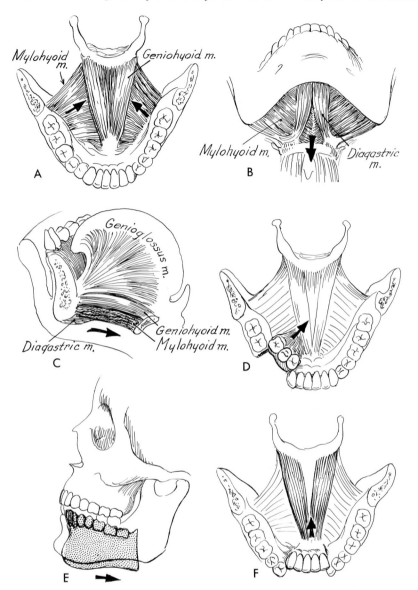

FIGURE 24–82. The anterior or depressor group of the muscles of mastication, the suprahyoid muscles. The arrows indicate the direction of pull and the displacement of fragments in fractures of the mandible. (From Kazanjian and Converse.)

ferentiates into an inner and outer layer. The inner layer, which is known as the synovial membrane, secretes a viscid fluid lubricant that minimizes friction and aids smooth functioning of the joint. The outer layer of connective tissue is intimately associated with the ligaments which surround the joint and provide an enveloping capsule within which the articular surfaces function. The temporomandibular joint is a compound joint. It is separated into two distinct chambers, one above and the other below an articular disc of fibrocartilage known as the meniscus. Movement of the articular disc is controlled by the attachments of the lateral pterygoid muscle which insert, through the capsule, into its anterior edge and by attachment of the disc to the posterior portion of the joint capsule. The hinge, rotating, and gliding movements of the temporomandibular joint are controlled by the muscles attached to the mandible.

Factors Influencing Displacement of Fractured Mandibular Segments. The direction and extent of displacement of fragments depends upon the site of the fracture, the direc-

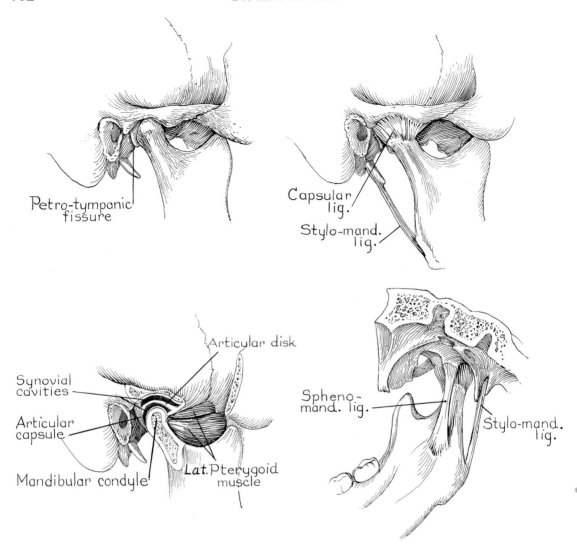

FIGURE 24–83.   The temporomandibular joint. (From Kazanjian and Converse.)

tion of the fracture, the direction of pull of the strong muscles attached to the mandible, the direction and intensity of force, and the presence or absence of teeth in the fragments. In fractures of the mandible, the segments may be displaced in the direction of the strongest muscle action.

DIRECTION AND ANGULATION OF THE FRACTURE LINE. Fry, Shepard, McLeod, and Parfitt (1942) pointed out that fractures may be favorable or unfavorable for displacement according to their direction and bevel. The muscular force in some fractures pulls the bone into a position favorable for healing, whereas in other fractures the muscle pull is unfavorable and separation of the bone fragments occurs.

Mandibular fractures that are directed downward and forward are classified as horizontally favorable (H. F.) because the posterior group of muscles and the anterior group of muscles pull in antagonistic directions favoring stability at the site of fracture. Fractures running from above downward and posteriorly are classified as horizontally unfavorable fractures (H. U.). The bevel of the fracture may influence the displacement medially. If the fracture runs from posteriorly forward and medially, displacement will take place in a medial direction because of the medial pull of the elevator muscles of mastication (V. U.). A fracture that passes from the lateral surface of the mandible posteriorly and medially is a favorable fracture because the muscle pull tends to prevent displacement. It

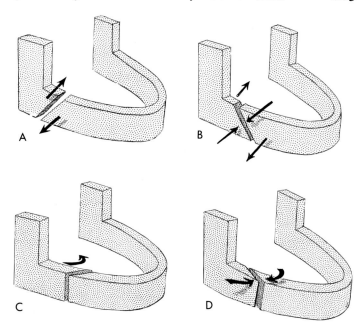

FIGURE 24–84. *A* and *C* demonstrate how the direction of bevel of the fracture line favors displacement due to muscular action. Arrows indicate the direction of muscle pull. *B* and *D* demonstrate bevels and direction of fracture that are unfavorable to displacement due to muscular action. The direction of the muscle pull in fractures beveled in this direction tends to prevent displacement by pulling the fragments together. (After Fry, W. K., Shepherd, P. R., McLeod, A. C., and Parfitt, G. J.: The Dental Treatment of Maxillofacial Injuries. Oxford, Blackwell Scientific Publications, 1942.)

is called a vertically favorable fracture (V. F.) (Fig. 24–84).

THE PRESENCE OR ABSENCE OF TEETH IN THE FRACTURED SEGMENTS. Upper displacement of the posterior segment is prevented by the occlusal contact of the lower against the upper teeth. The elevator muscles of the mandible pull the posterior fragment forward. The anterior group of muscles depresses the anterior segments of the mandible, separating the teeth anterior to the fracture from the upper

teeth. A single tooth in the posterior fragment may be extremely important and should be retained. Even if damaged, it will provide stability (Fig. 24–85).

SOFT TISSUE AT THE SITE OF FRACTURE. Fractures of the ramus of the mandible, even though extensively comminuted, have very little displacement because of the splinting action of the medial and lateral pterygoid and the masseter muscle attachments (Fig. 24–86). Some degree of stability is also provided by the

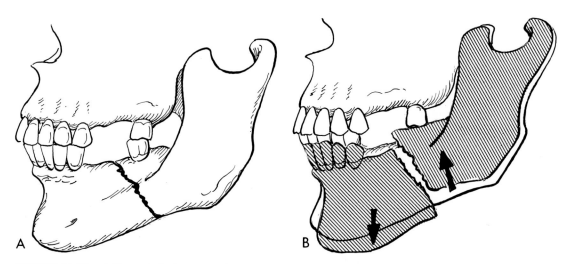

FIGURE 24–85. *A*, Upward displacement of the posterior segment can be prevented by the presence of a tooth on the posterior fragment. *B*, Displacement of the posterior fragment occurs because of the absence of an occluding tooth on the segment.

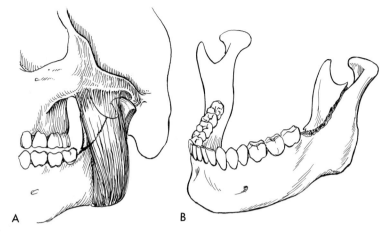

FIGURE 24–86. *A*, The heavy musculature and the periosteum surrounding the ramus of the mandible provide protection and tend to prevent displacement of fractured segments in this area. *B*, Fractures of the coronoid process are uncommon and displacement is usually minimal.

periosteum and soft tissue attachments surrounding the body of the mandible, but these are usually weak, and very little stability is offered by their presence. In extensive soft tissue wounds, such as gunshot injuries, no stability is offered from the torn tissues. Some degree of stability is provided to the fragments by the replacement of soft tissues and by suturing them carefully into position over the bone.

DIRECTION AND INTENSITY OF THE TRAUMATIC FORCE. The force on the mandible may directly or indirectly influence the site of fracture and the amount of displacement. Direct lateral force in the region of the premolar teeth may result in a fracture on the involved side and a fracture of the condyle on the contralateral side. Traumatic forces applied to the anterior portion of the mandible may break a segment between the canine or premolar teeth and drive it posteriorly into the floor of the mouth. Displacement will be aided by the muscles of the floor of the mouth which exert a downward and posterior force. Blows to the symphysis region may cause bilateral or unilateral condylar fractures or may force the condyle into the middle cranial fossa. The condyles may be forced into the external auditory canal by fracture of the tympanic plate.

FRACTURES OF THE ALVEOLAR STRUCTURES AND DAMAGE TO THE TEETH. Damage of the anterior teeth occurs more frequently than damage of the posterior teeth because of their forward position and single conical root structure.

Teeth may be completely avulsed from the bone or may fracture at the gingival line with the roots remaining in the bone, or segments of alveolar bone may be fractured with the teeth remaining firmly attached. The crowns and edges of the teeth may be fractured with exposure of the dental pulp.

Reimplantation of avulsed teeth may be successful in children, as the root apex is still open and the blood supply may be reestablished. Reimplantation sometimes is successful in adults if the pulp is removed and the root canal is filled and treated before the tooth is reimplanted. If the crown of a tooth has been fractured with exposure of the dental pulp, it is best to extract the tooth or remove the pulp prior to intermaxillary fixation. If this is not done, infection or severe pain may be troublesome. If segments of alveolus which contain teeth have been fractured and have an adequate blood supply by virtue of the soft tissue attachments, attempts should be made to replace the segments along with their contained teeth and wire them securely into position. Most of these tooth-bearing segments will survive and provide a satisfactory masticating surface.

Injury to the teeth without avulsion or fracture may result in devitalization owing to hemorrhage in the dental pulp. The teeth become insensitive and discolored as a result of infiltration of blood pigments into the tooth structure. If infection occurs, the teeth must be treated or extracted. Some of them, even though discolored and nonvital, remain as asymptomatic useful teeth.

As mentioned, teeth in the line of fracture should be retained if they offer any degree of stability to the bone fragments. Antibiotic therapy protects against infection. If teeth are loose or interfere with reduction, they should be removed. The retention of even one-half a tooth on the posterior segment may be helpful in maintaining the position of the proximal segment. After healing of the bone, the teeth can be given necessary attention by the patient's dentist.

PRINCIPLES OF TREATMENT

The primary consideration in the management of fractures of the mandible is to restore the function of the mandible and the masticating efficiency of the dentition. To accomplish this, the principles of fracture management must be applied. These are:

1. Reduction of the fractured bone segments to their anatomical position.

2. Fixation that will hold the fractured bone segments in position until healing takes place.

3. Control of infection.

Generally speaking, the simplest method of attaining and satisfying these requirements is the best method. Methods may vary with the age and general state of health of the patient, with the training and ability of the surgeon, and with the facilities and circumstances under which the patient is to be treated. A satisfactory end result may be accomplished by use of any one of several methods, but no method is acceptable that will jeopardize the function, appearance, or safety of the patient.

TREATMENT OF CLASS I FRACTURES OF THE MANDIBLE

Class I fractures are those in which there is a tooth on each side of the fracture (Fig. 24–87). They usually can be managed by dental appliances or intermaxillary fixation. Some can be managed best by open reduction and direct interosseous wiring in combination with dental appliances or intermaxillary fixation. The use of dental splints without intermaxillary fixation (monomaxillary fixation) is appealing to the patient because it is unnecessary to wire the teeth in occlusion. This permits the intake of solid foods and early return to work. Convenience to the patient should not influence the treatment if a more satisfactory result can be obtained by intermaxillary fixation. Four to six weeks of complete immobilization is not too long a period to be tolerated by the patient if a better result can be obtained. The factor of solid food versus liquid food for a period of four to six weeks is not of great significance and should not influence the operator in the use of less effective methods.

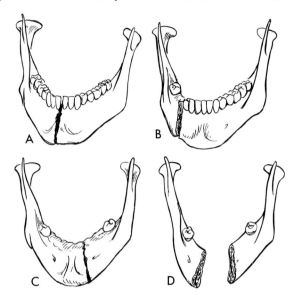

FIGURE 24–87. Class I fractures. Teeth are present on both sides of the fracture site. (From Kazanjian and Converse.)

Fixation of the fractured segments can be accomplished without intermaxillary fixation by use of a number of simple methods.

Horizontal Interdental Wiring. The fracture can be reduced manually and held together with 25-gauge stainless steel wire twisted around the necks of selected teeth on both sides of the fracture site and then twisted to a wire on the opposite side of the fracture site (Fig. 24–88). This method is simple and expedient and can be utilized on any Class I fracture in which there are stable teeth on each side of the fracture site. This may also be used in the lower anterior region when there is overriding of the fragments by passing the wire in such a way as to produce a leverage that will reduce and maintain the fracture (Fig. 24–89). It is inadvisable to use the teeth immediately adjacent to the fracture site, since their attachments are loosened and they may be dislodged by the force of the ligature wire.

Prefabricated Arch Bars. Winter type arch bars as modified by Erich are made of semi-rigid pliable metal and can be contoured to the dental arch and carefully fitted to the necks of the teeth without special equipment. Arch bars are generally used for intermaxillary fixation, but a single arch bar attached to the lower teeth for support of the Class I type of fracture may be used for monomaxillary fixation. This is done by shaping a bar long enough to pass

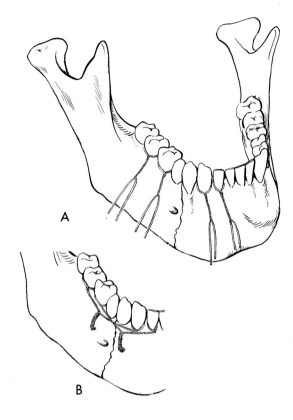

FIGURE 24–88. Horizontal wiring of mandibular fragments. *A*, In fractures with minimal displacement, wires may be placed around the teeth on each side of the fragment and twisted across the fracture site. *B*, Wires are twisted together across the fracture line. (From Kazanjian and Converse.)

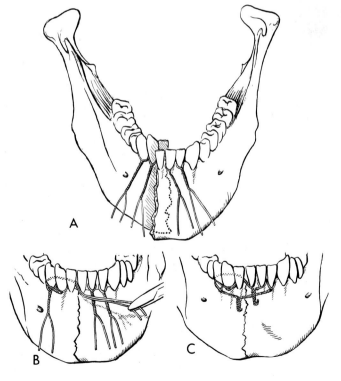

FIGURE 24–89. The wiring of an overriding fragment in a mandibular fracture. *A*, Wires are anchored to selected teeth on each side of the fracture site. *B*, The fracture is reduced by using the teeth on the overriding fragment to force the other fragment into apposition. *C*, The wires are twisted together across the fracture line. (From Kazanjian and Converse.)

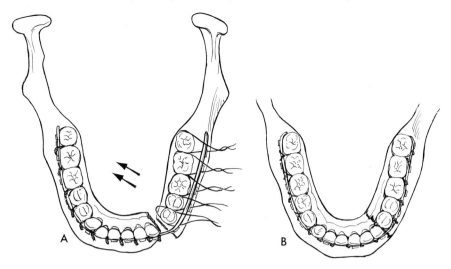

FIGURE 24–90. If maxillary teeth are not available for fixation of the mandibular fragments, a monomaxillary fixation can be accomplished by an arch wire attached securely to the teeth and bridged across the site of the fracture. *A*, Fracture of the mandible with medial displacement of the proximal segment. *B*, Fracture reduced and held with a single arch bar wired to the teeth on each side of the fracture site.

completely around the dental arch. This is securely ligated to the necks of the teeth on the larger fragment, and wires are loosely placed around the teeth and arch bar on the displaced fragment. The fracture is reduced manually and held firmly in position while an assistant tightens the wires (Fig. 24–90).

Sections of arch bars attached to the teeth of the posterior segment can be ligated in the anterior region after reduction of the fracture (Fig. 24–91). This provides adequate fixation and holds the fractured segments together. If maxillary teeth are present, supplementary fixation with intermaxillary rubber band traction will bring the teeth into optimum occlusion.

Cable Arch Wires. If no arch bars are available, a cable wire can be fashioned to provide stability across the site of the fracture and a means of intermaxillary fixation. This is fabricated by using a long length of 22-gauge stainless steel wire, which is passed around the last tooth on each quadrant of the dental arch and twisted up tightly to the teeth but left long. The wire from the right side is twisted to the wire of the left side at the midline and the excess is cut and removed. Ligature wires are then passed around the necks of the teeth and around the cable arch bar until all of the available teeth have been ligated (Fig. 24–92). The teeth can be wired into occlusion by passing small wires around the upper and lower cable and twisting these tightly to provide perpendicular intermaxillary fixation.

The Banded Dental Arch. Angle (1890) devised a banded arch wire for fixation of mandibular fractures (Fig. 24–93). These consist of prefabricated bands in sizes to fit the molar or bicuspid teeth. The bands are held with a jackscrew and nut attachment twisted tightly until the band is securely fixed to the tooth. A long section of 14-gauge annealed brass wire

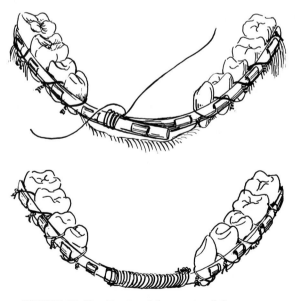

FIGURE 24–91. Fractured fragments of the parasymphyseal region may be supported by an arch bar attached to the segments on each side and wired together securely at the midline after reduction. (After Kazanjian and Converse.)

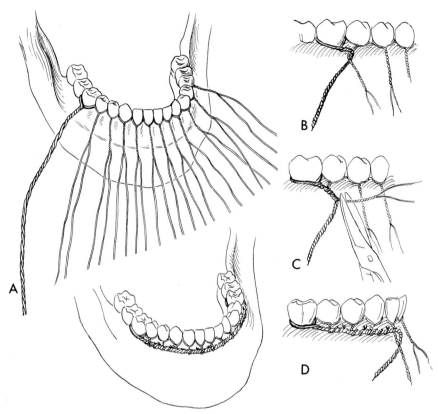

FIGURE 24–92. Cable arch wire (Kazanjian). *A,* Wires are twisted around each tooth. Note heavier gauge wire around molar tooth on right side. *B, C, D,* Heavier gauge wire is twisted successively with each of the thinner wires. Cable arch wire is completed. (From Kazanjian and Converse.)

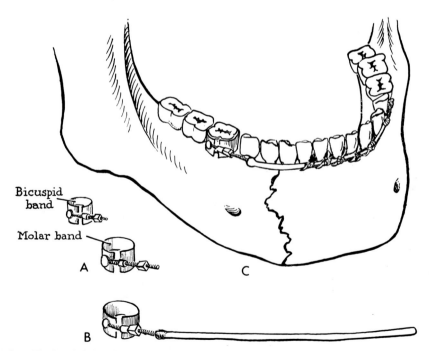

FIGURE 24–93. The banded dental arch. *A,* The banded arch wire for splinting the reduced mandibular fragments. *B,* A wire is soldered to the band to serve as an arch bar. The band is fixed securely to a lower molar on one side and then is bent to conform to the contour of the arch and is ligated to the necks of the teeth with fine wire ligatures. (Modified from Kazanjian and Converse.)

flattened to 19-gauge is soldered to the band. This malleable brass wire is then contoured along the lateral surface of the teeth to which it is ligated with fine stainless steel wire.

The orthodontist also may be helpful in applying a rigid lugged bar to several banded teeth. Banded appliances on upper and lower teeth serve well as fixation appliances for intermaxillary fixation but are complicated and expensive (Fig. 24–93). Usually simpler methods will suffice.

Cast Cap Splints. Cast cap splints are utilized extensively abroad but have not gained much favor in the management of fractures in the United States. These dental appliances are designed to cover the occlusal and exposed portions of the teeth and require the services of a skilled dentist and dental technician. Cast splints are especially useful when a strong appliance is needed. The cast cap splint is cemented to the occlusal surfaces of the teeth (see Fig. 24–79). This is a disadvantage inasmuch as the exact occlusion cannot be determined with the splint in position. Discrepancy in occlusion must be corrected orthodontically or by selective grinding of the teeth after the splint has been removed. Effective, equally useful, but less expensive appliances can be constructed by an orthodontist. The transparent acrylic splint is thin, strong, and easily fabricated by a prosthodontist and is an excellent alternate technique.

External Pin Fixation Appliances. External pin fixation or intramedullary wire pinning has little use in the management of Class I fractures in the presence of sound teeth at the site of the fracture (see Chapter 30).

Treatment of Compound Comminuted Anterior Mandibular Fractures. Comminuted fractures of the mandible, because of the very intimate attachment of the thin overlying periosteum and mucosa, are almost always compound, either through the skin or through the mucous membrane. With modern antibiotic therapy these fractures can be managed aggressively by open methods with an excellent chance of survival of the bone fragment. Conservative management will generally result in continuity of the bone upon healing if the fragments can be covered adequately by soft tissue with sufficient blood supply.

Fixation of the posterior segments is imperative. This may be accomplished by intermaxillary wiring between the retained mandibular teeth and the maxillary teeth or by constructing of a cast splint with an anterior retaining bar passed from one side to the opposite side (Fig. 24–94). If the posterior segments contain sufficient teeth, a commercially available arch bar can be used. The management of the segments depends upon the presence or absence of a satisfactory amount of soft tissue for coverage. If soft tissue is adequate, the fragment may be approached through the wound or through an external incision. The fragments are identified, aligned, and approximated by direct wiring technique (Fig. 24–95, *A*). Periosteal attachments should be retained, since even loose fragments may survive if stabilized and adequately covered with soft tissue with good blood supply. If the fragments are of sufficient size, they may be held by means of a Kirschner wire (Fig. 24–95, *B*) in a shish kebab fashion with the wire being attached to the solid proximal segments.

If there has been extensive loss of soft tissue of the lip, chin, and floor of the mouth along with bone, the posterior bone segments should be covered with skin and mucosa and properly splinted into position to prevent displacement by scar tissue contraction in the floor of the mouth. A vertical T bar soldered to the splint anteriorly will provide an attachment for an acrylic prosthetic mold to give support to the soft tissues during the period of reconstruction (see Fig. 24–107). These appliances are complicated and must be especially designed to fit the individual case. An acrylic splint made in a horseshoe fashion fitted over the remaining posterior segments and secured by means of circumferential wires is effective in maintaining the position of the posterior segments. It also

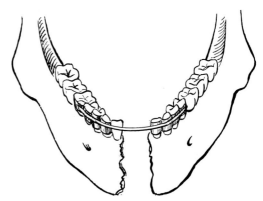

FIGURE 24–94. In Class I fractures with loss of bone or extensive comminution in the anterior region, the segments can be held in alignment by means of an arch bar attached to orthodontic bands on each side of the fracture site.

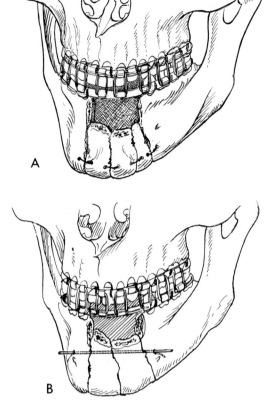

A

B

FIGURE 24–95. *A,* Comminuted mandibular fractures can be reduced and held by direct fixation supplemented with intermaxillary arch bar fixation. *B,* Satisfactory alignment may be maintained in some cases by use of transosseous wire pin fixation. (From Kazanjian and Converse.)

supports the soft tissue replacement during the phases of reconstruction (Fig. 24–96). Conservatism in the management of the fractured segments is important. Bone fragments should never be discarded if they can be used to help reestablish continuity of the bone or if they can be covered and salvaged under a soft tissue flap. These fragments of bone are invaluable in the reconstructive phase.

Open Reduction Techniques. It is impossible to reduce and adequately hold certain Class I fractures by closed methods, even though a satisfactory number of teeth are present in the dental arch. This applies especially to fractures in the region of the symphysis which run in an oblique direction downward and posteriorly, sometimes as far back as the molar teeth. The long splinter of the lingual segment has a tendency to telescope and override owing to pull of the muscles of the floor of

the mouth. Even though the teeth are brought into what appears to be satisfactory occlusion, there is medial rotation of the inferior border of the mandible. Fractures in the anterior region that run in an unfavorable direction require open operation for reduction and direct wire fixation. When sufficient teeth are present, interosseous wiring should be supplemented by intermaxillary fixation. Continuous moderate traction by rubber bands for a few days will result in anatomically correct occlusion (Fig. 24–97).

TREATMENT OF CLASS II FRACTURES OF THE MANDIBLE

In Class II fractures, teeth are present on only one side of the fracture site (Fig. 24–98). The fracture may occur in any portion of the body of the mandible. The problems of control of the edentulous fragment vary according to the direction and bevel of the fracture and the position of the teeth.

Open reduction and direct osseous wiring is indicated rather than the use of appliances in fractures with displacement and absent teeth in the posterior segment.

Fractures Horizontally and Vertically Favorable. If the fracture occurs from above downward and forward, the forces will resist separation and the fracture will be favorable from the standpoint of treatment (Fig. 24–99, *A*). If the fracture is directed as in Figure 24–99, *A* but is oblique along a frontal plane, upward displacement of the posterior fragment will occur. When the line of fracture is directed downwards and backwards (Fig. 24–99, *B*), the elevator (or posterior) muscles displace the posterior fragment upwards and medially. In this type of fracture, fixation of the teeth in intermaxillary occlusion alone does not suffice to give stability at the fracture site.

Fixation in favorable Class II fractures can be accomplished by the band and bar attachment (see Fig. 24–93), by the cable with intermaxillary wire ligatures (see Fig. 24–92), or by Erich arch bars with wire ligatures or rubber bands (see Fig. 24–73). The Kazanjian button (see Fig. 24–76) may be useful for fixation of fractured segments with isolated teeth.

Fractures in which the angle is unfavorable do not resist displacement. The pull of the elevator muscles attached to the posterior segment displaces it upward and medially and favors displacement. Wiring of the remaining

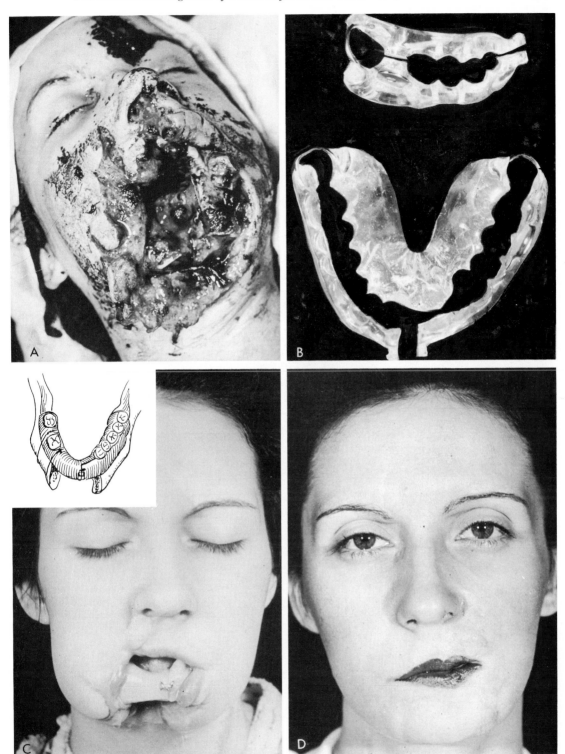

FIGURE 24–96.   *A*, Gunshot wounds with extensive destruction of soft tissue and bone. *B*, Acrylic splints made from a reconstructed model of the patient's dentition are used to stabilize the fractured mandibular segments after the method of Stout. *C*, Gunshot wound of the mandible with loss of bone from the right first molar to the left cuspid teeth. The segments of the mandible were held by an acrylic splint with circumferential wires around the mandible. *D*, Result obtained after restoration of soft tissues by cervicothoracic flap and iliac bone grafting. (See Chapter 30 for details on reconstruction following gunshot wounds.)

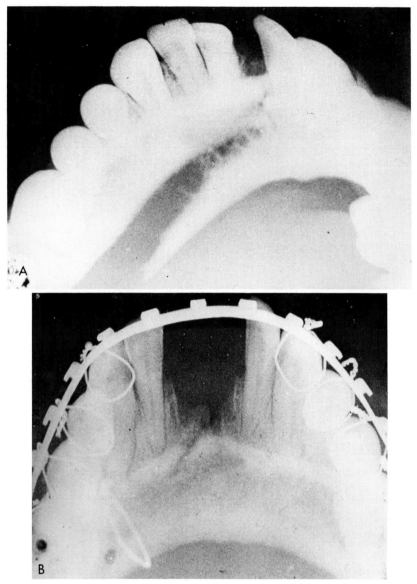

FIGURE 24–97. Oblique fracture through the symphysis region. *A*, Displacement from the pull of the mylohyoid muscle. This type of fracture does not respond well to intermaxillary fixation alone. *B*, Symphysis fracture fixation by interosseous wiring supplemented by arch bar intermaxillary fixation.

anterior teeth will not hold the posterior fragment in its normal position. A number of methods can be utilized to control the posterior fragment.

INTERLOCKING THE FRAGMENTS. Kazanjian and Converse (1974) describe the technique in which, by digital manipulation, fragments are placed in anatomical position and forced together; while they are in this position, the teeth are brought into intermaxillary fixation. Interlocking, if the fragments have the

proper contour, will hold the proximal segment in position.

USE OF A BITE BLOCK IN THE EDENTULOUS POSTERIOR SEGMENT. A bite block placed between the maxillary and mandibular teeth may serve to hold the proximal fragment in position during the course of healing. The bite block may be fabricated into an upper denture. This method is generally unsatisfactory because the posterior segment is difficult to control and the bite block causes irritation to the

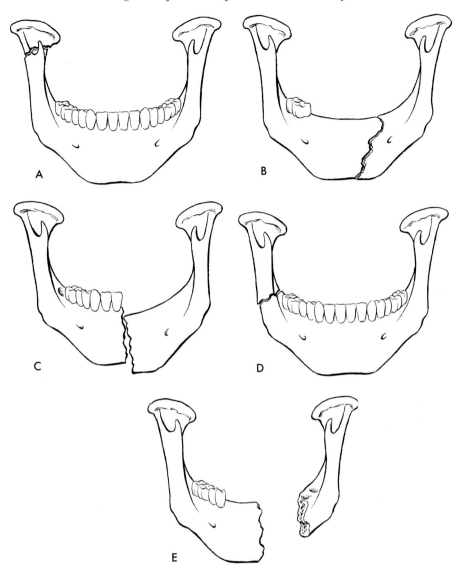

FIGURE 24–98.   Class II fractures. Diagram shows various types of fractures of the mandible with serviceable teeth on only one side of the fracture line. (From Kazanjian and Converse.)

gingival tissue and may result in pressure necrosis of the soft tissue and bone.

FORKED WIRE EXTENSION.   A band with a bar appliance attached to the teeth, with a 14-gauge wire prong projecting posteriorly across the fracture line and pressing down against the bony ridge of the posterior fragment, may prevent upward displacement. This type of appliance is usually ineffective. It provides questionable stability of the proximal fragment and may result in irritation of the soft tissues and the bone. The modern technique is open reduction and direct interosseous wiring (see Fig. 24–101).

USE OF A SPLINT OR THE PATIENT'S DENTURES WITH CIRCUMFERENTIAL WIRING.   If the patient is wearing a partial denture and the fracture is through the portion of the mandible below the saddle of the denture, it may be used to maintain fixation of the fractured segments. This is done by circumferential wiring on each side of the fracture and around the saddle portion of the denture (Fig. 24–100). One end of a 22-gauge wire passes through a 3-mm skin incision and through a wire-passing needle into the buccal vestibule. The other end is passed through a needle medial to the inferior margin of the bone, up through the lingual vestibule,

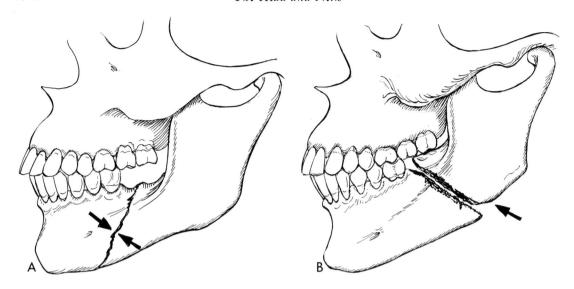

FIGURE 24–99. Favorable and unfavorable direction of the line of fracture. *A*, Line of fracture directed downward and forward: favorable; *B*, line of fracture directed downward and backward: unfavorable.

and through a drill hole in the denture. The two ends are twisted tightly at the lateral side of the denture (Fig. 24–100).

Open Reduction and Interosseous Wiring

INDICATIONS FOR INTEROSSEOUS WIRING IN MANDIBULAR FRACTURES

1. In complex fractures when the use of the teeth as points of fixation for appliances is not sufficient.

2. In fractures with a displaced posterior fragment.

3. In edentulous patients.

Under the protection of antibiotic therapy, satisfactory anesthesia, careful preparation of the mouth, and aseptic technique, open reduction for Class II fractures is expedient, positive, and safe (Fig. 24–101).

The most important precaution following direct interosseous wiring of bony fragments through the intraoral approach is the avoidance of hematoma. Infection follows hematoma formation and may require removal of the wire. Avoidance of hematoma is best achieved by placing at the fracture site a noncollapsible catheter connected to a suction aparatus. A

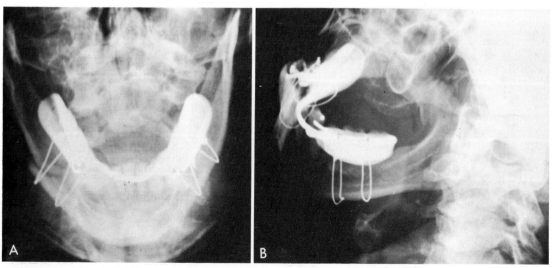

FIGURE 24–100. *A*, Stabilization of a fracture of the mandible by use of the patient's partial denture and circumferential wires around the mandibular segments. *B*, Lateral view of the circumferential wire around the patient's denture.

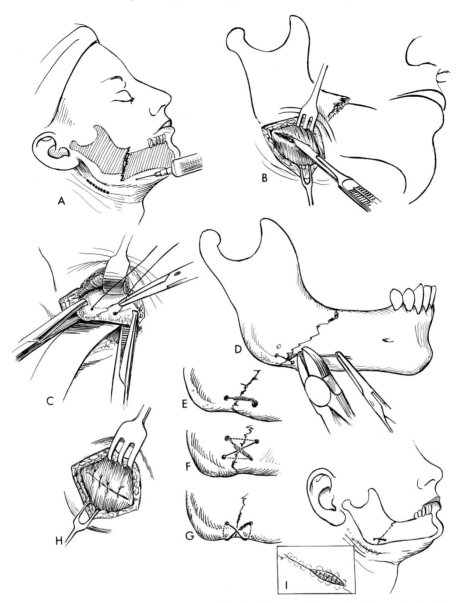

FIGURE 24-101. Open reduction and interosseous wiring for fracture of the angle of the mandible. *A*, Under local anesthesia the incision is made 1 cm below the border of the mandible. *B*, The attachments of the masseter muscle are divided and elevated. *C*, Small drill holes are passed through the bone on each side of the fracture site. *D*, Stainless steel wires used for fixation. *E*, The cut end of the wire is tucked into the drill hole on one side. *F, G*, A cross wire figure-of-eight type may be used if there is a tendency for dislocation of the fragments. *H*, The wound is closed in layers. *I*, A continuous subcuticular suture is an excellent means of wound closure.

sufficient time to ensure hematoma prevention is usually 48 hours. The catheter can be brought through the pressure dressing and pulled for removal.

Interosseous wiring results in anatomical reduction and positive fixation at the site of the fracture. The procedure may be performed under local anesthesia. An incision is made 1

to 2 cm below the inferior border of the mandible in or parallel to a skin crease in the neck and long enough to provide adequate exposure of the fracture site. The incision is extended through the skin, the subcutaneous tissues, and the platysma muscle. The dissection exposes the inferior border of the mandible, care being taken to identify and protect the mandibular branch of the facial nerve which lies along the inferior border of the mandible or slightly below it (Dingman and Grabb, 1962). The soft tissues are retracted, and by careful dissection the angle of the mandible and the anterior segment is identified. The fragments are grasped and reduced with the Dingman bone forceps (1954). With an electric drill and small drill points, holes are drilled on each side of the fracture site. Figure-of-eight or crisscross wires may be used through the drill holes, depending upon the difficulty encountered in maintaining the position. Usually two drill holes will suffice; if there is difficulty in maintaining position with one figure-of-eight wire, a single wire can be placed at a higher level. The twisted end of the wire is cut short and is forced into one of the drill holes alongside the wire passing through the hole. The musculature is secured by sutures at the inferior border of the mandible. This is accomplished by passing a suture from the fascial attachment of the masseter muscle to the fascial attachment of the medial pterygoid around the inferior border of the mandible. This holds both muscle insertions in position and favors healing of the bone. The wound is closed in layers with absorbable sutures in the deep structures, and nylon sutures are used to approximate the skin edges. Careful skin closure will give an acceptable inconspicuous scar within a few weeks (Fig. 24–101).

Intraoral Interosseous Wiring. Interosseous wiring may be done through the intraoral route in edentulous or partially edentulous patients. When the fracture line runs in a horizontally unfavorable direction, interosseous wiring at the alveolar ridge utilizes the muscle pull to advantage. The wire fixation provides a fulcrum at the crest of the ridge, and the muscle pull is in a direction that favors fixation of the segments (Fig. 24–102).

The authors have employed the intraoral approach for interosseous wiring of parasymphyseal (Fig. 24–103), body and angle fractures. After the fracture site is exposed, drill holes are made from the outer table through the bone. One 26-gauge wire is passed through each tunnel through the bone. One wire is doubled upon itself, and the loop thus formed threads the second wire from the medial to the lateral aspect of the bone. The wire is twisted, impacting the ends of the fractured bone (see Fig. 24–118). We agree with Paul and Acevedo (1968), who stated that intraoral open reduction can be achieved in most fractures of

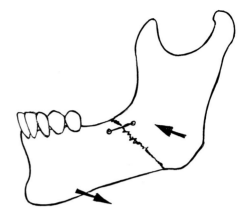

FIGURE 24–102. Fixation of the fracture with a wire near the upper border of the bone placed through an intra-oral approach.

the mandible in about half the time as extraoral open reduction.

External Fixation. If external pin fixation has a place in fracture management, it is in the control of the edentulous posterior fragment with extensive comminution at the fracture site. Pins in this area maintain the position of the posterior fragment by resistance against the elevator muscles of the mandible until consolidation of the fractured segments has taken place.

Kirschner Wire Fixation. Brown, Fryer, and McDowell (1949) favored intramedullary Kirschner fixation for immobilization of Class II and III fractures. The fracture is reduced manually. With the bones held in position by an assistant or by the operator, a three-sided, sharpened, pointed wire is passed through a small skin incision and driven through the bone into the medullary canal with an electric drill. It is driven across the fracture site and through the cortex of the opposite fragment, or it may be left in the fragment if it is solid before passing through to the outer cortical surface. The wire ends are cut at the skin level and left in place for six to eight weeks. Supplementary wiring of the teeth may be required. While alignment is achieved, impaction is not. Nerve damage and osteomyelitis are possible complications of this technique.

Comminuted Fractures

OPEN OPERATION AND BONE PLATE IN COMMINUTED FRACTURES AT THE ANGLE. The use of metal plating is preferable to direct wiring of the multiple fragments or to external

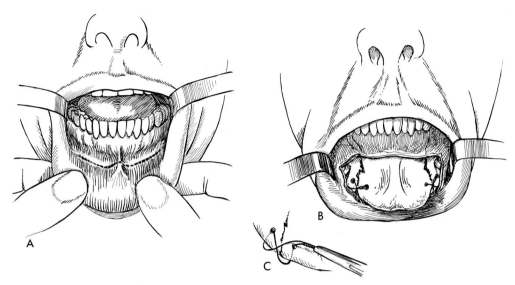

FIGURE 24–103. *A*, Location of the incision for the "degloving" technique (see Chapter 30). *B*, Direct subperiosteal exposure is obtained, and wire fixation after reduction will ensure accurate realignment of the fragments.

pin fixation for bridging areas of comminuted bone. The mandible is exposed through an incision below the inferior border. The main proximal and distal segments are identified and realigned. A thin metal plate is screwed or wired securely to the outer inferior margin, and the comminuted fragments are manipulated into a position of contact if possible (Fig. 24–104). A trough-shaped plate may be fashioned at the operating table from firm thin metal. This can be shaped to fit the inferior border of the mandible and will support the comminuted

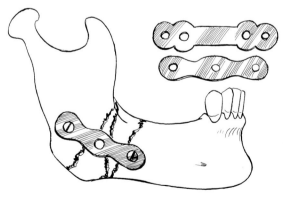

FIGURE 24–104. Bone plate fixation for fracture of the mandible. Fracture at the angle of the mandible fixed by interosseous wiring and reinforced with a thin metal bone plate held with screws. A bone plate is useful in bridging an area in which the comminution of bone fragments makes interosseous wiring impractical.

fragments until organized* (Hayward, (1962) (Fig. 24–105). The wound is closed in layers without drainage. This will maintain fixation of the fracture segments until healing takes place and the bone continuity is restored. If the splint causes reaction, it can be removed later.

EXTRASKELETAL WIRE TRACTION FOR CONTROL OF PROXIMAL SEGMENTS. Control of the proximal edentulous segment by an external wire attached to a rubber band and head cap was advocated by Lenormant and Darcissac (1927). This is said to be useful in cases of comminution at the angle of the mandible where other methods are not advised. The operation is done by exposing the angle of the mandible through a small skin incision. A hole is drilled through the angle with a bone burr, and a stainless steel wire is passed through the hole and both ends of the wire are brought out through the skin wound. The incision is closed around the wire, the two ends of which are twisted together in loop fashion for attachment of a rubber band. The plaster head cap technique has been largely replaced by the use of various types of external head frames maintained by direct fixation to the outer table of the skull. Georgiade's halo apparatus or "crown of thorns" is such an apparatus (Georgiade and Nash, 1966) (Fig. 24–106).

---

*Commercial tray, Titanium Mesh System, available from The Sampson Corporation, 214 S. Craig St., Pittsburg, Pa. 15213.

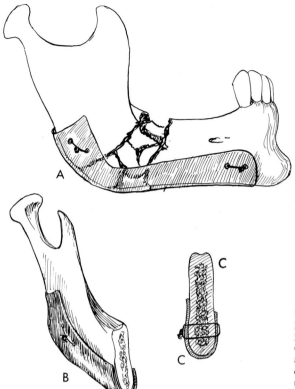

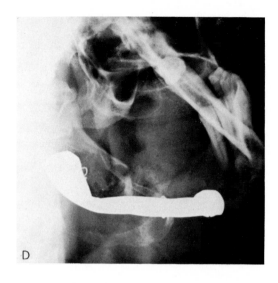

FIGURE 24–105. *A*, A thin metal plate may be shaped to fit the lower border of the mandible to support multiple comminuted fractures and maintain the position of the major segments of the fractured mandible. *B, C*, Method of contouring metal plate and fixation to the bone with wire suture. *D*, Roentgenogram of metal bone plate supporting extensively comminuted fractures of the mandible.

CONTROL OF COMMINUTED FRAGMENTS. If the bone is protected and supported by adequate adjacent periosteum and soft tissue, direct interosseous wiring techniques should be used in favor of complicated insecure dental appliances. If complicated by soft tissue loss, comminuted fractures of the mandible should be stabilized by adequate splints maintained by

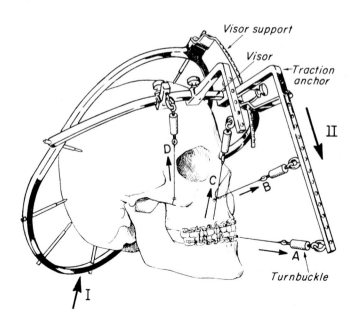

FIGURE 24–106. Georgiade's "crown of thorns" head frame is one of the numerous appliances developed in recent years. Attachments to the frame, which is held by pins penetrating the outer table of the skull, permit traction in various areas of the facial skeleton. (From Georgiade, N., and Nash, T.: An external cranial fixation apparatus for severe maxillofacial injuries. Plast. Reconstr. Surg., *38*:142, 1966. Copyright 1966, The Williams & Wilkins Company, Baltimore.)

circumferential wiring or with splints on the remaining teeth. This technique, together with intermaxillary fixation, if possible, will control the posterior segments and immobilize other segments until consolidation provides stabilization of the bone. All small segments of bone and soft tissue that might be useful in the reconstructive period should be saved.

The T bar of Kazanjian is used for attachment of an acrylic appliance to provide soft tissue support if full thickness lacerations or partial loss of the lower lip requires primary reconstruction (Fig. 24–107).

Fixation in Class II Fractures When the Maxilla is Edentulous. Fixation of the Class II

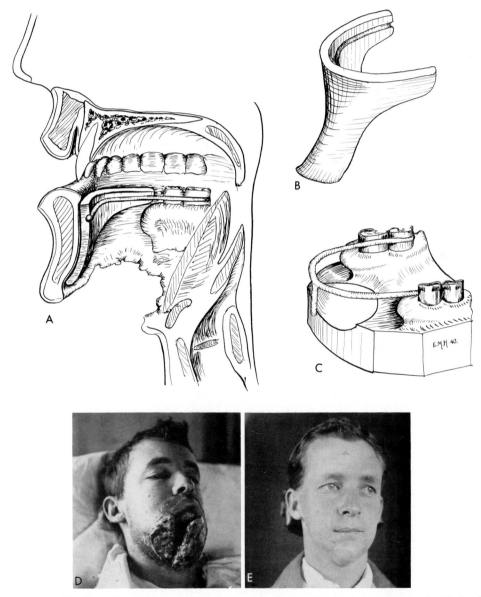

FIGURE 24–107. The Kazanjian T-bar attachment for a supporting prosthesis. *A*, Arch bar attached to bands on the molar teeth and prosthesis supporting soft tissues. *B*, Prosthesis. *C*, T-bar. This appliance is of considerable assistance in the treatment of compound fractures of the anterior portion of the mandible and of patients in whom a portion of the mandible has been destroyed. *D*, The soft tissues are repaired over the prosthesis, thus preventing their retraction *(E)*.

fracture with an edentulous maxilla may be accomplished by a bite-block against which the mandibular teeth occlude. The bite-block is maintained in position by internal wiring, the wires being looped around the zygomatic arch or attached to the frontal bone (Fig. 24–108). Fixation of the mandible to the bite-block is accomplished by means of a circumferential wire around the anterior portion of the mandible.

Open reduction and direct wiring techniques can be achieved by wiring through the nasal spine (see Fig. 24–71), through the edge of the pyriform aperture (see Fig. 24–72), looping a wire around the zygomatic arch, or wiring to the zygomatic process of the frontal bone (see Fig. 24–175).

Fractures of the Condyle

NICHOLAS G. GEORGIADE, M.D.

Fractures of the Condyle of the Mandible. The mandibular condyle is protected by the zygomatic portion of the temporal bone and is supported by the capsule, ligaments, and muscles around the joint. The condyle is most often fractured by indirect trauma. Although open reduction methods are indicated in some fractures of the mandibular condyle, the major- ity of condylar fractures will respond to simple conservative methods. Usually intermaxillary fixation will suffice. The temporomandibular joint will withstand long periods of fixation without ankylosis or dysfunction. One of our patients, a 65 year old man who had developed bony ankylosis of the mandible at age 5, decided to submit to condylectomy after 60 years of immobility. Condylectomy of the ankylosed joint was done, and within a few weeks the patient was able to open his mouth to the normal extent. He had a complete range of motion in the opposite normal joint which had been immobilized for 60 years.

The Condyloid Process. The condyloid process of the mandible consists of a broad, thick head with a narrow, thin supporting neck. The lateral pterygoid muscle attaches to a shallow depression just below the articular surface on the anterior border of the neck of the condyle. The upper fibers of the lateral pterygoid pass through the thin capsule and attach to the articular disc which separates the temporomandibular joint into two spaces. The insertion of the fibrous capsule which surrounds the condylar head of the joint attaches to the base of the glenoid fossa immediately above the lateral pterygoid insertion on the condyle. The posterior and lateral surfaces of the condylar head are surrounded by the firm, tough, ligamentous joint capsule. The capsule

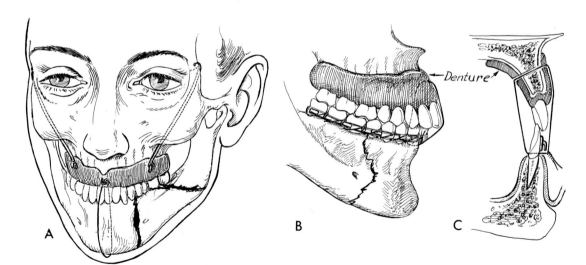

FIGURE 24–108. *A*, Fixation of the mandible in Class II fractures when the maxilla is edentulous. A bite-block has been constructed and is maintained by internal wiring to the frontal bone. Intermaxillary fixation between the bite-block and the mandibular teeth is then established. A circumferential wire has been placed around the mandible for stronger fixation. *B*, Fixation by transalveolar wiring. The denture and the alveolar process are penetrated above the level of the apices of the incisor teeth. A wire is then passed through the alveolar process, downward under the mandibular arch bar. *C*, The cross section shows the position of the transalveolar wire. A disadvantage of this technique is that the fixation of the denture is lost if the wire must be cut to allow opening of the mouth. (After Briggs and Wood-Smith, 1969.)

thins out medially and anteriorly, and its thin structure is a predisposing factor in its rupture. Anterior and medial displacement in fractures of the condyle is caused by the pull of the lateral pterygoid muscle.

The condylar neck is the thinnest portion and is most likely to be fractured by blows to the mandible. Blows to the lateral aspect of the mandible may cause a fracture of the condylar neck on the contralateral side. Violent force to the symphysis region may result in bilateral condylar fractures. The thinness of the condylar neck appears to be a safety mechanism which prevents the condyle from being driven into the middle cranial fossa or through the tympanic plate immediately behind the joint. When fracture of the condyle neck fails to occur, the head of the condyle may be forced into the middle cranial fossa or through the tympanic plate into the auditory meatus. Fortunately, the force is usually dissipated by a fracture at the condyle neck, and these injuries are rare.

CLASSIFICATION

Fractures above the level of insertion of the lateral pterygoid muscle. Fractures above the level of insertion of the lateral pterygoid muscle may be totally or partially within the capsule of the joint. The articular surface may be fractured or the break may extend from above downward and posteriorly. A fracture in this category shows little displacement because there are no muscle attachments to pull it out of position.

Fractures below the insertion of the lateral pterygoid muscle: subcondylar fractures. Fractures below the insertion of the lateral pterygoid muscle occur immediately below the lowermost muscle fibers or at the level of the sigmoid notch and extend downward along the posterior border of the ramus of the mandible. The short fragment is generally displaced more than the long fragment. Fractures below the insertion of the lateral pterygoid almost invariably are displaced forward and medially by the pull of the muscle. The fractured segment may be pulled out of position but remain within the intact capsule; this is classified as a "displacement" fracture. The condyle may be completely expelled from the disrupted joint capsule; this is classified as a "dislocation" fracture. The condylar head may be displaced in an anterior, posterior, medial, or lateral position, and in one of our cases it was displaced upward into the middle cranial fossa (Fig. 24–109). Upward displacement is relatively rare. The direction and degree of displacement of the remainder of the mandible depend upon the direction of the force of the blow, the presence or absence of teeth, and the direction and force of the muscles of mastication.

DIAGNOSIS. The diagnosis of fracture of the condyle is usually made on clinical examination and confirmed by roentgenographic findings. Clinically it will be noted that there is asymmetry of the face on the involved side due to shifting of the mandible posteriorly and laterally toward the affected side. Premature

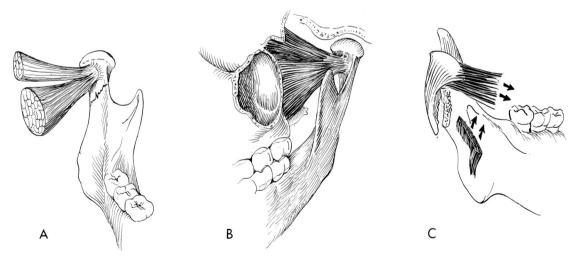

FIGURE 24–109. *A,* The insertions of the lateral pterygoid muscle on the condyloid process and condyle. *B,* The lateral pterygoid muscle arises by two heads: an upper from the inferolateral surface of the greater wing of the sphenoid and the infratemporal crest; a lower from the lateral surface of the lateral pyerygoid plate. *C,* In condylar fractures below the insertion of the muscle, the condyle is displaced medially and forward by the contraction of the lateral pyerygoid muscle.

occlusion on the involved side is caused by upward pull of the elevator muscles of the mandible. This results in a Class I lever with the fulcrum on the molar teeth on the involved side. An open bite deformity anteriorly and on the opposite side of the mandible is noted. Tenderness on palpation over the temporomandibular joint and in the external auditory canal is a common finding. Moderate to severe edema, ecchymosis, and occasionally hemorrhage may be noted in the external auditory canal. If both mandibular condyles are fractured, the patient will have a bilateral open bite deformity with occlusion only on the posterior teeth (Fig. 24–110).

Bilateral open bite deformity is caused by contraction of the strong elevator muscles of the mandible, upward displacement of the ramus, and telescoping of the fractured segments.

In bilateral subcondylar fractures which occur below the attachment of the lateral pterygoid muscle, the patient is unable to protrude the mandible. In unilateral fractures at the same level, the patient is unable to perform lateral motions to the opposite side. Lateral movements of the mandible can be made only toward the affected side, because the lateral pterygoid muscle on the unaffected side shifts the mandible medially and foward, while the muscle is completely out of function on the affected side.

The patient usually will have dysfunction and pain on attempting to open the jaw. If the posterior fragments have been displaced posteriorly, the mandible may shift forward as the segments of the ramus distal to the fracture ride upward and glide forward on contact with the condyle fragments. This may produce an open bite with protrusive relationships of the mandible (Fig. 24–111).

Fractures above the level of the lateral pterygoid insertion do not exhibit displacement because of the absence of the contracting muscles attached to the proximal segment. The patient may complain of severe pain in the temporomandibular joint, and it will be noted that there is tenderness on palpation over the joint and in the external auditory canal. It may be noted that the teeth are separated and do not come into occlusion on the affected side because of hemorrhage and edema in the joint which force the condyle downward. It may be several weeks before the teeth come into their normal occlusal relationships. In this type of fracture, especially in children, the parents should be warned about the possibility of the development of ankylosis owing to aseptic necrosis of joint surfaces and secondary bony proliferation (Fig. 24–112). In some cases, even though ankylosis does not occur, the head of the condyle (especially the cartilage) may be damaged, thus affecting growth, with subsequent maldevelopment.

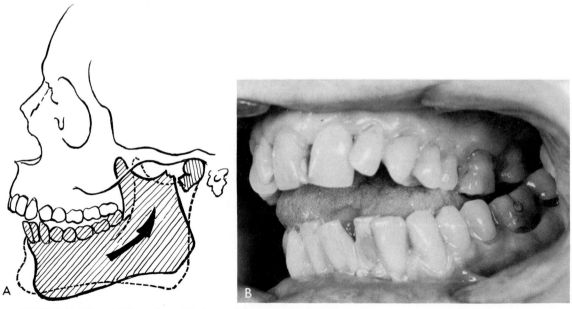

FIGURE 24–110. *A*, Bilateral mandibular condyle fractures result in upward and posterior displacement of the ramus of the mandible, premature occlusion of the posterior molar teeth, and an open bite deformity. *B*, Open bite deformity in a patient with bilateral mandibular condyle fractures.

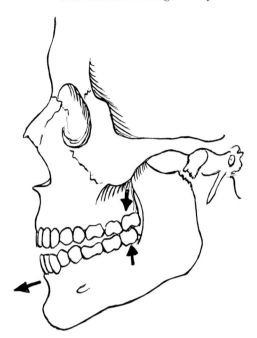

FIGURE 24–111. Forward shift of the mandible and bilateral condyle fractures. This occurs when the condyles are displaced posteriorly and the ramus below the fracture rides upward and glides forward.

ROENTGENOGRAPHY. A fracture of the condyle may be overlooked unless the fracture is demonstrated on roentgenography. If the fractures are linear without displacement or with minimal displacement, tomograms may be necessary to demonstrate the site of fracture. In most fractures of the condyle it will be noted that the condylar head is displaced anteriorly and medially. The head may be within the limits of the articular capsule, or it may be completely avulsed and dislocated. If the condyle fracture is very low in the region of the sigmoid notch or extends down along the posterior border of the ramus, the condylar head may be displaced medially, and the end of the posterior fragment will be noted protruding lateral to the site of the fracture. Stereoscopic views may demonstrate posterior displacement with fracture of the tympanic plate.

TREATMENT OF FRACTURES OF THE CONDYLE. Fractures of the mandibular condyle may be treated by closed reduction methods or by open reduction and direct wire fixation.

The nonoperative or closed reduction treatment has been the principal method of management of condylar fractures. This consists of immobilization of the mandible by means of intermaxillary fixation. Closed reduction was the only method known until a few years ago. In 1947 the combined efforts of the members of the Chalmers J. Lyons Academy of Oral Surgery produced a report on a study of 120 cases of fractures of the mandibular condyle treated by immobilization of the mandible. It was found that, without exception, the results were clinically acceptable, except for slight malfunction due to deviation of the mandible to one side on opening in seven cases.

In most centers closed reduction and intermaxillary fixation comprise the method or choice in the management of fractures of the mandibular condyle. Some surgeons prefer to manipulate the mandible prior to intermaxillary fixation in an attempt to improve the position of the fractured condylar segments. Some have manipulated the condyle head with a sharp pointed instrument passed intraorally or through the skin in an attempt to force the condyle head back into the fossa. These manipulations are generally unsuccessful, and X-ray examination following reduction usually shows no improvement in the position of the fragments.

There is evidence to indicate that subcondylar fractures with medial displacement of the head may finally heal in good alignment. This probably results from spontaneous or gradual movement of the condyle head back into the glenoid fossa rather than from resorption and

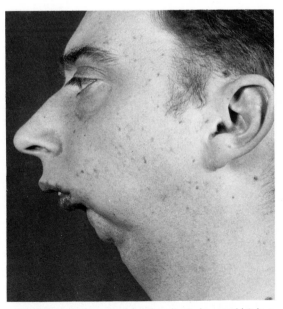

FIGURE 24–112. Facial deformity (micrognathia) in a patient with complete bilateral fibro-osseous ankylosis following injury to the mandible at age 2 years.

reconstitution of the condyle (Gregory, 1957). It is the opinion of MacGregor and Fordyce (1957) and of Walker (1960) that most fractures of the mandibular condyle with displacement, deviation, or dislocation undergo modeling resorption with ultimate reproduction of a comparatively normal articular process and normal or near normal function and appearance. Other observers believe this process of resorption and reconstruction occurs within 6 to 12 months in children whose mandibular condyle is under the stress and strain of mastication. The authors believe that this view is unrealistic and that the fractured displaced condyle returns to the fossa under the influence of functional forces after the spasm and inflammatory reaction subsides.

Undisplaced or displaced condylar fractures without dislocation are treated by reestablishment of normal dental occlusal relationships with intermaxillary fixation by means of arch bars or eyelet wiring of the teeth. Intermaxillary stabilization is thus maintained for a period of four to six weeks. In many instances, however, if the patient is able to reestablish or maintain adequate occlusal relationships, fixation is not necessary, and maintenance of the patient on a soft diet may be all that is necessary during the healing phase. This is particularly true in younger children who heal very rapidly. If there is moderate overriding of the condylar fragments, opening the bite posteriorly in the molar area on the side of the fracture for 1 to 2 mm, with interposition of a thin plastic wedge, will further reduce the malalignment of the fragments when a satisfactory occlusal relationship cannot be established by the usual conservative means. The great majority of condylar fractures respond well to such conservative therapy.

Intracapsular condylar fractures are difficult to diagnose and usually give rise to a number of complications many months later, including clicking in the joint space, pain, and, in some instances, ankylosis. The latter is caused by the inflammatory process resulting from the injury accompanied by partial degeneration of the joint surfaces and eventual fibrosis and ankylosis. Minimal restriction of motion for approximately three weeks, weekly intra-articular injections of steroid, a soft diet, and a gradual increase in excursions of the mandible constitute the best plan of treatment rather than complete immobilization for four to six weeks (Georgiade).

In some cases it is not possible to reduce the fragment manually, but orthopedic traction with rubber bands will bring the teeth into functional occlusion in a matter of a few hours. In patients appearing late for treatment, slow intermaxillary traction may be necessary over a period of three to four days before the teeth come into satisfactory occlusion.

Gregory (1957) and others have reported cases in which there was spontaneous repositioning of markedly displaced fractured condyle segments two or three years after treatment by intermaxillary fixation. In Gregory's case there was a subcondylar fracture on the right side with marked medial angulation. This was treated by intermaxillary fixation, and a few months after fixation the condyle remained angulated out of the fossa. It was noted three years later, however, that the condylar process had resumed an adequate vertical relationship and was in position in the glenoid fossa. The exact mechanism is unknown, but it must be assumed that certain forces of mastication favor drifting of the condyle head back into its normal position.

Leake, Doykos, Habal, and Murray (1971) reported 20 cases of condylar fractures in children who had subsequent normal growth, occlusion, and function without any treatment. Fractures varied from greenstick to severe displacement with anteromedial positioning and angulation of the condyle neck. Thirteen patients were followed for from 2 months to 17 years. Fifteen fractures were unilateral and five were bilateral condylar fractures. Intracapsular fractures in children, however, may lead to aseptic necrosis of the condylar head, fibroosseous ankylosis of the temporomandibular joint, and loss of the condyle growth center (see Fig. 24–112).

Open reduction. Because of the deep position of the mandibular condyle, the proximity of the branches of the seventh nerve and the internal maxillary artery, and the strong action of the lateral pterygoid muscle causing displacement, open operation for the reduction of mandibular fractures may be a complicated procedure.

Indications for open reduction. In condylar fractures with displacement of the condylar head out of the glenoid fossa, the head can usually be found in the pterygoid space, and consideration in these situations should be given to surgical replacement of the head in the fossa when there is an approximately 90 degree angle of the displaced condylar head from its normal position. An absolute anatomical alignment is not necessary, since it is often impossible to obtain. However, an end-to-end stabilization of the condylar neck fracture when the condylar head is replaced into the fossa is felt to be desirable, particularly in children and in patients who are edentulous and who, as a result, have a loss of the vertical dimension of the ramus because of the malposition of the condyle and overriding of fragments. Maintenance of the condylar head in the glenoid fossa with slight overriding of the fragments usually results in satisfactory bony union and the re-establishment of a normal bite pattern (Henny, 1951; Heurlin and coworkers, 1961; Georgiade, 1964).

Two types of roentgenograms are obtained before a decision is made whether to perform an open reduction of the displaced condylar fracture. A posterior-anterior view of the mandible or modified Towne view is helpful in establishing the position of the condyle in a frontal plane. Tomograms of the joint area are essential in order to locate accurately the relationship of the condylar head to the glenoid fossa.

Techniques of open reduction. Prior to extraoral reduction, arch bars or suitable wiring must be applied to the teeth if present. If the patient is edentulous, the patient's own dentures or a similar type of prosthetic appliance is used for immobilization following reduction of the condylar fracture; fixation can be obtained by means of nasomandibular wires. In children with a deciduous dentition, immobilization has been adequately achieved by attaching bilateral nasomandibular wires to a lower mandibular prosthesis, with circum-mandibular wires around the prosthesis or circum-mandibular wires around the mandible attached to the nasomandibular wires. Associated fractures are managed according to their type and the areas involved.

The indications for operation in the treatment of fractures of the condyle in children are not specific. The surgeon must rely upon his judgment and experience in making the decision.

The surgical approach to the fracture areas is preferably accomplished by some type of preauricular incision, usually an inverted "hockey stick" type of incision. The branches of the facial nerve are outlined by the use of a nerve stimulator and are retracted inferiorly and medially. Reduction of the condylar fracture is aided at this time by the use of muscle relaxing agents. The condylar head is usually found to have been displaced medially into the pterygoid space. A curved elevator and tracheotomy hook is employed to obtain leverage

on the medial aspect of the condyle so that it can be displaced laterally and back into the glenoid fossa (Georgiade). While the condyle is being displaced laterally, traction is maintained on the ramus of the mandible in order to allow sufficient room for the displaced fragment to be brought into an appropriate position. A Kocher type of clamp is useful in grasping the displaced condylar head in order to stabilize it and replace it in the condylar fossa. The articular disc is usually not sufficiently damaged to warrant its removal and is replaced into the fossa to minimize the danger of ankylosis. If possible, the lateral pterygoid musculature which attaches along the medial aspect of the condyle is left intact, as the blood supply to the condylar head enters in this area. This caution minimizes the chances of necrosis of the condylar head. The use of a single 28-gauge wire threaded through the condylar fragment and ramus and immobilization of the fractured fragment in an end-to-end position will usually be sufficient.

If the fractured condyle cannot be maintained in the glenoid fossa, a 28-gauge stainless steel looped wire is used to maintain the condylar fragment in satisfactory position (Messer, 1972). Other types of fixation have been described by Thoma (1954), Henny (1951), Georgiade and coworkers (1956), and Heurlin and coworkers (1961).

An alternate method is to stabilize the condylar head in the fossa when the pull of the pterygoid muscle continuously dislocates the condylar head. This technique involves the use of two or three stainless steel pins fixed to the zygoma, the condylar head, and the ramus. Wire fixation of the fragments is accomplished, and the pins can be removed three weeks after the initial fixation of the fragments. This procedure is required only when stabilization cannot be maintained by the simplified wiring technique previously described (Georgiade and coworkers, 1956).

Reduction through the Risdon Approach (1925). This approach is useful only when the condylar fragment is long owing to a fracture extending downward through the sigmoid notch to the posterior border of the mandible (Fig. 24–113). A 5-cm incision is made about 1 cm behind and below the angle of the mandible. The masseter muscle insertion is raised from the bone and elevated to expose the site of the fracture. A 22-gauge wire is passed through a small drill hole at the angle of the mandible for use in retracting the bone and identifying the posterior fragment. The poste-

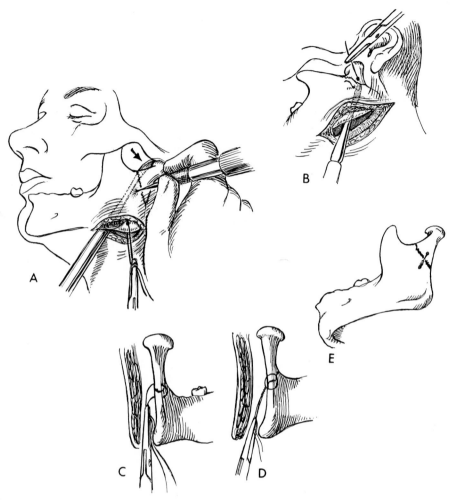

FIGURE 24–113. Open reduction of a fracture of the mandibular condyle through the Risdon approach. The incision is made below and behind the angle of the mandible. The masseter attachments and periosteum are elevated from the lateral surface of the bone to expose the site of the fracture. To place right-angled drill holes through the bone, the skin of the cheek may be punctured with the bone drill. The drill is not set into motion until the point comes in contact with the bone. (After Georgiade.)

rior or condylar fragment is the closest to the articular surface of the condyle; the anterior fragment is the main mandibular fragment. When the fracture site is identified, a drill hole is made through the anterior fragment and a wire is passed through it and looped out of the wound, where it can be used to further distract the ramus. The posterior fragment is identified and a drill hole passed through it. The operator is looking up through a long narrow wound to the fracture site which does not permit drill holes to be made at right angles to the bone surface. By puncturing through the soft tissues lateral to the fracture site, the tip of the bone drill can be placed perpendicular to the bone in order to drill holes in the desired direction. The fragments are held together with a 25-gauge stainless steel wire which is twisted, cut

short, and flattened against the bone. The wound is closed without a drain. Intermaxillary fixation for four to six weeks is indicated (Fig. 24–114).

Reduction through a preauricular approach. The preauricular incision is preferable in most instances for the approach to the region of the temporomandibular joint. The incision begins at the anterior border of the lobule and is extended upward over the posterior portion of the tragus and the anterior attachment of the helix into the temporal area, where it sweeps in a curve anteriorly for 3 cm. The tissues are dissected downward over the temporalis fascia to the joint area (Dingman and Constant, 1969). The dissection must be carefully done to avoid injury to the branches of the seventh nerve in the region of the joint. After iden-

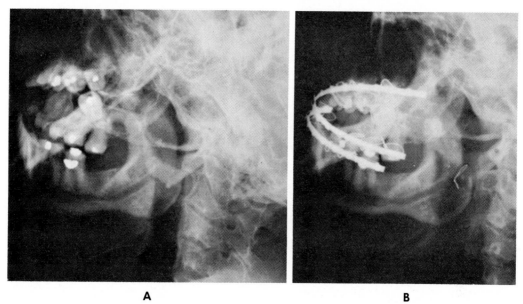

A **B**

FIGURE 24–114. *A,* Fracture of the mandibular condyle with telescoping of the fragments and forward positioning of the proximal segment. *B,* After open reduction and direct wiring through the Risdon approach.

tification and retraction of the branches of the nerve, the fascia overlying the temporomandibular joint is divided and the fractured segments identified. It may be extremely difficult to reduce the posterior fragment because of the strong pull of the lateral pterygoid muscle. Fixation is attained by means of drill holes passed through the bone fragments and securely wiring the neck of the condyle in position. Hoopes, Woolfort, and Jabaley (1970) reported a four-year follow-up of two children who underwent surgery at 2½ and 8 years of age involving a postauricular incision and transauditory canal approach to the temporomandibular area for reduction and fixation of severe fracture-dislocation. Both showed excellent results, and the authors stated that the surgical approaches provided satisfactory exposure.

Hendrix, Sanders, and Green (1959) and Georgiade (1960) advocated removal of the condyle head and replacement in the glenoid fossa as a free bone graft. They reported good results using this method.

COMPOUND COMMINUTED SUBCONDYLAR FRACTURES. This type of fracture results from penetrating injuries over the region of the temporomandibular joint or from gunshot wounds in this area. Treatment consists of repair of soft tissue wounds and fixation of the remaining portion of the mandible. If the joint is completely comminuted or infection is imminent, it is advisable to remove the condyle to control infection and prevent fibro-osseous ankylosis. Removal of the condyle results in a flail joint, generally with satisfactory function.

DISLOCATION OF THE CONDYLE OF THE MANDIBLE. Dislocation of the condyle of the mandible without fracture may be caused by opening the mouth too widely or by sudden violence. The head of the condyle may be dislocated out of the glenoid fossa anterior to the articular eminence, where it is held securely by contraction of the muscles of mastication. Dislocation of the mandible may be unilateral or bilateral.

In many instances mandibular dislocation can be reduced by the patient without difficulty. In some cases, reduction is not possible except by the use of muscle relaxing drugs and general anesthesia. Most dislocations can be reduced by grasping the mandible with the thumbs in the region of the mandibular molars and applying downward pressure on the posterior border of the mandible while simultaneously pressing upward and backward on the anterior portion. With this type of forceful movement the condyle usually snaps back into its proper position.

Johnson (1958) reported excellent results in obtaining spontaneous reduction of the dislocated mandibular condyle by injection of a local anesthetic solution into the joint area. He theorized that interruption of the reflex arc releases the muscle spasm and permits the condyle to slip back into position. Johnson stated that it is necessary to inject only one side to give relief in bilateral dislocations.

Recurrent dislocation may be frequent and chronic so that dislocation may occur whenever the patient opens his mouth too widely or bites too firmly. Dislocation lasting several months to two years has been reported by Gottlieb (1952). In a review of the literature he found only three cases of long-standing dislocation of the jaw reduced by manual methods. He stated that the dislocations had been present for three months as reported by Müller (1946), two months by Berg, and two months by Bouisson. Ginestet, Desorthes, and Houessou (1948) reported the presence of ankylosis three years after a forceful open reduction. Gottlieb treated his three cases successfully by condylar resection. Litzow and Royer (1962) reported a unilateral dislocation of six months' duration which was successfully treated by condylectomy. The condyle was cut with bone burrs and chisels through a Risdon (1925) approach at the angle of the mandible. Dislocation of the condyle is also discussed in Chapter 31.

Fractures of the Coronoid Process of the Mandible. This portion of the bone is so well protected by the overlying zygoma, the dense temporalis fascia, and the attachments of the temporalis muscle that fracture is a rare occurrence. Penetrating wounds or gunshot wounds may result in fracture of this area. Generally, the fracture shows little displacement by the insertions of the temporalis muscle and fascia. Treatment is usually not necessary, as the displacement is minimal.

N.G.G.

TREATMENT OF CLASS III FRACTURES OF THE MANDIBLE

Fractures in the Edentulous Mandible. Fractures of the edentulous mandible are seen less frequently in older persons than in the younger age group, since the older patient is less frequently exposed to hazardous situations in industry, sports, or travel. The fractures usually occur through the portion of bone in which the atrophy is the most advanced, and the bone is thin and weak. Quite often fractures occur bilaterally with moderate displacement. Because of the loose tissues over the bones, the fractures are less liable to be compound than they are in the mandible with teeth. Deformity is obvious when there are displacement and overriding of the bone fragments. Complications due to infection are infrequent, and healing generally takes place without difficulty (Fig. 24–115).

The usual methods of fixation of the mandibular fragments are not applicable in the case of the edentulous mandible. Treatment is lim-

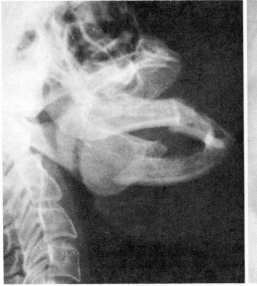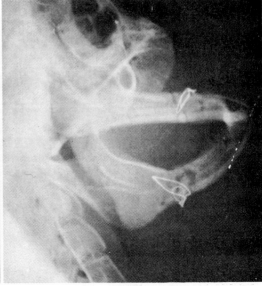

FIGURE 24–115. Bilateral fracture in an edentulous mandible. *A,* Preoperative roentgenogram shows overriding of fragments and downward and forward displacement of the anterior segment. *B,* Postoperative view following open reduction and direct wire fixation.

ited to the use of intraoral appliances, circumferential wiring, interosseous wiring, and pin fixation appliances.

INTRAORAL APPLIANCES. Intraoral appliances are useful in the simple fracture in which displacement is minimal or absent. The patient's dentures or specially made bite-blocks prepared by a prosthodontist are fitted to the upper and lower jaws to maintain stability of the mandibular segments. If displacement is minimal, the patient's own dentures, if undamaged, may be placed in the mouth and support against the mandible is applied with a head cap and chin strap. Relining the denture with softened dental compound or soft acrylic will compensate for the change of contour of the alveolar process caused by the fracture and avoid pressure necrosis. Fixation for a week to ten days will result in sufficient organization at the fracture site to prevent displacement. Broken dentures can be repaired, and all fragments of dental appliances should be saved until it is determined that they are no longer useful.

Impressions of the alveolar ridges are required for the construction of bite-blocks to fit the upper and lower jaws. When brought into occlusion, the bite-blocks provide the same stability as the patient's dentures.

CIRCUMFERENTIAL WIRING. Baudens (1840) was the first to use circumferential wiring for reduction of a mandibular fracture. His wire went around the mandible and was tied over a molar tooth. Robert (1852) used a single circumferential wire for reduction of a mandibular fracture. The wire was twisted close to the bone (Fig. 24–116).

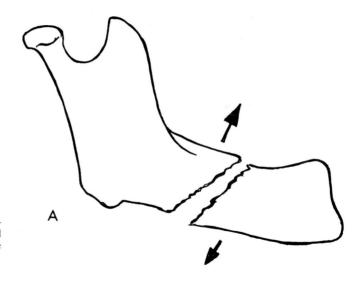

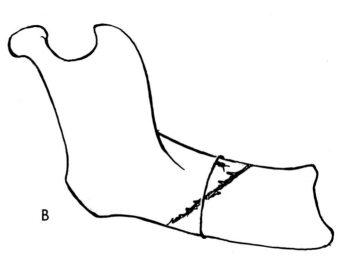

FIGURE 24–116. Fixation of a mandibular fracture with a single circumferential wire. Arrows indicate the direction of the muscle pull. (Robert, 1852.)

According to Ivy (1922), Black (about 1896) was the first American to employ circumferential wiring of the mandible. This consisted of passing a wire around the mandible and over a bite-block on the alveolar ridge to give stability to the fractured segments after reduction. Circumferential wiring can be used with an acrylic bite-block or the patient's dentures or around the bone without splints to hold oblique fractures in position after reduction (Fig. 24–117).

DIRECT INTEROSSEOUS WIRING. Interosseous wiring is indicated in the management of displaced fractures in the edentulous mandible in which there is overriding of the fragments. It may be used in compound or comminuted fractures. The intraoral or extraoral route may be employed.

The extraoral route. The approach is through an incision about 1 cm below the inferior border of the mandible. The incision is made long enough to give adequate exposure to the fractured segments. The fracture is identified, reduced, and held in position with bone forceps. Drill holes are placed through the bones on each side of the fracture site. The bone is securely fixed by interosseous 24-gauge stainless steel wire to provide positive fixation at the site of the fracture (Fig. 24–118). The wound is closed in layers.

The intraoral route. Intraoral interosseous wiring is an effective technique in fractures of the edentulous mandible. The fracture line is exposed through an incision lateral or medial to the crest of the alveolar ridge. The muco-

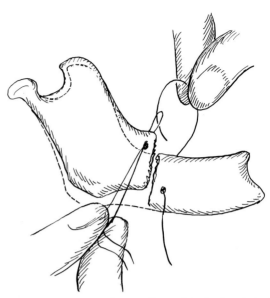

FIGURE 24–118. Diagram illustrating the location of holes in the mandible for open reduction and interosseous wiring and the technique of passing the interosseous wire through the prepared hole. The posterior fragment is pulled up by muscular action. To overcome the force, the hole on the displaced posterior fragment is made near the upper portion of the bone, whereas the one on the anterior fragment is made somewhat lower. When the fragments are approximated, a greater pull is thus exerted on the posterior fragment. (After Kazanjian and Converse.)

periosteum is raised on both the buccal and lingual surfaces of the mandible. In thin mandibles, the attachment of the mylohyoid muscle is near the crest of the alveolar ridge, and dissection should not be as extensive on the lingual surface as it is on the buccal surface. Interference with the muscle attachments will result in edema of the floor of the mouth and postoperative pain and discomfort on swallowing. The motor- or turbine-driven bone drill is used to make small holes through the bone near the end of each fragment (Fig. 24–119). A 24-gauge stainless steel wire is passed from the buccal to the lingual surface and back through the other hole to the buccal surface. The two ends are twisted so that the fragments are firmly and positively fixed into position. The wires are cut short, and the cut end is pressed against the bone. The soft tissue is closed over the fracture site. The wires may remain permanently and cause little, if any, reaction. It may be necessary, occasionally, to remove the wire several months later if pressure from the denture causes discomfort in the mucous membrane overlying the ridge. Removal can be done easily under local anesthesia as an outpa-

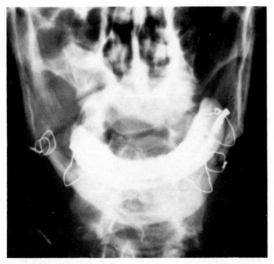

FIGURE 24–117. Direct interosseous wiring and circumferential wiring around the mandible and a prosthodontic appliance for treatment of a fracture of the edentulous mandible.

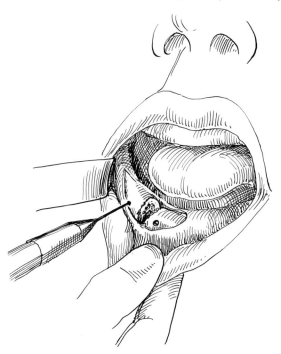

FIGURE 24–119. In the edentulous mandible, reduction and interosseous wiring can be accomplished effectively through an intraoral incision over the aveolar ridge.

COMPOUND AND COMMINUTED FRACTURES OF THE EDENTULOUS MANDIBLE. Kazanjian and Converse (1974) reported management of severe gunshot wounds of the anterior portion of the mandible in which only fragments of bone remained with no teeth in any of the fragments. The ends of a horseshoe-shaped heavy wire conforming to the dental arch were embedded in drill holes in the proximal segments of bone. This gave stability to the proximal segments and provided an opportunity for fixation of the small fragments by suspension with fine steel wires to the arch wire. This procedure is useful in those cases in which there is adequate soft tissue with a good blood supply to cover the bone fragments.

Similar cases are treated by direct wiring of the bony fragments to each other in order to reestablish the contour of the arch. The repair of soft tissues over the bone fragments will usually provide an adequate blood supply for reconstitution of the mandibular arch.

If large segments of the anterior mandible are missing, it is important to stabilize the

tient procedure by reopening the area and cutting the wire.

Interosseous wiring through the intraoral route is relatively simple and provides a mechanical advantage at the fracture site. The wire placed near the upper border of the fracture provides a fulcrum against which the muscle forces are favorable for stabilization (Fig. 24–120). The upward pull of the posterior muscles and the downward pull of the anterior group create forces that favor reduction. If the wire is placed low at the site of the fracture, an unfavorable situation is present, and the fragments have a tendency to become separated.

Infection following intraoral surgery is uncommon, and adequate antibiotic therapy provides additional protection.

The advantages of the intraoral approach are:

1. It is simple to accomplish.

2. There is no danger of surgical damage to the mandibular branch of the seventh nerve, the submaxillary gland, or the external maxillary artery.

3. It can be done with a minimal amount of instrumentation.

4. Healing takes place quickly and without complication.

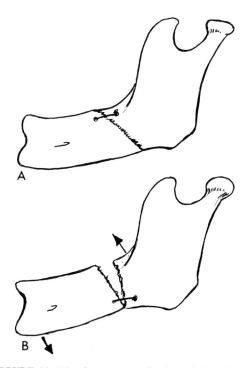

FIGURE 24–120. Interosseous fixation of the edentulous mandible. *A*, Correct location for interosseous wire. The fulcrum is near the upper portion of the fracture, and the muscular forces favor bony contact. *B*, With the interosseous wire near the inferior border of the mandible, displacement may occur through the pull of the muscles (indicated by arrows).

remaining posterior segments so they will not be submitted to medial displacement by scar formation in the floor of the mouth. Stabilization can be obtained by acrylic splints fixed to the posterior segments by circumferential wiring. In certain favorable cases, a perforated metal tray appliance (Titanium), fastened to the inferior border of the proximal segments and extended around the anterior portion in the form of an arch, may be used to hold the posterior fragments in position and to support the anterior fragments and soft tissue. It is desirable to utilize all the fragments of bone to aid in the reconstruction of the mandibular arch.

Obwegeser and Sailer (1973) have advocated the placing of bone grafts over the mandibular ridge to aid in the healing of the fractured atrophic edentulous mandible. The bone grafts are maintained by circumferential wiring around the mandible. This technique has the advantage of providing the patient with an alveolar ridge capable of supporting a denture, as well as helping to consolidate the fracture.

External Fixation in Mandibular Fractures. External pin fixation was used for fractures of the long bones by Lambotte (1913) but was not popularized for use in other areas until Anderson (1936) developed an appliance which was extensively utilized in the fixation of fractures of the facial bones (Fig. 24–121). This appliance gained popularity from 1936 until about 1942, when the use of pin fixation appliances largely gave way to open reduction

and direct wire fixation methods. Numerous variations of the pin fixation appliances were devised and described by Stader (1937), Berry (1939), Haynes (1939), and Griffin (1941).

The indications for external fixation are:

1. Those cases which cannot be treated by simpler methods, such as interosseous or circumferential wiring.

2. Fractures of the angle of the endentulous mandible when there is loss of bone immediately anterior to the posterior segment.

3. Cases in which control of the fragments during reconstructive bone grafting procedures is required.

4. Rare cases when wiring of the jaws is contraindicated.

At the present time the most popular technique involves the use of the Morris biphasic fixation appliance (Morris, 1949), which has been employed extensively for the fixation of bone fragments in bone grafting for defects of the mandible (see Chapter 30).

(see Chapter 30)

COMPLICATIONS IN MANDIBULAR
FRACTURE TREATMENT

Early Complications

PRIMARY HEMORRHAGE. Extensive bone and tissue injury may result in severe blood loss. Usually there is little hemorrhage in closed fractures in which the soft tissues are not extensively involved. Clamping and ligation of major vessels and secure packing of the wounds with pressure dressings are effective treatments for control of hemorrhage. External carotid ligation is seldom necessary unless the vessel has been severed.

RESPIRATORY COMPLICATIONS. These are seen in bilateral fractures of the body of the mandible with posterior displacement of the bone, which permits the tissues of the floor of the mouth and the tongue to fall back into the airway. Protraction of the tongue, repositioning of the anterior mandibular bone segments, or tracheotomy will establish the airway. Following intermaxillary fixation, the patient may have airway problems due to vomiting and aspiration of stomach contents (if the stomach contents have not been evacuated, an essential precaution), but this is a rare occurrence. It may be necessary to remove the intermaxillary rubber bands or wires to establish an airway or provide an improved airway. Usually a satisfactory airway can be established by insertion of an intranasal pharyngeal soft rubber tube, or large-bore rubber tubing can be placed along

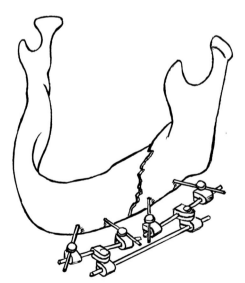

FIGURE 24–121. External pin fixation for stabilization of mandibular fracture. (From Kazanjian and Converse.)

the teeth in the buccal sulcus and between the last molar teeth.

INFECTION. With modern methods of fracture treatment, infections are relatively rare. Most complications from infection can be avoided by elimination of foreign material from the wound, accurate fixation, and antibiotic therapy. Foreign bodies such as infected teeth, portions of fractured teeth, dirt, metal, glass, and other materials in the line of fracture predispose to infection.

Inadequate fixation may be the cause of infection owing to movement and a pumping action at the site of fracture which forces foreign material into the fracture site. Continuous damage to the young granulation tissue from movement in the line of fracture prevents healing, invites bacterial invasion, and interferes with the process of repair. Nonvital or abscessed teeth in the line of fracture may lead to infection of the bone or the adjacent soft tissues. However, it is desirable to retain teeth or root fragments in the line of fracture if they aid in the stabilization of the fragments, and with antibiotic therapy it is safe to retain these structures until they have served a useful purpose. If teeth or roots are present in the line of fracture but have no value in maintaining the position of the fracture segments, they should be removed.

Preexisting disease in the area of fracture, such as an abscessed tooth, osteomyelitis, a dental cyst, or partially devitalized irradiated bone, predisposes to infection.

Once established, a purulent collection is incised and drained, making sure that the fixation of the fragments is secure. Procrastination in instituting drainage of an abscess with fluctuation leads to spread of the infection through the spongiosa of the bone or along the periosteum, resulting in extension and more serious infection. Drainage may be established by intraoral or extraoral incision and insertion of a rubber drain. Antibiotic therapy is no substitute for the surgical establishment of adequate drainage.

Infection and buried stainless steel wires. Stainless steel wire may be placed through the ends of bone fragments via both the extra- and intraoral routes. Hematoma must be avoided. Continuous suction, using noncollapsible silicone tubing, of the operative site prevents hematoma formation and possible consequent infection and abscess formation. Once infection has become established, the wire usually prolongs the suppuration, and removal of the wire is indicated.

Avascular necrosis and *osteitis* of bone may occur when bone has been denuded of its periosteal and muscular attachment. When bone is exposed, it is deprived of its blood supply from the covering soft tissues. Osteitis and avascular necrosis are the fate of loose, denuded bone fragments. These complications can be minimized by early coverage of exposed bone with well-vascularized soft tissue containing a sufficient blood supply. Undermining of the adjacent mucoperiosteum or skin and muscle usually will provide adequate soft tissue for covering exposed bone. If adjacent tissues do not suffice, rotation of a local flap over the bone may prevent osteitis and aseptic necrosis.

Osteomyelitis of the mandible is relatively uncommon as a complication in the management of facial fractures. Before the use of antibiotics and modern surgical techniques in fracture treatment, approximately one-third of all patients with fractures developed osteomyelitis. Many times this was extensive, with loss of large segments of bone. Incision and drainage, fixation of the bone segments, and intensive antibiotic therapy are indicated in cases of osteomyelitis. Sequestra should be removed as they form. In general, conservative management in osteomyelitis gives the best end result with the least amount of deformity.

Ankylosis of the temporomandibular joint may complicate compound comminuted fractures of the mandibular condyle or the coronoid process of the mandible. Ankylosis may also develop in intracapsular fractures of the articular head of the condyle in which there is aseptic necrosis with loss of the articular surface and destruction of the meniscus. Fibro-osseous ankylosis may occur following extensive comminuted compound fractures of the condyle. If it appears that infection is a complicating factor resulting in loss of bone with scar tissue formation, the devitalized head of the condyle should be removed.

Late Complications. The late complications include nonunion, malunion, delayed union, ankylosis of the temporomandibular joint, anesthesia of the inferior alveolar nerve, scar tissue contractures of the mouth, and facial deformity.

NONUNION. Healing at the site of fracture in most instances is accomplished in a period of four to eight weeks, depending upon the degree of fracture and the age and general condition of the patient. Healing is determined by clinical examination, as roentgenograms can show a radiolucency at the fracture site even in the presence of bony union. Nonunion may occur as a result of interposition of foreign substances, of muscle or soft tissue, improper immobilization, poor position of the fractured segments, loss of portions of the bone, sequestration of bone fragments, the presence of infection, or the debilitated condition of the patient. In one of our patients, union at the site of fracture of the mandible had not occurred after three months of fixation. It was found that the patient had lost approximately 30 pounds during this period because she did not like liquid foods and refused to take enough to provide an adequate nutritional intake. When she was placed upon a therapeutic feeding schedule, healing rapidly occurred.

On roentgenographic examination in nonunion, dense eburnated bone is noted covering the ends of the fractured segments.

The management of nonunited fractures is surgical. The bone ends should be exposed through an extraoral approach and the eburnated bone removed with bone burrs or rongeurs. If it is possible without shortening the mandible, the freshened bone ends are placed in apposition and held by interosseous wiring supplemented by intermaxillary fixation. In most cases of nonunion, there is insufficient bone to bridge the gap without forming a defect in the dental arch, and bone grafts are necessary. Before placing the bone graft, eburnated bone should be excised and the outer table partially decorticated. In small losses bone chips may be adequate to bridge the gap. In larger defects it is advisable to use solid segments of iliac bone as grafts. These should be fitted into the space between the segments of the mandible and securely fixed by direct wiring. The graft should be covered with adequate soft tissue to provide a blood supply for healing. Accurate intermaxillary fixation is imperative.

The mandible may be used as a donor site for small size bone grafts. These can be removed from the inferior border or angle of the mandible.

MALUNION. Malunion occurs as a result of inadequate reduction and healing of the bone in an abnormal position. Malunion may also result from inadequate fixation in which the fragments slip out of position and heal out of alignment, or from rotation of segments of the bone or overlapping of segments. Telescoping of the bone segments in the ramus of the mandible may result from the strong muscle pull of the muscles of mastication. If they are permitted to remain in this position, malunion will occur with open bite deformity in the anterior portion of the mandible. In early cases in which ossification is not complete, malunion may be overcome by strong orthopedic traction with arch bars and rubber band traction between the mandible and maxilla. This is effective if there is partial fibrous union but incomplete calcification.

The treatment of malunion consists of osteotomy at the site of malunion, repositioning of the bones, and fixation by direct bone plating or interosseous wiring. If bone segments have been lost, it may be necessary to supplement with bone grafts.

Fractures of the Maxilla

Fractures of the maxilla are less common than fractures of the mandible. The ratio of frequency appears to be changing from that of 4 to 1 stated by Rowe and Killey (1955) and Converse (1974). Recent series indicate a higher incidence of maxillary fractures in relationship to mandibular fractures.

The maxilla forms a large part of the bone structure of the middle third of the face and is attached to the cranium by a system of strong buttresses. The architectural and structural arrangement of these bones forms a mass capable of resisting considerable violence and is an important factor in protecting the brain case and intracranial structures. Violent forces in injuries of the anterior face are dissipated and absorbed by the maxilla and other facial bone structures, thus protecting the brain and spinal cord.

ANATOMICAL CONSIDERATIONS

The maxilla is formed by the midline junction of two irregular, pyramidal component parts. It contributes to the formation of the midportion of the face and forms part of the orbit, nose, and palate, and its hollow interior comprises the maxillary sinuses (Fig. 24–122). A large portion of the orbit, the nasal fossa, the oral cavity, and most of the palate, the nasal cavity, and the pyriform aperture are formed by the maxilla. The frontal processes of the maxilla support the nasal bones and nasal cartilages. As previously stated, the maxilla is attached to the cranium by a strong system of buttresses formed by the nasal bones and the frontal processes medially and by the zygoma lat-

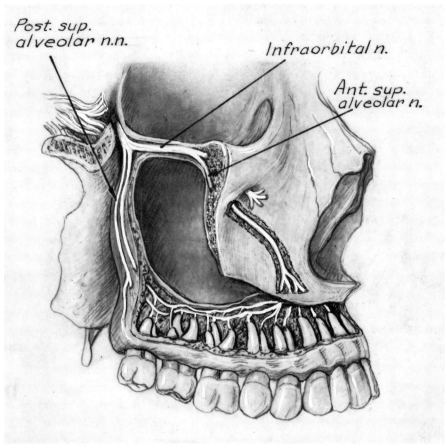

FIGURE 24-122. The maxilla. The maxillary sinus is opened, showing the relationship with the floor of the orbit. Note also the interface between the pterygoid plates and the tuberosity of the maxilla. The nerves are outlined. (From Kazanjian and Converse.)

erally. The maxilla obtains its stability by intimate association with nine other bones of the face (Fig. 24-123).

The maxilla consists of a body and four processes — the frontal, zygomatic, palatine, and alveolar processes. The body of the bone contains the large maxillary sinuses. In childhood the sinuses are small, but in the adult they are large with the overlying bone thinned to eggshell thickness.

When teeth are present in the maxilla, the alveolar process is a strong and thick bone giving excellent support to the horizontal processes and protection to the upper portion of the bone. In old age, when the teeth have been lost, there is marked atrophy of the alveolar process and thinning of the bone. The entire alveolar portion of the bone may recede to the nasal spine and as far as the floor of the maxillary sinuses.

The nerves to the teeth pass through the anterior wall of the bone, and the infraorbital nerve passes through the infraorbital canal of the maxilla to supply the soft tissues of the upper lip and lateral aspect of the nose. The mucosa overlying the bony palate and the mucosa of the soft palate are innervated by the palatine branches of the second division of the fifth nerve which pass through the palatine canal between the maxilla and the palatine bones. The nasopalatine nerves traversing each side of the vomer pass from the nasal cavity through the small incisive foramen to contribute to the innervation of the mucoperiosteum of the anterior portion of the hard palate.

Surgical Anatomy. The maxilla is designed to absorb the shock of mastication and of the occluding teeth and to distribute the load over the craniofacial skeleton. Forces are distributed through the arch of the palate and the articulation of the maxilla against the frontomaxillary, zygomaticomaxillary, and ethmoidomaxillary sutures. The palatine bone and pterygoid plates of the sphenoid give sta-

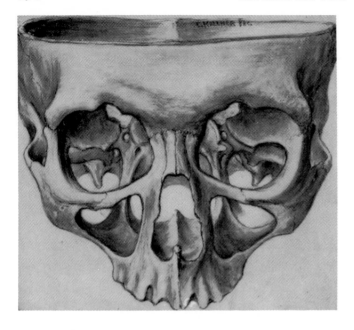

FIGURE 24-123. Drawing of a dissected skull. The thinner bony portions have been removed, leaving the heavier parts intact. (From Shapiro, H. H.: Applied Anatomy of the Head and Neck. Philadelphia, J. B. Lippincott Company, 1947.)

bility posteriorly. The vomer, the perpendicular plate of the ethmoid, and the zygoma distribute the load to the temporal and frontal bones. The upper half of the nasal cavity, situated below the anterior cranial fossa and between the orbits, is designated as the interorbital space (Fig. 24–124).

Fractures of the maxilla are usually caused by a direct impact to the bone and vary from simple alveolar fractures and fractures involv-

ing only the maxillary bone to extensive fractures of the entire midfacial skeleton.

Muscle contraction does not play an important role in displacement of maxillary fractures. The muscles of expression have no influence upon displacement of fractured maxillary segments. The pull of the pterygoid muscles exerts a backward displacement in high maxillary fractures. When maxillary fractures are associated with fractures of the zygoma, mas-

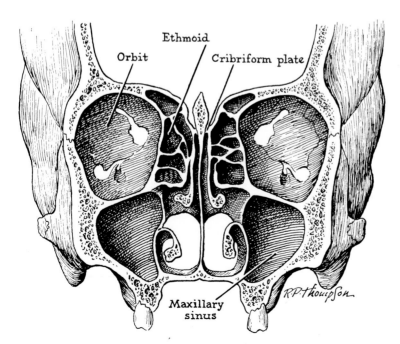

FIGURE 24-124. Frontal plane section through the skull showing the interorbital space. (From Kazanjian and Converse.)

seter muscle action may be a factor in displacement.

Injuries of the nasolacrimal system may occur in fractures of the maxilla as the lacrimal groove is formed partially by the maxilla. The roof of the ethmoid sinuses and the cribriform plate contribute to the anatomy of the anterior cranial fossa, and fractures of the maxilla at a high level (Le Fort III fractures) are occasionally associated with fractures of these structures. Dural laceration, cerebrospinal fistula, and brain damage may result.

Shapiro (1947) has emphasized that the heavier portions of the maxilla give strength to the bone, and the thinner portions are the areas through which fractures are most likely to occur (see Fig. 24–123). Le Fort's (1901) experiments determined the areas of structural weakness of the maxilla and led to the Le Fort classification of fractures of the maxilla (Figs. 24–125 and 24–126).

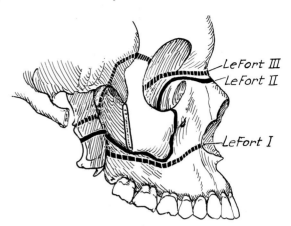

FIGURE 24–125. Le Fort's lines of fracture. (From Kazanjian and Converse.)

CLASSIFICATION

Alveolar Fractures. The dentoalveolar portion of the maxilla may be fractured by direct force or by indirect force against the mandible, which may shatter the maxilla. This may occur

from a blow to the undersurface of the mandible with transmission of upward and outward forces against the maxillary teeth, causing alveolar fractures with lateral displacement.

Transverse Fractures (Le Fort I). Fractures above the level of the apices of the teeth may include the alveolar process, the vault of the palate, and the pterygoid processes in a single block. This type is known as the Le Fort I, or Guérin's, fracture (Fig. 24–126, *A*).

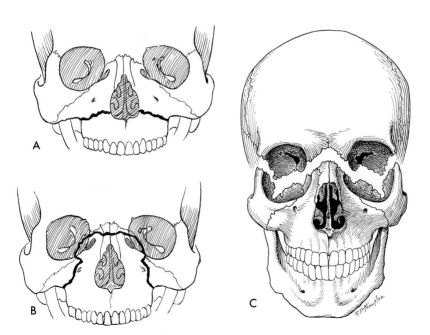

FIGURE 24–126. Le Fort's classification of midfacial fractures. *A*, Le Fort I, horizontal fracture of the maxilla, also known as Guerin's fracture. *B*, Le Fort II, pyramidal fracture of the maxilla. *C*, Le Fort III, craniofacial disjunction. (From Kazanjian and Converse.)

Pyramidal Fractures (Le Fort II). Blows to the upper maxillary area may result in fractures through the thin portion of the frontal process, extending laterally through the lacrimal bones, the floor of the orbit, through the zygomaticomaxillary suture line, along the lateral wall of the maxilla, and through the pterygoid plates into the pterygomaxillary fossa. This fracture, because of its general shape and configuration, is known as the pyramidal fracture. With marked posterior displacement, damage may occur to the ethmoidal area, to the septum, and to the lacrimal area with lateral splaying of the interorbital space (Fig. 24–126, *B*).

Craniofacial Disjunction (Le Fort III). Craniofacial disjunction may occur when the fracture extends through the zygomaticofrontal suture and the nasofrontal sutures and across the floor of the orbits to effect complete separation of the structures of the middle third of the face. In these fractures, the maxilla may not be separated from the zygoma or from the nasal structures, the entire midfacial skeleton being completely detached from the base of the skull and suspended only by soft tissues (Fig. 24–126, *C*).

Vertical Fractures. Fractures of the maxilla may occur in a vertical direction in which the maxilla is split along a sagittal plane (Fig. 24–127). This usually occurs just to one side of the midline, which is reinforced by the vomer. The bone is thin at the site of fracture.

Vertical fractures are usually associated with other fractures of the maxilla. Displacement depends upon the direction and the degree of force.

ETIOLOGY

The most common cause of fractures of the maxilla is the force sustained from the so-called "guest passenger" type of injury. This injury occurs in automobile, airplane, and other high-speed accidents when the patient is thrown forward and strikes the middle third of his face against the instrument panel, the back of a seat, or the head of another individual. If the force is sustained low on the maxilla, in the region of the upper lip, an alveolar fracture or a transverse fracture is most likely to occur. If the force is more violent and sustained at a higher level, comminuted fractures of the maxilla of the pyramidal type may be expected.

Although most traumatic forces are directed from the anterior or lateral direction, upward forces on the anterior portion of the maxilla may occur. Displacement is generally posteriorly and downward, giving the patient a "dish face" appearance in the middle third of the face and overall elongation of the facial structures. The posterior and downward displacement may be aided by the forces of the pterygoid musculature. Partial fracture of the maxilla or the alveolar process with displacement of the segments into the sinus or the region of the palate may occur from lateral forces. In sagittal fractures due to upward

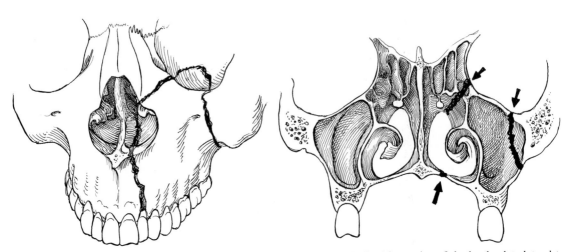

FIGURE 24–127. Sagittal fractures of the maxilla usually occur through the thin portion of the hard palate lateral to the vomer and are associated with fractue of the thin portion of the orbital floor and lateral maxillary wall. (From Kazanjian and Converse.)

forces, the fragments may be displaced outward on one or both sides. Vertical fractures are caused by forces transmitted through the mandible to the maxilla or by direct upward force to the anterior maxilla. Impacted fractures are infrequent, but in some cases the entire maxilla is driven upward and backward into the interorbital space or pharyngeal region and may be so securely impacted that no movement can be elicited on clinical examination.

EXAMINATION AND DIAGNOSIS

Inspection. Epistaxis, periorbital, conjunctival, and scleral ecchymosis, edema, and subcutaneous hematoma are suggestive of fractures of the maxillary-nasal area (Fig. 24–128). Malocclusion with anterior open bite is suggestive of fracture of the maxilla. A maxillary segment may be displaced downward and posteriorly, resulting in premature occlusion in the poste-

rior region. On intraoral examination, tearing of the overlying soft tissues of the labial vestibule or the palate generally indicates underlying fractures. The face will have a long, donkey-like appearance, suggestive of a fracture of the maxilla, and particularly of a craniofacial disjunction (Le Fort III fracture).

Palpation. Simultaneous bilateral palpation may indicate a steplike defect at the zygomaticomaxillary suture, indicating fractures of the pyramidal type. Intraoral palpation may reveal fractures of the anterior portion of the maxilla or fractured segments of alveolar bone. Fractures at the junction of the maxilla and zygoma may be detected by digital palpation along the inferior rim of the orbit. Movement of the nasal bones by palpation suggests that nasal fractures may be associated with fractures of the maxilla.

Digital Manipulation. Force applied by grasping the anterior portion of the maxilla between the thumb and index finger will elicit

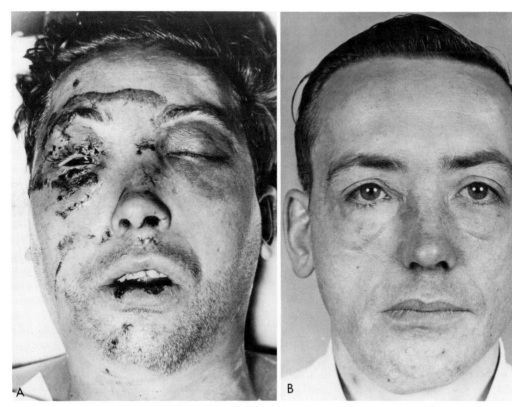

FIGURE 24–128. Extensive injury sustained in an automobile accident. *A,* Multiple facial fractures including the mandible, maxilla, zygoma, and nasal and ethmoid bones. These fractures were treated by mandibular open reduction, intermaxillary fixation with upper and lower Erich arch bars, open reduction and interosseous wiring of the zygomatic fractures bilaterally, and internal wire fixation from the frontal bone for suspension of the maxillary-zygomatic nasal compound. (See section on Midfacial and Panfacial Fractures: The Direct Approach.) *B,* Two months following treatment of multiple facial fractures.

mobility of the maxilla or the entire zygomaticomaxillary complex (see Fig. 24–13, *C*). The manipulation test for mobility is not entirely reliable, because impacted fractures may be extensive and exhibit no movement. These may be overlooked unless the occlusion is carefully checked. Manipulation of the anterior maxilla may show movement of the entire middle third of the face, including the bridge of the nose (Le Fort III fracture). Crepitation may be heard when the anterior maxilla is manipulated.

Cerebrospinal Rhinorrhea or Otorrhea. These complications involve the leaking of cerebrospinal fluid from the nose or ear. This signifies the presence of a fistula extending from the intracranial arachnoid space through the skull into the nose or ear. Clear fluid drainage from the nostrils, ears, or pharynx may be noted in fractures of the maxilla involving the cribriform plate and base of the anterior cranial fossa, or the middle cranial fossa in the case of otorrhea.

Malocclusion of the Teeth. With the mandible intact, malocclusion of the teeth is highly suggestive of maxillary fracture. It is possible, however, to have a high craniofacial dislocation and still have fair occlusion of the teeth. If the maxilla is rotated or markedly displaced backward and downward, there is complete disruption of the occlusal relationships.

Roentgenographic Findings. The clinical diagnosis of fractures of the maxilla should be confirmed by careful roentgenographic examination. Fractures of the maxilla may be difficult to demonstrate on roentgenographic examination because of the superimposition of other structures. The Waters view is excellent for demonstrating fractures of the maxilla and associated structures. Unless there is displacement, fractures may not be demonstrated by roentgenographic examination. The presence of an opaque maxillary sinus suggests fracture of the maxilla. The opaque shadow represents serum or blood in the sinus resulting from disruption of the sinus mucosa incident to the fracture. Separation in the nasofrontal area may be noted if the fracture is associated with nasal fractures. Steplike irregularities may be noted in the infraorbital margins, and the zygomaticomaxillary junction will be widened. Irregularity of the lateral wall of the maxillary sinus is usually noted. Vertical and alveolar fractures are best determined by the occlusal X-ray technique.

TREATMENT OF FRACTURES OF THE MAXILLA

Emergency Treatment. Treatment should be directed toward the establishment of the airway and control of hemorrhage.

THE AIRWAY. If considerable displacement of the fractured maxilla has occurred, the upper airway may be blocked by structures forced into the pharyngeal region or by blood clots, loose teeth, bone, broken dentures, or other foreign material. These should be removed and, if an adequate airway cannot be established, endotracheal intubation or tracheotomy should be done.

CONTROL OF HEMORRHAGE. Some maxillary fractures are associated with deep lacerations of the overlying skin and oral mucosa. Shearing fractures may tear the greater palatine vessels, or wounds may involve the internal maxillary artery, resulting in severe hemorrhage in the nasal and pharyngeal area. The bleeding may threaten exsanguination and may respond only to clamping of the deep vessels and packing of the wounds. Posterior nasal tamponade may control bleeding in the posterior pharyngeal region. In gunshot or avulsing wounds of the maxillary area, ligation of the external carotid artery may be indicated.

Definitive Treatment

ALVEOLAR FRACTURES. Simple fractures of portions of the maxilla, including the alveolar bone and teeth, usually will respond to digital manipulation and reduction. If the occlusion is satisfactory, the position of the teeth may be maintained by ligating the teeth in the fracture segment to the adjacent teeth. The segments can also be stabilized by ligation of an arch bar to adjacent normal segments of the maxilla and ligation of the teeth of the fragments to the arch bar. Individual teeth or segments containing several teeth may be stabilized by a splint fabricated at the operating table with quick curing acrylic resin moulded to the teeth and alveolus. If the fragments cannot be adequately reduced and there is premature contact between the teeth of the mandible and the teeth of the fractured segment, the application of upper and lower arch bars and intermaxillary rubber band traction for a few days will usually force the segment into position (Fig. 24–129). Fixation should be maintained for approximately three to four weeks.

TRANSVERSE FRACTURES. Fractures of the Le Fort I or Le Fort II type, in which there is an adequate complement of teeth and an intact

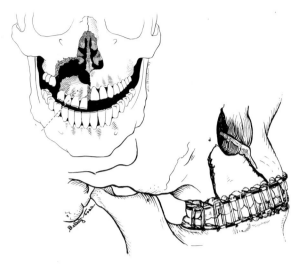

FIGURE 24–129. *A*, Fracture-dislocation of a large segment of alveolar bone and palate. *B*, Reduction and fixation is accomplished by rubber band traction between the mandibular teeth and maxillary teeth. The force of the traction results in reduction of the fracture and restoration of adequate occlusion of the teeth.

mandible with teeth, may be treated by intermaxillary fixation with arch bars and rubber bands and the application of a simple head cap with a chin support (Fig. 24–130).

The primary consideration is the reestablishment of functional dental occlusion, and this should be accomplished before upward traction is applied. The force of the mandible against the maxilla will reduce the fractured maxilla and hold it in position until consolidation takes place. In utilizing this method, care must be used to avoid necrotizing pressures against the soft tissues along the inferior border of the mandible. Ulcers may occur if pressure is intensive.

Head caps are usually unreliable and uncomfortable; more positive fixation of fractures of this type can be obtained by suspension of the mandible and maxilla by internal wire fixation to the first solid structure immediately above the fracture site. This is usually the pyriform margin, the infraorbital rim, or the frontal bone just above the frontozygomatic suture (Fig. 24–131).

Infraorbital fixation is achieved through percutaneous lid or transconjunctival incisions to expose the bony margin. Small drill holes are made through the infraorbital rim on both sides. A fine stainless steel wire is passed through each hole and looped over the infraorbital margin. The ends of the wire are led into the mouth through a needle and passed around the superior arch bar. After the teeth

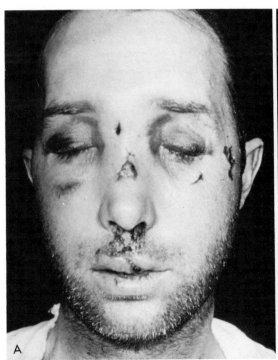
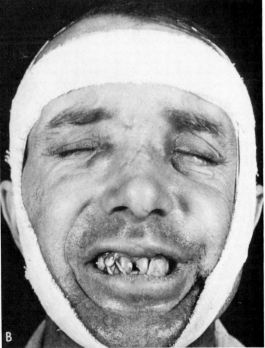

FIGURE 24–130. *A*, Pyramidal fracture of the maxilla. Note the elongated appearance of the face due to the downward displacement of the maxilla and nasal structures. *B*, Correction was by intermaxillary fixation forcing the mandible and maxilla upward by manual pressure and fixation with a plaster headcap.

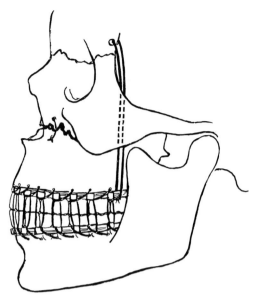

FIGURE 24–131. Fixation for a fracture of the maxilla by internal wire suspension to the zygomatic process of the frontal bone and direct wiring to the frontal process of the maxilla. The concept of internal wire fixation of facial fractures was introduced by Adams (1942) and elaborated upon by Adams and Adams (1956).

of the rubber bands. If advancement and downward rotation of the impacted maxilla is required, the rubber bands are placed obliquely between the maxillary and mandibular arches: the mandibular points of purchase of the rubber bands are further forward than the maxillary. Once reduction has been achieved, as judged by adequate occlusal relationships, intermaxillary fixation is established. A bandage may be adequate in simple fractures; internal suspension wiring may be required in more severe cases to provide cranial fixation.

When consolidation is more advanced, more energetic methods of disimpaction can be obtained by forceps, such as Rowe's (Fig. 24–135, *A*) or Hayton-Williams' (Fig. 24–135, *D*). Continuous traction can be exerted by means of an extraoral appliance attached to a cranial fixation appliance, such as a head frame (Georgiade's "crown of thorns") or a plaster head cap, are required. Extracranial orthopedic traction has also been employed in the past (Fig. 24–136).

are secured in occlusion by rubber band traction, the assistant applies pressure against the mandible, which repositions the maxilla. The wires are then securely twisted around the upper arch bar. The maxilla is guided into proper occlusal relationship with the mandible and is held by the suspension wires. This method provides positive fixation with minimal effort and maximal comfort to the patient. The concealed wires and arch bars permit early return to productive activity (Fig. 24–132).

Pyramidal fractures of the maxilla and fractures of the maxilla associated with the nasal bones can be reduced and maintained by open reduction and interosseous wire fixation (Figs. 24–133 and 24–134).

Malunited Fractures or Fractures Partially Healed in Malposition. Impacted fractures or those seen two or three weeks after injury and partially healed fractures may be impossible to reduce manually or by the usual methods.

Intermaxillary traction by means of rubber bands placed between an arch bar or Kanzanjian buttons placed on the maxillary dental arch and similar appliances on the mandibular dental arch will reposition the displaced maxilla if consolidation is not too advanced. An open bite will be closed by the vertical traction

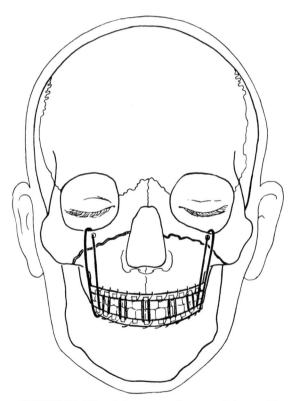

FIGURE 24–132. A transverse fracture of the maxilla treated by intermaxillary fixation and suspension from the infraorbital ridges by wires passing into the mouth and attached to the lower arch bar. The wires can also be attached to the upper bar.

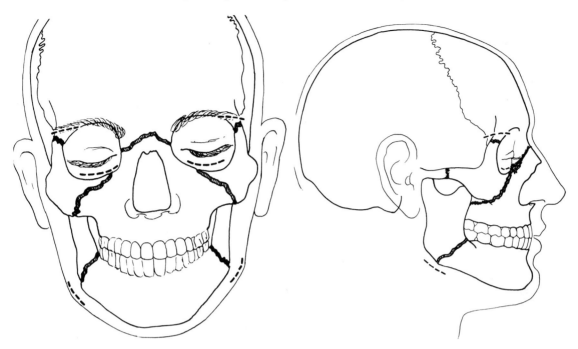

FIGURE 24–133. Common sites of fracture in multiple facial injury. Dotted lines demonstrate incisions and locations through which these fractures can be treated by open reduction and interosseous wire fixation.

Such methods have progressively been replaced, in many cases, by the direct surgical approach. Experience gained in craniofacial surgery has shown that such an approach can be employed safely and efficiently.

In malunited fractures of the maxilla, whether completely or partially consolidated, the direct approach, either through a transcutaneous or an intraoral approach, or both, is indicated. The Le Fort I malunited fracture is approached through an oral vestibular incision, and the line of fracture is exposed. The bone is liberated after transection of the fracture line, and the lower maxillary segment is replaced in the corrected occlusal relationships with the mandibular teeth.

The LeFort II and LeFort III fractures are also approached through appropriate cutaneous and intraoral incisions, and the malunited portions of the facial skeleton are disengaged and repositioned according to the principles established in craniofacial surgery. In some cases an intracranial approach may be required.

FRACTURES OF THE EDENTULOUS MAXILLA. Fractures of the edentulous maxilla are seen infrequently unless associated with extensive fractures of the other bones of the mid-third of the face. The absence of teeth, through which

fracturing forces are usually transmitted, provides a measure of protection for the edentulous patient. Older edentulous patients are not exposed to the traumatic hazards of younger age, which also reduces the incidence of maxillary fractures. Dentures give protection from fracture by absorbing traumatic forces which are dissipated by the breaking of the denture.

Fractures of the edentulous maxilla with minimal displacement. If the displacement is minimal, causing little facial deformity, it is reasonable to expect that the discrepancy in the maxillary-mandibular relationships will be corrected by means of adjustment or reconstruction of the patient's denture. Treatment is therefore unnecessary. Fractures of this type heal within a matter of two to three weeks. As soon as the edema and hematomas have disappeared, the patient may have a new denture constructed.

Edentulous fractures with significant displacement. If the displacement is such that it results in deformity of the midthird of the face and a problem for denture construction, efforts should be made to reduce and immobilize the fractured segments. If the fracture is transverse (Le Fort I type) and the patient has a usable upper denture, the fracture may be re-

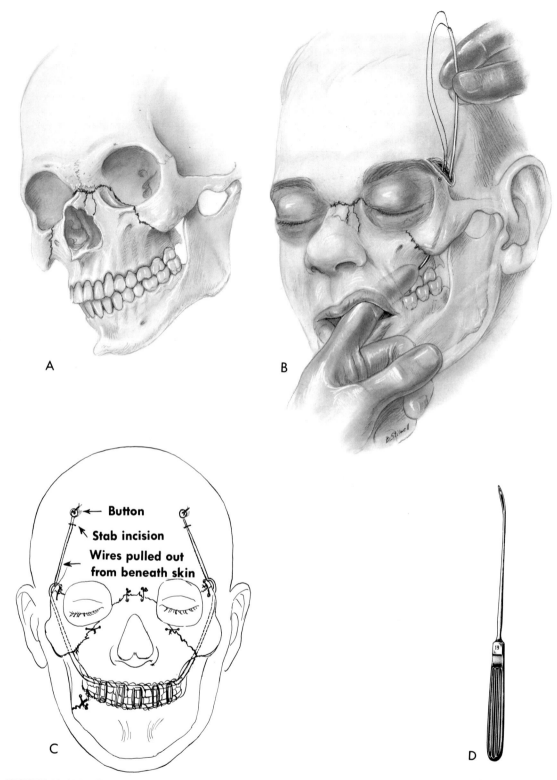

FIGURE 24–134. Craniofacial suspension and internal wire fixation. *A,* Pyramidal (Le Fort II) fracture. *B,* The suspension wire is passed through a spinal puncture needle (or a special wire-passer with a perforated tip) which is inserted through the brow incision, traverses the area medial to the zygomatic arch, and enters the oral cavity opposite the maxillary first molar tooth. The needle is withdrawn through the mouth. *C,* The areas of direct interosseous fixation and the direction of the wires used for craniofacial suspension. The suspension wires are removed after healing has taken place by cutting the wires in the mouth and pulling them out by traction on the pull-out wires in the forehead area. *D,* Wire-passer.

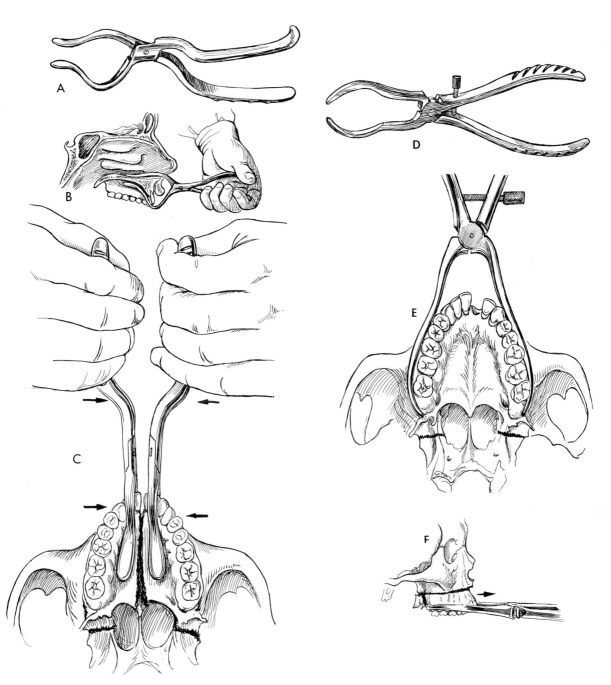

FIGURE 24–135. *A,* Rowe's disimpaction forceps. *B,* Forceps in position. *C,* Two forceps may be employed to exert greater force and approximate the edges of a paramedian sagittal fracture. *D,* Hayton-Williams forceps for maxillary disimpaction. *E,* Position of forceps which embraces maxillary tuberosities. Screw which penetrates the branches of the forceps permits regulation of the pressure exerted against the bone. *F,* Use of forceps in a low maxillary fracture. (From Kazanjian and Converse.)

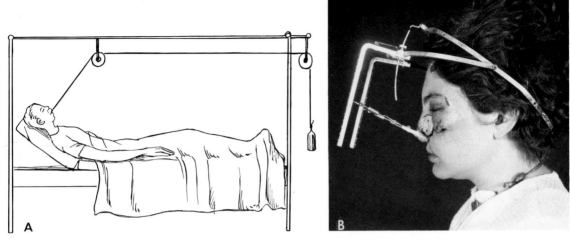

FIGURE 24–136. Extracranial orthopedic devices. *A*, Balanced suspension to overhead frame. *B*, Extracranial halo apparatus (Georgiade).

duced manually. The denture is inserted and brought into occlusal relationship with the lower teeth or the patient's lower denture, and a head bandage or plaster bandage (see Fig. 24–130) is applied. After a week to ten days, the fracture segments will remain in position without further fixation.

If the displacement is moderate and the patient has no upper denture, open exposure of the fracture site and wiring to the edge of the pyriform margin will provide fixation (Fig. 24–137).

In the pyramidal or Le Fort II fracture, the patient's upper denture may be wired to the fractured segment anteriorly and posteriorly. The denture is brought into occlusal relationship with the patient's teeth or lower denture; this then determines the position of the maxillary segment, which is advanced and rotated into the denture. The denture is secured by internal wire fixation through the infraorbital margins, to the zygomatic process of the frontal bone or by a wire looped around each zygomatic arch.

If the fractured maxilla is associated with other fractures, the patient's dentures or prepared splints and internal wire fixation (Fig. 24–138) are necessary for reduction and fixation.

Comminuted displaced fractures of the anterior maxillary wall with penetration of the maxillary sinus require reduction by the open method through an incision in the canine fossa. The maxillary sinus cavity is packed with rubber dam drain or gauze strips impregnated with petrolatum to maintain contour of the anterior maxillary wall and support the fractured segments. The end of the gauze may be brought out through a nasal antrostomy under the inferior turbinate for ease of removal. Fixation and support with the gauze packing for five to seven days will permit the fractured segments to consolidate into position.

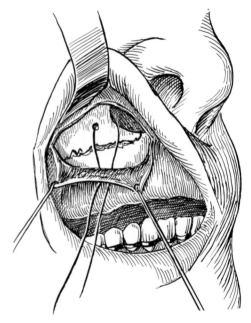

FIGURE 24–137. Intraoral exposure of the pyriform aperture for fixation of fractures of the maxilla. (From Kazanjian and Converse.)

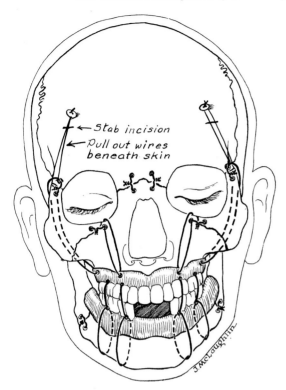

FIGURE 24–138. Method of interosseous wire fixation and internal wire suspension utilizing the patient's own dentures in an edentulous patient with multiple facial fractures. The lower front teeth are removed from the denture to facilitate feeding.

POSTOPERATIVE CARE OF MAXILLARY FRACTURES. Postoperative management of fractures of the maxilla consists of the usual general care, including adequate nutrition and antibiotics when indicated. The nasal cavity is usually involved, and it may be difficult to maintain an adequate nasal airway. Frequent suctioning of the nasal cavity will keep the airway free of mucus and blood clots. Vaso-constricting drugs may be helpful in keeping the airway open and may provide ventilation to the maxillary sinuses so that disintegrating clotted blood in the sinuses will have an opportunity to escape readily. Oral hygiene should be maintained by frequent use of mouthwashes and proper toothbrushing technique. This is especially important when the patient's dentures are fixed by circumferential wiring to the mandible and maxilla. Food particles under the denture or around the fixation appliances increase the possibility of infection and may give a foul odor to the breath.

COMPLICATIONS OF FRACTURES OF THE MAXILLA

Early Complications

HEMORRHAGE. The early complications are those associated with acute trauma incident to the injury. Extensive hemorrhage due to laceration of the overlying soft tissues or to fracture and tearing of major vessels passing through the maxilla may be serious and should be managed by clamping and tying vessels, by tamponade, or by packing the wounds with gauze.

AIRWAY OBSTRUCTION. The maxilla forms a large portion of the boundary of the nasal cavities and in almost all cases of extensive fracture of the maxilla, the airway will be compromised owing to displacement of fragments or edema of the soft tissues of the nasal cavity. Segments of bone may be forced into the oropharyngeal area, further interfering with the airway. Blood clots and fragments of bone and tooth structure should be removed from the upper pharyngeal and nasal area as early as possible. A soft rubber nasopharyngeal tube passed through the nostril may help in establishing an airway.

INFECTION. Maxillary wounds may be complicated by infection caused by contamination at the time of injury, by loose teeth or bone fragments in the maxillary sinus, or by fractures through a sinus with preexisting chronic infection. The appropriate methods of management of local infection must be instituted; this may require opening and drainage of the maxillary sinus, removal of foreign bodies, bone fragments, or teeth from the maxillary sinus or the nasal cavity, and the administration of antibiotics. Fractures of the maxilla may be associated with fractures of the cribriform area and cerebrospinal fluid rhinorrhea. Treatment consists of antibiotic therapy and reduction of the fractures. Blowing of the nose and nasal packing should be avoided.

BLINDNESS. Bilateral total blindness is fortunately rare as a complication of severe LeFort III facial fractures. It has been suspected that bone fragments projected backward into the apex of the orbit could sever the optic nerve, a cause of unilateral blindness. Ketchum, Ferris and Masters (1976) had the opportunity to witness the mechanism of bilateral blindness in the course of a craniotomy in a patient with bilateral blindness following a LeFort III fracture. The backward displacement of the fragments resulting from the orbital fractures had shredded the optic nerve, "as a piece of glass would shred twine, fraying it on one side and completely transecting it on the other."

Late Complications. Late complications of fractures of the maxilla include nonunion, malunion, lacrimal system obstruction, infraorbital anesthesia, and extraocular muscle imbalance.

NONUNION. Nonunion of fractures of the maxilla is rare unless there has been considerable destruction of bone as a result of comminution. Usually nonunion indicates failure to provide even the most elementary type of fixation. Should nonunion occur, the treatment consists of exposure of the fracture site, resection of fibrous tissue in the fracture site, placement of cancellous autogenous bone chips, and adequate fixation after restoration of adequate occlusal relationships.

MALUNION. In multiple, complex (panfacial) fractures, malunion may result from inadequate diagnosis of the fracture. The toothbearing segment of the maxilla may be placed in adequate occlusal relationships with the mandible, but other segments of the bone may remain unreduced. The treatment of panfacial fractures is discussed at the end of this chapter. Secondary osteotomies to restore contour and dental occlusion are discussed in detail in Chapter 30.

LACRIMAL SYSTEM OBSTRUCTION. The nasolacrimal duct may be severed or obstructed in transverse comminuted fractures extending across the facial skeleton at the level of the nasolacrimal duct. A dacryocystorhinostomy is usually indicated. In Le Fort II fractures, when they are associated with naso-orbital fractures, the lacrimal sac and canaliculi may be injured by displacement of bone fragments (see Chapter 28).

EXTRAOCULAR MUSCLE IMBALANCE. The inferior oblique muscle may be injured at its point of insertion at the medial portion of the orbital floor formed by the maxilla. Disturbances of the oculorotary mechanism of the eye are more frequent in maxillary fractures associated with orbital, naso-orbital, and zygomatic fractures.

FRACTURES OF THE ZYGOMA

The zygoma (Fig. 24–139) is a buttress of the facial skeleton and the bone of the face that gives prominence to the cheek area. The zygoma, commonly known as the malar bone, is a quadrilateral bone with frontal, maxillary, temporal, and orbital processes. It articulates with the frontal bone, the maxilla, the temporal

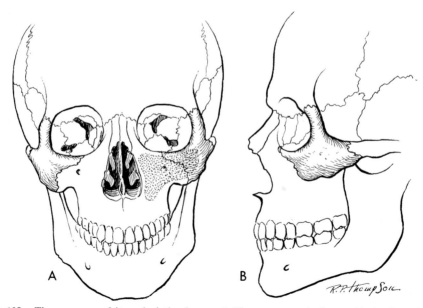

FIGURE 24–139. The zygoma and its articulating bones. *A,* The zygoma articulates with the frontal, sphenoid, and temporal bones and the maxilla. The dotted area shows the portion of the zygoma and maxilla occupied by the maxillary sinus. *B,* Lateral view of the zygoma. (From Kazanjian and Converse.)

bone, and the greater wing of the sphenoid. On its outer surface it is convex, forming the prominence of the cheek; on its inner surface it is concave and participates in the formation of the temporal fossa. The bone has its broadest and strongest attachment with the maxilla, a thin, weak attachment with the sphenoid, a moderately strong attachment with the frontal bone, and a weak attachment with the thin zygomatic process of the temporal bone. The zygoma forms the greater portion of the lateral orbital floor. In most skulls, it forms the lateral superior wall of the maxillary sinus and may be pneumatized with air cells connecting with the maxillary sinus. The bone furnishes attachments for the masseter, temporalis, zygomaticus, and zygomatic head of the quadratus labii superioris muscles. The zygomaticotemporal and zygomaticofacial nerves pass forward through small foramina in the zygoma to innervate the soft tissues over the malar prominences.

Surgical Pathology

Although sturdy, the zygoma is in a prominent location and is frequently subjected to injury. Moderately severe blows will be absorbed by the bone and its buttressing attachments. Severe blows, such as from a fall or a fist, may cause separation of the zygoma at its articulating surfaces. It is usually separated and displaced in a downward, medial, and posterior direction. Violent shattering injuries to the region of the zygoma may result in extensive comminution as well as separation at the suture lines.

The zygoma is the principal buttressing bone between the maxilla and the cranium. Fractures usually involve the orbital rim, resulting in hematoma or extravasation of blood into the tissues near the lateral canthus. Direct lateral force may result in fractures of the temporal portion of the zygoma and the zygomatic process of the temporal bone which make up the zygomatic arch. Fracture with medial displacement of the arch may cause impingement of the bone fragments against the temporal muscle attached to the coronoid process of the mandible (Fig. 24–140). This may result in difficulty in or inability to open the mouth because of interference with the forward and downward movement of the coronoid process. Fragments of bone driven through the temporal muscle into contact with the coronoid process may be the causative factors in the formation of a fibro-osseous ankylosis, necessitating excision of the coronoid process.

Fracture-dislocation of the zygoma with sufficient backward displacement to impinge on the coronoid process will interfere with mandibular motion (Fig. 24–141). Fracture-dislocation of the zygoma results in separation of the zygomaticofrontal suture line, which is palpable through the skin overlying the lateral orbital margin. Separation with a steplike deformity of the infraorbital margin can often be detected clinically. The lateral superior wall of the maxillary sinus is involved in fractures of the zygoma, resulting in a tear of the maxillary sinus lining and accumulation of blood in the sinus with unilateral epistaxis, which may last a short time. The lateral canthal ligament is attached to the zygomatic portion of the orbital rim; displacement of the bone carries the lat-

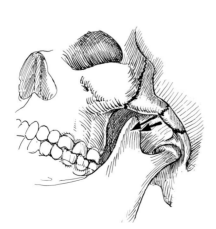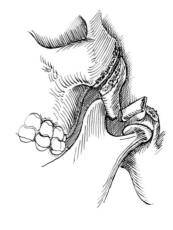

FIGURE 24–140.   Fracture of the zygomatic arch with medial displacement against the coronoid process of the mandible limiting the motion of the mandible.

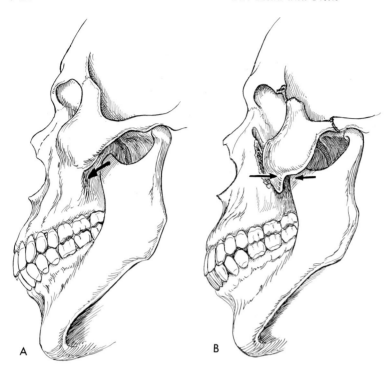

FIGURE 24–141. *A,* The intimate anatomical relationship between the zygoma and the coronoid process. *B,* If the fractured zygoma is displaced backward sufficiently to impinge on the coronoid process, movement of the mandible will be impaired.

eral canthal attachment with it, producing a visible deformity (Fig. 24–142). Dysfunction of the ocular globe may be noted as a result of disruption of the floor and lateral wall of the orbit. The septum orbitale, which attaches to the inferior orbital margin, may be displaced, causing retraction and shortening of the lower lid. Displacement of the globe and orbital contents may occur as a result of downward displacement of the suspensory ligament of Lockwood attached to the lateral wall in its zygomatic portion immediately behind the lateral canthal ligament. When there is fragmentation of the bony floor, the orbital contents may

herniate into the maxillary sinus, where they become incarcerated between the fractured bone segments. Although diplopia is usually transitory in uncomplicated fractures of the zygoma, it may persist when the fracture extends to the maxillary portion of the orbital floor (see Chapter 25).

The orbital fracture may also be complicated by a fracture of the inferior rim of the orbit. When the lower rim of the orbit is displaced backward by fracture, the septum orbitale attachment to the orbital rim is also displaced backward. A downward pull upon the lower eyelid and a tendency to eversion are the

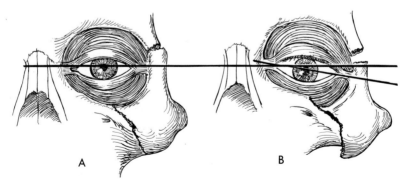

FIGURE 24–142. When the frontal process of the zygoma is depressed downward, the lateral canthal ligament and the canthus of the eye follow. *A,* Normal position of the lateral canthus in a fracture without displacement. *B,* Downward displacement of the globe and lateral canthus as a result of frontozygomatic separation and downward displacement of the zygoma and the floor of the orbit.

results of this anatomical derangement by the fracture.

The infraorbital nerve runs through a canal in the maxilla, but the close proximity of the zygoma usually causes damage by impingement against the nerve when the zygoma is fractured (Fig. 24–143). Laceration of the nerve in the canal or fragments of bone impacted into the area may result in permanent anesthesia. Infraorbital nerve anesthesia usually disappears progressively. Persistent anesthesia is an indication for exploration and decompression of the infraorbital nerve.

Knight and North (1961) proposed a classification of fractures of the zygoma based on the anatomy of the fracture. This is helpful in predicting the clinical features and planning treatment.

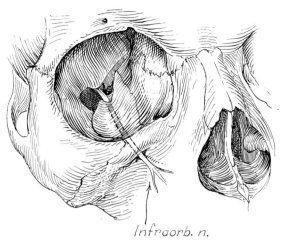

Infraorb. n.

FIGURE 24–143. The infraorbital nerve has an intimate relationship with the floor of the orbit and is almost always damaged in fracture-dislocation of the zygoma. The resultant anesthesia of the lower lid, lateral nasal area, and upper lip usually disappears progressively. (From Converse, J. M., and Smith, B.: Enophthalmos and diplopia in fractures of the orbital floor. Br. J. Plast. Surg., 9:265, 1957.)

CLASSIFICATION OF 120 CASES OF FRACTURE OF THE ZYGOMA

Group I. No significant displacement—fractures visible on roentgenogram but fragments remain in line 6%

Group II. Arch fractures—inward buckling of the arch—no orbital or antral involvement 10%

Group III. Unrotated body fractures—downward and inward displacement but no rotation 33%

Group IV. Medially rotated body fractures—downward; inward and backward displacement with medial rotation 11%

Group V. Laterally rotated body fractures—displacement is downward, backward and medialward with lateral rotation 22%

Group VI. Includes all cases in which additional fracture lines cross the main fragment 18%

Diagnosis of Fractures of the Zygoma

Clinical Evaluation. A history of the type of injury and the direction of force may be helpful in arriving at a diagnosis. A blow from a fist, a fall against a hard object, or a shattering wound to the side of the face from an automobile accident is likely to result in fracture of the zygoma.

A few hours after an injury resulting in fracture, the clinical picture may be obscured by edema and hematoma. Inspection may show ecchymosis of the lids, conjunctiva, and sclera, swelling of the face in the cheek area, displacement of the lateral canthal ligament, depression of the globe, retraction of the lower lid, a deeply sunken upper lid, unilateral epistaxis on the involved side, and inability to open the mouth as presumptive signs of fracture of the zygoma.

The patient may complain of pain on trying to open the mouth and will note that the mandible can move only a short distance. Anesthesia of the upper lip, lower lid, and lateral nasal area is usually present. Diplopia may not be noted after the onset of edema but may be a prominent feature when swelling subsides.

Bimanual palpation of the bone and the structures of the face may be helpful. With the patient seated or lying in a semirecumbent position, the bony prominences on both sides of the face are palpated simultaneously. With the fingers passing around the orbital rim, fractures of the zygomaticofrontal or zygomaticomaxillary suture area may be palpated. Fractures of the zygomatic arch may be detected by flatness or indentation over the infraorbital rim (Fig. 24–144, *A, B*) or zygomatic arch. Intraoral palpation with the finger passing along the lateral and anterior wall of the maxilla, over the region of the zygomatic process of the maxilla and tuberosity, may permit the surgeon to feel irregularities over the bone; the index finger, when palpating the buccal sulcus beneath the zygoma, will note a depression of the fractured zygoma, as the groove between the undersurface of the zygoma and the maxilla is absent if the bone is displaced downward, medially, and posteriorly (Fig. 24–144, *C*).

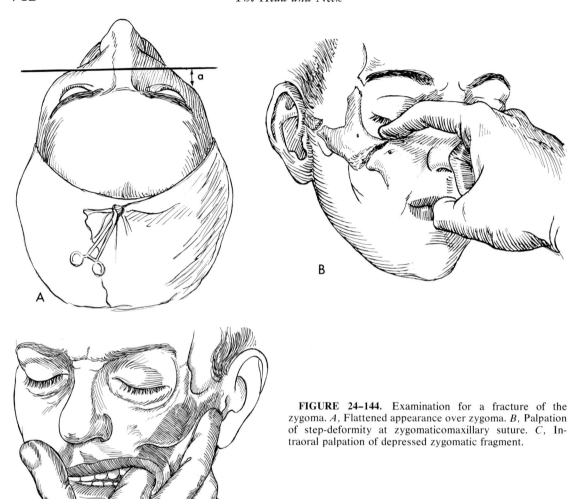

FIGURE 24–144. Examination for a fracture of the zygoma. *A*, Flattened appearance over zygoma. *B*, Palpation of step-deformity at zygomaticomaxillary suture. *C*, Intraoral palpation of depressed zygomatic fragment.

Roentgenographic Evaluation. The usual findings of disjunction at the zygomaticofrontal, zygomaticomaxillary, or zygomaticotemporal suture line are noted. The maxillary sinus is usually opaque owing to the presence of blood in the cavity. The Waters view (Fig. 24–145) will demonstrate the orbital margins and the body of the zygoma. The zygomatic arches can be demonstrated by the Titterington position, the semiaxial superoinferior projection. Tomograms are especially useful for detection of fractures of the orbital floor and orbital walls.

Treatment of Fractures of the Zygoma

The degree of fragmentation and the direction and amount of displacement may influence the management of fractures of the zygoma. Numerous approaches for reduction of the fractured zygoma have been described. Fixation may be obtained by impaction against the adjacent articulating bones, by support from normal muscle and fascial attachments, by the use of cranial fixation appliances, by direct fixation with interosseous wiring, or by the use of gauze packing in the maxillary sinus and the infratemporal region.

Disappointment and frustration in the management of zygomatic fractures after use of the usual closed methods of reduction have been experienced. In many cases of simple fracture without comminution, in which reduction was easily accomplished by the usual methods, late complications were observed in the form of diplopia, malunion, and residual deformity. It

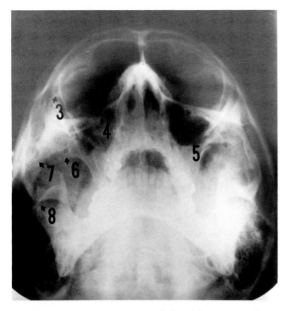

FIGURE 24–145. Fracture of the right zygoma shown in Waters' projection. Note the multiple fracture sites with displacement of the zygoma and clouding of the right maxillary sinus.

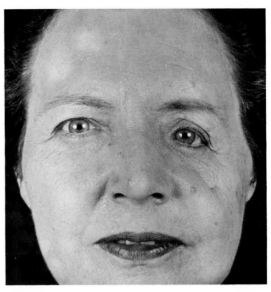

FIGURE 24–146. Malunited fracture of the left zygoma following treatment by the temporal approach without direct interosseous fixation. At the time of operation, clinical reduction seemed satisfactory.

was obvious that either the reduction had not been complete or dislocation of the fracture was recurring in the postoperative period. A careful study of the problem indicated that the fracture-dislocation was usually more severe than it appeared to be from the radiologic and clinical evaluation. Edema often obscured the true condition. Intraorbital edema gave support to the globe during the early stages, and after the edema subsided, diplopia was present. Displaced fractures and blowout fractures of the orbital floor were often overlooked, and the action of the masseter muscle in the face of a tear of the temporalis fascia resulted in postoperative displacement of the zygoma (Fig. 24–146).

These observations led to investigation. In a number of cases, fractures of the zygoma were treated in the usual manner by elevation in what appeared to be a satisfactory position clinically. The fracture sites were then exposed surgically in the zygomaticofrontal and zygomaticomaxillary areas. In many instances, the fractures actually had not been adequately reduced. Investigation of the orbital floor in some cases showed depressed fractures with herniation of orbital contents into the maxillary sinus. (See Chapter 25.) From these clinical studies, it is suggested that almost all fracture-dislocations of the zygoma should be treated by open reduction and direct wire fixation. This

has proved to be an effective program resulting in a high degree of satisfaction.

Methods of Reduction

INTRAORAL APPROACH. Keen (1909) described the intraoral approach for reduction of fractures of the zygoma. General anesthesia is preferable. With the cheek retracted by an assistant, the operator passes a sharp elevator up through the buccal vestibule behind the tuberosity of the maxilla. An incision may be made, but with a sharp, pointed, sturdy elevator the mucosa can be punctured and the instrument introduced on the posterior aspect of the zygoma beneath the zygomatic prominence (Fig. 24–147). Pressure applied in an upward, forward, and outward direction will elevate the zygoma, which snaps back into its position and remains in position without fixation. Infection following this method is unlikely. It is not necessary to suture the opening in the buccal mucosa. Because of the heavy masseter attachments, this method is not applicable to fractures of the zygomatic arch.

REDUCTION THROUGH THE MAXILLARY SINUS. Lothrop (1906) employed an antrostomy approach under the inferior turbinate and passed a curved trocar into the maxillary sinus, contacted the lateral superior wall, and rotated the depressed fractured zygoma in an upward and outward direction into position.

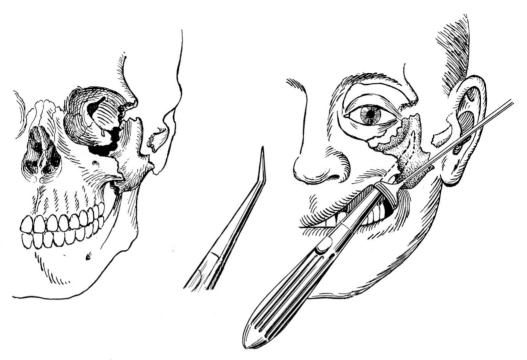

FIGURE 24–147. A method of reduction of fractures of the zygoma by means of a sharp elevator which penetrates the buccal mucosa and passes on the temporal side of the zygoma. The force applied is in an upward and forward direction. (After Kazanjian and Converse.)

TEMPORAL APPROACH. A temporal approach for reduction of zygomatic fractures was described by Gillies, Kilner, and Stone (1927). The temporal approach is useful and effective, especially for impacted fractures or those of several weeks' duration. Through this approach, strong leverage can be placed against the zygoma in the desired direction (Figs. 24–148 and 24–149).

The operation is accomplished through a

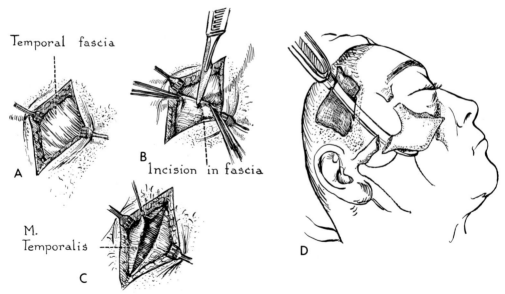

FIGURE 24–148. Temporal approach for reduction of a fractured zygoma. *A,* Incision through the scalp exposing the temporal fascia. *B,* The fascia is incised and a cleavage plane is found between the temporal fascia and the temporalis muscle *(C). D,* An elevator is inserted beneath the zygoma. (From Kazanjian and Converse.)

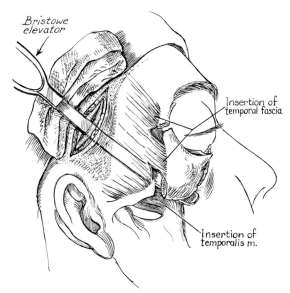

Bristowe elevator

Insertion of temporal fascia

Insertion of temporalis m.

FIGURE 24–149. The temporal fascia is inserted into the margin of the zygoma. In order to penetrate the temporal fossa, the elevator must be inserted deep to the temporal fascia. Forces are applied in an upward and forward direction. (From Kazanjian and Converse.)

vertical temporal incision about 2 cm long above and behind the hairline. The incision is extended through the skin and the subcutaneous and superficial temporal fascia. After the latter is incised, the glistening temporal fascia can be easily identified. A sturdy elevator is slipped down along the temporal fascia, underneath the temporal surface of the zygoma. A towel or sponge is placed over the scalp area, which provides a fulcrum against which considerable leverage may be applied to elevate the bone. Care must be taken to pass the instrument between the superficial and the deep layers of the temporal fascia; otherwise the elevator will pass lateral to the zygomatic arch instead of into the temporal fossa. Palpation of the bone with the other hand will guide the bone into position and guard against overcorrection. The wound is closed in layers with absorbable sutures in the fascia and nylon in the skin.

THE DINGMAN APPROACH.   Under general anesthesia, a solution containing epinephrine 1:100,000 is injected into the tissues of the lateral brow area and the infraorbital area. An incision is made in the lateral brow about 1.5 cm in length. Another incision is made in the lower lid. By means of a periosteal elevator, the zygomaticofrontal and the zygomaticomaxillary suture lines are exposed. Fracture separation will usually be found at these sites. A

moderately heavy periosteal elevator is passed through the upper incision behind and lateral to the orbital margin into the temporal fossa (Fig. 24–150, *A*). Excellent control of the zygoma is obtained through this approach, and by an upward, forward, and outward movement, depending upon the displacement of the fractured segments, the bone can be elevated into position. During elevation the zygoma is palpated through the skin and guided into position.

At this time, if indicated, the orbital floor can be explored (see Chapter 25 for details). Any herniation of orbital contents can be reduced and the defect in the orbital floor corrected.

Drill holes are placed through the bone on each side of the fracture site at the zygomaticofrontal and zygomaticomaxillary sutures (Fig. 24–150, *B*). Wires are passed through the holes and twisted to maintain the bony fragments in position.

The zygomatic arch can also be elevated through the supraorbital approach (Fig. 24–150, *C*). Usually the heavy fascial and muscular attachments to the arch will hold it in position, and direct wire fixation is not indicated.

Comminuted Fractures of the Zygoma.   Violent blows to the zygoma result in shattering of the bone into multiple fragments. The methods of management of this type of fracture include the intraoral approach through the anterior wall of the maxillary sinus with packing of the sinus, intraoral exposure with direct wire fixation, the suspension method, interosseous wiring, and packing of the temporal fossa.

PACKING THE MAXILLARY SINUS.   The maxillary sinus approach to comminuted fractures of the zygoma may be effective but is infrequently used by the authors for zygomatic fractures because of the small part of the zygoma contributing to the maxillary sinus. If the fracture is associated with maxillary fractures involving the orbital floor, maxillary sinus packing may be effective. Manipulation of the orbital floor through the maxillary sinus should be done in conjunction with exposure of the orbital floor to lessen the opportunity for bone fragments to damage the globe or nerves of the orbit. Packing is done through a Caldwell-Luc intraoral incision. The mucoperiosteum over the canine region of the maxilla is elevated, and if there is no fracture of the anterior wall of the maxilla, an opening is made with chisels, bone drills, or biting forceps. Through this opening it may be possible to

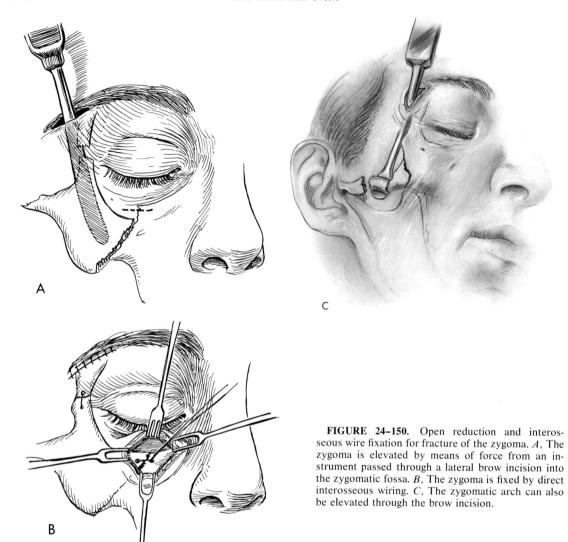

FIGURE 24–150. Open reduction and interosseous wire fixation for fracture of the zygoma. *A,* The zygoma is elevated by means of force from an instrument passed through a lateral brow incision into the zygomatic fossa. *B,* The zygoma is fixed by direct interosseous wiring. *C,* The zygomatic arch can also be elevated through the brow incision.

reduce the fragments of the zygoma by upward and outward pressure. Any fragments of the orbital floor that may have been herniated into the maxillary sinus are elevated into position and held by packing the sinus firmly with salvage-edge gauze permeated with petrolatum (Fig. 24–151). Blood clots and hematomas should be aspirated from the sinus, and the walls, floor, and roof of the sinus should be inspected and examined with a palpating finger to determine the presence of comminution in the orbital floor and possibly herniation of orbital contents into the maxillary sinus. A Penrose gauze-type rubber drain may be utilized to pack the sinus, or gauze impregnated with a suitable antibiotic and petrolatum may be used. An antrostomy opening is made beneath the inferior turbinate, and the end of the packing is brought into the nasal cavity. This provides adequate drainage to the sinus and a route through which the packing may be removed gradually after it has served its purpose. The oral wound is securely sutured. The packing is removed gradually in a week or ten days. Sinus infection is an unlikely complication with this method.

THE INTRAORAL APPROACH. Reduction of malposed zygomatic fractures can be accomplished by reflecting a large mucoperiosteal flap from the lateral wall of the maxilla to expose the zygomaticomaxillary junction. Impacted or partially healed fractures are dislodged by an elevator or an osteotome passed through the line of fracture (Fig. 24–152). Direct wire fixation may be used here. This approach may be useful in conjunction with another, the lateral brow approach, but alone it is not an effective method because of difficulty

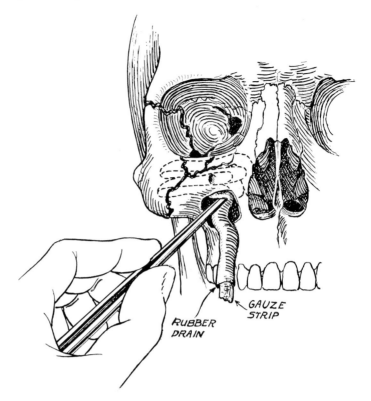

FIGURE 24–151. Packing of the maxillary sinus for support of multiple comminuted fragments of the oribital floor and lateral maxillary wall. The packing is introduced into a Penrose drain and brought out into the nasal cavity through an antrostomy window. (From Kazanjian and Converse.)

in visualizing the posterior extent of the fracture. It is possible to reduce a fracture in this manner, but additional fixation is necessary.

THE SUSPENSION METHOD. This method was suggested by Kazanjian (1933) and was employed in fractures which, after reduction, tended to relapse. Direct exposure of the infraorbital margin is obtained, and a small drill hole is made through the infraorbital margin in its zygomatic portion; the lower border of the zygoma may also be exposed through an intraoral approach and a drill hole is made, pass-

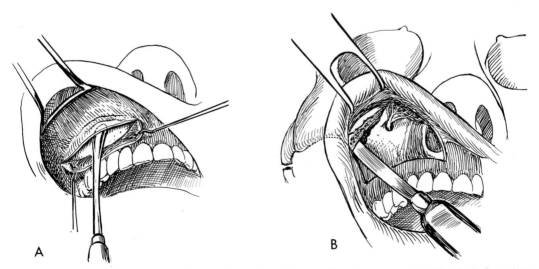

FIGURE 24–152. Intraoral approach to the anterior surface of the maxilla and zygoma. *A*, Incision in the buccal vestibule and elevation of the periosteum with an elevator. *B*, Verification of the site of fracture and reduction by means of an elevator. Direct interosseous wiring may be used for fixation.

ing the burr through the skin when the zygoma is rotated backward. A stainless steel wire is passed through the drill hole, and both ends are brought out through the wound and twisted

into a small loop. The wire is then attached by a rubber band to an ingenious appliance (Fig. 24–153) placed on the forehead and imbedded in dental compound with an outrigger, which

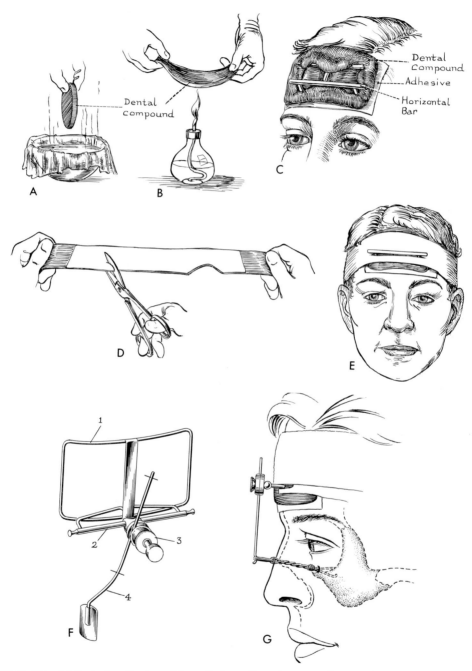

FIGURE 24–153.   Method of application of Kazanjian's appliance for external suspension. *A,* Dental compound is softened in hot water. *B,* The dental compound is passed over an open flame to make it more adherent. *C,* Frame of the splint is embedded into dental compound on the forehead, leaving a horizontal bar exposed. *D,* Method of preparing the adhesive tape to be placed around the head. *E,* Adhesive tape anchoring the frame of the splint on the forehead. Plaster bandage may also be used to hold the frame in position. *F,* Kazanjian's appliance consists of a metal frame (1), and a horizontal bar, (2), to which is attached a joint (3); the arm (4) is held by the joint and may be placed in the desired position by manipulating the joint. *G,* A hole has been drilled through the orbital rim, and a stainless steel wire is connected to the suspension appliance by an elastic band. (From Kazanjian and Converse.)

passes in front of the cheek area and is used to suspend the zygoma. Upward and outward traction is maintained for a period of two to three weeks, after which time the bone stays in position without support.

This is indicated (a halo frame appliance or plaster head cap may also be used) in cases that will not respond to other methods of management. In some patients, in spite of what seems to be adequate mobilization with no difficulty in reducing the fragment, the fragment has a tendency to relapse posteriorly and downward. In this type of case, suspension is most useful.

OPEN REDUCTION AND DIRECT WIRING. This technique is effective in obtaining accurate reduction and positive fixation and is effective in the simple as well as the complex comminuted type of fractures. Incisions 1.5 cm in length through the eyebrow and a subciliary eyelid incision will provide adequate exposure and access to the inferior and lateral orbital margins. The tissues can be shifted so that the entire inferior and lateral orbital margins can be inspected through these two incisions. The fragments are reduced, and small drill holes are placed, using motor-driven drills, through the bone wherever indicated. Fixation is provided with 28-gauge stainless steel wire. It is possible to reconstruct the entire orbital margin by wiring several small fragments of bone together (see Fig. 24–150).

Compound Comminuted Fractures of the Zygoma. Fractures of the zygoma may be compounded intraorally or extraorally when the force is severe enough to cause soft tissue wounds extending into the bone. Removal of foreign bodies, debris, and blood clots should be the first step in the treatment of the compound fracture. The fractured zygoma can be reconstituted by joining the comminuted fragments by interosseous wiring through the wound. Careful debridement and closure of the soft tissues over the comminuted fragmented bone usually results in satisfactory healing.

If medial displacement is a problem in zygomatic arch fractures, the segments may be supported after reduction by placing packing under the medial surface of the zygoma (Natvig, 1962). The fragments are elevated through the Gillies approach. If the fragments do not remain in position, a Penrose drain is packed into the infratemporal space beneath the zygoma to give it support. This is left in the wound for a week to ten days, at which time consolidation is completed.

OPEN REDUCTION AND DIRECT FIXATION. Open reduction and fixation with direct interosseous wiring may be done quickly, safely, and effectively. Open reduction with direct fixation is supplanting the older methods, which depended upon closed or blind operations and complicated gadgets for fixation (see Figs. 24–150 and 24–154).

PIN FIXATION. Brown, Fryer, and McDowell (1949) devised a technique utilizing one or more stainless steel pins (Kirschner wire or Steinmann pin) for fixation. Through the use of a hand-driven or electric drill, stainless steel pins are driven through the zygoma in a transverse direction and into the bones of the maxilla or zygoma on the contralateral side. The pins are cut off at skin level and are left in for a period of four weeks during consolidation of the fragments. This appears to be an effective method in the hands of experienced surgeons. Lange (1965) developed an instrument for holding the fractured segment of the zygoma in position during pin insertion and made other significant refinements in the technique. Complications in the form of osteomyelitis, malunion, nonunion, and facial deformity have been seen following use of this method by inexperienced operators.

Delayed Treatment of Fractures of the Zygoma. The best results are seen in cases treated relatively early. Fixation by organized fibrosis at the site of fracture occurs within two to three weeks, after which time it is difficult to mobilize and reposition the bone. This can be done, however, after several years (see Fig. 24–156). It requires exposure of the bone through the zygomaticofrontal area and through the oral route. The malunited bone may be mobilized by osteotomes through the old fracture lines and fibrous tissue. This can usually be done successfully if exposure is adequate. After mobilizing the bone, it is reduced and held with direct interosseous wiring.

The procedure must be done under direct vision: exposure of the floor of the orbit, of the zygomaticofrontal junction, and of the anterior surface of the maxilla is required through an intraoral approach. The Gillies technique provides strong leverage for reduction. Blind reduction carries the risk of radiating fracture lines extending into the apex of the orbit and loss of vision.

Complications of Fractures of the Zygoma

Early complications are relatively rare. Bleeding into the maxillary sinus is usually of short duration. It is unnecessary to remove the

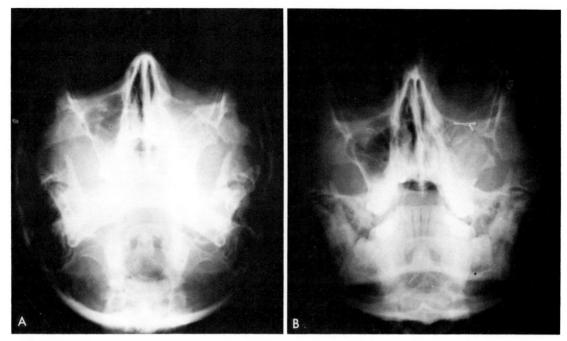

FIGURE 24–154. Fracture of the left zygoma. *A*, Preoperative. *B*, Postoperative. Fixation by interosseous wire method.

blood clots from the sinus. Clots disintegrate and drain spontaneously from the sinus without producing untoward results. Infection may be an immediate complication in compound fractures. This should be managed by adequate debridement of soft tissue and bone structure, establishment of drainage, and the administration of antibiotics. Acute exacerbation of a preexisting chronic sinus disease may be a complicating factor. Malfunction of ocular muscles as a result of damage from fractured fragments or injury of the cranial nerves has been seen. Kazanjian and Converse (1959) reported two cases of blindness following zygomatic fracture, in which segments of bone presumably were driven into the optic nerve.

Late Complications. The late complications of zygomatic fracture are nonunion, malunion, diplopia, persistent infraorbital nerve anesthesia, and chronic maxillary sinusitis. Gross downward dislocation of the zygoma may result in diplopia and require repositioning by open reduction (Figs. 24–155 and 24–156).

Orbital blowout fractures and the ocular complications resulting from such fractures, which occur concomitantly with fractures of the zygoma, are discussed in Chapters 25 and 28.

The late complications result mainly from malunion. In many cases correction can be obtained by osteotomy and replacement of the

zygoma with direct wire fixation. In those cases that cannot be managed by osteotomy, restoration of contour and elevation of the orbital floor can be accomplished by means of bone or cartilage grafts (see Chapters 25 and 28).

Impacted fracture of the zygomatic arch against the coronoid process may result in fibro-osseous ankylosis. If the zygoma cannot be adequately repositioned, resection of the coronoid process through the intraoral route will usually free the mandible and permit normal function.

Persistent anesthesia in the area of distribution of the infraorbital nerve after a period of six months should be an indication for exploration and decompression of the infraorbital canal. Bone splinters or constricting portions of the canal should be removed so that the nerve will have an adequate opportunity for regeneration. Permanent anesthesia is temporarily annoying, but the patient finally becomes accustomed to it.

FRACTURES OF THE NASAL BONES AND CARTILAGES

The external nose is a triangular pyramid composed of cartilaginous and osseous structures which support the skin, musculature, mucosa,

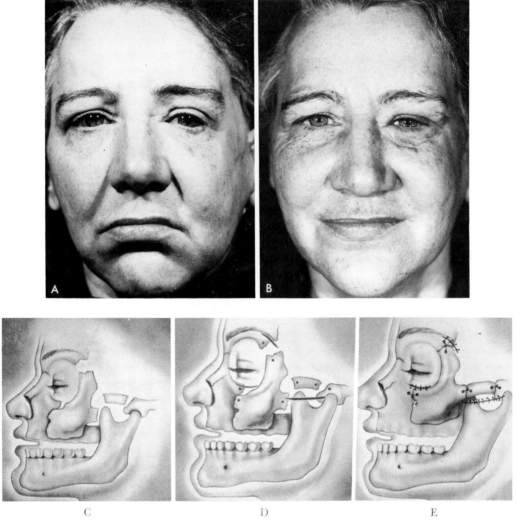

FIGURE 24–155. *A*, Patient with malunited fracture two years after fracture of the left zygoma. *B*, One month following osteotomy, open reduction and repositioning of the fragments and fixation with direct interosseous wiring technique. *C*, Drawing made from roentgenogram showing malunion and malposition of the fractured zygoma two years after injury. *D*, Incisions for approach to the fractured segments. *E*, Direct interosseous wire fixation of zygomatic segments by stainless steel wires passed through small drill holes on either side of the fracture sites.

nerves, and vascular structures. The upper third of the nose is supported by bony structures, while the lower portion gains its support from cartilaginous tissues. The skin in the upper part of the nose is freely movable, but in the lower portion it is thick, rich in sebaceous glands, and intimately attached to the cartilages. The excellent blood supply permits extensive dissection with safety and results in early rapid healing with minimal scar formation.

The supporting framework of the nose is made up of semirigid cartilaginous structures which are attached to the solid, inflexible bony structure of the nose (Fig. 24–157). The carti-laginous tissues include the lateral nasal cartilages, the alar cartilages, and the septal cartilage. There are several sesamoid cartilages in the lateral portions of the ala and in the base of the columella. The cartilaginous structures support the overlying subcutaneous tissue, skin, mucosa, and lining of the nose. The cartilages are intimately attached to the bony structures, which consist of the frontal process of the maxilla and the nasal spine of the frontal bone, the paired nasal bones and the bones of the septum, the vomer, and the perpendicular plate of the ethmoid (Fig. 24–158).

The paired nasal bones articulate in the

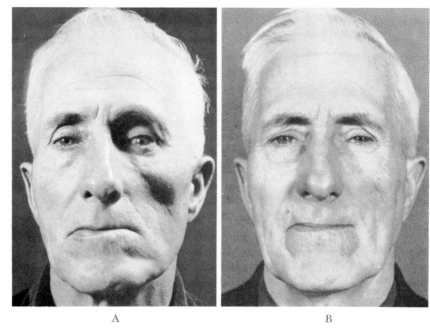

A   B

FIGURE 24–156. Zygomatic fracture associated with a blowout fracture of the orbital floor. *A,* A 67 year old man with an untreated fracture of the left zygoma and blowout deformity of the orbital floor six months after injury. *B,* One year postoperatively. Treatment consisted of osteotomy, open reduction, direct wire fixation of the fractured segments, and insertion of a preserved, irradiated, costal cartilage allograft to the floor of the orbit.

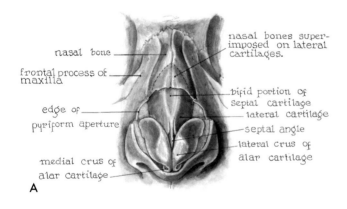

nasal bone

frontal process of maxilla

edge of pyriform aperture

medial crus of alar cartilage

nasal bones super-imposed on lateral cartilages.

bifid portion of septal cartilage

lateral cartilage

septal angle

lateral crus of alar cartilage

A

FIGURE 24–157. Anatomy of the nasal framework. *A,* Anterior view. *B,* Lateral view. (From Converse, J. M.: Cartilaginous structures of the nose. Ann. Otol. Rhinol. Laryngol., *64:*220, 1955.)

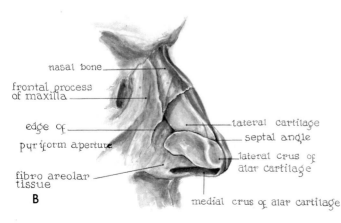

nasal bone

frontal process of maxilla

edge of pyriform aperture

fibro areolar tissue

B

lateral cartilage

septal angle

lateral crus of alar cartilage

medial crus of alar cartilage

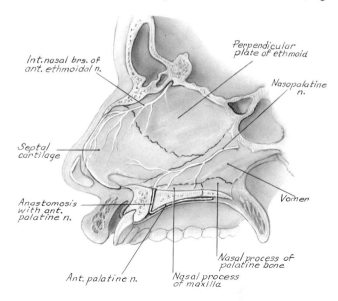

FIGURE 24-158. The bony and cartilaginous nasal septum and its innervation. (From Kazanjian and Converse.)

midline and are supported laterally by the frontal process of the maxilla and superiorly by the nasal spine of the frontal bone. The lower third of the nasal bones is thin and subject to fracture, but the bones are thicker in their upper portion and are supported by the nasal spine of the frontal bone. The nasal bones seldom fracture in the upper portions, where they are thick and firmly supported by their articulations, but frequently they fracture in the thinner lower half. For additional details of nasal anatomy, see Chapter 29.

Types and Locations of Fractures

Fractures in adults vary with the site of impact and the direction and the intensity of the force. Direct frontal blows over the nasal dorsum result in fracture of the thin lower half of the nasal bone or, if more severe, may result in separation of the nasofrontal suture. The margin of the pyriform aperture may also be fractured and dislocated into the nasal cavity, obstructing the airway (Fig. 24–159).

Lateral forces account for most nasal fractures and may produce a wide variation, depending upon the age of the patient and the intensity and direction of force. Younger patients tend toward fracture-dislocation of larger segments, whereas in older patients with dense, brittle bone, comminution may be observed more frequently.

The usual fracture occurs through the lower thinner portion of the nasal bone, the upper portion being thicker and more resistant to traumatic forces. Kazanjian and Converse (1959) reported that 80 per cent of nasal fractures occurred at the junction of the thick and thin portions of the nasal bones in a series of 190 nasal fractures. A direct force of moderate intensity from the lateral side may fracture only one nasal bone, with displacement into the nasal cavity. The frontal process of the maxilla may be associated with fracture of the nasal bones and be depressed on one side, or the entire bony structure of the nose may be fractured and dislocated to the side opposite the injuring force.

Violent frontal blows result in fracture of the nasal bones, the frontal processes of the maxilla, the lacrimal bones, and the septal cartilage, with all the components being driven into the ethmoid area. These displaced fractures are usually associated with damage to the nasolacrimal system, the perpendicular plate of the ethmoid, the ethmoid sinuses, the cribriform plate, and the orbital plate of the frontal bone. Displacement in severe comminuted fractures results in broadening and widening of the interorbital space and traumatic telecanthus (Fig. 24–160).

Fractured bone segments may be driven into the nasolacrimal system at various levels, resulting in dacryocystitis, interference with drainage of the tears, and permanent epiphora. The telescoping comminuted nasal fracture involving the nasal-ethmoidal-frontal area is commonly seen in the automobile crash injury,

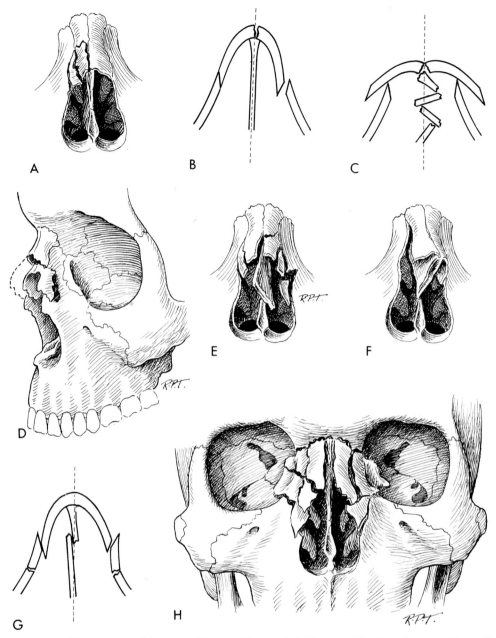

FIGURE 24–159. Various types of fractures of the nasal bones. *A, B,* Depressed fracture of one nasal bone. *C,* Open-book type of fracture seen in children. *D,* Fracture of the nasal bones at the junction of the thick upper and thin lower portions. *E,* Comminuted fracture. *F, G,* Fracture-dislocation. *H,* Comminuted fracture of the nasal bones involving the frontal processes of the maxilla. (From Kazanjian and Converse.)

in which the middle third of the face strikes against the instrument panel or other projecting objects inside the automobile.

Fractures and dislocations of the septal cartilage may occur independently or in association with fractures of the nasal bony framework. Because of their intimate association, it is unusual to observe fractures of the bony structures without damage to the cartilaginous structures. The caudal portion of the septum has a certain degree of flexibility and will bend to absorb moderate blows. More severe direct blows may result in fracture with dislocation of the septum from the vomer groove, with displacement into the adjacent airway. The cartilage may be fractured in any direction, the

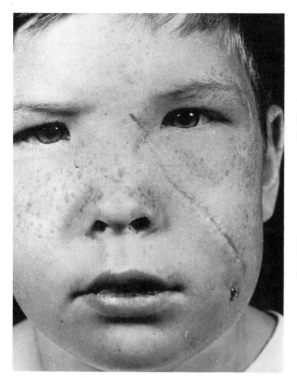

FIGURE 24–160. Traumatic telecanthus and widening of the interorbital space due to fracture of the nasal bones and frontal processes of the maxilla (see Chapter 25).

most frequent being in a vertical plane, but it also may be torn or fractured in a horizontal plane parallel to the crest of the vomer.

Fractures of the septum may be associated with a telescoping type of displacement. In the vertical fracture, the anterior portion of the septal cartilage may be driven backward to telescope over the posterior segment, which remains in its normal position owing to firm attachments to the vomer and to the perpendicular plate of the ethmoid. The cartilage may be fractured posteriorly and may be driven back under the mucoperiosteum of the perpendicular plate. This results in shortening of the nose, retraction of the columella, and deepened nasolabial folds. Septal fractures may be overlooked in children only to become evident with adolescent development.

Septal fractures result in angulation of the anterior portion of the septum with dislocation into one of the nostrils, deflection of the nasal tip, and separation of the alar cartilages with a flat and broad-tipped nose (Fig. 24–161).

Diagnosis of Fractures of the Bones and Cartilages of the Nose

Diagnosis is made on the basis of the history of injury, which may provide information concerning the direction and intensity of the force. Diagnosis may be difficult because of edema and hematoma, which occur within a few hours after the injury. Edema, periorbital ecchymosis, and subconjunctival hemorrhage are usual findings. Obstruction due to displacement of nasal structures, edema, blood clots,

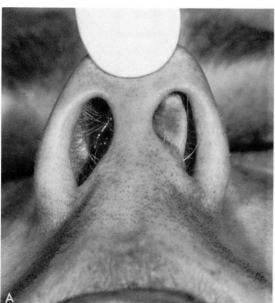
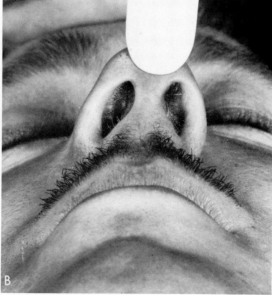

FIGURE 24–161. *A,* Nasal deformity due to lateral dislocation of the caudal portion of the nasal septum. The caudal edge of the septum shows in the left nasal airway. This deformity followed a fracture in early adult life. *B,* Result following septal reconstruction and repositioning of the cartilaginous segment of the nasal septum and tip.

or swelling of the mucosa and turbinates is present. Subcutaneous emphysema from blowing the nose and forcing air through the lacerated mucoperiosteum is seen occasionally. Increased mobility and crepitation on palpation along with tenderness are usually prominent signs except in the infected or displaced telescoped type of fracture. Fractures of the intranasal structures and lacerations of the mucosa are difficult to see in the presence of edema and dislocation of tissues. To evaluate the intranasal damage accurately, the mucosa should be shrunk if possible with vasoconstricting drugs, blood clots should be removed, and the hematoma of the septum should be evacuated or aspirated.

Roentgenograms are helpful in the diagnosis of nasal fracture but may frequently be negative in the usual views. Gillies and Millard (1957) recommended increasing the backward tilt of the occipitomental view from 15° to 30° to 45° to illustrate fractures not apparent in the usual occipitomental projection. Soft tissue techniques on profile views demonstrate fractures of the thin anterior edge of the nasal bones (Fig. 24–162). (See section on Roentgenographic Positions, p. 611.)

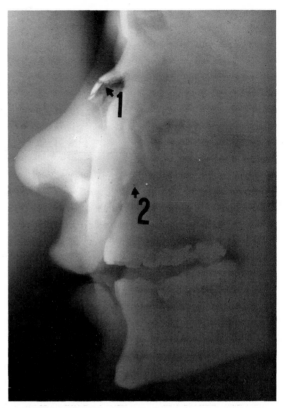

FIGURE 24–162. Lateral low density, soft tissue roentgenograms are best to demonstrate the small bones of the nasal dorsum.

Treatment of Nasal Fractures

When seen early before edema of the soft tissues becomes a complicating factor, fractures of the nasal bones are easily reduced. Most simple fractures can be managed on an outpatient basis in the emergency room by closed reduction methods. The more extensive comminuted compound fractures require special management.

If, when first seen, the patient has severe edema with no open wounds, treatment should be deferred until the edema subsides and a more accurate evaluation can be made. This requires postponing treatment for five to seven days.

Anesthesia. Nasal fractures in children are best managed under general anesthesia. Even if a short procedure is anticipated, it is best to anesthetize the patient completely. Endotracheal intubation is the technique of choice. This gives the operator an opportunity to assess the damage accurately and to obtain adequate reduction and fixation.

In both children and adults, the operation can be facilitated by packing the nose with cotton pledgets, soaked in vasoconstricting drugs for 10 to 15 minutes. The packs should be wrung out carefully before insertion. This will reduce the edema and result in less bleeding from manipulation. Ten per cent cocaine solution with an equal amount of epinephrine 1:1000, or 1 per cent xylocaine with epinephrine (1:100,000) will provide anesthesia and vasoconstriction. Cocaine packs should be avoided over raw areas to avoid excessive absorption of the drug. If severe edema is present, it may be necessary to spray the nose two or three times over a period of 15 to 20 minutes before the passages can be opened satisfactorily to permit intranasal inspection.

Most nasal fractures in adults can be successfully reduced with the aid of intranasal topical and infiltrative anesthesia. Adequate preoperative medication and intraoperative intravenous injection of tranquilizing drugs such as diazepam (Valium) facilitate the procedure.

Instrumentation for Reduction of Simple Nasal Fractures

A headlight is necessary for good intranasal illumination. Intranasal specula of various sizes and lengths are essential for adequate intranasal examination, reduction of fractures, and placement of packs. Almost all nasal fractures can be reduced by upward and outward forces, with an instrument placed in the nose under the nasal bones. A small nasal elevator upon which a rubber tubing is stretched or around which cotton has been twisted makes an excellent instrument for this purpose. The cotton should be covered with a layer of petrolatum.

Forceps designed for intranasal use, such as the Asche (Fig. 24–163) and the Walsham types, are useful, as force can be applied through both nasal cavities at one time.

Care must be exerted to place the instrument under the fracture site in a position not too high in the nose, lest it impinge under the nasal portion of the frontal bone and cause damage to the mucosa without being effective in reducing the fracture (Figs. 24–164 and 24–

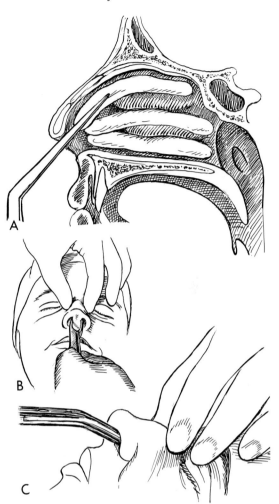

FIGURE 24–164. *A*, Method of placing cocaine-soaked cotton packs in the nose to obtain anesthesia for reduction of nasal fractures. *B*, *C*, Use of the Asche forceps to elevate the nasal bones and straighten the septum.

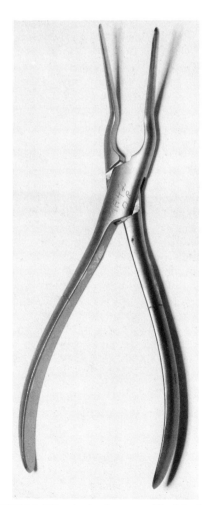

FIGURE 24–163. Asche forceps, utilized in the reduction and fixation of nasal fractures.

165). As the nasal structures are manipulated upward and forward with the instrument in one hand, the other hand is used to apply external digital pressure to mold the bones into position. The dislocated nasal septum will often be replaced in position by elevation of the nasal bones.

Intranasal fractures should be carefully examined after elevating the bones, and, if they are not in position, the Asche forceps should be used to straighten the septum.

Many fractures can be reduced and will remain in position without the need for nasal packing or nasal splints. If the bones are comminuted and loose, it is preferable to support the fractured nasal bones and septum by means of intranasal gauze packing impregnated with petrolatum. Gauze impregnated with a

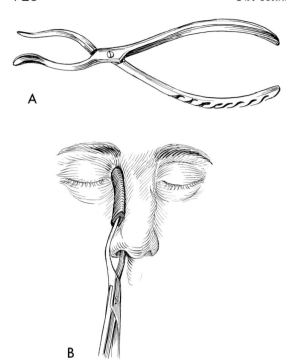

FIGURE 24–165. *A*, The Walsham forceps. *B*, Reduction of fractured bone. Note rubber tubing over blade of forceps.

waxy lubricant provides an excellent material for packing the nose or maxillary sinus. It will not adhere to the mucosa and can be removed without bleeding.

After the nasal bony and cartilaginous structures have beeen reduced and manipulated into position, they are usually held by the intranasal packing and an external splint. The use of small Silastic tubing as an airway in each nasal floor adds considerably to the comfort of the patient. The tubes do not provide a satisfactory airway but permit equalization of pressure in the nasopharynx during the act of swallowing and prevent the usual discomfort of negative pressures in the middle ear. The tubes are placed carefully in the floor of the nose on each side, and packs made up of several folds of gauze impregnated with petrolatum or strips of petrolatum-soaked gauze are carefully packed into the nasal cavity to give support to the fractured bone and cartilaginous structures.

The external nasal splint can be fabricated with Asche metal and dental compound (Fig. 24–166). A splint can also be fashioned from commercially prepared gauze impregnated with plaster, which is folded into a square four to six layers in thickness, soaked in water, and then cut to the desired shape (Fig. 24–167).

The plaster splint can be applied directly to the skin, where it will fit securely and cause no reaction. The plaster splint is held to the skin of the face with porous paper adhesive tape.

The rubber tubing is cleaned once or twice each day with a suction pipette. Intranasal packing and an external nasal splint are kept in place from five to seven days.

Treatment of Fractures and Dislocation of the Septal Framework

The septum should be straightened and repositioned soon after injury. The elevator used for the reduction of the nasal bones raises the nasal bones and also the lateral cartilages, which have an intimate anatomical relationship with the nasal bones as they extend under, and are adherent to, the undersurface of the nasal bones. Because the lateral cartilages also have an anatomical continuity with the septal cartilage, raising the lateral cartilage with an elevator may successfully reduce a horizontal fracture or replace the cartilage into the vomer groove from which it may have been luxated. Correction of the position of the septum is completed with Asche forceps. The realigned septal fragments are maintained by intranasal packing or Silastic or acrylic splints held by mattress sutures through the septum. The mucoperichondrium heals rapidly.

If correction is delayed, it may not be possible to obtain the desired result. When there is considerable displacement and overlapping of septal fragments, exposure of the septal framework by subperichondrial elevation, as for a submucous resection, may be the best approach. Such cases may require an immediate submucous resection of the nasal septum, but it is usually possible to realign the septal cartilage fragments and maintain their position by means of intranasal packing. These measures are indispensable if the surgeon is to be successful in reestablishing adequate nasal airways and realigning the external bony structures (see also Chapter 29).

Hematoma of the Septum. A hematoma develops between the septal mucoperichondrium and the cartilage in fracture or dislocation of the septum or simply as a result of excessive bending of the septal cartilage (Fig. 24–168, *A* to *D*). Hematoma of the septum is often bilateral, for fracture of the septum permits passage

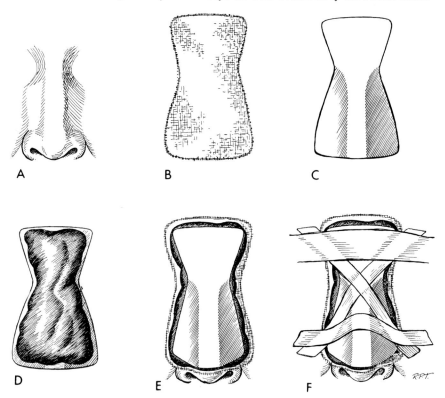

FIGURE 24–166. The nasal splint. *A,* The nose. *B,* A piece of fine mesh gauze is applied over the nose to protect the skin. *C,* A piece of soft metal, 22-gauge, is cut and shaped. *D,* Softened dental compound is spread over the metal splint. *E,* The splint is applied to the nose. *F,* The splint is retained with adhesive tape. (See also Chapter 29 for details on splinting the nose.) (From Kazanjian and Converse.)

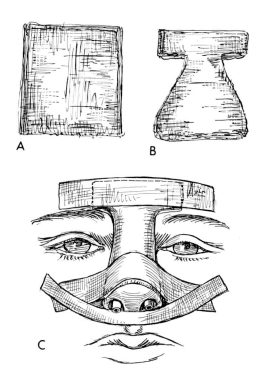

FIGURE 24–167. Method of making and applying a plaster splint. *A,* Four to six layers of plaster-impregnated gauze are folded. *B,* The splint is cut and dipped in warm water. *C,* It is applied to the nose and forehead area directly over the skin. Fixation after the plaster sets is accomplished by adhesive tape.

of the blood from one side to the other (Fig. 24–168, *E* to *G*).

Fibrosis may follow an untreated septal hematoma. Fibrosis of a long-standing hematoma results in permanent thickening of the septum, which blocks the nasal airway. This condition is similar to subperichondrial thickening of the auricle, commonly referred to as cauliflower ear, which is observed in pugilists. Necrosis of the cartilage can also be caused by a voluminous hematoma, even in the absence of infection. The authors have observed massive absorption of septal cartilage in patients who had been maintained under antibiotic therapy for two weeks; the hematoma had not been evacuated. After surgical intervention to evacuate the hematoma, fracture of the septal cartilage was discovered; in the absence of sepsis, the septal cartilage was partly absorbed and very soft. Infection of the hematoma and septal abscess usually results in complete necrosis of septal cartilage and collapse of the cartilaginous dorsum. In addition to surgical therapy, antibiotic therapy should be routine.

Septal hematoma is treated by incising the mucoperichondrium, and suction is employed to evacuate the blood clots and serum. A horizontal incision is made through the mucoperiosteum at the base of the septum to prevent refilling of the cavity with blood or serum, thus establishing a drainage incision in a dependent position. In bilateral hematoma, it is preferable to resect a portion of the septal cartilage to allow the two areas of hematoma to communicate. In comminuted septal fractures with hematoma, septal cartilage resection is also the best treatment. This approach affords a wide exposure between the mucoperichondrial flaps and permits removal of obstructing septal fragments and blood clots between the flaps. The horizontal incision through the mucoperichondrial flap along the floor of the nose insures drainage and prevents accumulation of blood between the flaps. Nasal packing is not necessary except to arrest epistaxis.

Comminuted Fractures. If seen within a few days after the injury, comminuted fractures can usually be reduced without difficulty.

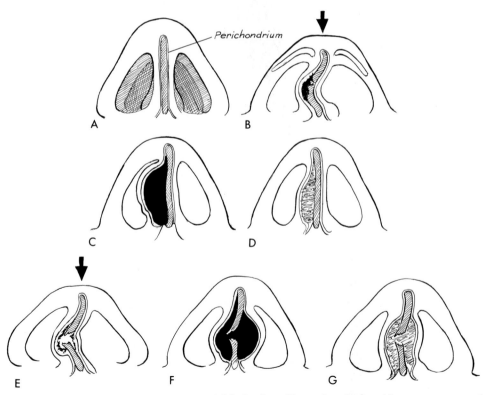

FIGURE 24–168. Hematoma of the septum. *A, B, C,* Mechanism of formation of a septal hematoma as a result of excessive bending of the septal cartilage without fracture. *D,* Thickening of the septum resulting from fibrosis when the hematoma is not evacuated. *E, F, G,* Fracture of the septal cartilage with formation of a bilateral hematoma and thickening of the septum from fibrosis. (From Kazanjian and Converse.)

Internasal packing and a nasal splint may not be sufficient to provide adequate fixation. If there is comminution and telescoping of the fragments, there is a tendency for the fractures to sink backward, and the patient may have a sunken or flat nasal dorsum following healing.

THROUGH-AND-THROUGH WIRING OVER ACRYLIC, SILASTIC, OR METAL PLATES. Support may be obtained by using plates on the side of the nose. Soft lead, Silastic, or acrylic plates 2 or 3 mm in thickness are satisfactory. These are held in position (Figs. 24–169 and 24–170) by passing a 25-gauge steel wire on a Keith needle through the plates and between the fractured segments. The wire is twisted over the plates to give support to the lateral aspect of the nose. The plates can be in contact with the skin without causing damage if the edges are everted so that no sharp edges contact the skin. The plates are effective only for treatment of fractures of the external nasal bone structures. More severe naso-orbital fractures require open reduction (see Chapter 25).

Compound Nasal Fractures. The bone and the cartilaginous structures of the nose may be observed through external wounds in compound fractures with open wounds. The bone fragments can be reduced and fixed through the external wound. The lining, muscle, and subcutaneous layers are approximated with fine absorbable sutures before closure of the skin. Careful attention to closure of soft tissue wounds will alleviate unsightly scars and prevent intranasal constricting scars and stenosis of the airway.

Delayed Treatment of Nasal Fractures. Purposeful delay in the treatment of nasal fractures is indicated in the presence of other injuries which contraindicate early management of the facial fractures. If this occurs and the patient is not seen until a week or ten days following the injury, the usual methods of manipulation and reduction of the nasal fractures may not be satisfactory. Open operations are required, but it is preferable to wait until the edema has subsided in order that the deformity can be fully evaluated. Septal hematoma or abscess should be treated and treatment delayed until reduction and fixation can be done conveniently and safely. Intentional delay is advisable to reduce the possibility of operative complications.

Complications of Nasal Fractures. Early complications are rare and consist of edema and ecchymosis of the skin and eyelids, epistaxis, hematoma of the nasal septum, and infection. The edema is temporary and disappears within a few days. Bleeding from the nose, usually of short duration, ceases spontaneously or may be controlled by intranasal packing. A large hematoma under the soft tissues of the nasal septum is controlled by evacuation or incision and drainage. Infection is best treated by adequate drainage, the use of hot packs, and the use of antibiotic therapy.

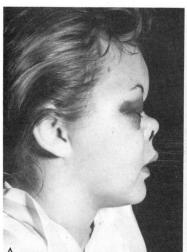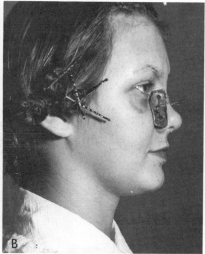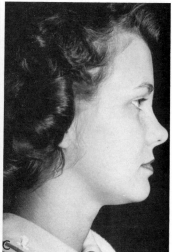

FIGURE 24–169. Wired plate method of fixation of comminuted nasal bone fractures. *A*, Backward and upward telescoping of the nasal bones into the ethmoid region due to a blow at the nasal tip. *B*, Reduction of fragments and fixation by means of wired plate method. *C*, Results after consolidation of the fractured segments and healing of the soft tissues. (From Kazanjian and Converse.)

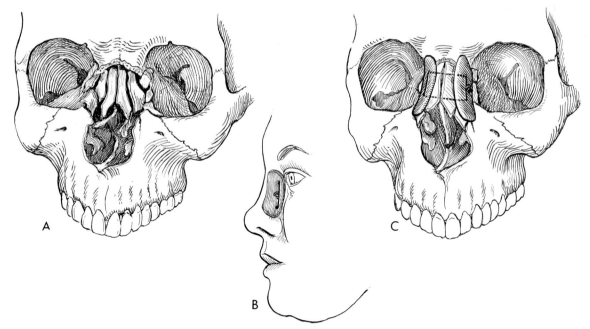

FIGURE 24–170. *A*, Wired plate method in comminuted nasal fractures (see Fig. 24–169). Diagrammatic illustration of a comminuted fracture of the nasal bone telescoping backward into the ethmoid area. *B*, Method of providing fixation of the comminuted fragments by the wired plate method. *C*, Frontal view of wired lead plates for support of the comminuted nasal bones. (From Kazanjian and Converse.)

Emphysema of the face and neck may occur from violent blowing in an attempt to dislodge blood clots from the lacerated nose but resolves spontaneously.

LATE COMPLICATIONS. An untreated hematoma of the nasal septum may become organized, resulting in subperichondrial fibrosis with thickening of the nasal septum and partial nasal obstruction. The septum may be as large as 1 cm in thickness, and in cases of repeated trauma the cartilaginous septum may be largely replaced with calcified material. Submucous resection of the thickened or deviated nasal septum may be required to produce a satisfactory airway (see Chapter 29).

Synechiae may form between the septum and the turbinates in areas where injured tissues are in contact. These are treated by cutting and placing an intervening nonadherent material between the cut surfaces for a period of five days. During this time, epithelization occurs.

Obstruction of the nasal vestibule may occur as a result of malunited fractures of the pyriform margin or scar tissue contracture from loss of vestibular lining. Osteotomy of the bone will correct the former; the scar tissue contractures may be corrected by Z-plasty procedures or by excision of scar and replacement with skin grafts in the nasal vestibule.

Osteitis is occasionally seen in compound fractures of the nose or in fractures associated with infected hematomas. The entire nasal bony framework may be lost as a result of infection. Appropriate antibiotic therapy, incision for drainage, and removal of sequestra from the wound constitute the regimen of treatment.

Nonunion is rare, but malunion of the nasal bone structures is a frequent complication resulting in external deformities which require secondary reconstructive operative procedures. These operative procedures are described in Chapter 29.

Naso-orbital fractures resulting from a strong impact over the nasal bony bridge, projection of the bony structures into the orbital space or the orbital cavities, and fractures of the frontoethmoidal region are discussed in Chapter 25.

MULTIPLE AND COMPLEX FRACTURES OF THE FACIAL SKELETON: PANFACIAL FRACTURES

In a treatise encompassing the entire field of reconstructive plastic surgery, space does not allow for a complete coverage of all aspects of the diagnosis and early treatment of facial injuries. A number of books entirely devoted to the subject have been published (Dingman and Natvig, 1964; Rowe and Killey, 1968; Schultz, 1970; Kazanjian and Converse, 1974).

In this chapter, the early treatment of fractures of individual bones of the face has been discussed singly for the sake of simplicity. Under the term "complex fractures," the authors designate multiple fractures of the facial bones. In some cases there are fractures of all facial bones (panfacial fractures), and these are often associated with multiple injuries in other areas of the body (Fig. 24–171).

Incidence

This type of injury is becoming more common with the advent of high-speed transportation; the magnitude of the traumatic force sustained and the greater number of survivors of such accidents are a result of improved methods of resuscitation and treatment of multiple systems injuries. The front seat "guest passenger" type of injury, which was described by Straith in 1948 and is characterized by extensive fractures of the middle third of the face, occurs as a result of the guest passenger being thrown against the windshield or instrument panel of

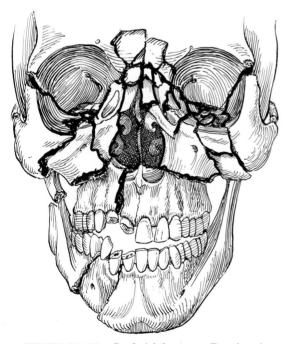

FIGURE 24–171. Panfacial fractures. Drawing shows multiple fractures involving all of the facial bones.

the automobile and is now commonplace. According to Georgiade (1969), 20 per cent of individuals who have sustained injuries to the facial skeleton have multiple facial bone fractures. McCoy and his associates (1962) reported a study of 855 patients with fractures of the facial skeleton. Forty per cent of these patients had fractures of the midfacial skeleton; the mandible alone was fractured in 38 per cent, and the nasal bones alone in 22 per cent. Of the 337 patients with middle-third facial fractures, 41 per cent had associated fractures of the mandible and 28 per cent associated nasal fractures. These figures may have to be revised in view of the considerable diminution in the number of injuries sustained in automobile accidents as a result of the 55 mile speed limit initiated in the United States in 1974.

Facial Fractures and Multisystem Injuries

Complex facial bone fractures are usually the result of a high-speed accident, such as the violent encounter of two cars traveling in opposite directions. In this type of accident, the maxillofacial component is only one manifestation of severe generalized trauma to which the victim is subjected. Craniocerebral injuries and associated orthopedic or thoracoabdominal injuries are frequently present and complicate the clinical management of the patient.

Because of the magnitude of the facial injuries, the plastic surgeon may be the first to be called and thus must assume the responsibility of immediate resuscitation of the patient and overseeing the overall treatment of the multiple systems injuries.

The treatment of complex fractures is best undertaken in a specialized center where plastic surgical and multidisciplinary specialists are present. The patient with multiple systems injuries must be given rapid resuscitation and treated for shock, ensuring that the patient is physiologically stabilized. The repair of multiple system injuries should be undertaken in the proper sequence, namely that the thoracic or abdominal injury be cared for as a first priority; brain injury in a comatose patient with multiple facial fractures requires that the trachea be intubated and that the necessary neurosurgical procedures be completed; fractures and soft tissue injuries of the extremities and hands are next in priority.

Treatment of multiple facial fractures must take second place until the above injuries are treated. The airway must be ensured by the insertion of an endotracheal tube or by tracheotomy. A tracheotomy is imperative in severe panfacial fractures with multiple fractures of the mandible. Routine use of gastric aspiration and lavage eliminates the dangers associated with emesis of recent meal contents and swallowed blood.

Facial injuries are not surgical emergencies. The only surgical emergency aside from the physiologic stabilization of the patient is the maintenance of the airway.

Clinical Examination. Except when the patient is seen within the first six hours after the accident, edema masks the magnitude of damage and skeletal displacement resulting from multiple facial bone fractures.

The patient's face is flattened, and the edema obliterates the bony contour of the facial skeleton. Traumatic telecanthus is often the outstanding deformity. These patients show distortion of facial form which is caused not only by the edema, which forms rapidly, or by hematoma but also by a flattening of the contour of the face. The eyes are closed by edema, and in naso-orbital fractures the telecanthus is evident. An elongation of the face may also be observed. Mobility of the tooth-bearing bones or other bones of the face may also be noted by palpation.

The classic lines of fracture observed by Le Fort (1901), which were described in the days of the horse-drawn carriage, have been complicated by fracture-dislocation and comminution of the maxilla and naso-orbital, zygomatico-orbital, and frontal skeletal structures as a result of increasing accelerating forces associated with automobile travel.

In many cases of "crash" and "crush" injuries, the soft tissue injuries may be minimal, and the magnitude of the facial bone fractures may not be recognized in the early stages, as it is masked by hematoma and edema, which often attains enormous proportions. An orbital fracture may not be diagnosed because of the extent of the edema, the eyelids being shut tight, and the patient cannot complain of diplopia. Examination of the eyes is possible by retracting the edematous eyelids and evaluating the intraocular damage, extraocular muscle derangement, and oculorotary disturbances. These findings are indicative of a blowout fracture or a massive disruption of the orbital framework.

Multiple fractures of the mandible, particularly when associated with multiple fractures of the midfacial bones, result in obstruction of the oropharyngolaryngeal airway. Some idea of the number of and extent of displacement of the fractures may be obtained by observing the disruption in the occlusal relationships of the teeth.

Complex facial fractures may also be compound, resulting from lacerations by an incisive object, such as the windshield of an automobile; bursting of the soft tissue may also be produced by a blunt force (Fig. 24–172).

Radiologic Examination. Radiologic investigation has been discussed earlier in the text. It is obvious that additional information will be gained by careful tomographic diagnosis done in both frontal and sagittal planes. Thus a picture may be assembled of the location and number of fractures and of the extent of osseous displacement.

Treatment

GENERAL CONSIDERATIONS. There are certain considerations in managing panfacial fractures. The first is the timing of the operative interventions. The optimal time for treatment is within six hours after the accident, before the development of the massive edema which follows these injuries. Such early treatment is possible only when other systems are not involved and the facial fractures are not too severe.

In patients with multiple fractures of the midfacial area and in patients with panfacial fractures which also involve the mandible, clinical evaluation of the extent and number of fractures is essential if the structural architecture of the facial skeleton is to be reestablished.

There is an argument, therefore, for waiting until the edema has subsided and until a thorough roentgenologic examination can be completed. This should include tomograms, which will show the extent of the fractures and the fracture-dislocations, and should be completed by a panoramic radiographic film of the mandible.

THE DIRECT APPROACH. At the present time, one-stage restoration of the architecture of the face is the preferred method of treatment of severely comminuted multiple facial bone fractures.

Open reduction and interosseous wiring of severe multiple fractures of the facial bones is the keystone to success. This may be combined with cranial fixation by internal wiring and orbital floor replacement (usually different modalities of treatment in various combina-

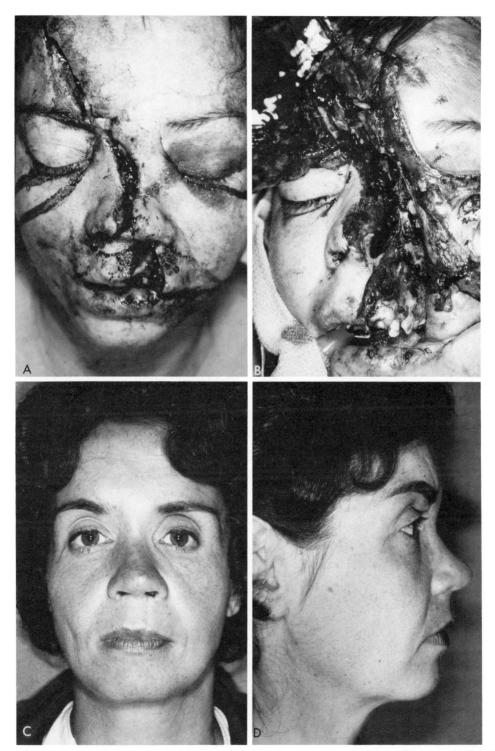

FIGURE 24–172.   Compound complex facial fracture resulting from an auto accident. In addition to the facial lacerations, there were fractures of the frontal bone, nasal bones, zygoma, frontal and ethmoid sinuses, medial wall and floor of the left orbit, and left maxillary sinus. *A*, Appearance in the emergency room. Note traumatic telecanthus. *B*, Appearance during exploration of the wound. *C, D,* Following open reduction and external wire fixation of the fractures and insertion of cartilage graft on the left orbital floor. The frontal lobe was debrided and dural tears were approximated.

tions). Adams (1942) originated the concept of treatment of facial fractures by internal suspension wires, and considerable emphasis has been placed on internal suspension wiring, which is adequate for fractures of moderate severity.

In "crush" and "crash" multiple fractures, in addition to permitting internal wiring, the direct approach through selective cutaneous and intraoral incisions offers other advantages (Fig. 24–173). The direct approach and interosseous wiring of the fragments after realignment have proved to be the best techniques for preventing the development of traumatic telecanthus, for verifying the integrity of the lacrimal apparatus, for treating orbital fractures, and, generally, for restoring the architecture of the facial skeleton (see Chapter 25, Figs. 25–46 to 25–48; Fig. 24–174).

When a considerable number of teeth and portions of the dentoalveolar process have been lost, early prosthetic restoration should be provided to support the lips and cheeks, particularly if these structures have been subjected to full thickness lacerations. This approach requires the application of a certain number of principles heretofore not entirely recognized.

ORDER OF PROCEDURE

1. The mandibular fragments are realigned and fixation is obtained by arch wire appliances (Fig. 24–175, *A, B*). Interosseous wiring should also be employed for difficult and unfavorable fractures or for stabilization of edentulous fragments of the mandibular arch. The intraoral degloving approach (see Chapter 30, Fig. 30–30) is employed.

2. The realigned mandibular arch serves as a guide for the assembly and realignment of the maxillary fragments.

3. The maxillary fragments are often best reassembled and maintained in fixation by direct interosseous fixation (Fig. 24–175, *B*), as the traumatic force which has comminuted the maxilla is often strong enough to avulse or damage the teeth, which are no longer available for fixation. When the teeth are present, fixation of the dentoalveolar fragments by an arch and wire appliance is possible.

4. Once the maxillary fragments have been realigned and intermaxillary fixation has been established, internal wires are placed and will eventually be tightened to suspend the maxillary arch (or the mandibular arch) to the frontal bone (Fig. 24–175, *B, C*) or will be looped around the zygomatic arch if it is intact. In edentulous patients, intermaxillary fixation is established by means of the patient's dentures, which are lined with dental compound and maintained by circumferential wires. The tightening of the wires for cranial fixation by internal wires is postponed until the bones of the midface have been realigned and maintained in fixation. The wires should extend obliquely backward and upward. In this manner the condyles are maintained in the glenoid fossae; the lateral pterygoid muscle propulsive movements are thus neutralized, and adequate forward projection of the maxilla is maintained.

The tooth-bearing segments of the maxilla having been realigned and intermaxillary fixation established, attention is directed to the midfacial fractures.

5. Cutaneous incisions placed in the lateral portion of the eyebrow, in the lower eyelid, and along the lateral wall of the bony nose provide exposure of the frontozygomatic junction, the infraorbital rim and orbital floor, the major portion of the anterior surface of the zygoma, the lateral wall of the orbit, the nasal bones, and the medial wall of the orbit (Fig. 24–175, *D*). Orbital fractures are treated by

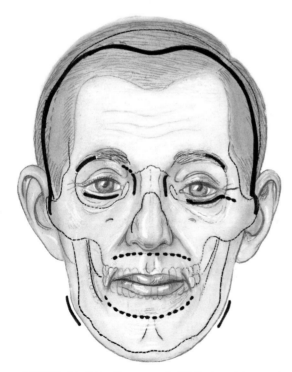

FIGURE 24–173. Cutaneous (solid line) and intraoral (dotted line) incisions available for open reduction and interosseous wiring of facial fractures. The conjunctival approach also gives access to the orbital floor and anterior aspect of the maxilla.

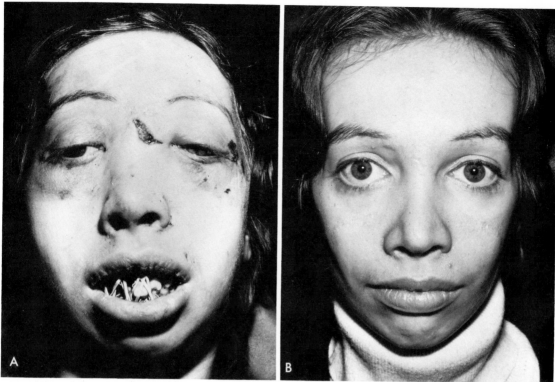

FIGURE 24–174.   Multiple midface fractures treated by one-stage direct approach. *A*, Appearance of patient on admission to the hospital. Note the traumatic telecanthus. *B*, One year after single procedure by the direct approach. The telecanthus was reduced from 45 mm to 30 mm. (From Merville, L. C.: Multiple dislocations of the facial skeleton. J. Maxillofac. Surg., *2*:187, 1974.

restoration of the continuity of the rim and floor of the orbit (see Chapter 25).

A wide exposure of the midfacial area can be obtained by raising a coronal flap, as advocated by Tessier and his associates (1967) in craniofacial operations. This exposure, supplemented by lower eyelid incisions for exposure of the orbital floor, is indicated in the most severe fractures.

In panfacial fractures associated with extensive soft tissue wounds, after the appropriate debridement and removal of glass and other foreign debris (steering wheel fragments, ingrained road grit and dirt), the wounds serve as a direct approach to the fracture sites, thereby obviating the necessity for separate incisions (see Fig. 24–173).

Interosseous fixation of multiple fractures should be initiated by establishing cranial fixation of the zygoma at the frontozygomatic junction by interosseous wiring (Fig. 24–175, *D*). This procedure restores the lateral wall of the orbit. Other zygomatic fragments are wired to the larger zygomatic fragment, and the inferior orbital rim is restored by realigning the fragments and wiring them to each other. The individual fragments are held with forceps, a small hole is drilled in each of the fragments, and they are aligned and joined by the stainless steel interosseous wire which is twisted upon itself and cut. The remaining end of the twisted wire is buried in the hole through one of the fragments (Fig. 24–176). Attention should then be directed to an orbital fracture if it is present. The next step is the reduction of a nasal bone or naso-orbital fracture (see Fig. 24–175, *E*). Transosseous wires reattach the medial canthal tendons to the medial orbital walls, and acrylic plates reapply the skin of the naso-orbital valley against the restored bony framework.

The facial structures are now realigned, and the facial architecture is reestablished; the last procedure is the tightening of the internal wires to maintain cranial fixation.

The basic principle, therefore, is to provide interosseous fixation to a stable bone in the midfacial area: the zygoma if it is not fractured, the frontal bone if both zygomas are fractured. The application of this principle leads to an order of procedure: *provide fixation of the larger bone fragments; these provide points of fixation for the smaller fragments.*

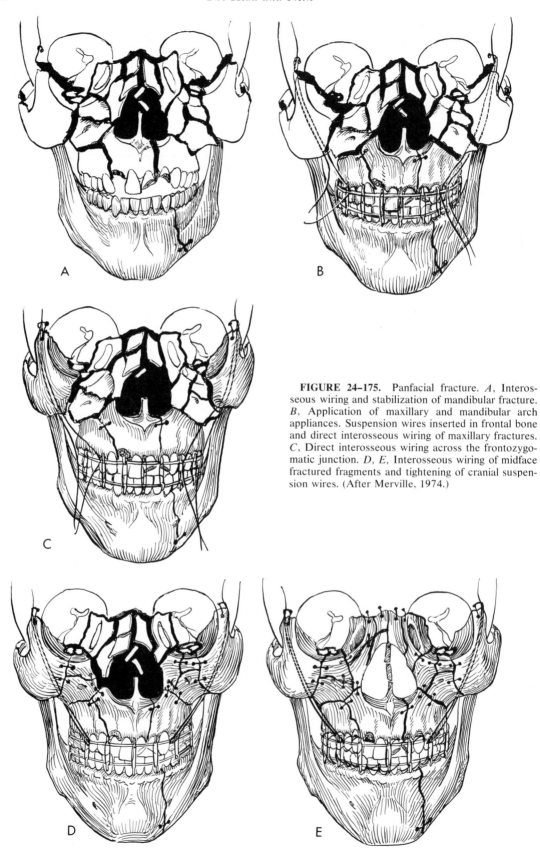

FIGURE 24–175. Panfacial fracture. *A*, Interosseous wiring and stabilization of mandibular fracture. *B*, Application of maxillary and mandibular arch appliances. Suspension wires inserted in frontal bone and direct interosseous wiring of maxillary fractures. *C*, Direct interosseous wiring across the frontozygomatic junction. *D, E*, Interosseous wiring of midface fractured fragments and tightening of cranial suspension wires. (After Merville, 1974.)

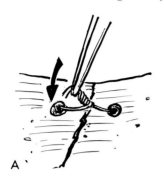

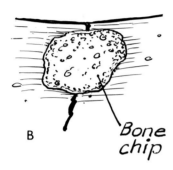

FIGURE 24–176. Wires are cut sufficiently long to bury the end in one of the drill holes. Bone chips *(B)* are often applied over the fracture lines.

Usually it is best to proceed from lateral to medial, reconstructing the midface piece by piece.

ORDER OF PROCEDURE WHEN THE MANDIBLE IS SEVERELY MUTILATED. If the mandible is severely comminuted and the continuity of the bone is interrupted, it cannot be employed as a guideline for the replacement of the maxilla (Fig. 24–177, *A*). The approach to the architectural restoration of the facial skeleton must be reversed, and reconstruction must proceed *from above downward.*

Fixation of the zygoma to the zygomatic process of the frontal bone should be first established; this usually requires elevation of the zygoma and the lateral portion of the floor of the orbit prior to interosseous wire fixation (Fig. 24–177, *B*). If the zygoma is fragmented, each fragment should be wired to its neighbor and to the maxilla (Fig. 24–177, *B, C*). The maxillary fragments are realigned and fixation is established by an arch bar and wire appliance (Fig. 24–177, *D*). The floor of the orbit is then explored and continuity restored if necessary. The naso-orbital fractures are approached through either cutaneous nasal incisions or the bicoronal flap, the main fragments being wired to the frontal bone (Fig. 24–177, *E*). Through-and-through transosseous wiring not only maintains the contour of the nasal skeletal framework and the medial orbital walls but also reattaches the medial canthal tendons to the medial orbital wall. The remaining mandibular fragments are placed into fixation with the maxilla after realignment and fixation, and cranial suspension is established by means of internal wiring extending upward through the zygomatic fossa to the frontal bone (Fig. 24–177, *F*).

FRACTURES INVOLVING THE ANTERIOR CRANIAL FOSSA. In patients with frontoethmoidal fractures involving the anterior cranial fossa, a dual approach is required from above, through a craniotomy which exposes the anterior cranial fossa, and from below, by means of the techniques of exposure described earlier in the chapter. These patients may have penetration of the brain by a bone fragment or destruction of dura or a portion of the frontal lobe (see Fig. 24–172). The destroyed brain should be removed and the dura sutured or repaired by a graft of temporalis fascia. Cerebrospinal fluid leakage is arrested by suture of the dura or by a graft of fascia or dermis, and bone defects of the anterior cranial fossa, including the roofs of the orbit, should be repaired by primary bone grafting (see Chapter 25).

CONSIDERATIONS ON PRIMARY BONE GRAFTING. Primary bone grafting has been performed for the restoration of the floor of the orbit for the past 20 years. Bonanno and Converse (1974, 1975) have also reported the use of primary bone grafting in the management of severely comminuted maxillary fractures to assist in maintaining the projection of the fractured maxilla, in the restoration of contour of the nose, and in reestablishing bony continuity when communition of certain areas of the facial skeleton reduces these areas to a state of pulp. A thin onlay bone graft of cancellous iliac bone will restore contour and assist in the consolidation of fractures.

Areas in which primary bone grafting is applicable are the nasal skeleton, the medial wall of the orbit, the orbital rims (see Chapter 25), the frontal bone, the canine fossa, and defects of the mandible. Experience gained from craniofacial surgery has shown that bone grafts are successful even though one surface of the bone graft lies exposed over a cavity, such as the maxillary sinus. The soft tissues,

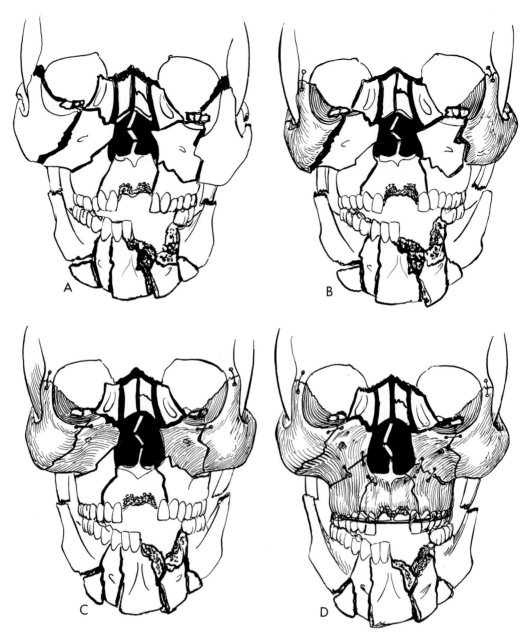

FIGURE 24–177. Panfacial fracture with comminution of the mandible. *A,* Fracture lines. *B,* Initially fixation of the zygoma is established by interosseous wiring to the frontal bone. *C,* Zygoma is also wired to the maxilla. *D,* Maxillary fragments are reduced and secured by interosseous wiring. Maxillary arch bar is applied.

Illustration continued on opposite page

however, must be well vascularized and provide adequate cover of the bone graft. It is obvious that in cases in which soft tissue has been destroyed, the soft tissue must be restored, and primary bone grafting is usually contraindicated. Primary bone grafting is also dependent on the general condition of the patient.

Primary bone grafting of the dorsum of the nose is often feasible through cutaneous lacerations or either transcutaneous or intranasal operative incisions. The addition of a bone graft at the primary stage of treatment when the nasal bones are comminuted and crushed will prevent saddling of the dorsum and shortening of the nose, often a difficult post-traumatic deformity to correct.

In severely comminuted midfacial fractures,

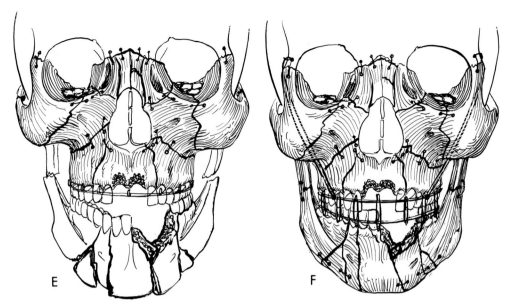

FIGURE 24–177 *Continued. E,* Interosseous wiring of naso-orbital fragments and exploration of the orbital floor. *F,* Mandibular fragments are reduced and secured by interosseous wires. Position is maintained by intermaxillary fixation and cranial suspension. (After Merville.)

after reduction and fixation by the usual methods (Fig. 24–178, *A* to *D*) (interosseous fixation of fragments, intermaxillary fixation, cranial fixation by internal wiring), if mobility is still present, the retromaxillary space should be explored by means of a curved hemostat. If there is indication of bony destruction in the pterygomaxillary area, a supportive bone graft placed in the pterygomaxillary interface and around the maxillary tuberosity is an important addition to conventional methods of treatment (Fig. 24–178, *E, F, G*). An incision is made through the mucoperiosteum anterior to the tuberosity of the maxilla, the periosteum is raised around the posterior aspect of the tuberosity, and a measured bone graft is wedged into the area. The procedure is repeated on the contralateral side. This technique is, at the present writing, subject to criticism as to its value. Although the tuberosities of the maxilla and pterygoid plates may be severely comminuted or even pulverized, a bone graft may be wedged between the comminuted fragments. The bone grafts provide buttresses maintaining the forward projection of the maxilla; more importantly, they also fill a void, and the additional bone may consolidate during the weeks of intermaxillary fixation, restoring the posterior buttresses and preventing secondary recession of the maxilla.

In naso-orbital fractures, the restoration of the medial orbital walls done in conjunction with the bone grafting of the nasal dorsum (Figs. 24–178, *H* to *L*) will assist in the correction of traumatic telecanthus (see Chapter 25).

The indications for primary bone grafting must be carefully evaluated. Panfacial fractures without soft tissue lacerations are particularly favorable for primary bone grafting. When extensive soft tissue wounds are present, bone grafting is a successful technique if the wounds are cleanly incised and if sufficient soft tissue coverage of the bone graft can be ensured. Contraindications are infected or severely contaminated soft tissue wounds.

POSTTRAUMATIC FACIAL PAIN

D. A. Crockford, F.R.C.S.

Pain persisting after the primary treatment of facial trauma is a relatively uncommon complication that can be disabling to the patient and can lead even to drug addiction. This problem has been considered by Crockford (1975a).

Pathogenesis

Seddon's well known triple classification (Seddon, 1942) of neurapraxia, axonotmesis, and neurotmesis is used to correlate the degree of injury and the characteristic clinical symptomatology. Although there has been little research into the effects of trauma on cranial nerves, it seems likely that facial pain is ex-

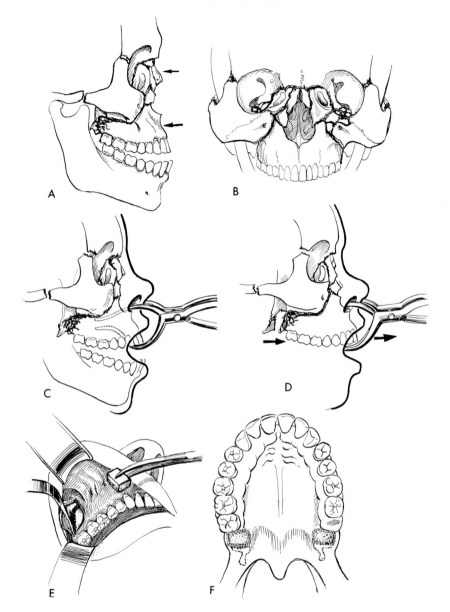

FIGURE 24–178. Primary bone grafting in the management of complex fractures. *A, B*, Complex midface fracture. *C, D*, Reduction of the impacted maxillary fragment. *E, F*, Insertion of measured block of iliac bone graft in the pterygomaxillary space.

Illustration continued on opposite page

perienced by mechanisms similar to those of spinal nerves (Wilson, 1974).

Peripheral nerves may be cut, crushed, or subjected to some form of traction injury at the moment of trauma. Subsequently, infection, compression by scar contracture, or callus formation may occur. The infraorbital nerve is damaged in about 80 per cent of the fractures of the zygoma (Barclay, 1960), infraorbital sensory disturbance being one of the classical symptoms of this injury. As is well known, after reduction of a displaced fracture, recovery of sensation in the ensuing weeks or months is usual; neurapraxia or axonotmesis has occurred as the nerve passes through the infraorbital canal. The supraorbital and supratrochlear nerves are particularly at risk where they lie just superficial to the unyielding surface of the superior margin of the orbit and the frontal bone. In this location, laceration or contusion are not uncommon. The external nasal nerve may be crushed as it emerges between

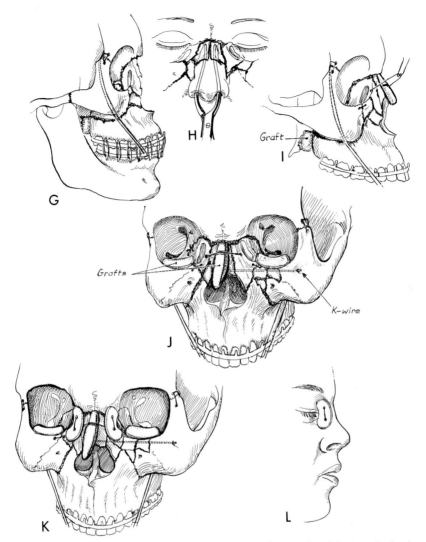

FIGURE 24–178 *Continued.* *G,* Suspension wire between the frontal bone and arch bars. *H,* Reduction of nasal bones. *I,* Addition of bone graft secured to nasal dorsum by transosseous wiring. *J,* Further stabilization with K wire. Note bone grafts on floor of orbit. *K, L,* Canthal buttons are used to reinsert the medial canthal tendons into the medial orbital walls and reapply the soft tissue in the naso-orbital area.

the nasal bone and upper lateral cartilage (McNeill, 1963).

The crude mechanisms of the nerve injuries described above are not in dispute. The wonder is, however, that overt injury in such anatomical situations is not more frequent. In fact, it is probable that damage to these nerves does occur much more often than is clinically apparent, as histologically demonstrable intraneural fibrosis and axonal disturbance following trauma give little indication of the presence or severity of clinical symptoms (White and Sweet, 1969). As yet, there is no universally accepted explanation of the mechanisms of

peripheral or central pain, although the "gate theory" of Melzak and Wall (1965) is considered to be nearest the truth. In particular, there is no good electrophysiologic explanation of the pain generated by amputation neuromas or nerve entrapment (Wilson, 1974), but it has been suggested that a possible mechanism for the persistence of pain is ascending constriction of sensory axons by collagen. Nerves so affected are often tender and swollen several centimeters proximal to the site of injury, and microscopic examination shows an ascending neuropathy with infiltration of collagen between individual axons (White, 1968).

It is generally recognized that in certain cases, pain at the periphery that is not controlled within a few months spreads centrally to become established in an apparently self-perpetuating way, making relief much more difficult.

Clinical Symptoms

The patient usually gives a history of facial trauma, although the late onset of pain after a forgotten or apparently trivial injury may cause diagnostic difficulty (Henry, Michelet and Loiseau, 1972). The great majority of patients with overt sensory nerve damage will also give a history of an anatomically recognizable area of resolving hypoesthesia or paresthesia.

In the small group of patients to be considered, the symptoms are worse. In their mildest form, dysesthesia will still be anatomically localized but of sufficient severity to prevent adequate toilet of the part. Pain may develop in the area, precipitated by physical or psychogenic stimuli. Analgesics may be regularly required, and significant interference with social activities will occur. The attacks of pain may become spontaneous, and radiate beyond the original area of involvement. Associated secretomotor and vasomotor activity may develop, thus culminating in a state analogous to the dreadful but rare complication of causalgia. These severe syndromes may occur within hours of injury, or onset may be so delayed that other causes of facial pain must be excluded. However, the majority of such patients experience a progressive increase in their painful manifestations as indicated above. It is the clinician's task to try and select the patients in this group, so that they may recieve the sympathetic and energetic care that can prevent the establishment of a recycling pain syndrome. Although the majority of the patients, because of their history and the presence of tenderness and paresthesia in an anatomically recognizable distribution, are relatively easy to assess, those with spontaneous pain radiating outside such an area can be more difficult. The help of an able and sympathetic psychiatrist may be invaluable in separating organic pain from an endogenous psychiatric state. If available, referral to the local pain clinic will obviously be considered, while no time should be lost in consulting an interested neurosurgeon if the simple measures to be described do not bring early relief. Finally, besides these medical factors, aggravating social, emotional and economic circumstances, together with the possibility of further financial compensation, may have to be considered.

Methods of Treatment

These may be broadly divided into nonsurgical (local and systemic) and surgical (peripheral and central). It is presumed that adequate primary care, including reduction and stabilization of fractures and the removal of obvious foreign bodies, has been carried out.

Nonsurgical Local Treatment. The single most helpful procedure is undoubtedly a local anesthetic block of the appropriate nerve. If successful, it may aid in making a diagnosis by localization, and may allow further examination of the part. Such an injection may also be prognostic, as variations in the response of the patient to an objectively successful block can indicate how much of the symptomatic reaction is psychologic or psychiatric. It often happens that pain relief occurs for a longer period than may be expected from the effects of the local anesthetic alone; relief may even be permanent after a single injection. This may be due to the interruption of a self-perpetuating pain cycle. The use of a long-acting local anesthetic such as bupivacaine, often with adrenalin, is worthwhile. To this may be added a relatively insoluble steroid such as triamcinolone hexacetonide. Although the mechanism of its anti-inflammatory action is not fully understood, resolution of hypertrophic skin scars by this drug is well documented. Crockford (1975b) has used it frequently in the hand for the relief of painful neuromas, usually with success. Recent work suggests, however, that it is not active against mature collagen (Rudolph and Klein, 1973), so that if indicated, a trial of its use should not be delayed. Injection of this "cocktail" into an intensely sensitive area can be extremely disagreeable inspite of its local anesthetic content; therefore, this is often done under a short general anesthesia. If the initial injection brings improvement, further injections may be given at monthly intervals until relief is obtained or a plateau of improvement is reached. Even if the first injection gives little improvement, a second will occasionally have a greater effect. If, inspite of adequate immediate anesthesia, such a course fails to bring permanent relief, and particularly if there are signs of secretomotor and vasomotor overactivity, a diagnostic trial of a stellate ganglion block is indicated. If complete pain relief occurs, a course of such blocks — four or five in 10 days — should be given. Interspersed with these, a placebo injection should be tried. Such a therapeutic course can be successful (Leriche, 1949); but, if only temporary relief occurs, excision of the superior cervical sympathetic ganglion may be indicated (Bingham, 1947). Stellate ganglion block sometimes followed by sympathectomy is a well recognized treatment for causalgia of the upper limb. Phenol and alcohol blocks of peripheral nerves for posttraumatic facial pain are no longer widely advocated because these drugs will cause further damage to the affected nerve.

Nonsurgical Systemic Treatment. Probably the most important factor in the successful use of systemic drugs is that they should be given as a course of treatment and not on demand. It takes at least a month for the full benefit of this treatment to develop. A "pain cocktail" containing minor analgesics such as aspirin and paracetamol, coupled with an antihistamine such as diphenhydramine, can be made up with a syrup base in such a way that its contents can be varied without the knowledge of the patient. Adequate sleep is, of course, essential, and regular use of an antidepresssnt with a strong hypnotic effect, such as amitriptyline, may be necessary. Full antidepresssnt therapy may also be indicated.

With regard to more specific therapy, carbamazepine, which is one of the drugs of election for trigeminal neuralgia and migraine, may be worth a trial in resistant cases, but unfortunately it can produce serious side-effects such as blood dyscrasias and liver damage.

Surgical Peripheral Treatment. Neurolysis alone seldom gives permanent improvement, but, if combined with decompression, e.g., of a painful infraorbital nerve crushed in its foramen, lasting relief can be achieved. This particular operation should always be considered in any patient in whom infraorbital sensory deficit persists for a year or more after trauma. It is theoretically reasonable to suggest that perineural triamcinolone should be instilled during neurolysis. No trial of this has been reported, but some initial success has been achieved with silicone rubber sheeting wrapped around the affected part of the nerve. White and Sweet (1969) from their considerable experience suggest that instead of neurolysis, excision of the damaged nerve and repair be done if possible. With recent advances in microsurgery and grafting of peripheral nerves, this approach may be worth trying. Neurotomy has, as is to be expected, a high recurrence rate, as the proximal end will inevitably develop a neuroma, which is again likely to be painful. Patakay, Graham and Mungar (1973) have shown experimentally that instillation of triamcinolone at the time of nerve division markedly reduces the inflammatory response; the integrity of the adjacent perineurium is preserved, thus preventing the outgrowth of axons, and hence reducing the chance of pain recurrence (Sutherland, 1968).

Surgical Central Treatment. Surgical sympathectomy has been mentioned in the previous section. More complex neurosurgical procedures, such as trigeminal rhizotomy and tractotomy, are beyond the scope of this treatise.

REFERENCES

Adams, W. M.: Internal wiring fixation of facial fractures. Surgery, *12*:523, 1942.

Adams, W. M., and Adams, L. H.: Internal wire fixation of facial fractures. A fifteen-year followup report. Am. J. Surg., *92*:12, 1956.

Anderson, R.: An ambulatory method of treating fractures of the shaft of the femur. Surg. Gynecol. Obstet., *62*:865, 1936.

Barclay, T. L.: Four hundred malar-zygomatic fractures. Trans. Int. Soc. Plast. Surg. 2nd Congress. Livingstone, Edinburgh, 1960, pp. 259–265.

Baudens, J. B.: Fracture de la machoire inférieure. Bull. Acad. Med., Paris, *5*:341, 1840.

Berry, H. C.: Fractures of the edentulous maxilla and mandible. J. Ark. Dent. Assoc., *10*:7, 1939.

Bingham, J. A. W.: Causalgia of the face. Two cases successfully treated sympathectomy. Br. Med. J., *1*:804, 1947.

Bonanno, P. C., and Converse, J. M.: Primary bone grafting in management of facial fractures. N. Y. State J. Med., *75*:710, 1975.

Braunstein, P. W.: Medical aspects of automotive crash injury research. J.A.M.A., *163*:249, 1957.

Brown, J. B., Fryer, M. P., and McDowell, F.: Internal wire-pin immobilization of jaw fractures. Plast. Reconstr. Surg., *4*:30, 1949.

Chalmers, J. Lyons Club (Prepared by): Fractures involving the mandibular condyle; post-treatment survey of 120 cases. J. Oral Surg., *5*:45, 1947.

Converse, J. M.: Fractures of the maxilla. *In* Kazanjian, V. H., and Converse, J. M.: The Surgical Treatment of Facial Injuries. 2nd Ed. Baltimore, The Williams and Wilkins Company, 3rd Ed., 1974.

Converse, J. M., and Bonanno, P. C.: *In* Kazanjian, V. H., and Converse, J. M.: Surgical Treatment of Facial Injuries. 3rd Ed. Baltimore, The Williams and Wilkins Company, 1974, p. 354.

Converse, J. M., and Smith, B.: Enophthalmos and diplopia in fractures of the orbital floor. Br. J. Plast. Surg., 9:265, 1957.

Crockford, D. A.: Posttraumatic facial pain. Paper read at the Sixth International Congress of Plastic Surgery. Paris, 1975a.

Crockford, D. A.: Unpublished data, 1975b.

Dingman, R. O., and Alling, C. C.: Open reduction and internal wire fixation of maxillofacial fractures. J. Oral Surg., 12:140, 1954.

Dingman, R. O., and Constant, E.: A fifteen year experience with temporomandibular joint disorders. Evaluation of 140 cases. Plast. Reconstr. Surg., 44:119, 1969.

Dingman, R. O., and Grabb, W. C.: Surgical anatomy of the mandibular ramus of the facial nerve based on the dissection of 100 facial halves. Plast. Reconstr. Surg., 29:266, 1962.

Dingman, R. O., and Natvig, P.: Surgery of Facial Fractures. Philadelphia, W. B. Saunders Company, 1964.

Dunphy, J. E., and Jackson, D. S.: Primary applications of experimental studies in the care of the primarily closed wound. Am. J. Surg., 104:273, 1962.

Eby, J. D.: Principles of orthodontia in the treatment of maxillofacial injuries. Internatl. J. Orthodontia, 6:273, 1920.

Fry, W. K., Shepherd, P. R., McLeod, A. C., and Parfitt, G. J.: The Dental Treatment of Maxillofacial Injuries. Oxford, Blackwell Scientific Publications, 1942.

Georgiade, N. G.: Personal communication, 1960.

Georgiade, N. G.: Disturbances of the temporomandibular joint. *In* Converse, J. M. (Ed.): Reconstructive Plastic Surgery. Philadelphia, W. B. Saunders Company, 1964.

Georgiade, N. G.: Complex and external fixation of multiple facial fractures. *In* Plastic and Maxillofacial Trauma. Symposium of the Educational Foundation of the American Society of Plastic And Reconstructive Surgery. St. Louis, Mo., C. V. Mosby Company, 1969.

Georgiade, N., and Nash, T.: An external cranial fixation apparatus for severe maxillofacial injuries. Plast. Reconstr. Surg., 38:142, 1966.

Georgiade, N. G., Pickrell, K., Douglas, W., and Altany, F.: Extra-oral pinning of displaced condylar fractures. Plast. Reconstr. Surg., 18:377, 1956.

Gillies, H. D., Kilner, T. P., and Stone, D.: Fractures of the malar-zygomatic compound, with a description of new X-ray position. Br. J. Surg., 14:651, 1927.

Gillies, H. D., and Millard, D. R.: The Principles and Art of Plastic Surgery. Vol. 2. Boston, Little, Brown and Company, 1957.

Gillman, T., Penn, J., Bronks, D., and Roux, M.: Closure of wounds and incisions with adhesive tape. Lancet, 2:945, 1955.

Gilmer, T. L.: A case of fracture of the lower jaw with remarks on treatment. Arch. Dent., 4:388, 1887.

Ginestet, G., Desorthes, P., and Houessou, J.: Luxation irreductible de la machoire suivie d'ankylose. Rev. Stomatol., 49:655, 1948.

Gottlieb, O.: Long-standing dislocation of the jaw. J. Oral Surg., 10:28, 1952.

Graham, J. R., and Scott, T. M.: Notes on the treatment of tetanus. New Engl. J. Med., 235:846, 1946.

Gregory, T. G.: Personal communication, 1957.

Griffin, J. R.: Treating fractures of the mandible by skeletal fixation. Am. J. Orthod., 27:364, 1941.

Hagan, E. H., and Huelke, D. F.: An analysis of 319 cases reports of mandibular fractures. J. Oral Surg. 19:93, 1961.

Haynes, H. H.: Treating fractures by skeletal fixation of the individual bone. South Med. J., 32:720, 1939.

Hayward, J. R.: Treatment methods for jaw fractures. J. Oral Surg., 20:273, 1962.

Hendrix, J. H., Jr., Sanders, S. G., and Green, B.: Open reduction of mandibular condyle. Plast. Reconstr. Surg., 23:283, 1959.

Henny, F. A.: A technic for the open reduction of fractures of the mandibular condyle. J. Oral Surg., 9:33, 1951.

Henry, P., Michelet, X., and Loiseau, P.: La néuralgie sous-orbitaire. Bord. Med., 19:2617, 1972.

Heurlin, R. J., Gans, B. J., and Stuteville, O. H.: Skeletal changes following fracture dislocation of the mandibular condyle in the adult rhesus monkey. Oral Surg., 14:1490, 1961.

Hoopes, J. E., Wolfort, F. G., and Jabaley, M. E.: Operative treatment of fractures of the mandibular condyle in children. Plast. Reconstr. Surg., 46:357, 1970.

Iverson, P. C.: Surgical removal of traumatic tattoos of the face. Plast. Reconstr. Surg., 2:427, 1947.

Ivy, R. H.: Observations of fractures of the mandible. J.A.M.A., 79:295, 1922.

Johnson, J. B.: Personal communication, 1962.

Johnson, W. B.: New methods for reduction of acute dislocation of the temporomandibular articulations. J. Oral Surg., 16:501, 1958.

Kazanjian, V. H.: Treatment of automobile injuries of the face and jaws. J. Am. Dent. Assoc., 20:757, 1933.

Kazanjian, V. H., and Converse, J. M.: The Surgical Treatment of Facial Injuries. Baltimore, Williams & Wilkins Company, 1949; 2nd Ed., 1959; 3rd Ed., 1974.

Keen, W. W.: Surgery, Its Principles and Practice. Philadelphia, W. B. Saunders Company, 1909.

Ketchum, L. D., Ferris, B., and Masters, F. W.: Blindness in midfacial fractures without direct injury to the globe. Plast. Reconstr. Surg. (in press, 1976).

Knight, J. S., and North, J. F.: The classification of malar fractures: An analysis of displacement as a guide to treatment. Br. J. Plast. Surg., 13:325, 1961.

Lambotte, A.: Chirurgie Opératoire des Fractures. Paris, Masson & Cie, 1913.

Lange, W. E.: Fractures of the orbit. Plast. Reconstr. Surg., 35:26, 1965.

Leake, D., Doykos, J., III, Habal, M. B., and Murray, J.: Long-term follow-up of fractures of the mandibular condyle in children. Plast. Reconstr. Surg., 47:127, 1971.

Le Fort, R.: Etude expérimentale sur les fractures de la machoire supérieure. Rev. Chir., Paris, 23:208, 360, 479, 1901.

Lenormant, C., and Darcissac, M.: Le procédé des "anses metalliques transosseuses" pour la contention des branches montantes, dans les fractures du maxillaire inférieur; son application dans un cas de fracture double retrodentaire de la machoire inférieure. Bull. Mém. Soc. Nat. Chir., 53:503, 1927.

Leriche, R. (1949): Cited by White, J. C., and Sweet, W. H.: In Pain and the Neurosurgeon. Springfield, Illinois, Charles C Thomas, 1969.

Litzow, T. J., and Royer, R. Q.: Treatment of long-standing dislocation of the mandible: Report of case. Proc. Staff Meet. Mayo Clin., 37:399, 1962.

Lothrop, H. A.: Fractures of the superior maxillary bone, caused by direct blows over the malar bone. A method for the treatment of such fractures. Boston Med. Surg. J., 154:8, 1906.

McCoy, F. J., Chandler, R. A., Magnan, C. G., Moore, J. F., and Siemsen, G.: Analysis of facial fractures and their complications. Plast. Reconstr. Surg., 29:381, 1962.

MacGregor, A. B., and Fordyce, G.: Treatment of fracture of the neck of the mandibular condyle. Br. Dent. J., *102*:351, 1957.

McNeill, R. A.: Traumatic nasal neuralgia and its treatment. Br. Med. J., *2*:536, 1963.

Melzack, R., and Wall, P. D.: Pain mechanisms: a new theory. Science, *150*:971, 1965.

Merville, L. C.: Multiple dislocations of the facial skeleton. J. Maxillofac. Surg., *2*:187, 1974.

Messer, E.: A simplified method for fixation of the fractured mandibular condyle. J. Oral Surg., *30*:442, 1972.

Miller, G. R., and Tenzel, R. R.: Ocular complications of midfacial fractures. Plast. Reconstr. Surg., *39*:117, 1967.

Morris, J. H.: Biphase connector, external skeletal splint for reduction and fixation of mandibular fractures. Oral Surg., *2*:1382, 1949.

Müller, G. M.: Long-standing dislocation of the mandible: manual reduction. Br. Med. J., *1*:572, 1946.

National Safety Council: Accident Facts. Chicago, 1975.

Natvig, P.: Personal communication, 1962.

Obwegeser, H. L., and Sailer, H. F.: Another way of treating fractures of the atrophic edentulous mandible. J. Maxillofac. Surg., *1*:213, 1973.

Patakay, P. E., Graham, W. P., III, and Mungar, B. L.: Terminal neuromas treated with triamcinolone hexacetonide. J. Surg. Res., *14*:36, 1973.

Paul, J. K., and Acevedo, A.: Intraoral open reduction. J. Oral Surg., *26*:516, 1968.

Risdon, F. E.: Arthroplasty of the temporomaxillary joint. J.A.M.A., *85*:2011, 1925.

Robert, C. A.: Nouveau procédé de traitement des fractures de la portion alvéolaire de la machoire inférieure. Bull. Gén. Thérap., *42*:22, 1852.

Rowe, N. L., and Killey, H. C.: Fracture of the Facial Skeleton. Baltimore, Williams & Wilkins Company, 1955; 2nd Ed., 1968.

Rudolph, R., and Klein, L.: Inhibition of mature ³H-collagen destruction by triamcinolone. J. Surg. Res., *14*:435, 1973.

Schultz, R. C.: Supraorbital and glabellar fractures. Plast. Reconstr. Surg., *45*:227, 1970.

Schultz, R. C.: *In* Facial Injuries. Chicago, Year Book Medical Publishers, 1970.

Seddon, H. J.: A classification of nerve injuries. Br. Med. J., *2*:237, 1942.

Shapiro, H. H.: Applied Anatomy of the Head and Neck. 2nd Ed. Philadelphia, J. B. Lippincott Company, 1947.

Stader, O.: A preliminary announcement of a new method of treating fractures. North Am. Vet., *18*:37, 1937.

Stout, R. A.: *In* Manual of Standard Practice of Plastic and Maxillofacial Surgery. Philadelphia, W. B. Saunders Company, 1942.

Straith, C. L.: Guest passenger injuries. J.A.M.A., *137*:348, 1948.

Straith, R. E., Lawson, J. M., and Hipps, C. J.: The subcuticular suture. Postgrad. Med., *29*:164, 1961.

Sutherland, S.: Nerves and Nerve Injuries. Livingstone, Edinburgh, 1968.

Tessier, P., Guiot, G., Rougerie, J., Delbet, J. P., and Pastoriza, J.: Ostéotomies cranio-naso-orbital-faciales. Hypertélorisme. Ann. Chir. Plast., *12*:103, 1967.

Thoma, K. H.: Treatment of condylar fractures. J. Oral Surg., *12*:112, 1954.

Walker, R. V.: Traumatic mandibular condylar fracture dislocations: Effect of growth in the Macaca rhesus monkey. Am. J. Surg., *100*:850, 1960.

White, J. C., and Sweet, W. H.: Pain and the Neurosurgeon. A 40 year experience. Springfield, Illinois, Charles C Thomas, 1969.

White, J. C.: *In* Soulairac, A., Cahn, J., and Charpentiér, J. (Eds.): Pain, New York, Academic Press, 1968, pp. 503–519.

Wilson, M. E.: The neurological mechanisms of pain. A review. Anaesthesia, *29*:407, 1974.

CHAPTER 25

ORBITAL AND NASO-ORBITAL FRACTURES

John Marquis Converse, M.D., Byron Smith, M.D., and Donald Wood-Smith, F.R.C.S.E.

Orbital fractures may occur independently or may be associated with other facial fractures. One should obtain specific details as to where and how the accident occurred, and if there was a period of unconsciousness, loss of vision, or diplopia. A history of prior medical or surgical treatment is also important.

Prior to the primary treatment of the fracture, an ophthalmologic examination should be done routinely to verify visual acuity and check the possibility of intraocular or corneal injury. Obviously, if the patient is unconscious, the examination is limited. In the conscious patient, a delay of the operative procedure for a few days will allow the edema to subside and permit a more thorough examination. Facial bone fractures are not surgical emergencies unless the airway is obstructed and a tracheotomy is indicated. Treatment of an orbital fracture should not be delayed more than necessary, however, as fibrosis of the entrapped extraocular musculature, loss of orbital fat, and organization of the fracture occur rapidly and complicate the treatment.

When feasible, extraocular muscle movements should be checked at far and near distance and in all cardinal fields, as ocular muscle imbalance is often associated with

fractures. A fundus examination often uncovers congenital anomalies or macula or optic nerve injuries that may limit the postoperative result because of diminution or loss of vision and may reduce the probability of satisfactory extraocular muscle fusion.

In trauma involving the medial canthus, when there is an associated naso-orbital fracture, an evaluation of the lacrimal system should be obtained, if feasible, depending on the magnitude of the injury. Irrigation of the secretory system showing drainage of the fluid into the nose demonstrates that the continuity of the lacrimal apparatus has not been interrupted.

Orbital fractures occur in association with zygomaticomaxillary, naso-orbital, and high maxillary (Le Fort III) fractures, as well as in pyramidal (Le Fort II) fractures, where the line of fracture traverses the orbital floor (see Chapter 24). The backward displacement of the fractured thick inferior orbital rim comminutes the thinner portion of the orbital floor. The downward displacement of the zygoma results in a separation at the frontozygomatic junction and a lowering of the orbital floor.

Orbital fractures complicated by diplopia are frequently associated with midfacial fractures.

748

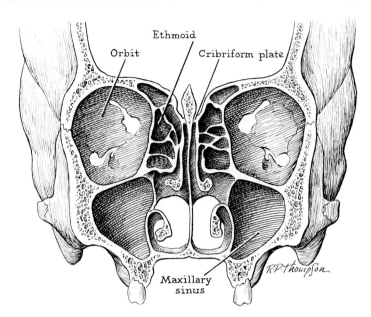

FIGURE 25-1.   The interorbital space.

McCoy, Chandler, Magnan, Moore, and Siemsen (1962) found an incidence of 15 per cent of ocular complications in a series of 855 patients with facial fractures. Morgan, Madan, and Bergerot (1972), in a review of 300 cases of midfacial fractures, found persistent diplopia in 11 per cent of the patients.

THE ORBIT: ANATOMICAL CONSIDERATIONS

The orbits are paired bony structures separated in the midline by the interorbital space (Fig. 25–1). The interorbital space, the portion of the nasal cavity situated between the orbits, is delimited above by the floor of the anterior cranial fossa, formed in this portion by the roof of each ethmoid sinus laterally and by the cribriform plate medially. The orbits are situated immediately below the floor of the anterior cranial fossa, a portion of the fossa being formed by the roofs of the orbits (see Chapter 56).

The orbital contents are protected by strong bony abutments: the nasal bones, the nasal spine of the frontal bone, and the frontal processes of the maxilla medially; the supraorbital arch of the frontal bone above; the frontal process of the zygoma and zygomatic process of the frontal bone laterally; and the thick infraorbital rim formed by the zygoma and maxilla inferiorly (Fig. 25–2).

The Skeletal Anatomy of the Orbit. The skeletal components of the orbital cavity are the frontal bone, the lesser and greater wings of the sphenoid, the zygoma, the maxilla, the lacrimal bone, and the ethmoid.

The bony orbit has been described as cone-shaped or pyramidal in shape. Both of these analogies are somewhat inaccurate. The widest orbital diameter is not located at the orbital rim but approximately 1.5 cm within the orbital cavity. The medial wall has a quadrangular rather than a triangular configuration. The optic foramen lies on a medial and slightly superior plane in the apex of the orbit. In children, the orbital floor is situated at a lower

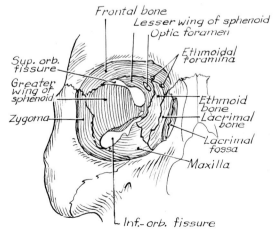

FIGURE 25-2.   Frontal view of the right orbit.

level in relation to the orbital rim because the maxillary sinus has not reached full development.

The orbits are protected anteriorly by the orbital rims formed of thick bone, whereas the orbital walls consist of relatively thin bone. Although it represents an artificial division, it is helpful in studying the bony orbit to divide it into four component parts: the roof, lateral wall, medial wall, and floor (Fig. 25–2).

The *floor of the orbit* (Fig. 25–3), a frequent site of fracture, has no sharp line of demarcation with the medial wall because the orbital floor tilts upward in its medial aspect, while the lower portion of the medial wall has a progressively lateral inclination. The floor is separated from the lateral wall by the inferior orbital (sphenomaxillary) fissure. The floor of the orbit (the roof of the maxillary sinus) is composed mainly of the orbital plate of the maxilla, a paper-thin structure medial to the infraorbital groove, and partly by the zygomatic bone anterior to the inferior orbital fissure. The infraorbital groove (or canal) traverses the floor of the orbit beginning at about the middle of the inferior orbital fissure. Anteriorly it penetrates the thick inferior orbital rim as the infraorbital canal, which opens on the anterior surface of the maxilla as the infraorbital foramen.

The orbital floor has a general upward inclination; the anterior portion is concave and the posterior portion is convex. In the blowout fracture mechanism, the force transmitted to the orbital contents tends to fracture the floor at its weakest point and may be nature's way

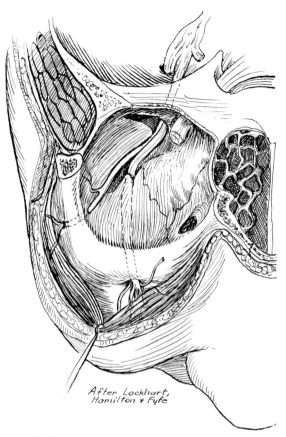

After Lockhart, Hamilton & Fyfe

FIGURE 25–4. The trajectory of the maxillary nerve, which takes its origin as the second division of the trigeminal nerve (fifth cranial nerve). When it enters the infraorbital canal (or groove), it assumes the name "infraorbital" nerve and exits at the infraorbital foramen.

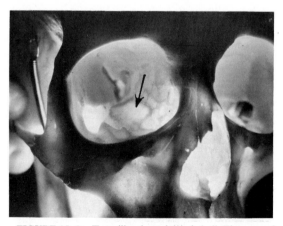

FIGURE 25–3. Transilluminated dried skull. The area of thin bone in the floor of the orbit is indicated by the arrow. Note the inferior orbital fissure posterolaterally, the lacrimal groove and lamina papyracea medially, and the wide angle of junction between the floor and the medial wall. The weak area is further weakened by the infraorbital groove or canal.

of protecting the ocular globe from rupture by decompressing the orbit. In the posterior portion of this inclined plane there is an area of thin bone. This "weak area" (Fig. 25–3) represents the thinnest bone of the orbit; its medial extension is the lamina papyracea of the ethmoid, a portion of the medial orbital wall which, as its name implies, is a plate of bone of paperlike thinness. The medial half of the orbital floor is also weakened by the canal (or groove) for the passage of the infraorbital nerve (Fig. 25–4).

The inferior oblique muscle arises from the medial aspect of the orbital floor, lateral to the lacrimal groove, near the anterior margin of the orbit.

The *medial wall*, reinforced anteriorly by the frontal process of the maxilla, is relatively fragile and is formed from the frontal bone, the lacrimal bone, the lamina papyracea of the ethmoid, and part of the lesser wing of the sphenoid around the optic foramen (Fig. 25–5). The lamina papyracea is the largest component and accounts for the structural weakness of the medial wall. The lesser wing of the sphenoid and the optic foramen are posterior to the lamina papyracea. Thus the optic foramen is located close to the posterior portion of the ethmoid sinus, not at the apex of the orbit (Fig. 25–5). Consequently, in severe fractures involving the medial wall in its posterior portion, the optic nerve can be injured.

The groove for the lacrimal sac is a broad vertical fossa lying partly on the anterior aspect of the lacrimal bone and partly in the frontal process of the maxilla; the anterior and posterior margins of the lacrimal groove form the respective lacrimal crests. The groove is continuous with the nasolacrimal duct at the junction of the floor and medial wall of the orbit, passing down into the inferior meatus of the nose.

Between the roof and medial wall of the orbit are the anterior and posterior ethmoidal foramina which lead into canals communicating with the medial part of the anterior cranial fossa.

The *lateral wall* (Fig. 25–6) is relatively stout in its anterior portion. It is formed by the greater wing of the sphenoid, the frontal process of the zygomatic bone, and the lesser wing of the sphenoid lateral to the optic foramen. The superior orbital fissure is a cleft which runs forward and upward from the apex between the roof and lateral wall (see Fig. 25–2). The fissure, which separates the greater and lesser wings of the sphenoid, gives passage to the three motor nerves to the extraocular muscles of the orbit and leads back into the middle cranial fossa. The lateral wall of the orbit is situated in an anterolateral and posterior medial plane (Fig. 25–7). It is related to the temporal fossa; posteriorly a small part of the wall lies between the orbit and the middle cranial fossa and temporal lobe of the brain. Between the floor and lateral wall of the orbit is the inferior orbital fissure which communicates with the infratemporal fossa.

The *roof of the orbit* is composed mainly of the orbital plate of the frontal bone, but posteriorly it receives a minor contribution from the lesser wing of the sphenoid. The fossa lodging the lacrimal gland is a depression situated along the anterior and lateral aspect under shelter of the zygomatic process of the frontal bone. The anterior portion of the roof can be invaded by the supraorbital extension of the frontal sinus or by an extension of the ethmoid sinus, a frontoethmoidal cell (see also Chapter 56). The roof separates the orbit from the anterior cranial fossa and from the middle cranial fossa on the posterolateral aspect.

Often consisting of brittle bone, the orbital roof varies in thickness and may be quite thin in its medial portion.

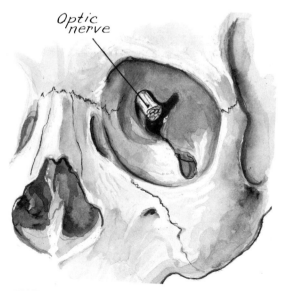

FIGURE 25–5. The relationship of the optic nerve and the orbital cavity. Note the high position of the optic foramen in relation to the floor of the orbit and the close proximity of the optic foramen with the posterior portion of the medial wall of the orbit.

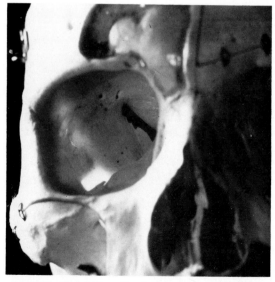

FIGURE 25–6. Transilluminated orbit demonstrating the thin posterior portion of the lateral orbital wall, contrasting with the strong abutment of its anterior portion and rim.

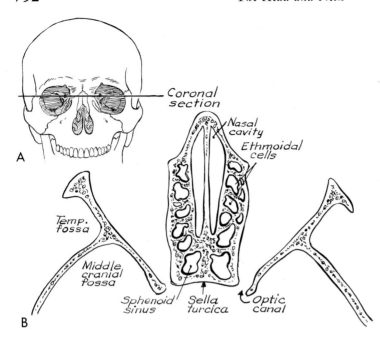

FIGURE 25-7. Coronal section showing the relationship of the orbit to the temporal fossa and the middle cranial fossa. *A*, The level of the coronal section is indicated by the horizontal line. *B*, Note that the lateral wall is inclined from lateral to medial as far as the optic foramen; it is thus situated along an oblique frontosagittal plane.

The supratrochlear and supraorbital nerves and, more medially, the trochlea of the superior oblique muscle are located along the superior rim of the orbit. The tendon of the superior oblique muscle functions in a cartilaginous pulley or trochlea, which is fixed by ligamentous fibers immediately behind the superomedial angle of the orbital margin. Fractures involving the superior rim of the orbit may result in compression of the supraorbital nerve, with consequent anesthesia of its area of distribution. Diplopia may also result from injury to the pulley of the superior oblique muscle, thus affecting the balance of the extraocular musculature (Fig. 25-8).

The Orbital Fat and the Ocular Globe. The ocular globe is surrounded by a cushion of orbital fat within the orbital cavity. The ocular globe occupies only the anterior half of the orbital cavity; the posterior half of the orbital cavity is filled with orbital fat, muscles, vessels, and nerves supplying the ocular globe. The two halves of the orbital cavity, anterior and posterior, are separated by Tenon's capsule, which subdivides the orbital cavity into an anterior or precapsular segment and a posterior or retrocapsular segment.

The Septum Orbitale. The orbital contents are maintained in position by the septum orbitale (orbital septum), a fascia inserted on the inner aspect of the rim of the orbit. The septum orbitale attaches to and blends with the levator aponeurosis in the upper eyelid for a

distance of a few millimeters above the upper border of the tarsus; in the lower eyelid, the septum orbitale is attached to the lower border of the tarsus.

The Periorbita. The periosteum lining the periphery of the orbit is known as the periorbita. The periorbita is continuous with the dura at those sites where the orbit communicates with the cranial cavity, e.g., the optic foramen, the superior orbital fissure, and the anterior and posterior ethmoidal canals.

The Optic Foramen and the Optic Canal. The optic foramen is situated at the junction of the lateral and medial walls of the orbit (see Fig. 25-7). The foramen is not located on a horizontal plane with the orbital floor but above it.

The optic canal, 4 to 10 mm in length, is the passage through which the optic nerve and ophthalmic artery pass from an intracranial to an intraorbital position. The canal is framed medially by the body of the sphenoid and laterally by the lesser wing and is thus in close approximation to the sphenoid sinus and the posterior ethmoidal cells.

BLOWOUT FRACTURES OF THE FLOOR OF THE ORBIT

A blowout fracture is caused by a sudden increase in the intraorbital pressure, resulting from the application of a traumatic force to the

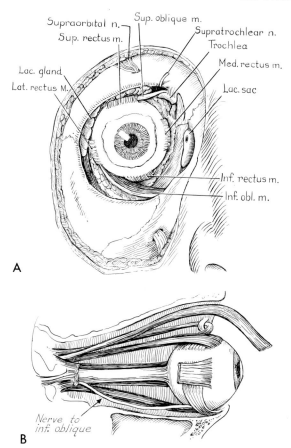

A

B

Nerve to
inf. oblique

Supraorbital n. Sup. oblique m.
Sup. rectus m. Supratrochlear n.
Trochlea
Med. rectus m.
Lac. gland
Lat. rectus M.
Lac. sac
Inf. rectus m.
Inf. obl. m.

FIGURE 25–8. Extraocular muscles. *A*, Frontal view; position of the inferior rectus and inferior oblique muscles on the undersurface of the ocular globe. *B*, Sagittal view; relation of the nerve to the inferior oblique muscle. This nerve may be injured in blowout fractures. (From Converse, J. M., and Smith, B.: Blow-out fracture of the floor of the orbit. Trans. Am. Acad. Ophthalmol. Otolaryngol., *64*:676, 1960.)

soft tissues of the orbit (Converse and Smith, 1957, 1960). The fracture is often complicated by diplopia, which is caused by a vertical muscle imbalance secondary to entrapment of the orbital contents which may include the inferior rectus and inferior oblique muscles and the surrounding fascial expansions into the dehiscence in the orbital floor. The escape of orbital fat through the blowout dehiscence is a major cause of enophthalmos.

One of the first descriptions of a blowout fracture was given by King and Samuel in 1944: "We would like to add one other type of fracture of great importance, which is not infrequent. In this there is a downward displacement of part of the orbital floor, unassociated with any damage to the margin of the orbit surrounding the facial bones. The cause of such a fracture is difficult to visualize. The most ready explanation is trauma transmitted through the eye to the orbital floor."

After the application of a traumatizing force over the orbital contents by a nonpenetrating object, such as a tennis ball (Fig. 25–9) or the human fist (Fig. 25–10), the orbital contents are forced backward into the narrower portion of the orbit (Table 25–1). The increased intraorbital pressure thus exerted causes a blowout at the weakest area of the orbital floor without fracturing the orbital rim. This type of fracture may be referred to as "pure" blowout fracture (Table 25–2) (Converse and Smith, 1957). The strong rim of the orbit protects against objects with a radius of curvature greater than 5 cm (Fig. 25–11); an object having a curvature of less than 5 cm may penetrate this protective barrier and damage the globe. Such objects are golf balls, hockey pucks, and the tip of a football. Damage to the globe leading to blindness may occur.

A champagne bottle cork may damage the globe, because its radius is less than 5 cm. However, its lesser propulsive force also makes it a frequent cause of blowout fracture. Such an accident has marred many festive occasions.

Larger objects cannot enter the orbital opening and cause direct injury to the eye unless

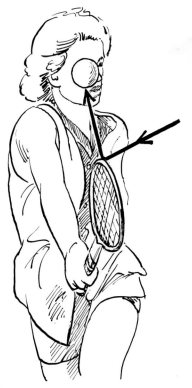

FIGURE 25–9. The tennis ball has a diameter and a curvature greater than 5 cm and thus does not penetrate the protective barrier of the orbital rim.

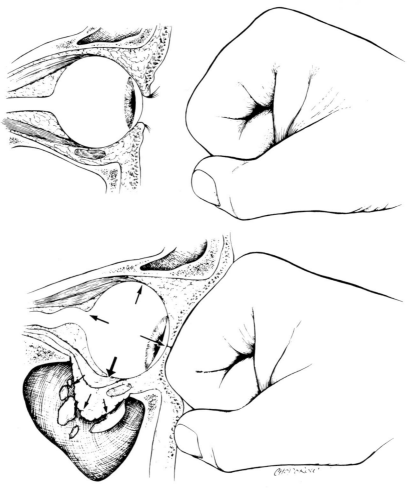

FIGURE 25-10. A frequent cause of blowout fracture is the human fist, which penetrates the protective barrier formed by the rim of the orbit, causing increased intraorbital pressure and a blowout at the weakest portion of the orbital floor.

fragile spectacle lenses, which can shatter, are interposed between the traumatizing object and the eye.

Blowout fractures are more frequent on the right side than on the left because most individuals are right-handed and many blowout fractures are caused by the human fist. One should beware of the patient with a "black eye" who complains of visual disturbances: he may have suffered a blowout fracture of the orbital floor.

Mechanism of Production of a Blowout Fracture

Following the clinical findings of fracture of the orbital floor, entrapment of the structures, and diplopia without fracture of the rim (Converse and Smith, 1957), the mechanism of

production of the orbital blowout fracture was demonstrated experimentally. It was verified in a cadaver by duplicating a force similar to that which had produced a blowout fracture in one of our patients, who had been hit by a ball used in the Irish game of hurling (Smith and Regan, 1957). The dried out condition of the cadaver globe was corrected by the intraocular injection of normal saline solution. A hurling ball was placed over the closed lid of the cadaver orbit, and the ball was struck sharply with a mallet. A cracking sound was heard and was interpreted as having been caused by fracturing bone. An exploratory incision through the skin of the infraorbital margin and elevation of the orbital contents from the floor exposed a depressed comminuted fracture of the floor of the orbit. Exenteration of the orbital contents exposed the fracture in its entirety. There was also a comminuted fracture without displace-

TABLE 25-1. *Etiologic Factors in 100 Blowout Fractures**

Automobile	49
Human fist	18
Human elbow	4
Wooden plank	1
Ball	5
Snowball	2
Ski pole	2
Edge of table	1
Hit by blunt object	1
Shoe kick	2
Steel bar	1
Hit by machinery	2
Boxing glove	1
Mop handle	1
Human buttock	1
Airplane accident	1
Water ski accident	1
Ice bank	1
Fall on face	4
Iatrogenic (surgical)	1
Military casualty (shell fragment)	1

*From Converse, J. M., Smith, B., Obear, M. F., and Wood-Smith, D.: Orbital blowout fractures: A ten-year study. Plast. Reconstr. Surg., *39*:20, 1967. Copyright 1967, The Williams & Wilkins Company, Baltimore.

margin from a height of 15 cm, produced a linear fracture of the orbital floor. When the weight was dropped from a height of 20 cm, a punched-out fracture in the convex portion of the orbital floor was produced. Both of these fractures occurred without fracture of the orbital rim.

While Rény and Stricker's statement is obviously conjectural, Fujino's experiments, performed with mathematical precision, fail to demonstrate the most important clinical consequence of the blowout fracture: the entrapment. How does he explain the entrapment of the orbital contents without the increased intraorbital pressure forcing the tissues into the site of fracture? And how is it possible for the increased intraorbital hydraulic pressure to occur without contact of the orbital contents with the traumatizing object?

Whatever the theory of the mechanism of the blowout fracture, the fact remains that, in the presence of diplopia due to entrapment and inability to rotate the globe by means of the forced duction test, release of the entrapment is the only means of relieving the patient of the extraocular muscle imbalance and diplopia.

ment involving the lamina papyracea of the ethmoid bone. No fracture of the orbital rim or zygomatic arch was observed. This experiment duplicated almost exactly the injury sustained by several of our patients.

In a second experiment, the opposite orbit of the cadaver was exenterated. The soft tissue covering the orbital rim was excised to allow direct contact of the bony orbital rim with the surface of the hurling ball. Repeated blows of similar force with the hammer failed to fracture either the floor or the rim of the orbit. However, when the striking force was sufficiently increased, the orbital rim and orbital floor were comminuted simultaneously.

The mechanism of blowout fracture (an increased hydraulic pressure) has been questioned by a number of authors (Rény and Stricker, 1969; Fujino, 1974a, b). Rény and Stricker suggested the following hypothesis: the traumatic force striking the inferior orbital rim, which is sufficiently resilient to transmit the force to the orbital floor, fractures the latter while the rim rebounds without fracturing. Fujino (1974a, b), in a series of experiments in collaboration with engineers, demonstrated on a dried human skull, without orbital contents, that a brass striker weighing 120 g with a flat silicone plate, when dropped on the infraorbital

TABLE 25-2. *Classification of Orbital Fractures**

1. Orbital blowout fractures
   A. Pure blowout fractures: fractures through the thin areas of the orbital floor, medial and lateral wall. The orbital rim is intact.
   B. Impure blowout fractures: fractures associated with fracture of the adjacent facial bones. The thick orbital rim is fractured, and its backward displacement causes a comminution of the orbital floor; the posterior displacement of the orbital rim permits the traumatizing force to be applied against the orbital contents, which produces a superimposed blowout fracture.
2. Orbital fractures without blowout fracture
   A. Linear fractures, in upper maxillary and zygomatic fractures. These fractures are often uncomplicated from the standpoint of the orbit.
   B. Comminuted fracture of the orbital floor with prolapse of the orbital contents into the maxillary sinus is often associated with fracture of the midfacial bones.
   C. Fracture of the zygoma with frontozygomatic separation and downward displacement of the zygomatic portion of the orbital floor and of the lateral attachment of the suspensory ligament of Lockwood.

*From Converse, J. M., Smith, B., Obear, M. F., and Wood-Smith, D.: Orbital blowout fractures: A ten-year study. Plast. Reconstr. Surg., *39*:20, 1967. Copyright 1967, The Williams & Wilkins Company, Baltimore.

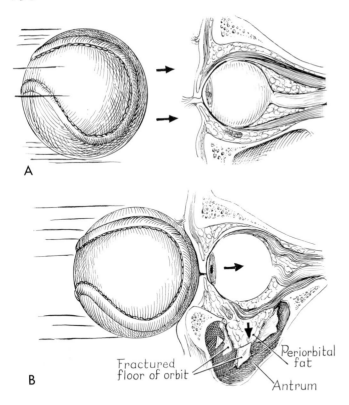

A

B

Fractured
floor of orbit

Periorbital
fat

Antrum

FIGURE 25–11. External pressure producing a blowout fracture of the orbital floor with entrapment of the inferior oblique and inferior rectus muscles and fascial expansions. Our first patient, in whom a diagnosis of blowout fracture was made, was hit by a hurling ball, here represented. (From Converse, J. M., and Smith, B.: Enophthalmos and diplopia in fractures of the orbital floor. Br. J. Plast. Surg., 9:265, 1957.)

"Impure" Blowout Fractures

According to Garrett (1963), ocular-orbital damage occurs in approximately 10 per cent of all head injuries sustained in automobile accidents in the United States. In the typical automotive injury in which the passenger's face is projected against the dashboard, the thick orbital rim is fractured and backwardly displaced, resulting in an eggshell comminution of the orbital floor. The continuing momentum and the pressure against the orbital contents produce a superimposed blowout fracture. It is to this type of orbital fracture that the term "impure" blowout fracture, as suggested by Cramer, Tooze, and Lerman (1965), may be applied (Table 25–2 and Fig. 25–12). The human fist was the principal factor in the causation of pure blowout fractures in the series studied by Emery and his associates (1971). In the series studied by Converse and his associates (1967), automobile accidents caused the largest proportion of fractures; most of these were impure and complicated fractures (see Table 25–1). Impure blowout fractures often occur in association with midfacial fractures.

Pyramidal maxillary fractures (Le Fort II) and craniofacial disjunction (Le Fort III) are characterized by fracture lines extending through the orbital floor, findings which further contribute to the comminution of the bone produced by the fractured orbital rim. Massive prolapse of the floor into the maxillary sinus may occur.

Not All Orbital Floor Fractures Are Blowout Fractures! The term "blowout" fracture (Converse and Smith, 1957) has been used to refer to all orbital floor fractures. Not every fracture of the floor of the orbit is a blowout fracture (see Table 25–2). The term "blowout" fracture defines a particular type of fracture mechanism. Orbital floor fractures, as stated earlier in the text, occur in fractures of the zygoma and in upper maxillary fractures, and comminuted fractures of the floor may result in a downward sagging of the orbital contents into the maxillary sinus.

Blowout Fracture in Children. The maxillary sinus is undeveloped in children. As a result, the floor of the orbit is situated in a low position, dipping downward from the orbital rim. Despite the resiliency and elasticity of young bones, blowout fractures are not infrequently seen in children. The mechanism of entrapment is similar to that seen in adults (Fig. 25–13).

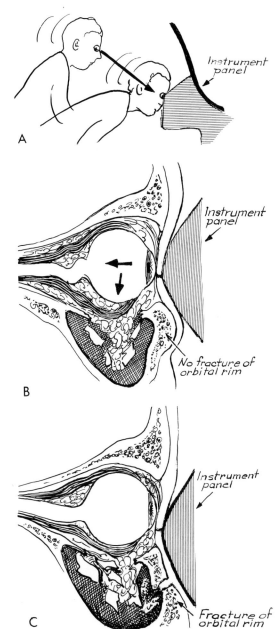

FIGURE 25–12. The pure and the impure blowout fracture. *A,* An automobile passenger's face striking the dashboard. *B,* If a protrusion in the dashboard does not fracture the orbital rim, a pure blowout fracture occurs. *C,* The mechanism of the impure blowout fracture. The inferior orbital rim is fractured, thus comminuting the weak portion of the orbital floor. Continuing pressure against the orbital contents produces a superimposed blowout fracture.

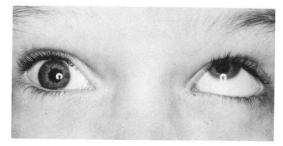

FIGURE 25–13. Blowout fracture in a child produced by the striking force of a snowball. Note the near complete fixity of the ocular globe and the enophthalmos.

tissue structures in the blowout fracture area, a finding which explains the constancy of vertical muscle imbalance (Table 25–3). These soft tissue structures may include the inferior rectus muscle, inferior oblique muscle, suspensory ligament of Lockwood, periorbita, and fascial expansions (see Fig. 25–8).

A downward displacement of one ocular globe does not always result in diplopia. Massive comminution of the orbital floor will cause a downward displacement of the ocular globe without entrapment: there is no diplopia.

The most common site of the blowout fracture is the portion of the floor that is weakened by the infraorbital canal or groove. The inferior oblique muscle arises from the maxillary portion of the orbital floor lateral to the lacrimal groove, and the inferior rectus muscle is situated immediately above the infraorbital canal on the undersurface of the orbital contents (see Fig. 25–8, *A*). It is not surprising, therefore, that these two muscles are frequently involved in the blowout fracture. Absence of elasticity in the impounded inferior

Surgical Pathology

Diplopia. Extraocular muscle imbalance and subjective diplopia are the result of deviation of the visual axes. The deviation has several causes: the major one is entrapment of the soft

TABLE 25–3. *Diplopia and Enophthalmos in Orbital Fractures*

1. *With diplopia, with enophthalmos.* This condition results from incarceration of the orbital contents into the area of the fracture and from tearing of the periorbita and escape of the orbital fat.
2. *With diplopia, without enophthalmos.* This condition may occur with fixation of the orbital contents in a linear fracture. There is no escape of orbital fat, no enlargement of the orbit, and no enophthalmos.
3. *Without diplopia, with enophthalmos.* There is no fixation of the inferior orbital contents into the area of the fracture. The periorbita is torn, and an opening has occurred which allows escape of orbital fat, or the orbital cavity is sufficiently enlarged to result in enophthalmos.
4. *Without diplopia, without enophthalmos.* This condition occurs when the fracture does not cause fixation of the orbital contents or disturb the anatomy of the periorbita or orbital cavity.

rectus muscle restricts rotation in the field of action of its antagonist, the superior rectus. Because the inferior rectus and the inferior oblique muscles are intimately connected at the point where the inferior oblique crosses beneath the inferior rectus, disturbance of function of the inferior oblique muscle is usually observed in blowout fractures. When the fracture is located lateral to the infraorbital groove or canal, the inferior rectus and inferior oblique muscles may not be involved. These variations in the site of the blowout fracture explain variations in the symptoms and clinical signs in these fractures.

NERVE INJURY. Injury to the motor nerves of the inferior oblique and inferior rectus muscles must also be considered. The inferior oblique and the inferior rectus muscles are innervated by the inferior division of the third cranial nerve. The branch to the inferior rectus muscle passes along its upper surface to pierce it at the junction of the posterior and middle thirds of the muscle. The branch to the inferior oblique muscle runs along the lateral edge of the inferior rectus muscle, enters the ocular surface of the inferior oblique muscle (see Fig. 25–8, B), and is exposed to injury in blowout fractures. The relatively short course of the nerve to the inferior rectus muscle renders it less vulnerable to injury. Electromyographic examination will assist in determining whether nerve conduction has been interrupted by the injury.

OTHER CAUSES OF DIPLOPIA. Other causes of diplopia are injury to the third, fourth, or sixth cranial nerves, direct injury to the extraocular muscles, laceration of the muscle by bone fragments, disruption of the muscle attachments, hemorrhage into the muscle, or muscle imbalance caused by a change in orbital shape. Secondary muscle imbalance occurs when ptosis of the globe is associated with enophthalmos. Secondary deviations are commonly due to overaction of the yoke or conjugate muscles of the opposite eye. A factor to be remembered is that no extraocular muscle acts singularly to produce ocular movements. Ocular rotation is the sum of the action, counteraction, and relaxation of 12 extraocular muscles (6 per ocular globe). It is not within the scope of this chapter to discuss the complex subject of the physiology of oculorotary muscles; only the aspects which pertain to the problem under discussion are explained.

Not only do paralytic deviations occur, but also trauma may often uncover tropias (constant imbalance) or phorias (latent imbalance occurring only with disruption of fusion) after temporary immobilization of the injured eye. These are usually horizontal in nature.

The typical blowout fracture is usually not seen in fracture-dislocation of the zygoma if the bone is displaced as a single fragment. In such a fracture, the site of impact is lateral to the orbital cavity and the orbital contents are usually not directly involved. In zygomatic fractures which are severely comminuted following an exceptionally strong impact, the lateral orbital wall and the rim and floor of the orbit may also be severely comminuted; the ocular globe is injured to the extent that enucleation may be required. A blowout with entrapment may have occurred, and release is necessary, even if the ocular globe is enucleated, to permit movement of the ocular prosthesis for purely esthetic reasons.

Enophthalmos. Enophthalmos, the second major complication of the blowout fracture, is the result of a number of causative factors. The first, the escape of fat from the orbital cavity, occurs when the periorbita is ruptured and the orbital fat escapes into the maxillary sinus (Fig. 25–14, A). A second cause of enophthalmos is the retention of the ocular globe in a backward position when the structures are entrapped in the fracture site (Figs. 25–14, B and 25–15). A third causative factor is the enlargement of the orbital cavity resulting from the fracture and the downward displacement of the orbital floor; the orbital fat is distributed in a large cavity (Fig. 25–14, C) and is no longer sufficient in quantity to prevent a sinking in of the globe (Fig. 25–16). A fourth factor is orbital fat necrosis resulting from pressure caused by orbital hematoma and a low grade inflammatory process.

The mechanism opposite to a blowout fracture is the "blow-in" fracture, in which penetration of bone fragments into the orbit diminishes the size of the orbital cavity, resulting in exophthalmos.

Enophthalmos, when it is conspicuous and particularly when orbital contents are downwardly displaced, results in a pseudoptosis of the upper eyelid, a deepening of the supratarsal fold (see Fig. 25–15, A), and a shortening of the horizontal dimension of the palpebral fissure. The deformity becomes more complex in orbital fractures associated with fractures of adjacent bones, especially a concomitant naso-orbital fracture.

Lower animals possess an orbital muscle which spans the floor of the orbit, covering the

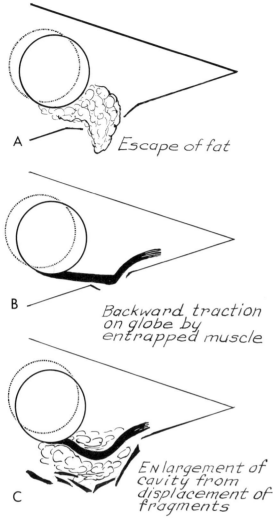

FIGURE 25-14. Three causes of enophthalmos in blowout fractures. *A*, Escape of orbital fat into the maxillary sinus. *B*, Entrapment maintaining a backward position of the ocular globe. *C*, Enlargement of the orbital cavity.

inferior orbital fissure; this muscle protrudes the eyeball for purposes of focusing vision. In man a vestige of this muscle has been designated as the orbital muscle. Some anatomists discount its importance; others claim that paralysis of the muscle is a factor in the production of enophthalmos in conditions such as Horner's syndrome, caused by paralysis of the third cranial nerve. Others feel that atrophic changes in the orbital fat due to injury of the sympathetic innervation may be responsible for the production of enophthalmos. Other factors which have been held responsible for the development of traumatic enophthalmos are dislocation of the trochlea of the superior oblique muscle, cicatricial contraction of retro-

bulbar tissue, and rupture of the orbital ligaments or fascial bands.

Enlargement of the orbital cavity as a factor in the causation of enophthalmos was suggested by Lang (1889): "I suggest that the injury may have produced a fracture and a depression of a portion of the orbital wall; the orbital fat would then be no longer sufficient in quantity to fill this enlarged postocular area without a sinking-in of the globe from atmospheric pressure and a resulting limitation in ocular movements."

The enlargement of the orbital cavity from the depression of the floor is a frequent factor in the production of enophthalmos. However, there may be no entrapment of the orbital structures and no diplopia (see Table 25-3).

ENOPHTHALMOS IN ORBITAL FRACTURES WITHOUT BLOWOUT FRACTURE. Fractures of

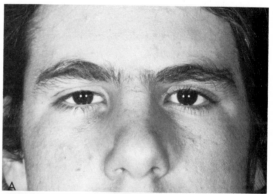

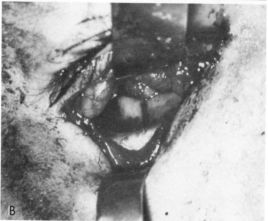

FIGURE 25-15. Enophthalmos produced by entrapment. *A*, Typical appearance of enophthalmos produced by entrapment by the orbital contents. *B*, The inferior orbital rim is intact. A linear fracture was located in the posterior reaches of the floor of the orbit. The photograph shows the entrapment. Because the fracture occurred posterior to the infraorbital canal, the patient had no loss of conduction of the inferior orbital nerve. The cause of the blowout fracture was the striking force of the elbow of a fellow football player.

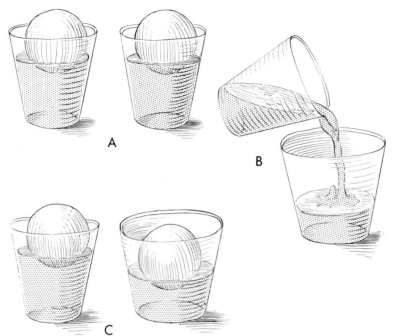

FIGURE 25–16. One of the mechanisms of production of enophthalmos: enlargement of the orbital cavity. *A,* Glass represents the orbital cavity, water represents the orbital fat, and the Ping-Pong ball represents the globe. An equal amount of water in each glass maintains the balls at the same level. *B,* Water is poured from one glass into a glass of larger size. *C,* The ball in the larger glass is at a lower level, although the amount of water is equal to that in the smaller glass. Thus, the ocular globe becomes enophthalmic not only when fat escapes from the orbit but also when orbital fat is in an orbital cavity enlarged by fracture. (From Converse, J. M., and Smith, B.: Enophthalmos and diplopia in fractures of the orbital floor. Br. J. Plast. Surg., *9:* 265, 1957.)

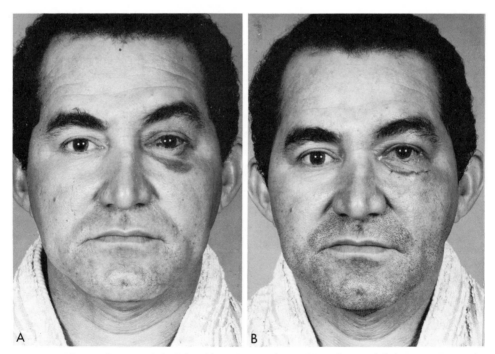

FIGURE 27–17. Blowout fracture of the left orbit. *A,* Forward gaze. Note the enophthalmos. *B,* Forward gaze after release of the herniated structures and restoration of the continuity of the orbital floor. Note the low eyelid incision (a higher incision is now preferred). The enophthalmos has been corrected.

Illustration continued on opposite page

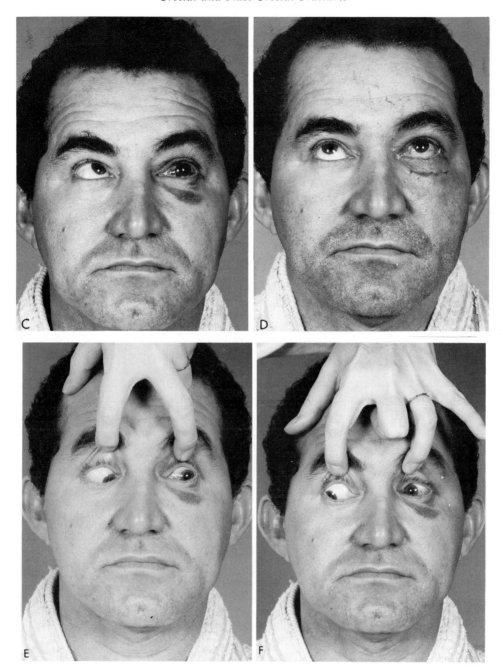

FIGURE 25–17 *Continued.* *C*, Restriction in the upward and lateral gaze before operation. *D*, Upward gaze after the operation, demonstrating the release of the entrapped orbital structures. *E*, The restriction in the dominant lateral gaze of the left ocular globe prior to operation. *F*, The restriction in the downward and inward gaze prior to operation. This patient was one of the first treated for a blowout fracture. (From Converse, J. M., and Smith, B.: Blowout fracture of the floor of the orbit. Trans. Am. Acad. Ophthalmol. Otolaryngol., *64*:676, 1960.)

the bones of the midfacial area often involve the orbital floor: Le Fort III fracture lines traverse the floor of the orbit; Le Fort II fractures also involve the orbital floor in its medial portion (see Table 25–2).

VARIATIONS IN DIPLOPIA AND ENOPHTHALMOS IN ORBITAL FRACTURES. Table 25–3 classifies the variations which occur in orbital

fractures according to the anatomical damage suffered by the orbit and its contents.

Examination and Diagnosis

Clinical Examination. In the typical blowout fracture, the patient complains of diplopia in the primary position which increases in the upward gaze. The patient may not recognize diplopia early if the eye is temporarily closed by edema of the lids or dressings or if there is an intraocular injury. When examined during the first hours after the fracture, the ocular globe appears displaced backward and downward (Fig. 25–17, *A*), and the supratarsal sulcus is deepened. Edema and hematoma may obscure such clinical findings when the patient is not examined during the first hours after injury. Ocular globe injury, eyelid damage, and lacerations and hematoma in the levator muscle or aponeurosis are not infrequently observed.

Diplopia is the most frequent complaint of the patient but is not necessarily an indication for operation; diplopia may be caused by hematoma and edema and may resolve spontaneously. Subjective diplopia is not an indication for surgical exploration.

When an object is held approximately two feet from the patient's eye and the patient is asked to look at the object, the affected eye is not able to rotate upward in the normal range as does the unaffected eye (Fig. 25–17, *C*); restriction in rotation in other directions is also observed (Figs. 25–17, *C, E, F* and 25–18). The function of the inferior rectus and inferior

oblique muscles is restricted by their entrapment in the floor of the orbit, and the superior rectus cannot rotate the globe because of the resistance offered by the short rein of the entrapped structures; when released, the globe is again able to rotate upward (see Fig. 25–17*D*). In a child, the authors have observed nearly complete fixity of the globe (see Fig. 25–13).

When the infraorbital rim is fractured (impure blowout fracture), one may observe that the lower lid is shortened vertically and everted. The infraorbital rim is displaced backward and in its forced retreat carries with it the insertion of the septum orbitale. This finding accounts for the vertical shortening of the lower eyelid (Fig. 25–19).

INDICATIONS FOR SURGICAL INTERVENTION. Although diplopia is the most frequent complaint of the patient, it is not an indication for operation, as diplopia may be caused by hematoma, edema, and neurogenic factors.

Indications for operation are: (1) limitation of forced rotation of the eyeball, (2) radiologic evidence of fracture, and (3) enophthalmos.

1. *Limitation of forced rotation of the eyeball.* This test, known as the "traction test" or the "forced duction test," provides a means of differentiating entrapment of the inferior rectus muscle from weakness or paralysis of

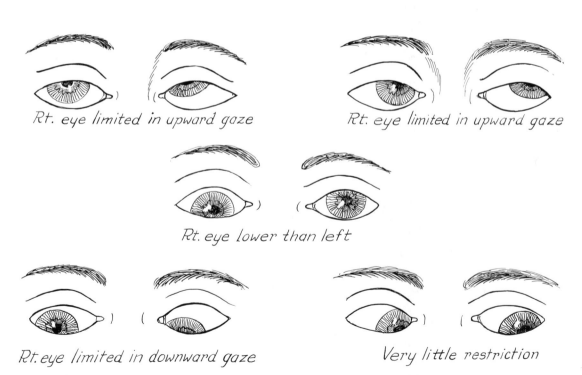

FIGURE 25–18. Diagrammatic representation of the limitation of oculorotary movements following a blowout fracture of the right orbit.

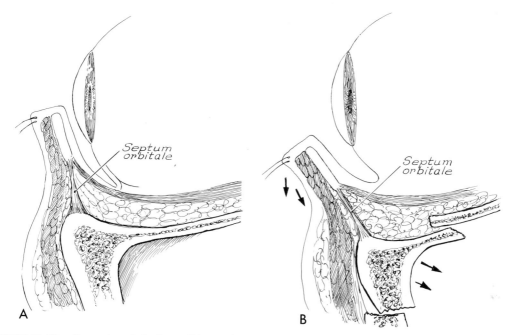

FIGURE 25–19. Shortening of the lower lid associated with orbital rim fracture. *A,* Sagittal section illustrating the insertion of the septum orbitale on the orbital rim. *B,* When the orbital rim is fractured and displaced backwards, the septum orbitale exerts a downward and backward traction upon the lower lid, causing vertical shortening and eversion.

the superior rectus, and *it is the pathognomonic sign of a blowout fracture of the floor of the orbit* (Fig. 25–20). A few drops of local anesthetic solution instilled into the conjunctival

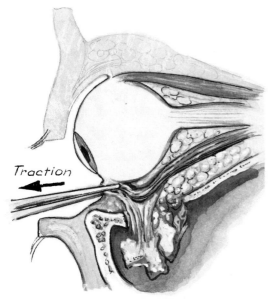

FIGURE 25–20. The forced duction test. Forceps grasp the ocular globe at the insertion of the inferior rectus muscle about 7 mm from the limbus.

sac provide sufficient anesthesia to permit grasping the eyeball with forceps at the insertion of the inferior rectus muscle at a point of approximately 7 mm from the limbus.

2. *Radiologic evidence of fracture.* Radiologic diagnosis is essential, and tomography is of additional assistance in locating the area of the blowout fracture. Careful roentgen examination will show a variety of findings and define the location, size, and type of the fracture site.

3. *Enophthalmos.* Clinically obvious enophthalmos is another indication for surgical exploration, as it suggests a gross derangement of the orbit — enlargement of the volume of the orbit resulting from the fracture of the floor or escape of orbital fat (Fig. 25–21).

SENSORY NERVE CONDUCTION LOSS. In a suspected orbital floor blowout fracture, anesthesia or hypoesthesia in the area of distribution of the infraorbital nerve is suggestive evidence of a blowout fracture involving the infraorbital groove or canal. This finding assists in locating the site of the blowout fracture. Absence of infraorbital anesthesia implies that the fractured area is either lateral, medial, or posterior to the infraorbital groove or canal and is not a sign that the orbital floor is not fractured. In the patient shown in Figure 25–15, *A,* a linear fracture occurred posterior to

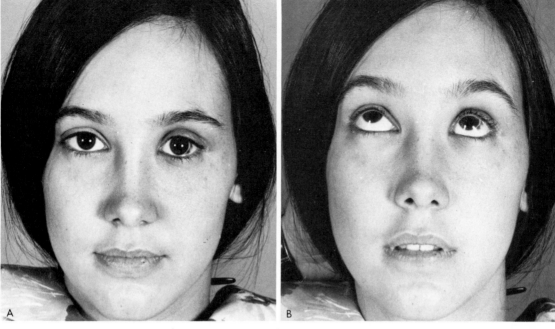

FIGURE 25–21. Orbital blowout fracture without gross entrapment. *A,* Appearance of the patient after receiving a blow over the left eye. Note the subconjunctival ecchymosis. *B,* Despite some restriction in the upward gaze, the forced duction test was negative. Exploration of the floor of the orbit showed comminution of a major portion of the orbit with collapse of the floor into the maxillary sinus. The floor of the orbit was reconstructed by an iliac bone graft. This is an example of a case in which the patient had no diplopia and a negative forced duction test; severe enophthalmos would have developed had the orbital floor and the architecture of the orbit not been restored by bone grafting.

the infraorbital canal, entrapping the soft structures (see Fig. 25–15, *B*).

Radiologic Examination. Because of the superimposition of both thick and thin bones, the roentgen picture is apt to be difficult to interpret. The diagnosis of orbital fracture by roentgenography is made by means of a variety of positions: the Caldwell position, the Waters position, the fronto-occipital position, the anteroposterior projection, the reverse Waters position, and the oblique orbital-optical foramen view.

Diagnosis of blowout fracture of the orbit is frequently missed if the radiologic examination is not comprehensive. Fracture lines may be mistaken for superimposed bony septa or suture lines, or they may be hidden by disease processes in the underlying maxillary sinus. The thin orbital floor, partially transparent on radiographs, may be obscured against the background of other bones of the skull. Tomography will often disclose the presence of a blowout fracture and its location (Zizmor and coworkers, 1962).

Polytomography, as well as hypocycloidal movement, is advocated in all skull radiography. It brings into focus a 1-mm thin layer

of tissue with reasonable clarity and sharpness. It is far superior to the curvilinear tomography formerly used.

With adequate technique, blowout fractures of the orbit can be diagnosed in over 90 per cent of the cases with conventional radiography (Fig. 25–22, *A*). Polytomography has a similar degree of diagnostic accuracy and, in addition, can delineate the location, depth, and extent of the fracture with a degree of clarity and accuracy not possible with conventional radiography (Fig. 25–22, *B*).

The type of blowout fracture varies: a lowering of the orbital floor; the "hanging drop," seen in the blowout fracture through which the orbital fat has extruded into the maxillary sinus (Fig. 25–23); the trapdoor fracture, one or two bone fragments hanging into the sinus on a periosteal hinge (Fig. 25–24); the massive extrusion of orbital contents into the maxillary sinus (Fig. 25–25); associated fracture of the medial wall (Fig. 25–25, *B*). Such positive radiologic signs, combined with positive clinical signs, are indications for surgical intervention. Crikelair, Rein, Potter, and Cosman (1972) have drawn attention to the danger of "overoperating" when only presumptive radiologic signs (such as opacity of the maxillary

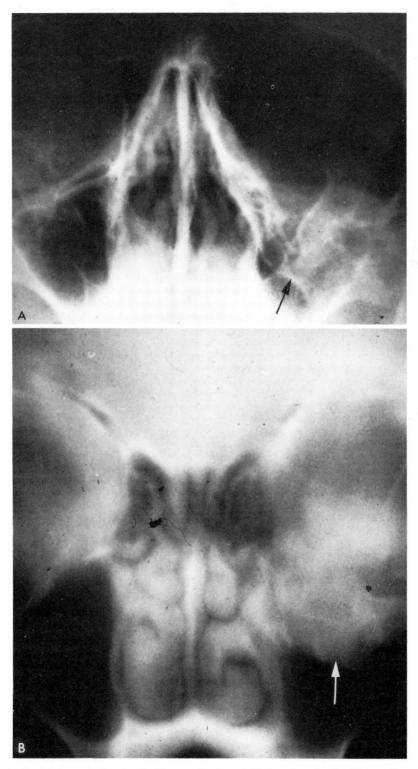

FIGURE 25–22.   Roentgenogram showing the blowout fracture. *A*, Waters view showing blowout fracture of the orbital floor (as indicated by the arrow). *B*, The tomogram shows the prolapse of the orbital contents into the maxillary sinus (arrow). (Figs. 25–22 to 25–25 courtesy of Dr. J. Zizmor.)

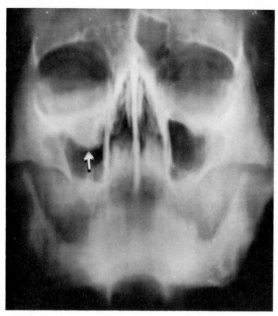

FIGURE 25-23. Tomogram shows prolapse of the orbital contents into the maxillary sinus (arrow).

sinus) are present. Certainly in the absence of positive clinical signs, surgical intervention should not be undertaken on the basis of presumptive radiologic signs alone.

Treatment

The three main purposes of surgical treatment are to (1) disengage entrapped structures and restore oculorotary function; (2) replace orbi-

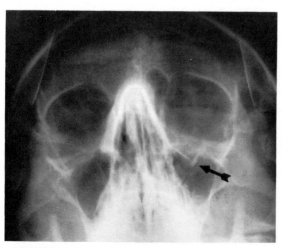

FIGURE 25-24. Roentgenogram showing blowout fracture (arrow) with fragments of bone hanging on periosteal hinges into the maxillary sinus.

tal fat into the orbital cavity if it has prolapsed into the maxillary sinus; and (3) restore orbital cavity size and form to minimize extraocular muscle imbalance and enophthalmos.

Once these primary objectives of treatment have been achieved and the bony architecture of the orbit is restored, additional surgery may be required to restore oculorotary function and to correct residual deformities or malfunction of the ocular adnexa.

Timing of Surgery. It is not necessary to operate immediately, particularly if post-traumatic edema is present. It is usually advisable to wait a few days, as subsidence of edema can be expected in this period of time. Delay beyond seven days is dangerous, particularly in children, as bone regeneration is rapid and the freeing of incarcerated orbital contents becomes more difficult. If treatment is postponed for two or three weeks, complications consisting of late motility problems as well as enophthalmos may be encountered. Undue delay, therefore, is not advocated.

In a large series of facial fractures studied by Hakelius and Pontén (1973), 21.8 per cent of the patients with midfacial fractures had double vision. By comparing a series of cases treated within two weeks after the accident and another series in which treatment was delayed, Hakelius and Pontén, in a follow-up study, found that 16 per cent of the patients in the first group reported the presence of diplopia only when they were tired (93 per cent were completely free of diplopia); in the second group, 24 per cent still had unchanged diplopia. As a result of the study an early, active surgical approach was recommended. It is significant that in a series of 50 patients with blowout fracture and other complications referred following unsuccessful, delayed treatment (mean time between trauma and surgery 3 1/2 weeks), 43 patients showed extraocular muscle imbalance (Converse and coworkers, 1967). Emery, von Noorden and Schlernitzauer (1971) also reported the clinical findings in 159 patients with orbital floor fractures. They reported late diplopia in 60 per cent of patients with untreated blow out fractures when the diplopia was still present 15 days after injury.

SURGICAL TREATMENT: YES OR NO? The authors have had a few patients in whom the entrapment was relieved by the forced duction test; these patients often do not require any further treatment. It is difficult to agree with Putterman, Stevens, and Urist (1974), who advocate the nonsurgical management of blowout fractures of the orbital floor. Putterman and

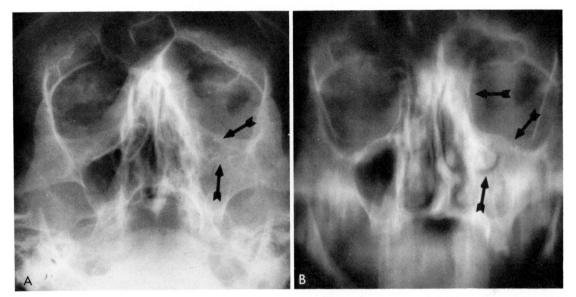

FIGURE 25–25.   Waters view showing fracture of the floor of the left orbit and tomogram showing fracture of the medial wall of the orbit. *A*, Prior to a radiologic examination, blood in the left maxillary sinus was aspirated and air was substituted. The Waters view shows a depressed fracture of the left orbital floor with downward herniation of orbital tissues (arrows). *B*, The tomogram shows the fracture and the downward herniation of the orbital tissues profiled by a trace of air in the opaque left maxillary sinus. The tomogram also showed a fracture of the medial orbital wall, as indicated by opacification of the ethmoidal cells. There is emphysema of the left orbit (arrows).

his associates reported 25 per cent residual diplopia in a retrospective study and 27 per cent residual diplopia in a prospective study. Enophthalmos occurred in 65 per cent of the patients in the retrospective study and in 36 per cent of the patients in the prospective study.

Each case should be considered individually, and the decision for or against exploratory surgery is made on the basis of the criteria set forth above. One must bear in mind that diplopia is not the only major consequence of a blowout fracture; enophthalmos can be a major complication if the surgeon is content to watch the ocular globe sink progressively into the orbital cavity.

Operative Technique.   A number of questions are usually asked concerning the method of treating blowout fractures. First and foremost is whether the method of approach to the orbital floor is through the eyelid or through the canine fossa and the maxillary sinus.

Although the eyelid or conjunctival approach to the orbital floor is preferred because it facilitates disengagement of the entrapped orbital tissues, the authors recognize that the approach to the orbital floor through the canine fossa and the maxillary sinus is indicated occasionally for the removal of bone fragments in the maxillary sinus and has merit in commi-

nuted fractures of the maxilla and other bones of the midfacial area. Indeed, the placing of gauze packing or an inflatable balloon may be the only method of maintaining the contour of the orbital floor when these bones are fragmented into small pieces. A trapdoor type of fracture can be supported by gauze packing once the entrapment has been relieved.

In the absence of a blowout fracture without entrapment, intramaxillary sinus packing may effectively support the comminuted orbital floor at a suitable level. However, maxillary sinus packing may be dangerous when it is excessive. In the patient shown in Figure 25–26, the globe was pushed upward under considerable pressure. Simultaneous observation of the floor of the orbit through the eyelid approach at the time of maxillary sinus packing would have prevented this complication. Suppuration has also been observed after gauze packing of the maxillary sinus, and blindness has been reported following this procedure. McCoy and associates (1962) reported a case in which packing of the maxillary sinus caused fragments of bone to damage the optic nerve with ensuing blindness. They condemn the method as dangerous, archaic, and ineffective in giving support to the fragments.

The maxillary sinus approach alone is not satisfactory for the release of the entrapped or-

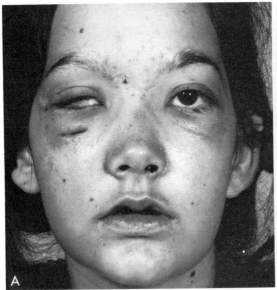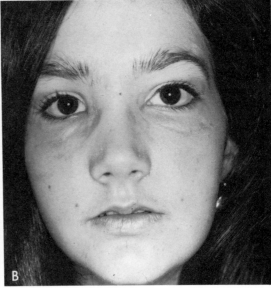

FIGURE 25–26. Excessive elevation of orbital floor after maxillary sinus packing. *A,* Blowout fracture of the right orbit treated by gauze packing placed in the maxillary sinus. The ocular globe has been pushed upwards to the point where the pupil is hidden by the upper eyelid. *B,* After removal of the maxillary sinus packing, exploration of the floor of the orbit through an eyelid incision and restoration of the continuity of the fractured orbital floor. This case demonstrates the danger of attempting to restore the level of the orbital floor by maxillary sinus packing without direct observation of the orbital floor through an eyelid incision. Excessive compression by packing may cause blindness.

bital soft tissues or for placing the orbital floor graft or implant. In a follow-up study of a series of 50 complicated cases, eight patients whose fractures had been repaired through the maxillary sinus alone required the trans-eyelid approach to release the incarcerated orbital contents from the surrounding impacted healed bony fragments (Table 25–4).

TABLE 25–4. *Analysis of Complications in Orbital Fractures Persistent after Floor Repair* (50 cases)†*

		POSTOPERATIVE	
	PREOPER-	*3*	*1*
COMPLICATIONS	ATIVE	*Months*	*Year*
Extraocular muscle imbalance	43	30	20
Enophthalmos	27	15	11
Ptosis	12	3	2
Medial canthal deformity	12	12	9
Lacrimal obstruction	3	3	0
Vertical shortening of the lower lid	4	4	2
Visual impairment	5	5	5
Trichiasis-symblepharon	2	1	0

*These complications were observed in patients referred to us after unsuccessful treatment.

†From Converse, J. M., Smith, B., Obear, M. F., and Wood-Smith, D.: Orbital blowout fractures: A ten-year study. Plast. Reconstr. Surg., *39:*20, 1967. Copyright 1967, The Williams & Wilkins Company, Baltimore.

The use of gauze packing or an inflated balloon is indicated when the orbital floor is comminuted and prolapsed into the maxillary sinus. Support of the comminuted fragments restores the floor of the orbit to the level of the floor on the contralateral side. The orbital floor should be explored, however, through an eyelid incision in order to check the level of the supported floor, to release an entrapment, if present, and to introduce an implant or transplant.

EXPOSURE OF THE ORBITAL FLOOR

The incision. Various types of incisions through the lower eyelid may be employed. The one stroke incision to the orbital rim has the disadvantage of causing a unified line of cicatricial tissue which may result in a retracted scar and vertical shortening of the lower lid.

Although the subciliary incision near the margin of the lid about 3 mm below the lashline (Fig. 25–27) leaves an inconspicuous scar, an incision through one of the skin folds of the lower lid is also inconspicuous after healing and requires less dissection. The subciliary incision is made through the skin and orbicularis muscle until the tarsus is reached. At this point, the muscle (pretarsal portion of the orbicularis) is raised from the tarsus, the septum orbitale comes into view below the tarsus, and the dissection over the septum orbitale is con-

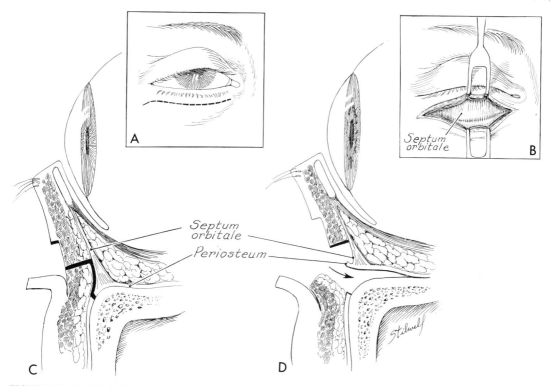

FIGURE 25–27. Technique of exposure of the orbital floor. *A,* Outline of the eyelid incision. *B,* Septum orbitale exposed. *C,* Sagittal section showing skin incision through orbicularis oculi muscle and path of dissection over the septum orbitale to the orbital rim. *D,* Periosteum of the orbit (periorbita) is raised from the orbital floor. (From Converse, J. M., Cole, J. G., and Smith, B.: Late treatment of blowout fracture of the floor of the orbit. Plast. Reconstr. Surg., *28*:183, 1961.)

tinued to the rim of the orbit. An incision below the tarsus obviates the need for as much dissection and is less liable to cause vertical shortening of the lid.

The conjunctival approach is another incision which has been advocated by Tessier (1973) in craniofacial anomalies and by Converse, Firmin, Wood-Smith and Friedland (1973) in post-traumatic deformities. If careful dissection is done according to the technique shown in Figure 25–28, it permits the surgeon to avoid perforating the septum orbitale with consequent extrusion of the orbital fat.

A simplified technique employed by Tenzel and Miller (1971) consists of a direct incision in the fornix which reaches the orbital rim and a retroseptal approach which exposes the orbital fat. A Desmarres retractor is used to retract the lower eyelid away from the globe. A malleable retractor placed posterior to the orbital rim gives adequate exposure (Fig. 25–29). The incision is made through the conjunctiva to the orbital rim and includes the periosteum. This incision of necessity penetrates through the

septum orbitale and exposes orbital fat. Tenzel and Miller have employed this type of incision in patients with small blowout fractures without restriction of ocular rotary movements of the globe. They did not employ the incision in patients with massive fractures with herniation of the orbital contents into the maxillary sinus.

The conjunctival incision avoids an external scar, albeit inconspicuous, and claims have been made that it prevents postoperative lower lid lagophthalmos in the upward gaze.

Because of the need to preserve the orbital fat and recuperate fat which has extruded into the maxillary sinus, it is preferable to avoid extrusion of fat through the septum orbitale, whenever possible.

When the orbital rim has been reached by following the septum orbitale downward (see Figs. 25–27, *B*, *C* and 25–30), an incision through the periosteum is made immediately below the orbital rim (see Fig. 25–27, *C*, *D*). Subperiosteal elevation is extended backward until the area of the blowout fracture is identified (see Fig. 25–27, *D*). The infraorbital

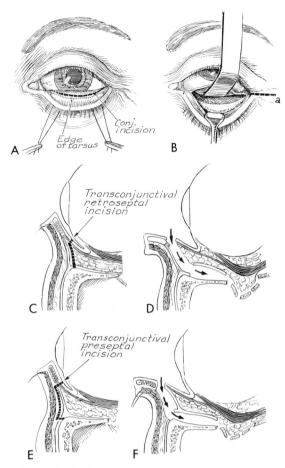

FIGURE 25–28. Transconjunctival approach. *A,* Conjunctival incision below the lower border of the tarsus. *B,* Subperiosteal exposure of the orbital floor. Dotted line shows the lateral canthal extension for additional exposure. *C,* Retroseptal approach. *D,* Sagittal view of retroseptal approach to the fracture. *E,* Preseptal incision. *F,* Sagittal view of the preseptal approach to the fracture.

displaced backward, it is essential that the fragments be realigned in their former position. This measure will prevent postoperative vertical shortening of the lower eyelid.

The inferior rectus muscle and orbital structures are liberated from the areas of the blowout. The floor must be explored sufficiently far back into the orbit until the posterior edge of the defect can be identified. Verification that the ocular globe is freed from the fracture site is obtained by the forced duction test (see Fig. 25–20); it is essential to demonstrate the full range of all oculorotary movements. The most common cause of failure to release the entrapped structures is inadequate exposure of the floor in depth. The fracture may be far back; in the patient shown in Figure 25–15, a linear fracture situated posteriorly had entrapped the structures.

RESTORATION OF THE CONTINUITY OF THE ORBITAL FLOOR. Restoration of the continuity of the orbital floor is required in all orbital floor fractures, except in small fractures in which the entrapped structures can be freed readily and the forced duction test shows that free rotation of the eyeball has been reestablished.

Bone grafts. An iliac bone graft (a split rib graft in children) taken from the smooth inner aspect of the ilium is preferable in fractures in which there is a wide area of communication between the orbit and the maxillary sinus (Fig. 25–32). The bone graft, as it becomes vascularized, is better able to resist bacterial invasion than an inorganic implant. The authors have given preference to the bone graft in all major fractures with disruption of the orbital

nerve should be respected; with the aid of visual magnification with binocular loupes, the nerve may be carefully dissected from the herniated and entrapped soft tissues.

The orbital structures should be raised using a caterpillar technique with two retractors. Dural pliable retractors with rounded edges minimize pressure on the ocular globe. Retraction of the intraorbital contents should be relaxed periodically. When necessary, a wide exposure can be obtained through the eyelid incision (Fig. 25–31).

If the infraorbital rim is also fractured (impure blowout fracture), the fragments are realigned and fixation is maintained by interosseous wiring. If the orbital rim has been

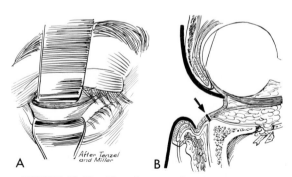

FIGURE 25–29. The direct conjunctival approach to the orbital floor. *A,* One retractor depresses the globe; another retractor depresses the lower lid. The infraorbital rim protrudes under the conjunctiva. *B,* The conjunctiva is incised, exposing the orbital rim.

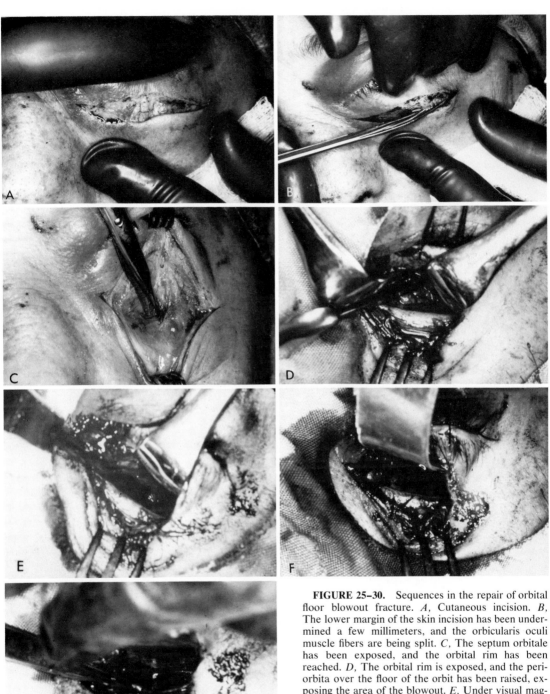

FIGURE 25–30. Sequences in the repair of orbital floor blowout fracture. *A,* Cutaneous incision. *B,* The lower margin of the skin incision has been undermined a few millimeters, and the orbicularis oculi muscle fibers are being split. *C,* The septum orbitale has been exposed, and the orbital rim has been reached. *D,* The orbital rim is exposed, and the periorbita over the floor of the orbit has been raised, exposing the area of the blowout. *E,* Under visual magnification using binocular loupes, the entrapped structures are released. Care is taken to avoid damage to the infraorbital nerve. *F,* The area of the blowout fracture can be seen after the entrapped structures are released. *G,* Continuity of the floor of the orbit is reestablished by the placement of a Teflon implant.

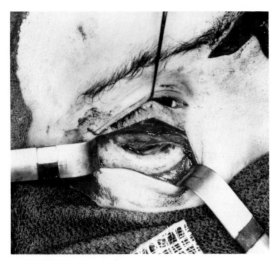

FIGURE 25–31. Exposure obtained through an eyelid incision.

floor. We have also used the anterior wall of the maxillary sinus in the area of the canine fossa, the perpendicular plate of the ethmoid, and the septal cartilage for the restoration of small defects of the floor. Costal cartilage has also been employed and constitutes an excellent, seldom used transplant. Irradiated cartilage allografts have been employed by Dingman and Grabb (1961).

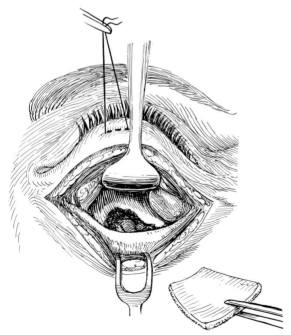

FIGURE 25–32. A thin iliac bone graft has been carved and shaped and is placed so as to straddle the area of the blowout.

The mucous membrane lining of the subjacent maxillary sinus, often ruptured, will repair itself and line the undersurface of the transplant.

Inorganic implants. Inorganic materials employed in the orbital region have included solids, sponges, gels, and liquids. Tantalum, stainless steel, Vitallium, Paladon, methylmethacrylate, polyvinyl sponge, polyurethane, polyethylene, Teflon, Silastic, and Supramid have been commonly used.

Ballen (1964) employed Cranioplast, a rapidly polymerizing methylmethacrylate, which is prepared by mixing powdered acrylic with a liquid catalyst. The material is molded in situ and hardens by a process of polymerization, which gives off considerable heat. Ballen has used this procedure in 31 patients but does not mention complications. Miller and Tenzel (1969) have employed prefabricated Cranioplast implants, which are prepared in various sizes and thicknesses, in over 300 patients (Tenzel, 1974). The prefabrication has the advantage of eliminating the time interval required for the polymerization of the methylmethacrylate.

Freeman (1962) implanted sheets of Teflon in 36 patients with orbital floor fracture, despite communication with the maxillary sinus in several; Browning and Walker (1965) have reported the successful use of Teflon in 45 patients with orbital blowout fractures. Our own experience confirms these findings. Teflon is available in sheets 1-mm thick, and Silastic may also be carved to fit the specific defect. Supramid sheets 0.3-mm thick are also available.

The inorganic implant offers the advantage of obviating the need for an additional concomitant operation for the removal of a bone graft, and it has been satisfactory in most simple fractures. The authors have also had successful results in large defects with a wide area of communication with the maxillary sinus. In the course of secondary operations, regeneration of the maxillary sinus lining under the implant and, in moderate-sized defects, bone regeneration have been observed.

The purpose of the orbital floor insert, whether bone graft or inorganic implant, is to reestablish the continuity of the floor, seal off the orbit from the maxillary sinus, and restore the volume of the orbital cavity. The orbital floor insert should bridge the defect and rest on the stable adjacent portions of the floor. Smooth materials such as Teflon tend to slide forward and protrude under the skin of the eyelid. A tongue is prepared by making two cuts in the implant (Fig. 25–33); the tongue is introduced under the anterior edge of the bony defect in the orbital floor, thus maintaining it in position and avoiding forward displacement and extrusion. Care should also be taken to avoid dead space between the inorganic implant and the bone of the orbital floor, as the accumulated fluid in the dead space constitutes a favorable medium for the growth of bacteria.

Blowout Fractures: Variations

A concomitant naso-orbital fracture suggests the possibility of an associated blowout fracture through the lamina papyracea of the medial orbital wall.

A major portion of the floor may be collapsed into the maxillary sinus. More limited blowout fractures are located medially, centrally, or laterally. The central blowout is typical of the pure blowout fracture. The medial blowout often occurs in the impure type associated with a naso-orbital fracture, a fracture of the medial orbital wall, and a blowout through the lamina papyracea. The lateral blowout occurs in the impure type associated with fracture of the zygoma.

There is no standard pattern in blowout fractures; fixity of the eyeball may be observed in massive blowout fractures as well as in small

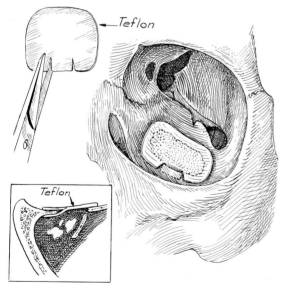

FIGURE 25–33. Technique to prevent forward displacement of a Teflon implant. The tongue slipped under the anterior border of the bony defect blocks the forward migration of the implant.

blowout fractures. In one case, the inferior orbital contents were pierced and pinned to the floor by a sharp bone fragment. The entire orbital floor may be fragmented and hanging hammocklike into the maxillary sinus, and the patient suffers no diplopia because oculorotary action is only slightly impaired (see Fig. 25–21). The prolapse of the orbital contents into the maxillary sinus may be extreme; in some of these cases, the ocular globe is difficult to find. The authors recall a patient in whom a long nasal speculum was necessary to retract the edematous eyelids in order to locate the ocular globe. The most dramatic case of this sort involved a fireman who inadvertently turned on the full power of his fire hose as he was inspecting the inside of the nozzle. The resultant blowout fracture was of such extent that the ocular globe disappeared from the orbital cavity and was presumed to have been enucleated by the force of the projected blast of water. The eyeball, which underwent several choroidal tears, was subsequently located in the maxillary sinus and replaced in position. After repair of the orbital floor and a normal postoperative course, the patient's vision was 20/20 for reading and 20/60 for distant vision.

Fractures of the Medial Orbital Wall. Medial orbital wall fractures usually occur in conjunction with an orbital floor fracture or a naso-orbital fracture. A special etiologic factor is the ski pole, the tip of which has struck the medial canthal area.

CLINICAL FINDINGS. Rougier (1965) reported tethering of the medial rectus muscle following a blowout fracture, strongly suggesting an associated fracture of the medial orbital wall into the ethmoid sinus with entrapment of the medial rectus by a blowout mechanism similar to that which occurs in the orbital floor. Fractures of the medial wall were also noted by Miller and Glaser (1966), Edwards and Ridley (1968), Trochel and Potter (1969), Dodick, Galin, Littleton and Sod (1971), and Rumelt and Ernest (1972). The clinical signs were progressively increasing enophthalmos, narrowing of the palpebral fissure, horizontal diplopia with restriction of abduction, and increasing enophthalmos on abduction.

It has been suggested that medial orbital wall fractures are associated with orbital floor blowout fracture in an incidence varying from 5 per cent to 50 per cent (Gould and Titus, 1966; Jones and Evans, 1967; Dodick and co-workers, 1971). The high percentage can be explained by the structural relationships between the orbital floor and the medial wall described in an earlier section of the chapter. Our own experience, as well as that of Prasad (1973), is that entrapment of the medial rectus muscle is rare and that many of these fractures are found on radiographic examination to be in association with a naso-orbital fracture. The cellular structure of the ethmoid bone offers resistance which the hollow maxillary sinus beneath the orbital floor does not. The possibility of a concomitant blowout fracture of the medial orbital wall should be suspected, however, if enophthalmos develops following adequate treatment of an orbital floor fracture.

RADIOLOGIC FINDINGS. The diagnosis is often made by radiography; the presence of air within the orbit, clouding of the ethmoid sinus (see Fig. 25–25), and medial displacement of the medial orbital wall or displaced fragments of bone (Fig. 25–34) often seen on tomography demonstrate a medial wall fracture. The radiologic examination is invaluable in verifying the integrity of the medial wall preoperatively so that adequate measures can be taken at the time of surgery.

TREATMENT. Depending on the severity of the fracture, exposing the medial orbital wall, freeing the medial rectus muscle if it is entrapped, and placing an inorganic implant over the area of fracture will usually suffice to restore the architecture of the orbit. Primary bone grafting may be required in massive com-

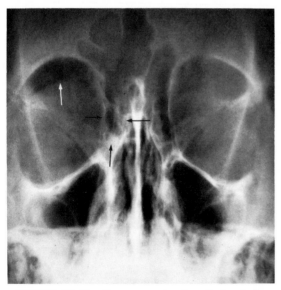

FIGURE 25–34. Tomogram showing displaced fragments (arrows) in the medial orbital wall, clouding of the ethmoid sinus, and medial displacement of a portion of the medial orbital roof. Note also fracture of the orbital roof (arrow).

minuted fractures. The treatment varies, therefore, according to the clinical and radiologic findings; abstention from surgical treatment is indicated when only a linear fracture is present.

Progressively developing enophthalmos may be the price to pay for the failure to diagnose a medial wall fracture.

Fractures of the Lateral Orbital Wall. The lateral orbital wall consists of a strong, resistant anterior frontozygomatic rim which is exposed to facial trauma and a thinner posterior portion (see Fig. 25–6) formed by the orbital process of the greater wing of the sphenoid.

The most severe fractures of the lateral wall of the orbit occur in conjunction with massive trauma to the zygomatic area with frontozygomatic disjunction and downward displacement of the lateral portion of the orbital floor. The lateral canthus is dislocated downward, with ectropion of the lower eyelid. This type of fracture requires a direct approach similar to that employed in multiple fractures of the midfacial skeleton (see Chapter 24, page 732). Direct interosseous wiring of the fragments and primary bone grafting to restore the orbital floor, lateral wall, and zygomatic osseous framework are indicated. In such severe fractures, the ocular globe suffers injury of varying degree, and loss of vision is not infrequent.

Lateral wall fractures are probably more frequent than is generally assumed. The authors have noted a number of such fractures during craniofacial operations performed for the correction of grossly malunited fractures. In some cases, orbital fat was found in the temporal fossa, suggesting a blowout fracture of the posterior portion of the lateral orbital wall. Behind the thick, lateral orbital rim is an area of thin bone; fracture of the rim may comminute this thin portion of the lateral orbital wall, facilitating a blowout of the area. Such a fracture may also be an unsuspected cause of persistent postoperative enophthalmos.

Fractures of the Orbital Roof. LaGrange (1918), in his classic monograph, showed that the thin medial portion of the orbital roof is fractured and displaced in its posterior part in the region of the superior orbital fissure and optic foramen (Fig. 25–35). A fracture of this type can lead to serious complications, such as optic nerve atrophy and injury to the nerves to the extraocular muscles which enter the superior orbital fissure. Dodick, Galin, Littleton and Sod (1971), in a series of 22 cases of suspected

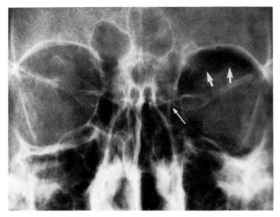

FIGURE 25-35. Roentgenogram showing evidence of fracture of the roof of the left orbit (two arrows). There is also a fracture of the medial wall, as evidenced by orbital emphysema and clouding of the ethmoid cells (one arrow). (Courtesy of Dr. J. Zizmor.)

blowout fracture of the orbit, obtained radiologic evidence of fracture of the orbital floor in 15 cases; in two cases there was a concomitant fracture of the orbital roof.

Fracture of the orbital roof may also occur in conjunction with naso-orbital fractures, as the medial portion of the orbital roof is thinner and more susceptible to fracture.

If the superior rim of the orbit is fractured and the trochlea of the superior oblique muscle is displaced, consequent impairment of the function of the superior oblique muscle may result in diplopia, which is usually temporary.

Fractures of the orbital roof usually occur in conjunction with fractures of the supraorbital rim and frontal bone. A combined craniofacial approach is required in these fractures. The dura, which may be torn or penetrated by comminuted fragments, is raised and retracted. In such cases, after exposure of the anterior cranial fossa and neurosurgical repair, the orbital roof is repaired by a suitable thin bone graft.

ORBITAL FLOOR FRACTURES WITHOUT BLOWOUT FRACTURE

Examination and Diagnosis

Clinical Examination. The symptoms and signs of fractures of the floor of the orbit without blowout fracture are similar to those of a blowout fracture, with the fundamental difference that the patient is able to effect ocu-lorotary movements in an essentially normal fashion. The forced duction test is negative. There may be transitory diplopia.

Roentgenographic Examination. Tomograms will fail to reveal the characteristic excrescence of the orbital contents into the maxillary sinus, although in crushing fractures the orbital rim and the floor of the orbit may have collapsed into the sinus. Maxillary and zygomatic fracture lines involving the orbital floor and irregularity of the contour of the infraorbital rim are noted on roentgenograms in these types of fractures.

Treatment

Fractures of the orbital floor occurring in zygomatic and maxillary fractures often do not require orbital intervention other than realignment and wiring of the fragments of the fractured orbital rim. The treatment is that required for the maxillary or zygomatic fracture. Verification should always be made, however, that the patient does not have a blowout fracture. Careful checking of the oculorotary movements and radiologic examination will eliminate this possibility.

In fractures with bony displacement, the risk of enlargement of the orbital cavity and of consequent enophthalmos is an important consideration. Treatment of an orbital fracture is done in conjunction with the reduction and fixation of fractures of other bones of the midfacial area. Measures are taken to restore the bony continuity of the displaced or fragmented bones. This is best done by direct exposure of the fractured area, reduction, and interosseous wire fixation.

When there is doubt as to the integrity of the orbital floor, exploration is indicated in order to eliminate an occult comminuted and depressed fracture.

Comminuted Fractures of the Orbital Floor. In cases of exceptionally severe "crush" and "crash" injuries seen following accidents in automobiles, helicopters, or airplanes and usually associated with other fractures of the midfacial skeleton, the orbital rim and floor may be completely demolished. The fragments of bone, most of them suspended hammocklike from the periosteum, and the orbital contents sink into the maxillary sinus. The bone is pulverized or reduced to small particles. If bone fragments can be salvaged, they are used to reconstruct the orbital rim. The lateral wall must be stabilized by interosseous fixation prior to reconstruction of the orbital floor. Ocular globe injury often requires enucleation. Opening the maxillary sinus through the canine fossa provides an approach to the fragmented orbital floor, which is elevated by packing the maxillary sinus with gauze impregnated with antibiotic ointment. Small portions of the orbital floor may remain laterally and medially and serve to support the bone graft used to restore the orbital floor and rim. Wire fixation is often required to stabilize the graft. In one of our patients whose eye was enucleated, a shelf of bone was found only in the posterior reaches of the orbit.

area of the facial skeleton. The bones of the middle third of the face are also in close anatomical relationship to the floor of the anterior cranial fossa and the frontal lobes of the brain through the frontal and ethmoid sinuses and the cribriform plate. The possibility of a concomitant blowout fracture of the orbital floor has also been discussed.

Because of the possibility of brain damage, patients suffering these fractures should be observed for neurologic complications, such as progressive loss of consciousness, and signs of epidural hematoma, aerocele, and chronic subdural hematoma. Fracture of the odontoid process, which requires early reduction, has been reported. Pulmonary edema is another complication of head injuries.

NASO-ORBITAL FRACTURES

Severe injuries of the midfacial area associated with fractures of the maxilla, nasal bones, zygomas, or orbits may also be complicated by fracture of the bones of the frontoethmoidal

Structural Aspects

The thin areas of the medial orbital wall transilluminate readily and thus contrast with the heavier abutments formed by the nasal process

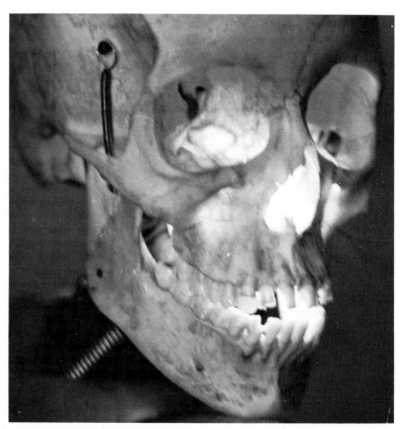

FIGURE 25–36.   Human skull photographed with a light source placed at the base of the skull behind the naso-orbital region. Thin bony areas of the medial orbital wall transluminate readily and thus contrast with the thick and heavier abutments formed by the nasal bones, frontal processes of the maxilla, and nasal process of the frontal bone. (From Converse, J. M., and Smith, B.: Naso-orbital fractures and traumatic deformities of the medial canthus. Plast. Reconstr. Surg., *38:* 147, 1966.)

of the frontal bone, the frontal processes of the maxilla, and the thick upper portions of the nasal bones (Fig. 25–36). Posterior to the frontal process of the maxilla, the thinner lacrimal bone and the delicate lamina papyracea are vulnerable to trauma. The anterior and posterior ethmoidal foramina are situated along the upper border of the lamina papyracea in the frontoethmoidal suture, where the orbital plate of the frontal bone and the lamina papyracea of the ethmoid are joined. The anterior ethmoidal foramen transmits the nasociliary nerve and the anterior ethmoidal vessels; the posterior ethmoidal foramen gives passage to the posterior ethmoidal nerve and vessels. The rupture of these vessels in naso-orbital fractures with backward penetrating fragments is one of the causes of orbital hematoma, a complication which may require immediate incision and drainage.

The most posterior portion of the medial orbital wall is formed by the body of the sphenoid immediately in front of the optic foramen. In severe skeletal disruption of this area, the fracture lines involving the optic foramen and the optic nerve may result in blindness.

The Interorbital Space. The term "interorbital space" designates an area between the orbits, beneath the floor of the anterior cranial fossa. The interorbital space contains the two ethmoidal labyrinths, one on each side (Fig. 25–37).

The interorbital space is roughly cuboidal, being wider anteriorly than posteriorly. It is limited above by the cribriform plate in the midline and by the roof of each ethmoidal mass on the sides and is divided into two approximately equal halves by the nasal septum. The interorbital space is limited below at the level of a horizontal line through the lower border of the ethmoidal labyrinth. The lateral walls of the interorbital space are the medial walls of the orbit. Anteriorly the interorbital space is limited by the frontal processes of the maxilla and by the nasal process and spine of the frontal bone.

The interorbital space contains cellular bony structures, the ethmoidal cells; spongy bony structures, the superior and middle turbinates (Fig. 25–37); and a median thin plate of bone, the perpendicular plate of the ethmoid bone which forms the posterosuperior portion of the nasal septal framework.

The Frontal Sinus. The size of the frontal sinus varies greatly; it may be that of an ethmoidal cell, or it may be a very large sinus,

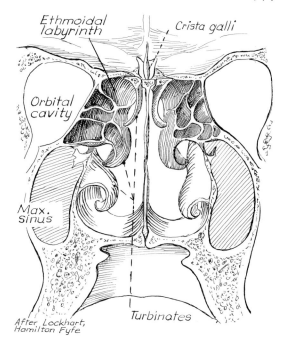

FIGURE 25–37. The interorbital space seen from behind. Frontal section through the ethmoids showing the relationship of the midportion of the orbits with the interorbital space.

pneumatizing the frontal bone. Occasionally it is absent.

The sinus has the shape of a pyramid with inferior, anterior, and posterior walls (Fig. 25–38). The inferior wall or floor of the frontal sinus corresponds to the roof of the orbit and is the thinnest portion of the frontal sinus. The anterior wall is thickest and is composed of cancellous bone. The posterior wall is thinner than the anterior wall and is entirely composed of compact bone which separates the sinus from the frontal lobe.

The Ethmoidal Sinus. The ethmoid bone occupies the lateral portion of the interorbital space. Below the interorbital space, the lower half of the nasal cavity is flanked by the maxillary sinuses (see Fig. 25–37). Each lateral mass of the ethmoid is connected medially to the cribriform plate; the roof of each ethmoidal mass is inclined upward from the cribriform plate and projects, in its lateral portion, about 0.25 cm above the cribriform plate.

The ethmoid is pyramidal or cuboidal, measuring 3.5 to 5 cm long and 1.5 to 2.5 cm wide. It is cellular in structure and contains eight to ten cells with thin lamellar walls; these cells drain into the middle meatus of the nose. The

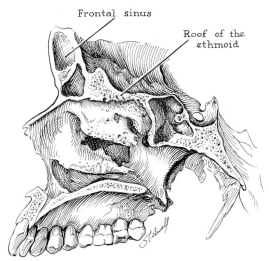

FIGURE 25–38. Sagittal section showing the lateral wall of the nose, the turbinates, and the frontal sinus with a frontoethmoidal cell beneath it.

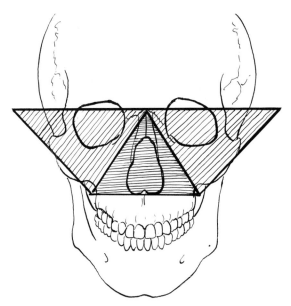

FIGURE 25–39. The bones forming the skeletal framework of the nose are situated in the upper and central portions of the midfacial skeleton. The diagram illustrates the concept by which the middle third of the face is divided into three triangles—a central nasomaxillary and two lateral orbitozygomatic triangles.

frontal sinus drains through the ethmoid, either through a distinct duct or by emptying into an anterior ethmoidal cell and into the middle meatus. Thus there is an intimate anatomical relationship with the frontal sinus through the frontonasal duct. It will be recalled that, in embryologic development, the frontal sinus is formed by an outcropping ethmoidal cell. A large ethmoidal cell, the frontoethmoidal cell, may be seen in the frontal bone between the frontal sinus and the roof of the orbit (Fig. 25–38).

Surgical Pathology

Situated in the upper and central part of the middle third of the face, anterior to the anatomical crossroads between the cranial, orbital, and nasal cavities (Fig. 25–39), the bones forming the skeletal framework of the nose may be projected backward between the orbits when they are subjected to a strong traumatic force. The term "naso-orbital" is employed to designate this type of fracture (Converse and Smith, 1963, 1964, 1966). A typical cause of naso-orbital fracture is an impact force applied over the upper portion of the bridge of the nose caused by the projection of the face against the dashboard (Fig. 25–40) or steering column of an automobile when it comes to a crash stop. A crushing injury with comminuted fractures is thus produced. Bursting of the soft tissues due to the severity of the impact and

penetrating lacerations of the soft tissue resulting from projection through the windshield may transform the closed fracture into a compound fracture (Fig. 25–41).

If the impact force suffered by the strong an-

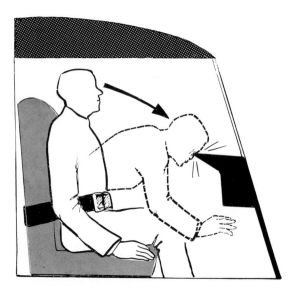

FIGURE 25–40. Dashboard injury producing naso-orbital fracture by projection against the protruding lip seen in many dashboards of present day automobiles. (From Converse, J. M., and Smith, B.: Naso-orbital fractures and traumatic deformities of the medial canthus. Plast. Reconstr. Surg., *38*:147, 1966.)

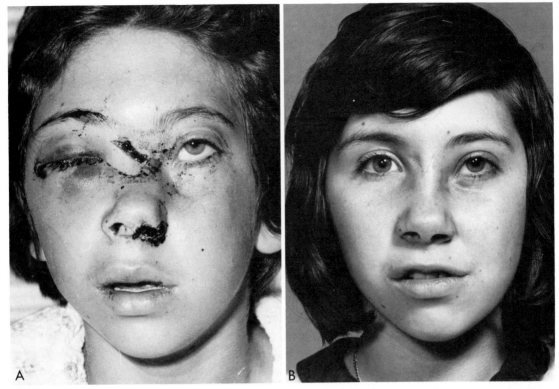

FIGURE 25–41. Naso-orbital fracture. *A,* A 12 year old girl victim of an automobile accident with typical naso-orbital fracture.The patient had cerebrospinal fluid rhinorrhea,which subsequent ceased spontaneously. Note the flattened nasal dorsum, hematoma of the right orbit, and displacement of the left medial canthus. The initial treatment consisted of through-and-through wiring to maintain the reduction of the comminuted bone fragments (see Fig. 25–47). *B,* After reconstructive surgery. A left medial canthoplasty was done. A large portion of the left nasal bone and frontal process of maxilla was extruded into the nasal cavity at the time of the accident. A bone graft was required to restore the nasal contour. Treatment of the naso-orbital fracture was postponed for a few days until the neurosurgical status of the patient could be established. (From Converse, J. M., and Smith, B.: Naso-orbital fractures and traumatic deformities of the medial canthus. Plast. Reconstr. Surg., *38*:147, 1966.)

terior abutments is sufficient to cause backward displacement of these structures, no further resistance is offered by the matchbox-like structures of the interorbital space; indeed, these structures collapse and splinter as would a pile of matchboxes struck by a hammer. The roof of the interorbital space is frequently involved in these fractures, and the anterior cranial fossa is penetrated, the fracture occurring either medially through the cribriform plate or laterally through the roof of the ethmoid sinus.

Some of the neurologic complications resulting from naso-orbital fractures are laceration of the dura covering the frontal lobes, laceration of the tubular sheaths enveloping the olfactory nerves as they perforate the cribriform plate, penetration of the brain by a sharp-edged ethmoidal cell wall, and necrosis of brain tissue.

An additional point of interest in the skeletal structure of this area is the continuity of the thin lamina papyracea of the medial orbital wall with the thin portion of the floor of the orbit. The splintering of the lamina papyracea facilitates a blowout fracture in this area and may occur in patients who suffer a blowout fracture of the floor of the orbit concurrently with a naso-orbital fracture (Fig. 25–42).

Lacerations of the soft tissues may sever the levator palpebrae superioris or penetrate through the medial canthal area, severing the medial canthal tendon and the lacrimal canaliculi or sac.

Fractures of the other facial bones, particularly of the midfacial skeleton, are frequently seen. In some of our patients, the frontal bone was also involved.

The Nasal Area: The Weakest Portion of the Facial Skeleton. Studies confirm that the nasal area is the weakest portion of the facial skeleton; fractures occur in this area with an impact load of 35 to 80 g. In Swearingen's study (1965), 45 impacts were made on cadaver heads to determine the fracture points of the

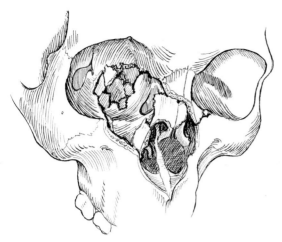

FIGURE 25–42. Naso-orbital fracture. Because of the backward displacement of the skeletal structures, the lacrimal bone and the lamina papyracea have been severely comminuted. Primary bone grafting may be indicated in such cases.

various portions of the facial skeleton. The comparative forces that can be tolerated over the various facial areas without fracture are illustrated in Figure 25–43. With the exception of the neck of the condyle, the zygomatic area is the next weakest area, being unable to sustain impact forces greater than 50 g. The upper portion of the middle third of the face, which includes both the nasal and orbital areas, is structurally susceptible to fracture. In contrast, the lower portion of the maxilla sustains impact forces of up to 100 g, and the major portion of the body of the frontal bone, with the exception of the central portion which is weakened by the frontal sinus cavities, sustains impact forces of up to 200 g.

Although padding of the rigid dashboard decreases the severity of the injuries sustained by the right front seat passenger, the padded dashboard lip in many automobiles has a contour suitable for the production of the "pushback" of the nasal structures between the orbits (Fig. 25–44). Such fractures occur even though the passenger is wearing a lap seat belt; they occur less frequently when he is protected by the shoulder harness type of belt. The passenger without a seat belt is often projected through the windshield and suffers various types of soft tissue lacerations, including penetrating lacerations of the naso-orbital tissues.

Traumatic Telecanthus. In many naso-orbital fractures, the patient has a characteristic appearance; the bony bridge of the nose is depressed and widened, and the eyes appear far apart as in orbital hypertelorism (see Fig.

25–41). The appearance of the patient is the result of traumatic telecanthus, an increase in the distance between the medial canthi (intercanthal distance) as a result of displacement by fracture of the bones forming the skeletal framework of the nose and medial orbital walls. Naso-orbital fractures may be unilateral but are most often bilateral following severe trauma. Traumatic orbital hypertelorism is a deformity characterized by an increase in the distance between the orbits and ocular globes and occurs in massive disruption of the midfacial skeleton and frontal bone (Converse, Smith and Wood-Smith, 1975).

Traumatic telecanthus is produced by two varieties of backward displacement of the bony structures. In the first, the frontal processes of the maxilla and the nasal bones penetrate the interorbital space, comminuting the ethmoid cells and out-fracturing the medial wall of the orbit (Fig. 25–45, *A*). The medial canthal tendon attachments are displaced with the bones, and the medial canthus is displaced laterally and deformed, assuming a rounded shape.

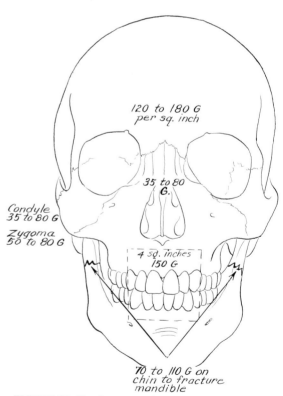

FIGURE 25–43. Summary of maximal tolerable impact forces on a padded deformable surface. This schema illustrates the comparable forces that can be tolerated over various facial areas without fracture. (After Swearingen, J. J.: Tolerances of the Human Face to Crash Impact. Oklahoma City, Federal Aviation Agency, 1965.)

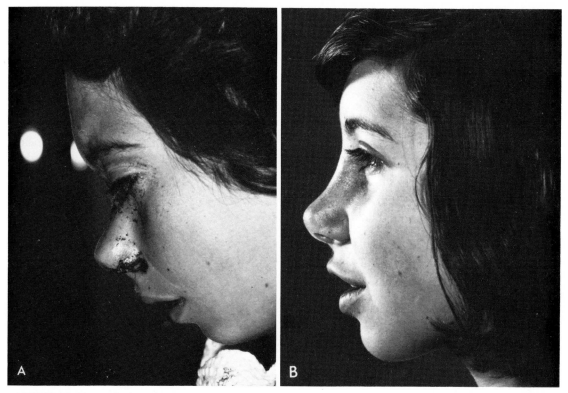

FIGURE 25–44. *A,* Patient shown in Figure 25–41. Backward displacement of the nasal skeletal structures into the interorbital space. *B,* After completion of the treatment.

In the second type of fracture, the nasal bones and frontal processes of the maxilla are splayed outward and projected backward into the medial portion of the orbital cavity along the lateral surface of the medial orbital wall, severing the medial tendon, transecting the lacrimal sac, or severing the canaliculi (Fig. 25–45, *B*). Thus traumatic telecanthus is also caused by increase in the thickness of the medial orbital wall from the overlapping of bone fragments (see also Fig. 25–49).

Loss of bone in the area may result from injudicious debridement and removal of bone fragments or the expulsion of bone fragments into the nasal cavity at the time of fracture.

Occasionally the medial portion of the inferior rim of the orbit is also fractured and displaced backward.

Examination and Diagnosis

Clinical Examination. The appearance of the patient who has suffered a naso-orbital fracture is typical (see Figs. 25–41 and 25–44): the nose is flattened, appearing to have been pushed between the eyes; the medial canthal areas are swollen and distorted, the caruncles and plicae semilunares being covered by the edematous and displaced structures; ecchymosis and subjunctival hemorrhage are usual findings.

Intranasal examination shows the findings observed in fractures of the nasal bones and septum. Fracture of the septum is suggested by septal hematoma. Naso-orbital fractures are often accompanied by signs of orbital blowout fracture or fracture of the maxilla or zygoma, which are frequently associated fractures. Edema and hematoma often mask the extent of the skeletal distortion of the area, particularly if the patient is not seen during the first hours after the accident.

The patient may be unconscious or have had loss of consciousness of long or short duration. Loss of consciousness is suggestive of brain injury. The patient may be irritable, restless, or even thrashing about after a severe injury. As in other fractures around the orbit, extensive edema of the lids and orbital structures may cause mechanical limitation of eyeball movements.

There may be little evidence of skeletal de-

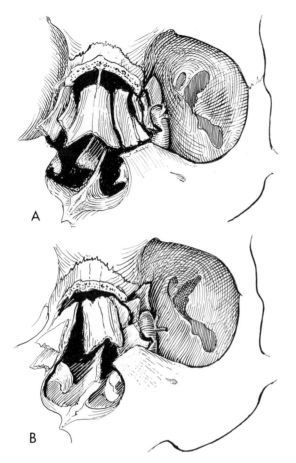

A

B

FIGURE 25–45. Two mechanisms of the production of
traumatic telecanthus resulting from backward telescoping
of the nasal skeletal structures and comminution of the
medial wall of the orbit. *A,* Backward displacement of
the nasal bones and frontal processes of the maxilla into
the ethmoid, resulting in displacement of the medial wall
of the orbit laterally. *B,* Bone fragments displaced backward, lateral to the medial wall of the orbit, penetrating
the lacrimal sac.

formity because of hematoma or swelling. In
some cases the deformity is evident when the
frontal bone has been crushed inward or the
nasal structures have been projected into the
interorbital space. The bones may be loose,
and crepitation may be felt when they are
mobilized. The entire upper jaw may be movable, and motion may be felt in the bones of
the interorbital space. A portion of the forehead skin may be avulsed in compound fractures, exposing the bone and revealing the site
of fracture.

Clear fluid escaping from the nose is
strongly suggestive of cerebrospinal fluid rhinorrhea. Patients with cerebrospinal fluid rhinorrhea show an initial escape of blood from the
fracture site; the fluid then becomes brownish

in color and finally clear. The fluid may be
seen to pulsate within the nose.

Roentgenographic Examination. Roentgenograms and tomograms are required
to estimate the amount of damage. As
stated earlier in the text, a fracture of the medial orbital wall may be associated with a
blowout fracture of the orbital floor. Careful
tomographic study will show suggestive signs
of medial wall fracture. Fractures of the cribriform plate may be impossible to detect by ordinary radiographic examination. The presence
of air in the subdural, subarachnoid space or in
the ventricle is a sign of communication with
the nasal cavity or sinuses, establishing a
direct pathway to infection, and is an indication for neurosurgical intervention. Air may
not be detected during the first 24 hours.
Roentgenograms should therefore be repeated
if the patient shows increasing signs of frontal
lobe dysfunction in the nature of mental
changes.

Fragmentation and a "buckled" appearance
of the cribriform plate are suggestive of penetration of fragments of ethmoidal cells into the
brain; this is an additional indication for neurosurgical operation. Tomograms may be of help
in evaluating the location of the damage and the
degree of displacement of the fragments.

Treatment

Brain injury should be suspected when the patient has been unconscious. Neurosurgical intervention is required in patients who have suffered destructive lesions of the brain or
penetration of bone fragments into the brain.
Careful neurologic and radiologic examination
is required. Cerebrospinal fluid rhinorrhea
should not be a contraindication for treatment
of the fractures. A delay of a number of days
may be required to allow for subsidence of
swelling and hematoma and clarification of the
neurosurgical status of the patient; such a
delay does not jeopardize an ultimate satisfactory result (see Fig. 25–41).

The technique of the treatment of naso-orbital fracture consists of the elevation of the
comminuted fragments by means of an instrument placed inside the nasal cavity. External
digital pressure and, if necessary, realignment
of the fragments restore the position of the
medial orbital walls. In naso-orbital fractures,
the wired plate technique and the figure-of-
eight wire suspension have their selective ap-

plications. In severe cases of naso-orbital fractures, the open-sky method is the treatment of choice.

The Open-Sky Technique (Converse and Hogan, 1970). In compound naso-orbital fractures, the external wound permits direct inspection of the area, and the comminuted fragments can be realigned under direct vision. In severely comminuted naso-orbital fractures that are not compound (Fig. 25–46), an open reduction is indicated (Fig. 25–47). Bilateral vertical incisions through the skin over the lateral wall of the nose provide exposure (Fig. 25–47, *A* to *C*); if additional exposure is required, the vertical incisions are joined by a transverse incision placed over the root of the nose (Fig. 25–48). The bilateral vertical incisions, if they are of adequate length, give adequate exposure in most cases, and the resulting scars are not conspicuous, usually being hardly perceptible. After the fragments are dissected one by one, each lacrimal sac and the nasolacrimal duct exposed and preserved, and the medial canthal tendon identified, subperiosteal exposure of the medial walls of the orbit is extended posteriorly behind the area of fracture. It is then possible, under direct vision, to replace the fragments in acceptable alignment, aided by an instrument placed intranasally (Fig. 25–48). Repair of the lacrimal apparatus in any of its sections can also be done under direct vision. Fragments of the nasal bones and the frontal processes of the maxilla may be joined to each

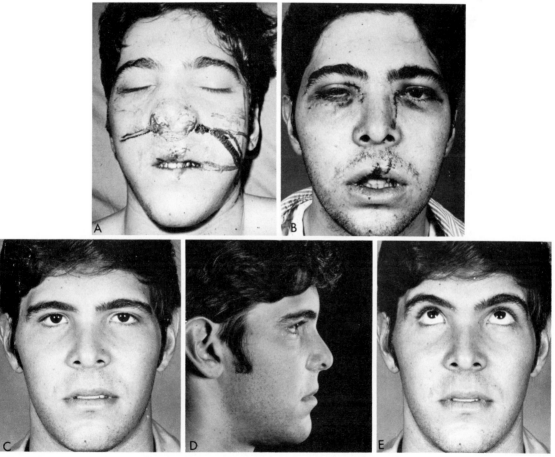

FIGURE 25–46. Open-sky technique in the treatment of naso-orbital fractures. *A,* Facial injury resulting from projection of the face onto the steering column of an automobile after a crash. Patient has suffered naso-orbital fracture, blowout fracture of the right orbital floor, and a pyramidal (Le Fort II) fracture of the maxilla. *B,* Forty-eight hours after treatment. Comminuted fragments of the naso-orbital fracture were reduced, realigned, and maintained in fixation by direct interosseous wiring through external incisions (see Fig. 25–47). Through a lower eyelid incision, the orbital contents, entrapped in the blowout fracture, were released, and an inorganic implant restored orbital floor continuity. Reduction of the maxillary fracture was postponed until 48 hours later, and an airway was maintained until the patient was fully conscious. *C, D,* One month later. *E,* Oculorotary movements of the right eye have been reestablished; the fractured maxilla was reduced by intermaxillary fixation. (*A* through *D* from Converse, J. M., and Hogan, V. M.: Open-sky approach for reduction of naso-orbital fractures. Case report. Plast. Reconstr. Surg., *46*:396, 1970.)

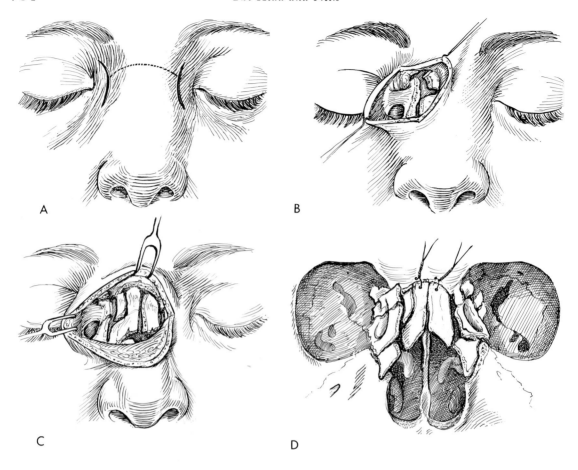

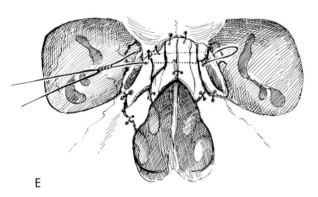

FIGURE 25–47. Open-sky technique in the treatment of naso-orbital fractures. *A,* The lateral nasal incisions can be joined, if necessary, by a transverse component. *B,* Exposure obtained through the external incisions. *C,* Comminuted fragments, the lacrimal sac, and medial canthal tendon are seen and examined. *D,* Interosseous wiring of the main fragments of the nasal bones established, providing initial stability. *E,* Other fragments have been joined by interosseous wiring, and a through-and-through wire maintains the anatomical position of the medial orbital walls. (From Converse, J. M., and Hogan, V. M.: Open-sky approach for reduction of naso-orbital fractures. Case report. Plast. Reconstr. Surg., *46:*396, 1970.)

other by interosseous wiring as well as to the frontal bone (see Fig. 25–47, *D, E*). Direct exposure of the fracture area is indispensable in fractures involving the cribriform plate with cerebrospinal rhinorrhea, as it permits inspection of the cribriform plate through the area of fracture.

The principle of the open treatment of naso-orbital fractures is the preservation of all fragments of bone, even where they are detached from soft tissues.

A frequent occurrence is the lateral displacement of the portion of the medial orbital wall containing the anterior lacrimal crest and the attachment of the medial canthal tendon (Fig. 25–49). The orbicularis oculi muscle exerts a

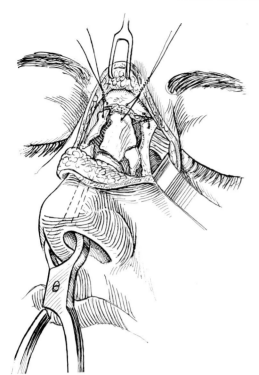

FIGURE 25–48. Elevation of retroposed comminuted fragments in a naso-orbital fracture by means of the Asche forceps. The position of the fragments is maintained by interosseous wiring.

lateral traction, deforming the medial canthal area; this is another mechanism in the production of traumatic telecanthus (see also Fig. 25–45).

Primary Bone Grafting. Primary bone grafting is indicated to restore bone continuity when the medial orbital wall is reduced to a pulp. The bone graft establishes an area of purchase for the attachment of the medial canthal tendon and also restores the medial orbital wall and the size and shape of the orbit (see Chapter 28, Fig. 28–155).

In the preceding chapter (see Chapter 24, page 739), certain indications for primary bone grafting were given—namely, when bone is destroyed, and when assistance is required in maintaining the projection of the maxilla by bone grafting in the pterygomaxillary area. Primary bone grafting has also been advocated for the repair of defects of the floor of the orbit, of the median and lateral walls, and of the orbital roof. Moreover, primary bone grafting in severely comminuted naso-orbital fractures is indicated when the clinical conditions are favorable (Figs. 25–50 and 25–51).

SUPRAORBITAL AND GLABELLAR FRACTURES AND FRACTURES INVOLVING THE FRONTAL SINUS

Either independently or in conjunction with naso-orbital fractures, fractures of the lower portion of the frontal bone in the supraorbital and glabellar regions are relatively infrequent. Schultz (1970) estimated the incidence of such fractures at approximately 5 per cent of those patients suffering fractures of the facial bones. Furthermore, he noted that patients suffering supraorbital and glabellar fractures require a longer average hospital stay than other facially injured patients irrespective of the cause.

Fractures of the supraorbital ridge are clinically evident by the observation of an area of local depression, especially in the early stages. In later stages, edema and periorbital ecchymosis may mask the deformity. The degree of depression of the supraorbital arch may depend on the size of the frontal sinus, which is extremely variable from one individual to another. Individuals with large frontal sinuses are more susceptible to fracture. When the depressed area involves the trochlea and the pulley of the superior oblique muscle, the patient may complain of diplopia, which is usually transitory. Some of our patients with supraorbital fractures had penetrat-

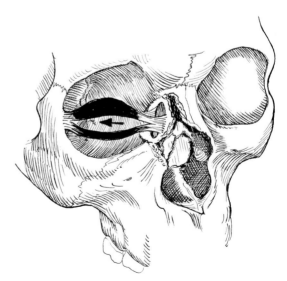

FIGURE 25–49. Diagram illustrating the displacement of a portion of the comminuted medial wall of the orbit as a result of the contraction of the orbicularis oculi muscle. The medial canthal tendon is still attached, and a fragment of bone is displaced laterally. This is one of the causes of traumatic telecanthus.

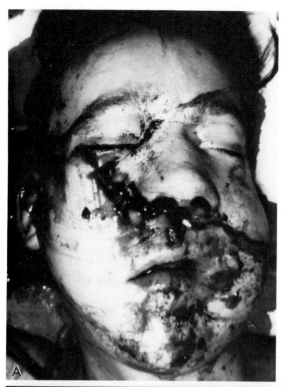

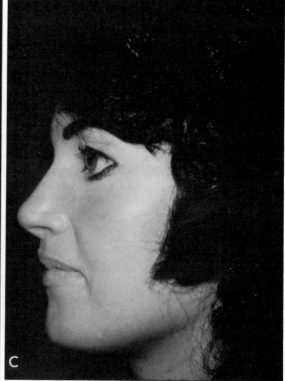

FIGURE 25–50.   *A*, Appearance of the patient following an automobile accident with naso-orbital and midfacial
fractures (Le Fort I and Le Fort II). The left ocular
globe had been penetrated by a piece of glass and required enucleation. The traumatic telecanthus was corrected by the open-sky method (see Fig. 25–47). There
was considerable loss of nasal skeletal structures due to
severe comminution; a primary bone graft was done. *B,
C*, Appearance of the patient after completion of the
repair. The patient was provided with a prosthetic ocular
globe. (From Converse, J. M., and Bonanno, P. C.: *In*
Kazanjian and Converse.)

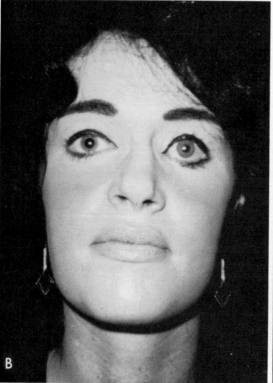

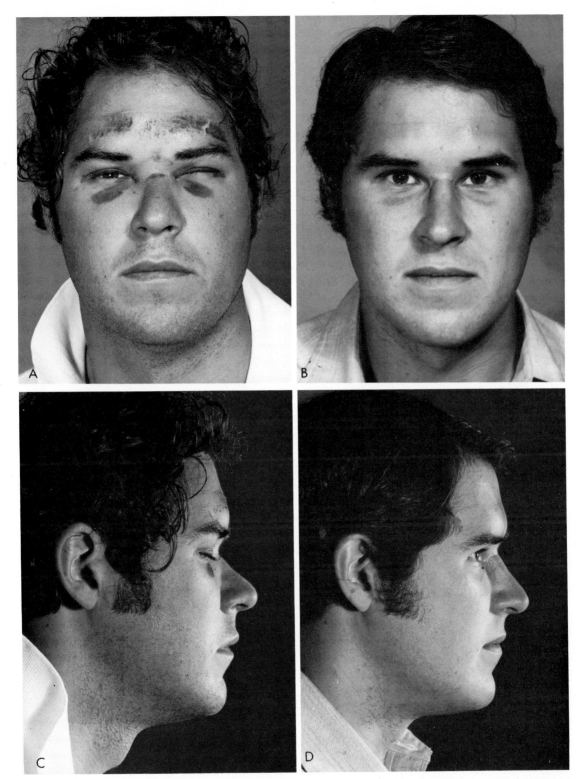

FIGURE 25–51.   Primary bone grafting following open sky treatment of naso-orbital fracture and concomitant bilateral blowout fractures of the orbital floor. *A* and *C,* Appearance of the patient nine days following trauma. The patient, an automobile racing driver, was involved in a crash. The helmet he was wearing descended over his face and the rim of the helmet struck the dorsum of the nose, causing a naso-orbital fracture with backward recession of the bones of the nasal framework into the interorbital space with a splaying apart of the medial orbital walls (telecanthus, *A*), depression of the root of the nose (*C*), and bilateral orbital floor blowout fractures. *B* and *D,* Appearance four months postoperatively. A trapdoor flap was raised and the comminuted fragments were reassembled and wired (see Fig. 25–47). The orbital fractures were treated by disentrapment of the orbital fragments and placing a Teflon implant over the blowout defects. A primary iliac bone graft restored the nasal contour.

ing injuries which severed the levator palpe-brae superioris. The resulting ptosis of the upper eyelid was masked in the early stages by edema and ecchymosis. Restriction of global movements secondary to the ecchymosis might lead one to the suspicion of a concomitant blowout fracture. If the lid, however, is care-fully raised with a small elevator, unrestricted upward rotation of the globe can be observed and can be confirmed by the forced duction test. These findings eliminate the presumptive diagnosis of blowout fracture of the orbital floor.

The authors have observed concomitant fracture of the supraorbital arch, depressed fracture of the glabellar region, and naso-orbi-tal fracture in the same patient. More frequently, however, the glabellar fracture is associated with a severe naso-orbital fracture, and the supraorbital arch fracture occurs inde-pendently.

When the causative impact is extremely vio-lent and when an associated brain injury is present, the fragmented bones may be so badly comminuted that their realignment is not possi-ble; some of them may even be ejected by the explosive force. In such cases, the type of de-formity illustrated in Figure 25–52 may be

seen, with loss of nasal, glabellar, and supraor-bital arch skeletal framework.

Roentgenographic diagnosis may be difficult, particularly in attempting to demonstrate a fracture of the posterior wall of the frontal sinus by lateral, Waters, or posteroanterior views. Tomograms, however, may be helpful in evaluating the extent of the damage and frac-ture.

Treatment nearly always involves open re-duction through the wound or through a surgi-cal incision. Exposure for supraorbital arch fractures can be achieved through the eyebrow if the incision is correctly placed. Objections have been made to such incisions because of subsequent hairless scars separating the upper and lower portions of the eyebrow. The hair follicles of the eyebrow are implanted in an oblique fashion; the incision should be slanted downward in order to parallel the direction of the hair follicles. In this manner, an inconspic-uous scar will result in a well-furnished eye-brow, particularly in male patients. In female patients with plucked eyebrows, it may be preferable to make the incision immediately below the orbital margin.

The approach to glabellar fractures, often as-sociated with the telescoping type of naso-orbi-tal fracture, can be achieved through the in-cisions made for the open-sky approach to naso-orbital fractures (see Fig. 25–47). If wider exposure is required, a transverse inci-sion at the root of the nose is extended lat-erally on each side immediately below the or-bital margin.

The best technique of exposure in major fractures involving the frontal bone is the coronal flap advocated by Tessier. In severe fractures involving the anterior cranial fossa, an intracranial approach and neurosurgical col-laboration are indicated.

Reduction and realignment of fragments de-pend essentially upon the type of fracture. When large fragments are present, they may be levered upward and will often remain in posi-tion without interosseous wire fixation. When smaller fragments are present, direct interos-seous wiring of the multiple fragments, as in the treatment of naso-orbital fractures, may be necessary.

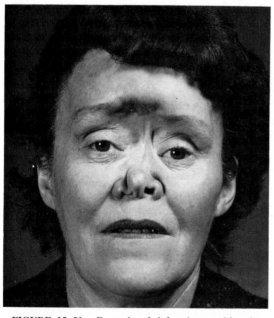

FIGURE 25–52. Example of deformity resulting from severe naso-orbital fracture and fracture of glabellar por-tion of the frontal bone. The patient suffered severe head injury and was in a coma for 72 hours; neurosurgical inter-vention was required for brain damage (removal of bone fragments penetrating into the frontal lobes and arrest of cerebrospinal rhinorrhea). (See Chapter 27, Fig. 27–34.)

Treatment of Fractures Involving the Frontal Sinus. Excluding the possibility of a concomi-tant head injury which may require crani-otomy, fracture with backward crushing of the anterior wall of the frontal sinus may not cause any functional disturbance, but it leaves the patient with a depression deformity if no treatment is applied.

Open reduction of the depressed anterior wall of the frontal sinus, in a manner similar to that employed in glabellar fractures, is the method of choice. The depressed bone is elevated and maintained by wire fixation. When the anterior wall of the frontal sinus is comminuted, the following approach can be practiced.

In fractures of the anterior wall of the frontal sinus, an incision is made along the upper portion of the lateral wall of the nose from the point where the root of the nose joins with the supraorbital arch to a few centimeters below. The incision is through the skin and periosteum, equidistant between the dorsum of the nose and the medial canthus of the eye. Subperiosteal elevation is extended upward to below the supraorbital arch. The lacrimal sac is temporarily elevated and retracted from the lacrimal groove. Posterior to the area of the lacrimal groove, the lamina papyracea of the ethmoid is cut through, and the ethmoidal sinus is penetrated. By working upward from the ethmoidal sinus with a small Kerrison punch, it is possible to follow the ethmoidal cells until the medial aspect of the frontal sinus is reached. Part of the floor of the frontal sinus is removed, and the frontal sinus is entered. The fractured anterior wall of the frontal sinus is pried forward with a blunt probe or a hard rubber catheter. Often, if the depressed fracture consists of one large fragment, the fragment will maintain its position after it has been repositioned.

If the anterior wall of the frontal sinus is severely comminuted and if the general condition of the patient is satisfactory, a thin iliac bone graft is resected and placed over the frontal sinus to restore contour, if a satisfactory soft tissue covering can be assured.

If clinical and radiologic examination shows intracranial injury and a posterior wall fracture of the frontal sinus, neurosurgical exploration and treatment should be undertaken.

COMPLICATIONS OF ORBITAL AND NASO-ORBITAL FRACTURES

The type of injury, the force of the impact, associated tissue damage, and inadequate or delayed treatment are the major causes of complications in orbital and naso-orbital fractures.

Early diagnosis and adequate repair of the orbital floor result in few late complications. Depending on the quality of the initial treatment and despite adequate treatment, some cases are subjected to an inexorable evolution toward late complications (see Table 25–4).

The sequelae and their treatment have been discussed in some detail (Converse and co-workers, 1967; Kazanjian and Converse, 1974), and enumeration of these sequelae follows: structural deformities; complications with the implant or transplant; muscular imbalance and enophthalmos; ocular complications; lacrimal system disturbances; hematoma and blindness; blepharoptosis; medial and lateral canthal deformities; vertical shortening of the lower eyelid; and infraorbital nerve anesthesia. These complications and their treatment will be discussed in Chapter 28. A discussion of a few of the early complications follows.

Structural Deformities. Deformities and functional impairment are late complications which can be reduced by early diagnosis and treatment, but often the diagnosis is obscured by more severe cranial and facial injuries which demand primary treatment. The unconscious patient cannot experience diplopia, and orbital edema, hemorrhage, and ptosis can mask the enophthalmos. After several weeks, fibrous cicatrization is established, and reconstruction of the orbital cavity and restoration of symmetrical ocular function in a malunited fracture must be undertaken in the presence of scarred, atrophic orbital fat and muscles.

Complications with the Implant or Transplant. Dead space between the inorganic implant and the bone of the orbital floor should be avoided, as the accumulated fluid in the dead space constitutes a favorable medium for the growth of bacteria. Orbital infection and suppuration are indications for incision, drainage, and removal of the implant, which is replaced after the infection has subsided. Antibiotic therapy should be routinely employed in all cases to avoid this complication.

In the average blowout fracture caused by a fist punch, a 1-mm Teflon implant is adequate to restore the continuity of the floor. Excessive thickness of the implant may cause the eyeball to be elevated. If the latter complications occurs, the implant should be removed and replaced by a thinner one. Furthermore, excessive overcorrection may result in elevation of the ocular globe and excessive compression on the orbital contents and the optic nerve.

Occasionally in severe trauma, hematoma may elevate the ocular globe. Gradual resorption of the hematoma will reduce the ocular globe to a level commensurate with the contralateral ocular globe.

An implant of excessive anteroposterior dimensions may compress the optic nerve and cause blindness. Extrusion of the implant by progressive forward migration can occur and can be avoided by the technique shown in Figure 25–33.

There is no perfect substitute for the orbital floor at the present time. The material used, however, should fit certain criteria. It should be well tolerated by the patient, sufficiently strong to support the orbital contents, relatively nonreactive to prevent adhesions to the orbital capsule, easily obtainable at the time of surgery, and workable into the desired shape. In early fracture repairs, the thin inorganic prosthesis is best, as exophthalmos can result from overcorrection. While autogenous bone is well tolerated by the patient and is the most physiologic substitute, it is not immune to absorption. Every effort should be made to ensure close contact of the bone graft with the bone of the orbital floor by carefully shaping the bone graft and eliminating dead space with small slivers of cancellous bone. Teflon, Silastic, Supramid, and Cranioplast implants are the preferred inorganic implants presently available. They can be shaped or carved and fitted to the floor of the orbit without preliminary preparation or delay.

Muscular Imbalance and Enophthalmos. Despite adequate early treatment of the orbital fracture, progressive ocular muscle imbalance and enophthalmos may ensue. Many adequately treated orbital floor fracture patients do not recover complete extraocular muscle function. Slight limitation in the upward gaze results in diplopia in this position, a relatively slight handicap. Extraocular muscle surgery on the affected eye or on the contralateral unaffected eye is a frequent requirement to restore eye muscle balance.

The complicated blowout fracture is often accompanied by multiple fractures of the facial bones and injuries of the soft tissues. Many of the fractures with complications treated by us have fallen into this category. These patients show impairment of oculorotary action and diplopia, enophthalmos, depression of the zygomatic prominence, ptosis of the upper eyelid, downward displacement of the orbital contents, medial canthal deformities, shorten-ing of the horizontal dimension of the palpebral fissure, shortening of the vertical dimension of the lower eyelid, saddle deformity and/or widening of the nasal bony bridge, and occasionally deformities of the supraorbital arch (see Table 25–4). Most complicated orbital fractures require extraocular muscle surgery during the months following the injury.

Ocular Complications. Ocular injury following orbital fractures has been reported as varying between 14 per cent (Milauskas and Fueger, 1966), 17 per cent (Miller and Tenzel, 1967), and 29 per cent (Jabaley and coworkers, 1975) in different series. Ocular globe injury also varies in severity from a corneal abrasion to loss of vision from a ruptured globe or a fracture involving the optic canal. Blindness or loss of the eye is remarkably infrequent, in view of the severity of some of the injuries sustained.

The importance of the ophthalmologic examination in all fractures of the orbit has already been discussed. Vitreous hemorrhage, dislocated lens, rupture of the sclera, traumatic cataract, choroidal rupture and hemorrhage, ruptured iris sphincter, glaucoma, retinal detachment, and diminution or loss of vision are some of the complications which may be avoidable if treatment is instituted early.

Verification of vision is essential in the course of an ophthalmologic examination. An excellent prognostic sign is the Marcus Gunn pupillary sign. A light is moved rapidly from one eye to the other alternately. If conduction of the optic nerve is lessened, the pupil on the involved side will appear to dilate as the light is brought from the sound eye to the involved eye. Monocular vision should also be considered.

The need for preliminary ophthalmologic examination is dramatically illustrated in a case reported by Miller (1968). Miller reported a patient with a midfacial fracture in whom vision in the left eye was 20/70 a few hours after the injury but dropped to no light perception by the fifth day. No surgery had been done. If the surgery had been performed before the fifth day, the resulting blindness could have been attributed to the operation.

Blindness has never resulted from repair of the orbital floor in any of the patients treated by the authors. We have seen patients whose vision was lost following repair by others. Nicholson and Guzak (1971) reported six cases in which vision was lost in a series of 72 patients who underwent orbital floor repair by means of silicone implants inserted by various surgeons in the same hospital. This high rate of visual loss, occurring in a reputable hospital, may be explained by the fact that the patients were operated upon by a number of different surgeons. It is preferable to place such patients under the care of specialized experienced surgeons.

Lacrimal System Complications. Interruption of the continuity of the lacrimal apparatus, a chronic inflammatory condition of the lacrimal sac, or cystic dilation (known as a mucocele) with ensuing epiphora requires dacryocystorhinostomy or other procedures (see Chapter 28).

Hematoma and Blindness. Hematoma is unusual. It occurs if continuous bleeding from the anterior and posterior ethmoidal arteries is not spontaneously arrested in fractures involving the medial orbital wall. Blindness may be the consequence of a hematoma occurring under a firm pressure dressing. The use of continuous suction drainage is recommended if bleeding is excessive at the end of the operation. The treatment of hematoma of the orbit is usually conservative (see Chapter 37).

Blepharoptosis. True ptosis of the upper lid is to be differentiated from pseudoptosis resulting from the downward displacement of the eyeball and enophthalmos. True ptosis results from loss of function of the levator palpebrae superioris. This may occur either as a result of transection of the levator aponeurosis or of intramuscular hematoma and subsequent fibrosis, or from an injury to the third cranial nerve. In most cases the levator aponeurosis is transected, usually not through its entire width. The levator aponeurosis can usually be successfully repaired (see Chapter 28, page 920).

Vertical Shortening of the Lower Eyelid. Vertical shortening of the lower eyelid with baring of the sclera below the limbus of the globe in the primary position (scleral show) may result from downward and backward displacement of the fractured inferior orbital rim. Release of the septum orbitale attachment from the orbital rim and restoration of the position of the orbital rim after osteotomy may be required. If such operative procedures fail, a tarsoconjunctival graft from the same or opposite upper eyelid will elevate the lower lid margin up to 4 mm. Often pseudoptosis and depression of the supratarsal fold accompany

vertical shortening of the lower lid; these three problems can also be at least partly resolved by means of a tarsoconjunctival graft.

The authors have received a number of personal communications concerning vertical shortening of the lower lid following the approach to the floor through a subciliary incision. We are now using a slightly lower incision, below the inferior tarsus, to eliminate such a complication.

Infraorbital Nerve Anesthesia. Infraorbital nerve anesthesia may be very disconcerting to some patients. The area of sensory loss usually extends from the lower lid over the cheek and lateral ala to the upper lip. Release of the infraorbital nerve from the pressure of bone fragments within the canal may be indicated (see Chapter 28, Fig. 28–137). Sensation may return spontaneously as late as one year after fracture.

Cerebrospinal Fluid Rhinorrhea. This complication occurs in naso-orbital fractures. The present trend is toward a conservative approach, influenced by a diminished fear of meningitis which results from the protection provided by antibiotic therapy. However, there have been reports of cases of traumatic cerebrospinal fluid rhinorrhea with recurring bouts of meningitis 15 years after injury.

When the radiologic examination fails to show evidence of damage other than a fracture line, the patient is treated conservatively while being observed for signs of impending complications, such as meningitis or extradural or intracerebral abscess. No packing is placed in the nasal fossae, smoking is forbidden, and the head of the bed is elevated to an angle of 60 degrees. The patient should be warned against blowing his nose, because the leakage might recur, or he might force tissue or air into the cranial cavity. If the cerebrospinal fluid rhinorrhea is prolonged, an operation to close the fistula should be considered; this is a decision to be made by the neurosurgeon. Collins (1973) stated that spinal fluid drainage is confirmed by the presence of glucose in amounts of more than 30 mg of glucose per 100 ml of fluid. The use of glucose oxidative paper is not reliable as a test for glucose. As high as 75 per cent positive reactions have been obtained when using the oxidative paper test in patients with normal secretions. The fistula may be located by isotope dyes or by dyes placed in the lumbar or ventricular cerebrospinal spaces.

As stated in Chapter 24, Collins (1973) advocated early reduction of facial fractures in the presence of cerebrospinal fluid rhinorrhea (Dingman, 1974). He stated that the objective is to obtain reduction and fixation of the fractured bones, thus providing support of the area of injury. In 19 patients treated by him in whom the facial bone fractures had been reduced in less than 48 hours, only two patients required operative repair of the dural fistulae, and in both the fistulae were not in proximity to the facial bone fractures.

REFERENCES

Ballen, P. H.: Further experiments with rapidly polymerizing methylmethacrylate in orbital floor fractures. Plast. Reconstr. Surg., *34*:624, 1964.

Browning, C. W., and Walker, R. V.: The use of alloplastics in 75 cases of orbital floor reconstruction. Am. J. Ophthalmol., *60*:684, 1965.

Collins, W. F.: *In* Youmans, J. R. (Ed.): Neurological Surgery. Vol. 2. Philadelphia, W. B. Saunders Company, 1973.

Converse, J. M., and Bonanno, P. C.: *In* Kazanjian, V. H., and Converse, J. M.: Surgical Treatment of Facial Injuries 3rd Ed. Baltimore, Williams & Wilkins Company, 1974, p. 394.

Converse, J. M., Cole, G., and Smith, B.: Late treatment of blowout fracture of the floor of the orbit. Plast. Reconstr. Surg., *28*:183, 1961.

Converse, J. M., and Hogan, V. M.: Open-sky approach for reduction of naso-orbital fractures. Case report. Plast. Reconstr. Surg., *46*:396, 1970.

Converse, J. M., and Smith, B.: Enophthalmos and diplopia in fracture of the orbital floor. Br. J. Plast. Surg., *9*:265, 1957.

Converse, J. M., and Smith, B.: Blowout fracture of the floor of the orbit. Trans. Am. Acad. Ophthalmol. Otolaryngol., *64*:676, 1960.

Converse, J. M., and Smith, B.: Naso-orbital fractures (symposium: midfacial fractures). Trans. Am. Acad. Ophthalmol. Otolaryngol., *67*:622, 1963.

Converse, J. M., and Smith, B.: Deformities of the eyelids and orbital region. *In* Converse, J. M. (Ed.): Reconstructive Plastic Surgery. Philadelphia, W. B. Saunders Company, 1964, pp. 645–661.

Converse, J. M., and Smith, B.: Naso-orbital fractures and traumatic deformities of the medial canthus. Plast. Reconstr. Surg., *38*:147, 1966.

Converse, J. M., Smith, B., Obear, M. F., and Wood-Smith, D.: Orbital blowout fractures: A ten-year study. Plast. Reconstr. Surg., *39*:20, 1967.

Converse, J. M., Firmin, F., Wood-Smith, D., and Friedland, J. A.: The conjunctival approach in orbital fractures. Plast. Reconstr. Surg., *52*:656, 1973.

Converse, J. M., Smith, B., and Wood-Smith, D.: Deformities of the midface resulting from malunited orbital and naso-orbital fractures. Clinics in Plastic Surgery, *2*:107, 1975.

Cramer, L. M., Tooze, F. M., and Lerman, S.: Blowout fractures of the orbit. Br. J. Plast. Surg., *18*:171, 1965.

Crikelair, G. F., Rein, J. M., Potter, G. D., and Cosman, B.: A critical look at the "blowout" fracture. Plast. Reconstr. Surg., *49*:374, 1972.

Dingman, R. O.: Personal communication, 1974.

Dingman, R. O., and Grabb, W. C.: Costal cartilage homografts preserved by irradiation. Plast. Reconstr. Surg., *28*:562, 1961.

Dodick, J. M., Galin, M. A., Littleton, J. T., and Sod, L. M.: Concomitant medial wall fracture and blowout fracture of the orbit. Arch. Ophthalmol., *85*:273, 1971.

Edwards, W. C., and Ridley, R. W.: Blowout fracture of the medial orbital wall. Am. J. Ophthalmol., *65*:248, 1968.

Emery, J. M., von Noorden, G. K., and Schlernitzauer, D. A.: Orbital floor fractures: long-term follow-up of cases with and without surgical repair. Trans. Am. Acad. Ophthalmol. Otolaryngol., *75*:802, 1971.

Freeman, B. S.: Direct approach to acute fractures of the zygomatic-maxillary complex in immediate prosthetic replacement of the orbital floor. Plast. Reconstr. Surg., *29*:587, 1962.

Fujino, T.: Experimental "blowout" fracture of the orbit. Plast. Reconstr. Surg., *54*:81, 1974a.

Fujino, T.: Mechanism of orbital blowout fracture. Jap. J. Plast. Surg., *17*:427, 1974b.

Garrett, J. W.: Ocular-orbital injuries in automobile accidents. Bull. #4. Automotive Crash Injury Research of the Cornell Aeronautical Laboratory, Inc. Buffalo, N.Y., 1963.

Gould, H. R., and Titus, O.: Internal orbital fractures: The value of laminography in diagnosis. Am. J. Roentgenol., *97*:618, 1966.

Hakelius, L., and Pontén, B.: Results of immediate and delayed surgical treatment of facial fractures with diplopia. J. Maxillofac. Surg., *1*:150, 1973.

Jabaley, M. E., Lerman, M., and Sanders, H. J.: Ocular injuries in orbital fractures: A review of 119 cases. Personal communication, 1975.

Jones, D. E., and Evans, J. N. G.: "Blow-out" fractures of the orbit: An investigation into their anatomical basis. J. Laryngol., *81*:1109, 1967.

Kazanjian, V. H., and Converse, J. M.: *In* Converse, J. M. (Ed.): Surgical Treatment of Facial Injuries. 3rd Ed. Baltimore, Williams & Wilkins Company, 1974.

King, E. F., and Samuel, E.: Fractures of the orbit. Trans. Ophthalmol. Soc. U.K., *64*:134, 1944.

LaGrange, F.: De l'anaplerose orbitaire. Bull. Acad. Med. Paris, *80*:641, 1918.

Lang, W.: Traumatic enophthalmos with retention of perfect acuity of vision. Trans. Ophthalmol. Soc. U. K., *9*:41, 1889.

McCoy, F. J., Chandler, R. A., Magnan, C. G., Moore, J. F., and Siemsen, G.: Analysis of facial fractures and their complications. Plast. Reconstr. Surg., *29*:381, 1962.

Milauskas, A. T., and Fueger, G. F.: Serious ocular complications associated with blow-out fractures of the orbit. Am. J. Ophthalmol., *62*:670, 1966.

Miller, G. R.: Blindness developing a few days after a midfacial fracture. Plast. Reconstr. Surg., *42*:384, 1968.

Miller, G. R., and Glaser, J. S.: The retraction syndrome and trauma. Arch. Ophthalmol., *76*:662, 1966.

Miller, G. R., and Tenzel, R. R.: Ocular complications of midfacial fractures. Plast. Reconstr. Surg., *39*:37, 1967.

Miller, G. R., and Tenzel, R. R.: Orbital fracture repair with methylmethacrylate implants. Am. J. Ophthalmol., *68*:717, 1969.

Morgan, B. D. G., Madan, D. K., and Bergerot, J. P. C.: Fractures of the middle third of the face — A review of 300 cases. Br. J. Plast. Surg., *25*:377, 1972.

Nicholson, H., and Guzak, S. V.: Visual loss complicating repair of orbital floor fractures. Arch. Ophthalmol., *86*:369, 1971.

Prasad, S. S.: Blow-out fracture of the medial wall of the orbit. *In* Bleeker et al. (Eds.). Second International Symposium on Orbital Disorders. Vol. 14. Basel, Karger, Stockholm, 1975.

Putterman, A. M., Stevens, T., and Urist, M. J.: Non-surgical management of blow-out fractures of the orbital floor. Am. J. Ophthalmol., *77*:233, 1974.

Rény, A., and Stricker, M.: Fractures de l'orbite. Indications ophthalmologiques dans les techniques opératoires. Paris, Masson & Cie, 1969.

Rougier, M. J.: Résultats fonctionnels du traitement chirurgical des paralysies oculaires secondaires aux tramatismes de la face. Bull. Soc. Ophthalmol. Fr., *65*:502, 1965.

Rumelt, M. B., and Ernest, J. T.: Isolated blowout fracture of the medial orbital wall with medial rectus entrapment. Am. J. Ophthalmol., *73*:451, 1972.

Schultz, R. C.: Supraorbital and glabellar fractures. Plast. Reconstr. Surg., *45*:227, 1970.

Smith, B., and Regan, W. F., Jr.: Blowout fracture of the orbit: Mechanism and correction of internal orbital fracture. Am. J. Ophthalmol., *44*:733, 1957.

Swearingen, J. J.: Tolerance of the Human Face to Crash Impact. Federal Aviation Agency, Oklahoma City, 1965.

Tenzel, P. R.: Personal communication, 1974.

Tenzel, R. R., and Miller, G. R.: Orbital fracture repair, conjunctival approach. Am. J. Ophthalmol., *71*:1141, 1971.

Tessier, P.: The conjunctival approach to the orbital floor and maxilla in congenital malformation and trauma. J. Maxillofac. Surg., *1*:3, 1973.

Trochel, S. L., and Potter, G. D.: Radiographic diagnosis of fracture of the medial wall of the orbit. Am. J. Ophthalmol., *44*:733, 1969.

Zizmor, J., Smith, B., Fasano, C., and Converse, J. M.: Roentgen diagnosis of blowout fracture of the orbit. Trans. Am. Acad. Ophthalmol., *66*:802, 1962.

CHAPTER 26

FACIAL INJURIES IN CHILDREN

JOHN MARQUIS CONVERSE, M.D.,
AND REED O. DINGMAN, M.D.

Facial injuries in children are considered separately in this text because of special problems which arise in their treatment. Children are subjected to injuries similar to those of adults. The automobilie is responsible for large numbers of deaths and injuries, and children, as victims, are no exception.

Children under 5 years of age account for 2 to 3 per cent of automobile occupant deaths; children under 14 years of age account for approximately 6 per cent of automobile deaths. Of children between the ages of 5 and 14 years who were injured in automobile collisions, 56 per cent were actual occupants of automobiles (Burdi and coworkers, 1969).

These figures relate to automobile accidents; there are other causes of accidents in children extending over a wide range from a fall to a thermal burn. Athletic activities are responsible for facial injuries in the older child. The vast canine population in the United States (it is estimated there are over 65 million dogs) subjects the child to dog bites, which often result in considerable soft tissue disorganization and loss.

Soft tissue injuries and fractures may require special therapeutic techniques owing to difficulties in obtaining the cooperation of young children. Another aspect of facial injuries in children that must be considered is the effect of trauma upon facial development. A posttraumatic facial deformity in a child is the result not only of the displacement of bony structures caused by the fracture but also of faulty or arrested development resulting from the injury. Developmental malformations seen in young adolescents and adults are often secondary to early childhood injury. A statement should always be made to the parents of a child, preferably in writing, that maldevelopment in growth may occur as a result of a facial bone fracture despite adequate remedial treatment, particularly in injuries involving the nasomaxillary complex and the condylar area of the mandible. This is an essential medicolegal precaution.

The Child and the Adult: Anatomical Differences

Infants and children are not small adults. They differ structurally from adults, particularly in the relation of the head mass to the remainder of the body. The child's head is proportionally larger than that of the adult; this heavier head mass may, in part, be the basis for a high frequency of head (and face) injury.

At birth the facial portion of the head is smaller than the cranium in a 1:8 ratio, as compared with the adult ratio of 1:2.5. Owing to the large size of the frontal lobes, the forehead is high and protrusive. Although half of the postnatal increase in brain volume occurs during the first year of life and the brain attains 75 per cent of its adult size by the end of the second year, disproportionate craniofacial size is noticeable even in children 7 or 8 years of age.

Vertical growth of the face progresses in spurts related to respiratory needs and tooth eruption, first during the first 6 months after birth, then during the third and fourth years, from the seventh to the eleventh years, and lastly between the sixteenth and nineteenth years.

Thus, it is obvious that during the period of growth and development the child differs structurally from the adult and that soft and hard tissue injuries consequently require special consideration.

Prenatal and Birth Injuries

Intrauterine compression is thought to be one of the causes of prenatal deformities, although evidence of this type of injury has never been substantiated.

Birth injuries may result from prolonged labor with difficult passage through the birth canal and delivery by obstetrical forceps. Most of the injuries due to obstetrical forceps are minimal, and recovery usually takes place without residual deformities. Infant and child skulls are pliable because of the segmental arrangement, flexibility, resiliency, and relative softness of the bones. The bones develop as a loosely joined system found in the matrix surrounding the brain. They are separated by fontanelles and sutures covered by a thin fibrous sheath. These characteristics explain the malleability of the cranial and facial bones and the fact that they are subject to distortion and crushing injuries which may have subsequent developmental repercussions.

Deviation of the septum has been attributed to forced deflection during birth. More severe injuries have been attributed to forceps compression of the soft tissues and bones of the face, which may cause permanent facial scars and osseous deformities in the region of the zygomatic arch and temporomandibular joint, resulting in temporomandibular ankylosis with subsequent developmental hypoplasia of the mandible. Because of the lack of development of the mastoid process at birth and the superficial position of the seventh cranial nerve, facial paralysis caused by injury of the nerve by delivery forceps pressure is not infrequently observed.

Injuries to the eye or its adnexa, such as damage to the extraocular musculature, may be caused by intraorbital hemorrhage. Fractures of the body of the mandible due to birth injury are rare. They are usually linear fractures with little, if any, displacement. Healing occurs in a short time without manipulative treatment.

Johnson (1962) reported the case of a newborn baby with separation of the two halves of the mandible at the symphysis following a maneuver in which the obstetrician placed his finger in the child's mouth and used forceful manipulation to deliver the baby.

Injuries in Infants

It has long been suspected that infants fall much more frequently than is generally known. Of 536 infants involved in a study sponsored by the National Safety Council (Kravits and coworkers, 1969), 47.5 per cent fell from a high place such as an adult bed, a crib, or an infant dressing table during their first year of life. Some of the infants in the series suffered cranial, intracranial, and facial injuries. It can be assumed that facial trauma occurring in such falls in infants, although not often resulting in fractures because of the elasticity of the neonatal bones, may be sufficient to interfere with growth centers and may explain some of the developmental malformations of the face observed in later years.

SOFT TISSUE INJURIES IN INFANTS AND CHILDREN

Soft tissue wounds in children heal rapidly and therefore require early primary suture. Fortunately, lacerations repaired at an early age tend to become less conspicuous with the passage of time. Pediatricians will often advise the parents to wait until the child has reached adolescence before effecting the repair; this is poor advice, because many scars repaired in infancy and childhood are inconspicuous if not invisible in adolescence.

Some wounds tend to heal with considerable hypertrophic scarring; discouraging results often require later repair of the scar (see Chapter 16). It is wise to mention this possibility to the parents, advising that secondary surgery may be necessary. Densely scarred areas may require reconstructive procedures, for such untreated areas may interfere with subjacent bony growth, particularly in the area of the mandible.

Loss of soft tissue of the face by avulsion or

thermal burns is remedied by skin transplantation. Defects of the nose are adequately repaired, in many cases, by composite auricular grafts, which show a high success rate in children. While subtotal or total loss of the nose has not been observed by the authors, Lewin (1955) has described reconstruction of the nose in a 2 month old infant.

EMERGENCY TREATMENT

Arrest of hemorrhage and provision of an adequate airway are emergency measures that are more important in the facially injured child than in the adult. The small size of the laryngotracheal airway in the child, edema of the laryngeal mucous membrane, or retroposition of the base of the tongue can contribute to sudden respiratory obstruction. Immediate relief of obstruction is obtained by means of a suture placed through the tongue for forward traction. Although humidification of the room by a vaporizer or administration of corticosteroids can relieve the symptoms of laryngeal obstruction, one should not hesitate to perform a tracheotomy in a child with a fractured mandible or maxilla who is unconscious or who is showing increasing respiratory distress. In doing a tracheotomy in a young child, one should avoid incising through the first tracheal ring because of the danger of causing tracheal stenosis. Caution must also be exercised to avoid the innominate vein in a low approach to the trachea. Expert intratracheal intubation may obviate the need for a tracheotomy.

FRACTURES OF THE FACIAL BONES IN CHILDREN

Incidence. Fractures of the facial bones are less frequent in children than in adults. Except in large medical centers, the total experience of any surgeon in the management of facial fractures in children is limited.

During their early years children live in a protected environment under close parental supervision. The resiliency of the developing bone, the short distance of the falls, and the thick overlying soft tissue enable the child to withstand forces that in the adult would result in extensive comminution rather than in the greenstick fractures seen most frequently in children. The tooth to bone ratio in the developing mandible is comparatively high, and the bone has a more elastic consistency. The rudimentary paranasal sinuses, the large cartilaginous growth centers, and the small volume ratio between the jaws and the cranium are all factors providing protection to the facial bone structures.

The incidence of facial bone fractures in children varies according to various reports. In a series of mandibular fractures reviewed by Kazanjian and Converse (1974), children between 4 and 11 years represented approximately 10 per cent. In a series reported by Panagopoulos (1957), fractures of all facial bones in children represented only 1.4 per cent of the entire series. Pfeifer (1966), reviewing a series of 3033 cases of facial bone fractures, noted that 4.4 per cent of these cases had occurred in children in the age group extending from birth to 10 years; in the age group extending to 14 years, the incidence was 11 per cent; in the age group from 11 to 20 years of age, the incidence was 20.6 per cent.

Rowe (1968) summarized the data by stating that 1 per cent of facial fractures occur before the sixth birthday, and a total of 5 per cent occur in children under the age of 12 years. Approximately 1 in 10 fractures in children under 12 years involves the midfacial skeleton; midfacial fractures are uncommon before the age of 8 years.

One of the principal causes for the rarity of fractures of the facial skeleton in children is the large size of the cranium in relation to the facial skeleton (Figs. 26–1 to 26–4). McCoy, Chandler, and Crow (1966), in an analysis of 1500 cases of facial fractures, reported 86 children of whom 35 (40.8 per cent) had associated skull fractures. This finding can be explained by the protrusion of the massive brain case; the large cranium-face proportion is noticeable even up to 7 or 8 years of age (Fig. 26–5).

A major portion of the cranial growth is achieved by the age of 2 years. In contrast, facial skeletal growth continues during childhood. The facial skeleton gradually becomes pneumatized by the accessory sinuses. Although the period of maximal growth of the maxilla is reached around the age of 6 years, the adult size of the orbit is attained during the seventh year (see Fig. 26–3). From birth until adult size is reached, the facial skeletal framework increases threefold in size compared with the cranium. The small facial skeleton, not yet weakened by the air sinuses and further pro-

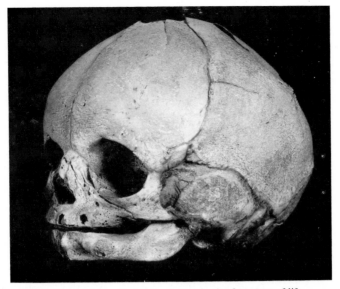

FIGURE 26-1. Skull of an infant in the first year of life.

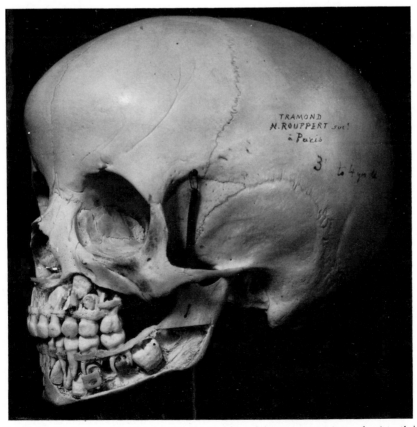

FIGURE 26-2. Skull of a 3 year old child showing the position of the permanent (secondary) teeth in relation to the deciduous (primary) dentition.

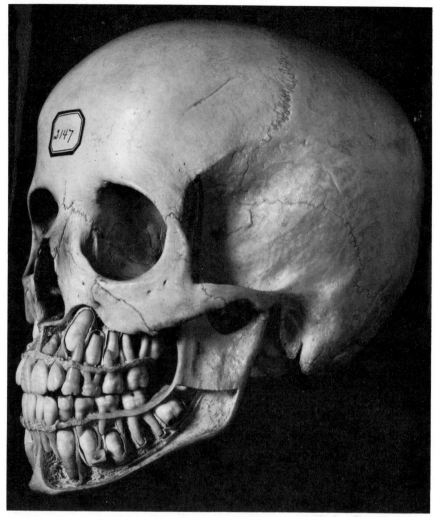

FIGURE 26–3. Skull of a child in the seventh year showing the position of the permanent teeth in relation to the deciduous dentition.

tected by the soft tissues with the thick adipose layer characteristic of young children, is less subject to fracture than the dominant cranium (Fig. 26–6).

MANDIBULAR AND FACIAL BONE FRACTURES IN CHILDREN: SPECIAL ASPECTS

1. Predisposition to greenstick fractures in developing bone is attributed to two factors. The first, as mentioned earlier in the text, is subcutaneous tissue, mainly adipose tissue, which increases rapidly in thickness during the nine months after birth. At the age of 5 years,

this subcutaneous tissue is actually only half as thick as in a 9 month old infant.

The second factor is the resiliency of the developing bone, which predisposes to the characteristic greenstick type of fracture. The line of differentiation between cortical bone and medullary bone is not sharply defined, and the resiliency of the young bone explains the higher frequency of such fractures in the child. When fractures do occur, however, fractures involving the body of the mandible frequently show a considerable degree of displacement, and the fracture lines tend to be long and oblique, extending downward and forward from the upper border of the mandible. The obliquity of the fracture line is quite different from that observed in the adult, in whom the

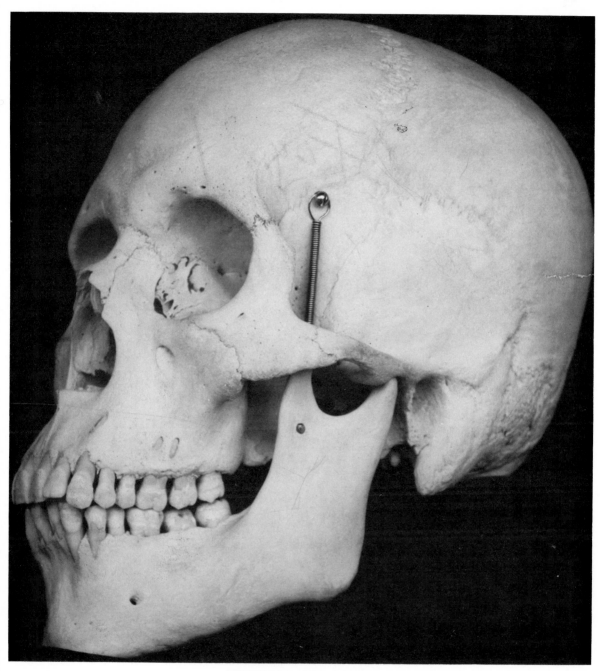

FIGURE 26–4.   The adult skull.

direction of the fracture line is usually downward and backward.

2. Prior to the eruption of the permanent (or secondary) dentition, the developing permanent teeth occupy most of the body of the mandible (see Figs. 26–2 and 26–3). This anatomical characteristic must be considered if interosseous fixation is to be employed, in order to avoid injuring the tooth buds of the permanent teeth. The wires must be placed near the lower border of the mandible. The roots of the deciduous teeth are gradually being resorbed, and between the ages of 5 and 9 years (the mixed dentition), because of the frequent ab-

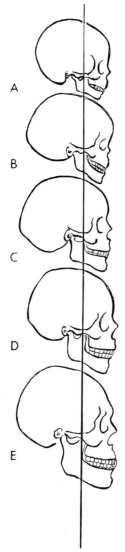

FIGURE 26–5. Tracings of a series of skulls showing changes in the size of the face as well as the position of the face in relation to the cranium. Growth of the face is associated with growth of the jaws and eruption of the teeth. (After Hellman, 1935. From Kazanjian and Converse.)

sence of teeth and the poor retentive shape of the crowns of the deciduous teeth, it is often difficult to utilize the dentition for fixation.

The teeth cannot be employed for fixation in the treatment of mandibular fractures in very young infants in whom the teeth are unerupted or only partly erupted. An impression of the mandible can be taken under light anesthesia and an acrylic splint fabricated. After realignment of the fragments, the splint is placed over the mandibular arch, lined with softened dental compound for better adjustment, and maintained in position by circumferential wir-

ing (see Chapter 24, Fig. 24–96). This type of monomaxillary fixation may be adequate. Intermaxillary fixation is obtained by circumferential wiring around the body of the mandible, and the wire is further passed into the floor of the nose and downward through the palate, thus surrounding the alveolar area of the maxilla without interfering with the tooth buds of the secondary dentition. Transalveolar wiring above the apices of the teeth can be used in the older child after the eruption of the secondary dentition. At this later age, however, the dentition may be adequate for intermaxillary dental fixation.

During the period when the deciduous dentition is being replaced by the permanent dentition, particularly in the period between the ages of 6 and 12 years, some difficulty may be experienced in obtaining interdental fixation. Acrylic splints may prove to be most useful in this age group.

In older children in whom the dentition is more retentive, various types of fixation can be employed. The cable arch wire (Fig. 26–7) is useful as an emergency fixation appliance. A band and arch appliance can be employed if the teeth permit retention of the appliance; circumferential wire will aid in stabilizing the mandibular appliance (Fig. 26–8). Eyelet wiring may also be feasible (see Fig. 26–13). Direct interosseous fixation, placing the wire near the lower border of the mandible in order to avoid injuring the tooth buds, is of considerable assistance in maintaining the fixation when only deciduous teeth are present for fixation. The interosseous wires may be placed through an intraoral approach after degloving the mandible. A circumferential wire around the mandible is also a useful adjunct in reinforcing the fixation established by the arch bar fixation (Fig. 26–8, *B*) and can be employed after exposing the ends of the fractured bone intraorally by the degloving procedure (see Chapter 24, Fig. 24–103).

When the deciduous teeth and alveolar process are avulsed, as shown in Figure 26–9, *A*, the deciduous teeth are discarded, the alveolar bone is replaced, and the mucous membrane is sutured (Fig. 26–9, *B*).

Figure 26–10 shows another example of a severe compound fracture of the maxilla treated by arch bars wired to the remaining teeth. Following the interosseous fixation, intermaxillary fixation is established whenever possible.

3. Fractures of the facial bones in children must be recognized and treated early because

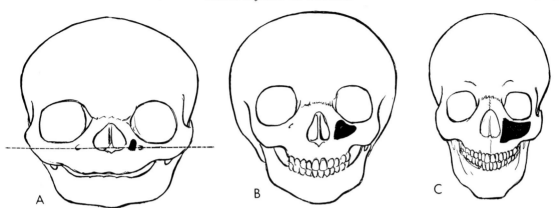

FIGURE 26–6. Skull at birth (*A*), at 5 years (*B*), and in the adult (*C*) has been drawn with the same vertical dimension to show the relative size increases of the maxillary sinus. Note the progressive increase in the size of the maxillary sinus, extending laterally beyond the infraorbital foramen (*B*) and descending below the level of the floor of the nose (*C*) after eruption of the permanent teeth. (From Kazanjian and Converse.)

the reparative process in children is rapid; loose, displaced fragments become adherent to one another within three or four days after injury. At this time, fragments are difficult to manipulate and must be loosened under general anesthesia before reduction of the fracture is possible.

Minor degrees of malunion can be tolerated in the growing facial bones, as corrective adjustment will take place with the erupting teeth under normal masticatory stresses.

4. Fractures involving the body of the mandible frequently involve the permanent tooth follicles, but it is seldom necessary to remove these. Eruption of the permanent teeth may be delayed, however, and the teeth may show varying degrees of damage after consolidation of the fracture.

5. Children are usually not as cooperative as adults because of fear, apprehension, and pain. Kindness, consideration, and tact are necessary in managing the child patient. Whenever

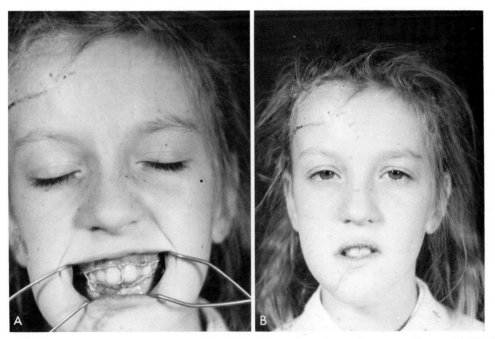

FIGURE 26–7. Cable arch wire appliance. *A*, Kazanjian's cable arch wire appliance (see Chapter 24, Fig. 24–92) employed for the reduction of a compound comminuted fracture of the mandible, which occurred when the child was struck by the revolving blades of a motor boat. *B*, Intermaxillary fixation has been established; the wounds are healing.

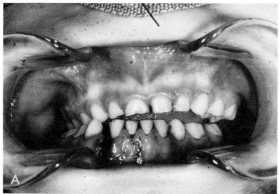

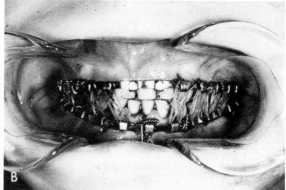

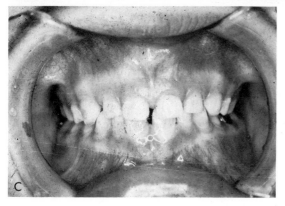

FIGURE 26–8.   Band and arch appliance. A, Compound fracture of the mandible between the right deciduous lateral incisor and cuspid tooth. B, Closed reduction with arch bar fixation and a circumferential wire around the symphysis of the mandible to stabilize the lower arch bar. Note the circumferential wire twisted at the top of the arch bar. C, Postoperative occlusion of the teeth two years later.

possible, the operative procedure or even minor manipulative work, such as intermaxillary wiring or the making of wire loops or buttons, should be performed under general anesthesia.

A few children, however, if the need for treatment is carefully explained to them, become remarkably cooperative, and these procedures can then be done under sedation, which may also be required before radiographic examination.

6. Fractures or injuries to the articular surface of the temporomandibular joint should be suspected in all children who have suffered a severe blow to the chin. Radiologic studies may demonstrate fractures of one or both mandibular condyles with or without displacement. Condylar fractures and injuries (see Chapter 24) should always be viewed with concern in the young child because of the possibility of secondary growth deformities resulting from damage to the condylar growth centers. Inju-

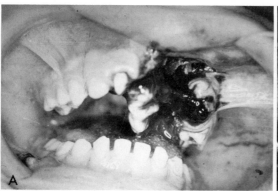

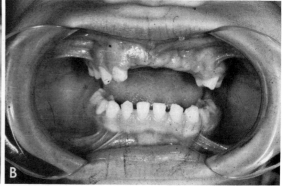

FIGURE 26–9.   Maxillary alveolar fracture with dislocation and avulsion of several teeth. A, Preoperative appearance. B, Postoperative healing after removal of the deciduous teeth, replacement of the alveolar bone, and suture of the soft tissues.

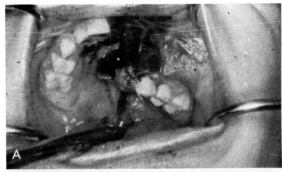
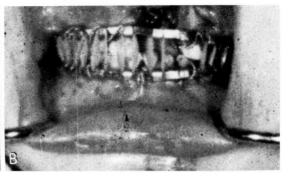
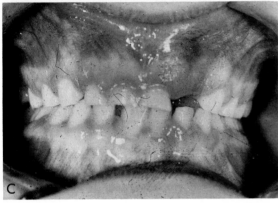

FIGURE 26–10. Compound maxillary fracture with displacement of fragments and avulsion of the teeth. *A*, Preoperative appearance. *B*, After reduction. The fractured segments were replaced, the totally avulsed teeth were removed, the remaining teeth were fixated with an arch bar and intermaxillary fixation was established. Note the circumferential wire reinforcing the lower arch bar. *C*, Satisfactory postoperative result with survival of the fragments and avulsed teeth.

ries to the articular surface of the joint may result in hemarthrosis with cicatricial organization and damage to the articular surface of the joint with subsequent bony ankylosis. This potential should always be considered and discussed with the parents in injuries of this type.

Temporomandibular ankylosis may follow injury to the condyle. An example of such a complication is the following: one of our patients, a 3 year old boy, was examined after a fall on the chin. No apparent injury could be found on clinical and radiologic examination. Six months later, the child had developed limitation of motion of the mandible due to partial ankylosis of the right temporomandibular joint. Resection of the head of the condyle restored mandibular function.

Topazian (1964) reported that trauma, most frequently a traumatic force applied to the point of the chin in children under 9 years of age, was responsible for approximately one-third of the cases of temporomandibular ankylosis in a personal series of 44 cases and in 185 cases surveyed in the literature.

Fractures of the condyle which involve the base of the neck of the condyle are often of the greenstick variety and are not usually accompanied by disturbance of the temporomandibu-

lar joint. Fortunately, many fractures in the condylar area of the mandible in children are not followed by ankylosis or growth disturbance.

A progressive straightening of the neck of the condyle is observed after fractures in which bony contact between the fragments has been maintained. Pfeifer (1966) noted that, in fracture-dislocation with loss of contact between the fragments, there was a shortening of the ramus on the affected side and asymmetry of the mandibular arch. In these cases, resorption of the condyle was observed, followed by the formation of a new joint. In none of these cases did ankylosis occur, although deviation upon opening of the mouth was frequent owing to the shortening of the ramus and dysfunction of the lateral pterygoid muscle.

A case referred to in Chapter 24 (see page 684) (Gregory, 1957) is that of a girl, aged 8 years, who sustained a subcondylar fracture of the mandible on the right side when she fell while riding on her bicycle. Roentgenographic examination showed a medial dislocation of the right condyle; the teeth were wired in occlusion by means of intermaxillary wire. Consolidation was completed with the head of the condyle at right angles to the ramus. The patient had no trouble in masticating food, but there was a deviation of the mandible to the affected side when the mouth was opened wide, indicating dysfunction of the right lateral pterygoid muscle. She was instructed to stand before a mirror and exercise her jaw daily in order to restore lateral pterygoid muscle function. Radiographs taken three years later showed a nearly normal position of the condyle and satisfactory growth, position, and function of the mandible.

Temporomandibular ankylosis (see Chapter 31) and mandibular hypoplasia are often attributable to damage to the articular cartilage of the condyle. Varying degrees of anatomical disruption of the condylar process, overriding of fragments and comminution do not seem to be the responsible factors in causing temporomandibular ankylosis. Before the age of 5 years the condylar neck is less developed, and the bony tissues are soft and more susceptible to a "crush" type of injury; after the age of 5 years, the condyle will, in all probability, fracture at the neck. The crush type of injury may cause the condylar cartilage to sustain the main damage. Because the condylar cartilage is one of the factors in mandibular growth, mandibular hypoplasia results when it is injured (Fig. 26–11). The degree of deformity seems to be inversely proportional to the age at which injury was sustained: the younger the patient at the time of injury, the more severe the deformity.

Condylar cartilage is first noted during prenatal life at the twelfth week. Blackwood (1965) has shown that large vascular channels appear during the twentieth week of fetal life and persist until the second or third year of postnatal life, when they progressively diminish in size. During this period the neck of the condyle progressively increases in length to form the long, slender condylar neck of the adult. Despite the fact that during the first three years of postnatal life the condyle is short and thick and thus less susceptible to fracture, it is also more vulnerable to a crushing injury because of its vascular trabecular structure. The crushing results in intra-articular and periarticular hemorrhage, and osteogenesis and progressive ossification results in temporomandibular ankylosis. Dufourmentel (1929) had noted that the condyle in the young child was more easily crushed than fractured.

There seems, therefore, to be a distinct difference in the results of a crushing injury in early childhood and a fracture of the neck of the condyle in later childhood. Whereas the crushing injury and the resultant damage to the condylar cartilage, as emphasized by Walker (1957), result in developmental arrest, the deformity resulting from the condylar neck fractures, when treated by simple intermaxillary fixation, is self-correcting (Gregory, 1957; Blevins and Gores, 1961; Rakower and coworkers, 1961; Kaplan and Mark, 1962; Mac-

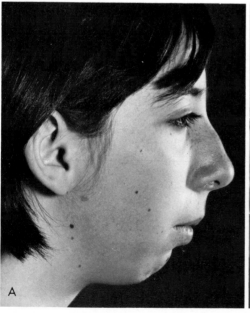 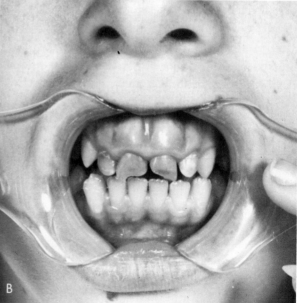

FIGURE 26–11.   Typical mandibular deformity resulting from condylar injury in early childhood. *A*, Underdeveloped mandible as seen in profile view in patient with temporomandibular ankylosis (see also Chapter 31). *B*, Maximum opening (1 to 2 mm) achieved by the patient. Note the poor condition of the teeth.

Lennan and Simpson, 1965; Rowe and Killey, 1968; Rowe, 1969). The advisability of intermaxillary fixation in fractures of the neck of the condyle in children has been questioned by Leake, Doykos, Habal, and Murray (1971), who observed spontaneous recovery of function and form in 20 children with unilateral or bilateral condylar neck fractures treated by early motion and no immobilization.

Fractures of the Alveolus

Injuries of the Teeth. In the young child, teeth may be dislodged along with a segment of alveolar bone which is subjected to a labial, buccal, and lingual displacement. Frequently the fragments of bone can be molded into alignment, and the teeth will survive if adequately supported for several months by wiring to an arch bar, by fixation with an acrylic splint, by threading wires between the teeth and wiring the fragment to solid teeth on either side of the fragment, or by use of a cable arch wire. In the child with incompletely developed roots, teeth may regain their blood supply and survive. In some instances, after root canal therapy the tooth can be replanted with success. If the teeth are fractured and the alveolar structures are hopelessly damaged so that they cannot retain tooth structures, it is best to remove the teeth, trim the alveolar process, and suture the soft tissues over the retained but injured bone (see Fig. 26–9). Bone fragments should not be dissected from attached soft tissue, and alveolar bone structure that has any opportunity to survive should be retained; even loose bone fragments, if covered with soft tissue, will survive as grafts.

Fractured crowns of teeth without exposure of the pulp should be protected by dental methods, as they can usually be successfully restored. If the crown of the tooth is fractured with the dental pulp exposed, the prognosis may be good if the tooth is capped or partial pulpectomy is done. This is most successful in the tooth with an open apex, but even in the more fully developed tooth, pulpectomy and root canal treatment may be effective in saving the tooth structures. Fracture of the root near the crown of the tooth usually requires extraction. If teeth can be retained only a few months, they may be useful in maintaining space until prosthetic replacement can be provided. Damage to the permanent tooth buds may result in deformed tooth structure, faulty eruption, or irregular arrangement of erupting teeth in the dental arch.

Delayed Treatment. If reduction of a fractured mandible has been delayed and cannot be achieved through simple manipulation, the fibrous tissue which forms rapidly in children between the ends of the fragments is excised and the fragments are loosened. A stout needle or trochar establishes a hole through the alveolar process of the distal and proximal fragments. Stainless steel wire is then passed from the buccal to the lingual side across the fracture line and returned from the lingual to the buccal side. The fragments are manipulated into alignment, and the ends of the wire are twisted. The twisted ends are bent close to the alveolar process and left long enough to protrude through the gingival tissue. The wire can then be removed as early as 14 days later, as consolidation occurs rapidly in children.

Although this procedure may occasionally cause injury to unerupted teeth, little damage has occurred in our cases. Even though one or more teeth must eventually be sacrificed, less harm ensues than would occur if the jaw fragments were permitted to heal in a distorted position, which may lead to greater deformity in children than in adults.

FRACTURES OF THE BONES OF THE MIDFACIAL SKELETON

The preceding pages have considered facial fractures in general and mandibular fractures in particular. Midfacial fractures in children up to the age of 12 years have constituted less than 0.5 per cent of all facial fractures; this figure may require revision in view of the greater number of children involved in automobile accidents. Because of the higher degree of elasticity of the facial bones in young children and the lesser degree of development of the midfacial skeleton in relation to the frontal and cranial area, middle-third facial fractures in children are less frequent than in the adult. Maxillary, naso-orbital, and orbital blowout fractures are not infrequent, and in children submitted to an unusually strong traumatic force, frontal bone and telescoping naso-orbital fractures can be associated with midfacial bone fractures.

Fractures of the Maxilla. The typical Le Fort lines of fracture are rarely seen in children's fractures. Low maxillary (Le Fort I) and pyramidal (Le Fort II) fractures are occasionally encountered.

Problems with fixation are similar to those encountered in the treatment of mandibular fractures because of the presence of poorly retentive teeth. In addition, alveolar fractures cause loosening, luxation, avulsion, or fracture of teeth, particularly the anterior teeth which are especially exposed to injury. A fixation appliance (cable arch, arch bar, or acrylic splint) may be attached to the remaining teeth and, in the older child, to selected erupted permanent teeth.

Internal wire fixation is an excellent means of fixation in the older child. In the young child, internal wire fixation to the frontal bone, to the orbital rim, or around the zygomatic arch may be unsatisfactory because the bone is soft and the wire, when placed under tension, tends to cut through the bone. Internal wire fixation to the edges of the pyriform aperture, which consists of thicker and stronger bone, is a preferable method.

Rapid fabrication of an acrylic splint in the operating room with quick-curing acrylic resin, while other fractures of the middle third of the face are being treated, will provide an appliance which is held by wire fixation to the edge of the pyriform aperture.

Because fractures of the facial bones in children consolidate readily and rapidly, a simple head bandage may be all that is required to provide cranial fixation of the fractured maxilla in the young child after occlusal relationships are established either with or without intermaxillary fixation.

Nasal Skeletal Fractures and Naso-orbital Fractures. Fractures of the nasal skeleton in children are more frequent than fractures of the maxilla or zygoma. In the early years of childhood, the nasal skeleton is proportionately more cartilaginous than bony, and diagnosis of nasal fracture is thus more difficult. The nasal bones in children are separated in the midline by an open suture line; thus the open-book type of fracture, with overriding of the nasal bones over the frontal processes of the maxilla, is a characteristic feature of nasal fracture in the child.

As with other types of childhood facial injuries, but particularly more so in nasal injuries, the complicating factor is that growth and development may be affected even after accurate diagnosis and adequate treatment.

The first five years of postnatal life are years of rapid facial growth. After a period of moderately active growth, a second period of rapid growth occurs between the ages of 10 and 15 years. Growth of the nasomaxillary complex may be affected by trauma during the early postnatal years. The work of Kravits and his associates (1969) suggests that injuries in infants are more frequent than generally suspected. Such injuries, as well as those suffered during delivery, may explain nasal deviation and nasomaxillary hypoplasia which have no other apparent cause.

The diagnosis of nasal injury in a young child is difficult and may often require general anesthesia in order to permit careful intranasal, extranasal, and skeletal inspection and palpation. Roentgenographic examination is a requisite for diagnostic and medicolegal purposes.

The nasal bones, which are relatively small, may not be fractured. Fractures, dislocations, and hematomas may be present, however, in the cartilaginous portion of the nose, which occupies a large proportion of the surface area of the nasal pyramid in the younger child.

The nasal bones are formed on the surface of the cartilaginous nasal capsule, and there is a considerable overlap between the lateral cartilages and the nasal bones. The lateral cartilages may be detached from the undersurface of the nasal bones because of their relatively loose attachment in the child and may collapse in conjunction with a fracture of the septum. A hematoma may form in this area between the lateral cartilages and the undersurface of the nasal bones; it should be evacuated through an intercartilaginous incision. A subperichondrial blood collection may also form over the alar cartilages and should be evacuated through a transcartilaginous incision.

Fractures and dislocations of the septal cartilage are frequent attendant injuries in fractures of the nasal bones, but they may occur independently. Hematoma of the septum, a collection of blood between the cartilage and the mucoperichondrium caused by rupture of the abundant vasculature of the area, manifests itself as a bluish-red bulging in the vestibule and nasal fossa. *Beware of the child who cannot breathe through his nose after a nasal injury!* Septal hematoma may also be caused by a simple traumatic bending of the septal cartilage without fracture or dislocation. Hematoma of the septum is always a serious complication in children, not only because of nasal obstruction which results from fibrous tissue increasing the thickness of the septum but also because of the possibility of collapse of the dorsum and saddling, as a result of loss of septal cartilage support through pressure necrosis from hematoma or a septal abscess.

Special care should be taken to drain the septal hematoma (see Chapter 24). An L-shaped incision, extending through the muco-periosteum over the vomer, is made along the floor of the nose and extends forward and then vertically upward through the mucoperichon-drium over the septal cartilage. The flap of mucous membrane thus outlined is raised, and the hematoma is evacuated. The dependent position of the incision assures drainage and thus prevents a recurring collection of blood. When the septal framework is fractured, the hematoma may collect bilaterally on both sides of the septal cartilage (see Chapter 24, page 730). A portion of the septal cartilage should be removed so that the two areas of hematoma communicate; a bilateral incision through the mucoperiosteum covering the vomer at the base of the septal framework provides depend-ent drainage and prevents recurrence of the hematoma.

Treatment of nasal bone fractures in chil-dren is similar to that of fractures in adults (see Chapter 24). Under general anesthesia, an ele-vator is placed into the nasal fossa, and the fractured fragments of nasal bones and frontal processes of the maxilla are elevated. Further realignment is obtained by external manual palpation. The septum, if fractured, is straight-ened, and if it is dislocated, the lateral carti-lages are realigned and repositioned. A splint of dental compound or plaster is placed over the nose for five to seven days. Intranasal packing is often necessary, in conjunction with the external splint, to assist in the realignment of the bony and cartilaginous fragments.

Naso-orbital fractures in which the bony structures of the nose are pushed backward into the interorbital space between the medial orbital walls, or lateral to the medial wall into the medial portion of the orbit, occur in au-tomobile accidents and can be treated by the wired plate technique (see Chapter 24). The open-sky method (Converse and Hogan, 1970) provides ideal exposure (see Chapter 25). Open reduction is achieved through bilateral vertical incisions over the frontal processes of the maxilla, exposing the comminuted bones, which are realigned and maintained by subcu-taneously placed transosseous wiring. An al-ternative approach is the bicoronal incision (Tessier and associates, 1967). This type of direct approach can prevent the subsequent sequelae of traumatic telecanthus, saddle-nose deformity, and lacrimal apparatus disturb-ances. Naso-orbital fractures are often asso-ciated with blowout fractures of the orbital floor.

Nasal bone fractures heal rapidly in chil-dren, frequently with overgrowth of bone and hypertrophic callus, resulting in widening of the bony dorsum of the nose. Children who have suffered comminuted nasal bone fractures may show developmental deformities years later, even though they received adequate treatment after the accident, an important con-sideration from a medicolegal viewpoint. The deformities are deviation and thickening of the septum, flattening of the nasal dorsum, widen-ing of the bony skeleton by hypertrophic callus, and varying degrees of nasomaxillary hypoplasia.

One should not hesitate to realign by osteot-omy the nasal pyramid or septum in children who have suffered an injury resulting in mal-united fracture and nasal obstruction. The risk of impairing growth is slight, as the damage to the growth potential has already been done by the causative trauma. The deformity, character-ized by depression of the dorsum with widen-ing of the nasal bridge, may require correction for psychologic as well as for functional rea-sons. A costal cartilage or bone graft may be required, with the understanding that definitive surgery will be required during adolescence. Nasomaxillary deformities are discussed in Chapter 30.

Zygoma and Orbital Floor Fractures. Zygoma fractures are rare in children and occur mostly in older children. Considerable force is required to fracture the resilient zygoma of the child, and the fracture usually takes the form of a fracture-dislocation. Lack of complete union at the frontozygomatic su-ture also explains the mechanism of this type of fracture. Treatment is similar to that of zygoma fracture in the adult (see Chapter 24).

Orbital fractures (see Chapter 25) in chil-dren are observed after automobile accidents and are often characterized by a separation of the frontozygomatic junction in the lateral or-bital wall with downward displacement of the floor. This type of unilateral craniofacial de-tachment is more frequent in the child than the Le Fort III bilateral craniofacial disjunction. Treatment consists of direct interosseous wire fixation.

The mechanism of production of orbital blowout fractures is similar to that of fractures in adults. The authors have observed blow-out fractures in children caused by the thrown snowball, another child's fist, tennis balls, and other objects. The maxillary sinus is small in the young child, and the floor of the orbit is concave, dipping downward behind the rim of the orbit, an anatomical characteristic that can mislead the surgeon into an erroneous diagnosis of orbital floor collapse. Despite the small size of the maxillary sinus, escape of orbital contents through the fractured floor occurs and may cause enophthalmos.

Restoration of the continuity of the orbital floor is the method of treatment, as it is in the adult. Comminuted fragments should be carefully preserved in children, as they consolidate very rapidly in a realigned position. The release of the entrapped orbital contents from the area of the blowout, which can then be covered by a small alloplastic implant, is followed by rapid return of ocular rotary movements. Children seem to have rapid recuperative ability after a blowout fracture, restoring the full range of extraocular muscle function, a recuperative ability which recalls that observed after flexor tendon repair in children.

Complications of Facial Bone Fractures in Children. Pulmonary complications were mentioned by McCoy, Chandler, and Crow (1966); aspiration of stomach contents or gastric dilatation occurred in 25.6 per cent of the children in their series. They noted that tracheostomy does not prevent this complication but suggested that a cuffed tube might prevent the problem. Early evacuation of stomach contents by nasogastric tube is indicated as a preoperative and postoperative measure.

Ocular injuries, damage to the lacrimal system, and cerebrospinal fluid rhinorrhea are observed in children and must receive the same consideration as those complications in the adult patient. Nonunion occurs infrequently. Osteomyelitis, which at one time was a serious complication in fractures, is rarely seen with modern antibiotic therapy.

Underdevelopment, maldevelopment, malocclusion, and ankylosis are all potential complications of facial bone fractures in children.

COMPOUND, MULTIPLE, COMMINUTED FRACTURES OF THE FACIAL SKELETON IN CHILDREN

In trauma of particularly severe violence, multiple lacerations with partial avulsion of the soft tissues and multiple fractures of the facial bones require careful surgical care. The reward for adequate primary management is the prevention of severe facial disfigurement.

Partly or nearly totally avulsed flaps of soft tissue and loose comminuted bone fragments should be preserved and replaced, as the blood supply of the facial area, and particulary of the child's face, ensures survival.

The following case history (Kostecki and coworkers, 1969) is an example of the satisfactory management of such a problem and is described in some detail, as it will serve to illustrate the application of many of the principles enumerated above.

Case History

A 5 year old boy was leaning through the open doors of a garage building elevator shaft when the elevator, on its descent, struck him on the right side of the face. On arrival at the Bellevue Hospital Center, he was conscious but was in respiratory distress. His blood pressure was 100/70, respiratory rate 20, and pulse rate 100.

Clinical Examination and Diagnosis. The injuries were confined chiefly to the head and, more specifically, to the right side of the face (Fig. 26–12). The most conspicuous defects were two major transverse soft tissue lacerations delimiting an area in which the soft tissues were avulsed from the bone and attached by small pedicles. One laceration extended from the midportion of the forehead to the upper pole of the right ear. The second laceration extended from the left side of the nose, across the dorsum of the nose and through the right lower eyelid, anterior to the right tragus, then downward toward the angle of the mandible. The second laceration extended into the nasal and oral cavities. There were also a laceration through the skin of the right upper eyelid and a full thickness laceration through the right portion of the upper lip, extending upward into the floor of the nose. Bilateral mandibular body fractures extending through the midportion of the body of the mandible were noted (Fig. 26–13). It was necessary to maintain foward traction on the loose anterior portion of the body of the mandible in order to keep the tongue from occluding the airway. There was no injury to the ocular globes.

A transverse laceration through the right upper eyelid raised concern as to whether it extended through the levator palpebrae su-

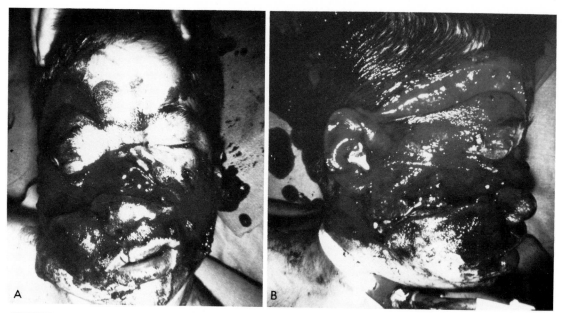

FIGURE 26–12. Five year old boy struck by a descending elevator. *A*, Extent of facial laceration. *B*, Avulsed flaps of soft tissue.

perioris muscle or aponeurosis. Levator function of the upper eyelid seemed to be intact as far as could be determined in the presence of severe edema. Orbicularis oculi and frontalis muscle function seemed adequate, a reassuring sign that the temporofacial portion of the seventh nerve was not severed. Exploration of the badly damaged tissues of the cheek area was postponed until the patient was under anesthesia.

An intravenous cannula was immediately inserted to facilitate fluid administration. Tetanus toxoid and antibiotics were given, and portable skull and chest roentgenograms were taken. The child was moved to the operating room where a tracheotomy was done under local anesthesia. A suitable airway was thus established, and inhalation anesthesia was administered through a cuffed intratracheal tube.

The child's face was cleansed with an antiseptic, and the injuries were evaluated by careful tissue manipulation and palpation. Ex-

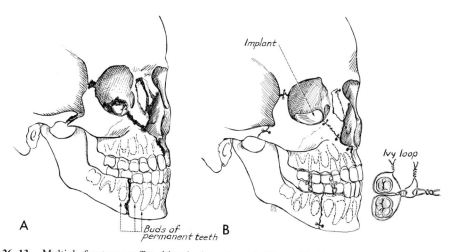

FIGURE 26–13. Multiple fractures suffered by the boy shown in Figure 26–12. *A*, Sites of fractures. Orbital blow-out fracture was repaired by a Silastic implant. Other fractures were treated by realignment and direct interosseous wiring. Note wire fixation of the mandible near the lower border.

amination of the soft tissues of the cheek denuded by the avulsion of the cutaneous flap
showed that Stensen's duct and the buccal
branches of the facial nerve had been severed
as they emerged from the parotid gland. Posteriorly, the proximal stump of the severed cervicofacial branch of the facial nerve was identified; the distal end was located with the aid of
a nerve stimulator. The right lower canaliculus
was divided approximately 3 mm medial to the
punctum.

Further examination showed a fracture of
the right half of the maxilla extending through
the center of the hard palate, the base of the
frontal process of the maxilla, the orbital floor,
and the right zygomaticomaxillary suture line
(Fig. 26–13). The right zygoma was mobile,
being separated by fractures through the frontozygomatic suture line and also through the
base of the frontal process of the maxilla.
There was also a fracture through the body of
the mandible on the right side.

The ocular globe moved freely, and the
forced duction test was negative, the eyeball
being readily rotated upward when the forceps
were applied to the inferior rectus tendon
through the sclera. The right infraorbital rim
and orbital floor were shattered, and it was obvious that the contents had collapsed into the
right maxillary sinus (Fig. 26–13). There was
also a fracture involving the right nasal bone,
which was separated from the left nasal bone
at the midline suture between the bones.

Treatment.   The mandibular fragments were
reduced, realigned, and stabilized by means of
stainless steel wire interosseous fixation near
the lower border of the mandible, thus avoiding injury to the tooth buds (Fig. 26–13).

Intermaxillary wires were applied using the
Ivy loop technique, and satisfactory occlusal
relationships were established between the
maxillary and mandibular teeth. The teeth
were in sufficiently good condition to retain the
eyelet (Ivy) loops. The maxillary and zygomatic
fractures were treated by realignment of the
fragments and direct interosseous wiring under
direct observation through the open wound.

The periorbita was raised over the orbital
rim and floor of the right orbit medial and lateral to the area of the comminuted fracture.
The continuity of the inferior orbital rim was
reestablished by realignment and wire fixation
of the fragments. The orbital contents were
then elevated from the maxillary sinus, and a
Silastic implant (Dow-Corning #600-802),
measuring approximately 20 × 20 × 2 mm.

was inserted over the orbital floor (Fig. 26–
13).

A PE–50 polyethylene catheter was
threaded through the punctum of the right
lower eyelid, through the distal end of the
divided canaliculus, and passed into the medial
portion of the canaliculus and lacrimal sac.
The protruding end of the catheter was sutured
to the lower lid, and the lid wounds were
closed with interrupted 6–0 nylon sutures.

The distal end of the parotid duct could not
be located in the midst of the badly damaged
tissue. As it seemed to have been destroyed
and restoration of the continuity of the duct
was not possible, the proximal stump was
ligated.

The facial nerve branches anterior to the
parotid gland were too fragmented for individual repair. Under magnification the proximal
stump of the severed cervicofacial branch was
sutured, using 8–0 nylon sutures, to the distal
stump, which has been located with the nerve
stimulator.

The remaining facial lacerations were closed
with subcutaneous plain catgut and fine nylon
skin sutures (Fig. 26–14). A pressure dressing
was applied over the face after an occlusive suture was placed through the right eyelid. A
feeding tube was inserted through the nose.

Postoperatively the patient took fluids by the
second day, and the feeding tube was removed.
The tracheotomy opening was closed on the
fifth postoperative day. The polyethylene catheter was removed from the right lacrimal duct
on the seventh day after the operation. The
child was discharged from the hospital on the
seventeenth postoperative day with the intermaxillary wires in place. Epiphora of the right
eye had subsided before the patient's discharge
from the hospital, and he was able to close the
right upper lid well enough to protect the cornea. Extraocular movements of the right globe
seemed to be close to normal on discharge
from the hospital. Contractions of the orbicularis oculi and frontalis muscles were weaker
than on the unaffected side. Paralysis of the
muscles innervated by the lower branches of
the facial nerve persisted.

During subsequent months, the postoperative result was considered to be satisfactory in
view of the severity of the initial injury (Fig.
26–15, *A*, *B*). Facial nerve function became
the main concern. Periodic clinical observation
and electrodiagnostic studies during the ensuing year showed a progressive reinnervation of
the muscles supplied by the right facial nerve
(Fig. 26–15, *C*). Serial electromyographic stud-

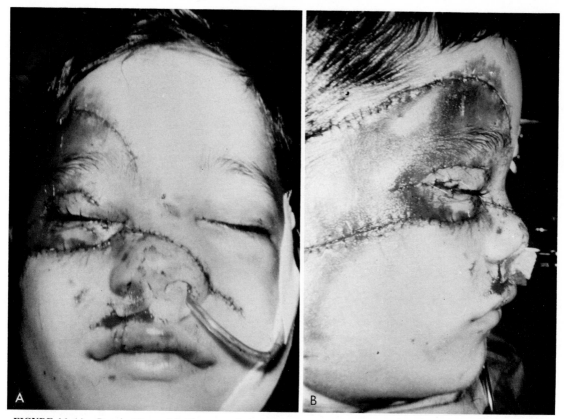

FIGURE 26–14. Boy in Figure 26–12 at completion of surgery. *A*, A feeding tube has been placed through the left nasal fossa. *B*, Profile view following approximation of flaps.

ies of the right orbicularis oculi muscle showed evidence of a partial lesion of the seventh nerve. Polyphasic potentials indicated that some regeneration was still occurring eight months after injury. Progressive return of movement was observed in the lower facial musculature with associated movements, movements of the mouth being observed when the child closed his eyes tightly. The synkinesis thus observed suggested that, in addition to the section of the cervicofacial division, the main trunk of the facial nerve had also been injured (Fig. 26–15, *C, D*). Weakness of the frontalis muscle had been observed soon after injury, also suggesting some degree of nerve injury. The "splitting" of regenerated axons and the resultant associated movements were evidence of injury to the main trunk of the facial nerve. One year after injury the patient was able to whistle without movements of the orbicularis oculi muscle, evidence of return of function of the buccal musculature through the repaired cervicofacial branch (Fig. 26–15, *C*). The patient's condition was relatively satisfactory in view of the severity of the injuries. Scar revision and a medial canthoplasty of the right eye will be required to improve the contour of the area.

Discussion of Management

TRACHEOTOMY. When treatment of the patient was begun in the emergency room, the major hemorrhage had ceased, and the patient was not in shock. Vital signs remained stable throughout the initial period of treatment. The immediate problem of impending airway obstruction, because of the unstable mandible, indicated the need for tracheotomy. The severe injuries to the nasal and oral cavities which might also cause airway obstruction were additional indications. Oliver, Richardson, Clubb, and Flake (1962), in a review of 294 tracheotomies in children under 18, stressed the importance of prior intubation. Difficulty with decannulation of the tracheostomy was encountered in 14 cases; seven formed fistulae requiring operative closure, and three developed tracheal stenosis.

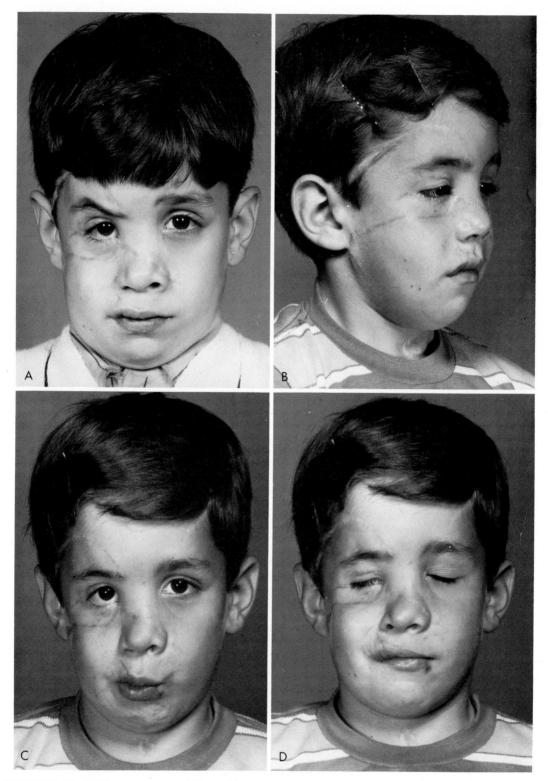

FIGURE 26–15. Follow-up views. *A, B,* Boy in Figure 26–12 one year after injury. *C,* Patient is able to whistle without associated movement of the eyelids. *D,* When patient closes the eyelids, associated movement of the right upper lip is noted.

In our patient, because of extensive wounds and fractures of the lower jaw, intubation prior to tracheotomy was not possible. Severe swelling of the oral and nasal airways combined with the intermaxillary wiring forced postponement of the decannulation until the seventh postoperative day.

‘TREATMENT OF FRACTURES. After the tracheotomy, the wounds were carefully explored, preserving all attached fragments of skin, while dirt and debris were removed. Reestablishment of the continuity of the mandible and maxilla by means of direct interosseous and intermaxillary wire fixation was first accomplished. The undamaged left maxilla acted as the fixed point for the restoration of near-normal occlusal relationships and the fixation of the mandibular and maxillary fragments.

The presence of the permanent tooth buds in a child 5 years of age left minimal space near the lower border of the mandible for drill holes and wires. Direct interosseous wiring of the fragments was done on each side of the body of the mandible (see Fig. 26–13). After the interosseous wiring, the fragments were still somewhat unstable. A number of deciduous teeth were loose, and some permanent tooth buds were dislodged at the fracture sites. The tooth buds were replaced in their sockets. There was a sufficient number of firmly fixed deciduous and permanent teeth to permit the application of Ivy loops on each side of the fracture lines on both the anterior and posterior fragments of the fracture of the body of the mandible. This wiring technique was selected because of its simplicity and easy adaptability with a minimum of special equipment. The other facial fractures were reduced through the open wounds and wired under direct vision with 26-gauge stainless steel wire.

REPAIR OF THE ORBITAL FLOOR FRACTURE. A massive comminuted fracture of the right orbital floor with ptosis of the orbital contents into the maxillary sinus does not usually result in restriction of ocular movements (see also Chapter 25). Indeed, in this case, the forced duction test was characteristically negative. Restoration of the continuity of the orbital floor was an essential requirement in order to reestablish the size of the orbit and avoid enophthalmos, which would have been massive had no treatment been instituted. The use of the alloplastic implant was justified as the simplest method of repairing the orbital floor in a severely injured child.

REPAIR OF THE CANALICULUS. Beard (1967) described a technique for canalicular repair with the Worst probe and the use of polyethylene tubing as a conformer left in place in the duct for two weeks (see also Chapter 28). Beard observed that, if the lower canaliculus alone is severed, the upper canaliculus usually can handle the normal flow of tears. If both canaliculi are severed, however, dacryocystorhinostomy should be done, with excision of the caruncle and placement of a Pyrex tube between the medial commissure and the nasal cavity.

Fortunately, in our patient, at the eighth-month follow-up visit, epiphora occurred only when the eye was irritated on a cold or windy day.

LIGATION OF STENSEN'S DUCT. When a repair of the parotid duct is not feasible, ligation of the proximal stump of the duct results in subsequent progressive atrophy of the parotid gland. In this manner, subsequent painful swelling of the gland is avoided.

REPAIR OF THE FACIAL NERVE. Restoration of the continuity of the branches of the facial nerve should be done; Maxwell (1954) first demonstrated the remarkable results obtained after reapproximation of severed branches and nerve grafting (see also Chapter 36). Because the orbicularis oculi and frontalis muscles seemed to be functioning, the temporofacial division of the facial nerve was thought to be intact. The severed nerve located in the posterior aspect of the wound was too large to be the mandibular marginal branch; it was felt to be the cervicofacial division and was reapproximated by suture. The buccal branches were badly damaged and could not be repaired. Converse and Goodgold (1959) have reported spontaneous regeneration of these nerves after section in adults and are of the opinion, as are Hanna and Gaisford (1965), that cross innervation occurs through the plexuslike connections between the peripheral branches of the facial nerve and also between branches of the fifth nerve. A review of the anatomy of the facial nerve branches anterior to the parotid gland (Hollingshead, 1958) shows numerous plexuslike interconnections. Despite some divergent views, there seems to be some clinical evidence supporting the opinion that the power of nerve regeneration is greater in children than in adults (Önne, 1962).

The associated movements observed during the period of return of function of the musculature can be explained by an undiagnosed lesion of the main trunk of the facial nerve; the weakness which was observed in the orbicularis oculi muscle reinforces this hypothesis.

Associated movements are attributed to misdirection of regenerating nerve fibers and can occur without section of the nerve (see Chapter 36). Associated movements are observed, for example, in cases of Bell's palsy (Ford and Woodhall, 1938), in which there is no loss of continuity of the nerve, but there is loss of conduction due to inflammatory edema of the nerve within the fallopian canal.

DEVELOPMENTAL MALFORMATIONS OF THE FACIAL SKELETON

Many facial developmental malformations can be attributed to trauma in early childhood. Trauma may have a deleterious effect on the growth and development of facial bone in postnatal life similar to that of a defective gene during prenatal development. In many cases it is difficult to ascertain whether the disturbance occurred before or after birth.

In order to provide an understanding of some of the developmental deformities resulting from prenatal or postnatal insult, a review of facial development follows.

Postnatal Growth of the Face

Knowledge regarding craniofacial growth has been determined by a variety of methods reviewed by Enlow (1968). The cross-section approach requires the utilization of large numbers of skulls of varying ages (Hellman, 1927; Keith and Campion, 1922; Krogman, 1930). Other methods can be employed which permit serial measurements on the same growing individual to evaluate the actual amount of growth. Four principal methods have been employed. The first involves the use of vital stains such as madder, as first practiced by John Hunter (1835–1837); the second involves vital staining of calcifying bones by means of a single intraperitoneal or intravenous injection a 2 per cent solution of alizarin red (Schour and coworkers, 1941). Thirdly, Björk (1955) was the first to study facial growth in man with the aid of metallic implants. Gans and Sarnat (1951) utilized implants of amalgam on each side of the frontozygomatic, frontomaxillary, zygomaticomaxillary, zygomaticotemporal, and premaxillomaxillary sutures. These implants were placed after incisions were made to expose bony areas. Finally, serial cephalometric roentgenograms were employed by Broadbent (1931, 1937), Margolis (1940,

1947), Higley (1936), Gans and Sarnat (1951), Krogman and Sassouni (1957), Moyers (1963), and Salzmann (1961).

The growth of the face is rapid and is best illustrated by the changes in facial size. At three months the face is less than half the size of that of the adult (approximately 40 per cent). At two years it has reached approximately 70 per cent; at 5.5 years it attains approximately 80 per cent of the adult size.

Earlier in the text it was reported that the proportions of the face change markedly during the period of postnatal growth. The skull at birth presents a relatively large cranial portion and a small facial component when compared with the skull of the adult; thus the proportions are 8 to 1 at birth in favor of the cranial portion over the facial portion, but they fall to 4 to 1 at 5 years, and 2 to 1 in the adult.

These changes are due to two factors: (1) the actual growth of the face, and (2) the modification of the proportions which brings forth characteristics, distinguishing the faces of males from those of females and establishing distinctive individual features.

1. **The Growth of the Face.** The facial skeleton is relatively small at birth. The nasal cavities and paranasal sinuses are also small (see Fig. 26–6, *A*); the nasal cavities are as wide as they are high. The pyriform aperture is broad, and its lower border and the floor of the nasal cavities are on a level slightly below that of the lower rim of the orbit and a horizontal line passing approximately through the two infraorbital foramina (see Fig. 26–6, *A*).

The growth of the maxillary sinus parallels that of the face. The maxillary sinus is narrow in the newborn and is not sufficiently developed to reach beneath the orbit (see Fig. 26–6, *A*); the sinus progressively increases in size. During the first year the medial-lateral dimensions have reached beneath the orbit, but no further laterally than the infraorbital foramen. During the third and fourth years the medial-lateral dimension of the maxillary sinus has increased considerably; at 5 years it extends to a point lateral to the infraorbital canal (see Fig. 26–6, *B*). The floor of the maxillary sinus remains above the level of the floor of the nose in the child up to the age of 8 years. It is only after the eruption of the permanent dentition in the twelfth year and the development of the alveolar process that the maxillary sinus descends below the level of the floor of the nose (see Fig. 26–6, *C*).

Increase in the vertical dimension of the face is due in part to the development and eruption of the dentition. In the newborn the crown portions of the upper and lower teeth or the alveolar processes do not contribute to vertical height, as the teeth have not yet erupted (see Fig. 26–1). A gradual facial change occurs at 7 years as a result of a general increase in size in all dimensions (see Fig. 26–3). The completion of facial growth varies, occurring from the eighteenth to the twenty-fifth year.

2. Changes in the Proportion of the Face. Increase in facial height is greater in the middle third of the face than in the lower third; the increase in the anterior-posterior direction is greater in the lower jaw than it is in the upper jaw; and the face widens more in the lower jaw than in the upper jaw.

The changes in the proportions of the face during the period of postnatal growth are well illustrated by comparing the face of a 3 month old infant with that of the same individual at the age of 23 years (Fig. 26–16, *A, B*). The growth of the middle and lower thirds of the face is striking.

At birth the portion of the nasal fossa occupied by the ethmoid bone is twice the height of the maxillary portion. During childhood the growth of the maxillary portion is accelerated, approximating the ethmoidal portion at the seventh year when adult proportions are attained. The growth of the maxillary portion of the nasal fossa is due in part to the increase in size of the maxillary sinus and to the eruption of the dentition and the supporting alveolar process. Changes in the maxilla and mandible result in characteristic changes of profile (Fig. 26–17).

The peak rate of growth in the head and face occurs between 3 and 5 years. After this period, growth proceeds slowly, but an acceleration occurs again between the thirteenth and fifteenth years. Growth is greatly diminished after the age of 15 years. Growth of the nose is completed between the eighteenth and twenty-fifth year. From a surgical standpoint, one may consider the growth of the nose completed at about the age of 16 years. Minor changes occur throughout life.

Postnatal Growth of the Mandible

The mandible is most frequently involved in developmental malformation. To explain the influence of extraneous factors upon the development of the mandible, one should recall the embryologic development of this bone.

The dorsal part of the first mandibular arch grows forward beneath the developing eye

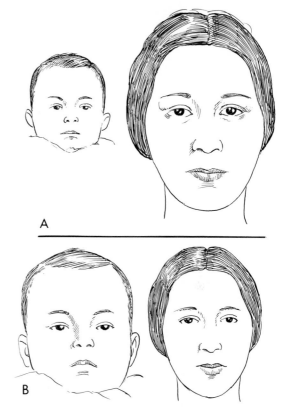

FIGURE 26–16. Growth of the face. *A*, Same individual at 3 months and 23 years of age showing transformation of the face from infancy to adulthood. *B*, Same individual at 3 months and 23 years of age showing similarity in size but difference in form. The photograph on the left has been enlarged so that the vertical dimension of the face is the same as that in the photograph on the right. Note the actual increase of the midfacial area in the adult. (After Hellman, M.: The face in its developmental career. *In* The Human Face—A Symposium. Philadelphia, The Dental Cosmos, 1935.)

region to the olfactory area, forming the maxillary process. As the result of the formation of this process, the mesenchymatous condensation, which gives origin to the first pharyngeal arch, becomes bent, and part of this dorsal portion becomes chondrified, forming a small cartilaginous mass which represents the pterygoquadrate bar of lower vertebrates. The remaining ventral and much larger portion of the pharyngeal arch chondrifies to form Meckel's cartilage (Fig. 26–18).

The posterior extremities of the pterygoquadrate bar of Meckel's cartilage articulate with each other. The intermediate portion of Meckel's cartilage retrogresses, and its sheath becomes ligamentous, forming the anterior ligament of the malleus and the sphenomandibular ligament. The dorsal portion, in contact with the pterygoquadrate cartilage, becomes recognizable as the definitive cartilaginous rudiment of the malleus, whereas the ventral por-

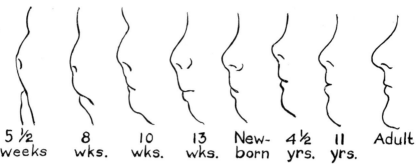

FIGURE 26–17. Series of profile outlines of the face from 5.5 weeks to adult. (After Peter and Schaeffer.)

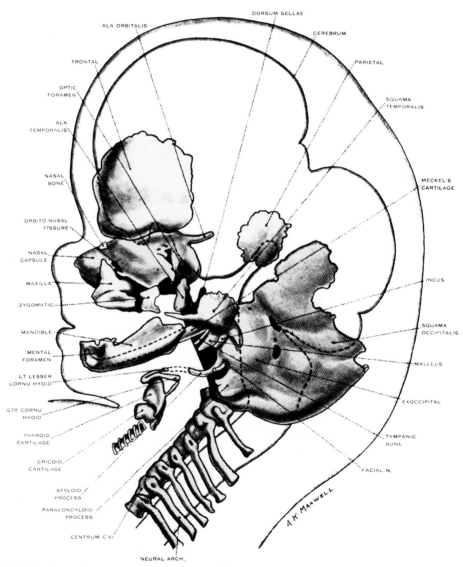

FIGURE 26–18. Lateral aspect of a model of the skull in a human embryo of about 40 mm. (Based on Macklin, 1914 and 1921.) Chondrocranium is colored blue, membrane bones yellow, and ala temporalis green. ×6. (From Hamilton, W. J., Boyd, J. D., and Mossman, H. W.: Human Embryology. Copyright 1945, The Williams & Wilkins Company, Baltimore.)

tion is involved in the development of the incus (Fig. 26–19).

Later in development, two membrane bones are laid down on the outer side of Meckel's cartilage (Fig. 26–20): (1) The anterior of these, which appears very early, is related to the lateral aspect of the ventral portion of the cartilage and forms the mandible. At first it is a small covering of membrane bone, but by growth and extension it soon surrounds Meckel's cartilage, except at its anterior extremity, where some endochondral ossification occurs. (2) Upward growth forms the mandibular ramus at the posterior end of the developing mandible (Fig. 26–20). This portion of the mandible comes into contact with the squamous part of the temporal bone to form the temporomandibular joint, in which a fibrocartilaginous articular disk develops. Part of the ramus of the mandible is transformed into cartilage before ossification occurs.

In mammals, as in many other vertebrates, arches of the membrane bone are laid down lateral to the cartilages of the first pharyngeal arch and in the substance of the maxillary and mandibular processes. In the maxillary processes of each side, four such ossification areas form the premaxilla, maxilla, and zygomatic and squamous temporal bones.

The mandible, small at birth (see Fig. 26–1), is destined to grow both by development of the alveolar process, which accompanies the development of the teeth, and by bone growth.

John Hunter (1835–1837) demonstrated the mode of growth of the mandible. He applied the discovery of Duhamel (1734), who had studied the growth of bone by feeding animals madder. The observation that madder, the root of a plant, had the property of acting as a vital stain for living bone cells had been described by Belchier (1738). Belchier fed some of his fowls with madder and noted that living bones were stained red by the madder.

Hunter fed two young pigs on a madder diet for a month. He sacrificed one of the pigs at the end of the month and retained the other for an additional month on ordinary food before sacrificing it. Hunter found that the appearance

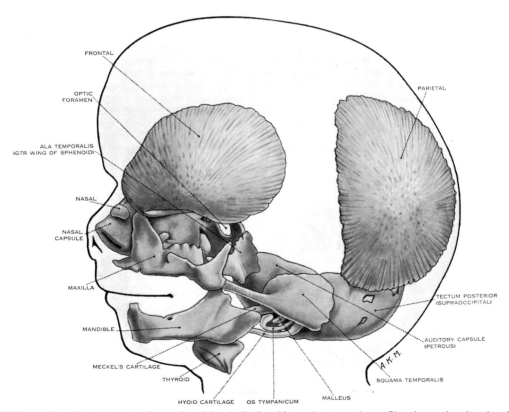

FIGURE 26–19. Lateral aspect of a model of the skull of an 80-mm human embryo. Chondrocranium is colored blue, membrane bones yellow, and ala temporalis green. (Based on Hertwig's model, from Kollmonn's Handatlas, 1907.) (From Hamilton, W. J., Boyd, J. D., and Mossman, H. W.: Human Embryology. Copyright 1945, The Williams & Wilkins Company, Baltimore.)

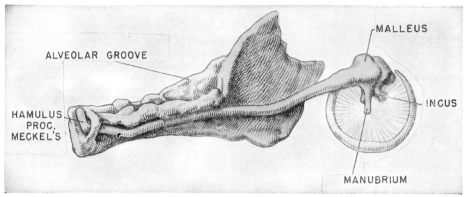

FIGURE 26–20. Mandible, Meckel's cartilage, malleus, and incus of a human fetus 80 mm long. (After Kollmann, Keibel, Franz, and Mall: Manual of Human Embryology. Philadelphia, J. B. Lippincott Company.) (From Shapiro, H. H.: Maxillofacial Anatomy. Philadelphia, J. B. Lippincott Company, 1954.)

presented by the bones of these two pigs met his expectation in the most exact manner. What had been the condyle and the posterior border of the mandible during the period of madder ingestion were now included in the substance of the ramus, which had grown during the period in which the pigs had not received madder. The madder-stained bone was almost completely removed by absorption from the anterior border of the ramus (Fig. 26–21). Hunter concluded that growth of the bone is due to the addition of bone on the extremity of the mandible, combined with absorption of bone in other areas (Keith, 1919).

The recognition of condylar growth centers

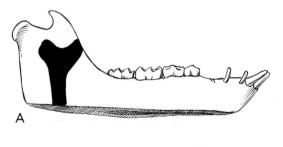

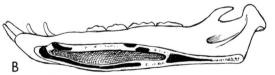

Figure 26–21. Copy of Hunter's drawing to show the manner in which growth takes place in the mandible. Drawings represent two views of the right half of the mandible of a pig, which was fed on a madder diet for one month and then on a normal diet for one month. Outline of the ramus at the end of the madder period is shown by the dark areas. (After Keith, 1919.)

(Charles, 1925; Brodie, 1941) confirmed Hunter's original findings and showed that the forward projection of the mandible is a consequence of this posterior growth. Elongation of the mandible involves continued additions of bone at each condyle and along the posterior border of the ramus. Posterior appositional growth is only one of the many major movements associated with total growth, as all of the different portions of the bone participate in the growth process (Enlow, 1968). In addition to the centers of growth, increase in size is the result of surface apposition, the local contours of the mandible constantly undergoing changes as a result of relocation and remodeling, and resorptive and depository activities.

Growth of the condyle is the result of endochondral ossification in the epiphysis. Microscopic examination of human material (Orban, 1944; Rushton, 1946) showed chondrogenic, cartilaginous, and osseous zones. The condyle is capped by a narrow layer of avascular fibrous tissue, which contains connective tissue cells and a few cartilage cells. The inner layer of this covering is chondrogenic, giving rise to hyaline cartilage cells which form the second or cartilaginous zone. Destruction of the cartilage and ossification around the cartilage scaffolding can be seen in the third zone. The cartilage of the head of the mandible is not similar to the epiphyseal cartilage of a long bone, for it differs from articular cartilage in that the free surface bounding the articular space is covered by fibrous tissue. Walker (1957) has emphasized the role of trauma to the condylar articular cartilage in producing mandibular hypoplasia, particularly if the trauma occurs before the age of 5 years.

Postnatal Growth of the Nasomaxillary Complex

The skeleton of the midfacial area is formed from membrane, with the exception of the nasal cartilaginous capsule. These bones grow in a complex manner in a variety of regional directions. The growth and development of the nasomaxillary complex has been studied by numerous anatomists. Among the early studies are those of Disse (1889), Peter (1913), Stupka (1938), who was concerned with developmental anomalies, and Negus (1958), who was concerned with comparative anatomy. More recent studies in animals and man, with the use of vital staining, anatomical sections, and cephalometrics, include those of Scott (1953, 1956–1959, 1963), Baume (1968), and Enlow (1968). The anteroposterior growth of the nasomaxillary complex is related in utero and also after birth to the growth of the basal cranial cartilages and their synchrondroses. The intersphenoidal and the septoethmoidal synchondroses show signs of activity until adulthood. At birth the nasal septum is continuous with the cartilages of the cranial base. Around the first year, the perpendicular plate of the ethmoid starts to ossify from the mesethmoid center. At 3 years of age there is bony union between the ethmoid and the vomer. The bony structures of the nasomaxillary area then follow a complex process of growth, which has been reviewed in detail by Enlow (1968).

There is not only a forward downward growth of the maxilla but also a constant remodeling of the multiple regional parts. The main steps in this development include a displacement away from the cranial base, a posterior enlargement corresponding to the lengthening of the dental arch, and an anterior resorption of the malar region. The nasal vaults grow forward and laterally, and the descent of the premaxillary area occurs by resorption on the superior and anterior surface of the nasal spine and by bony deposition on the inferior surface.

Considerable controversy has arisen over the role of the septum in the growth of the nasomaxillary complex and over the implications of trauma in causing abnormal growth of the area. Scott, reminding us that the midfacial area is formed of membrane with the exception of the cartilaginous nasal capsule, considered the septum to be the driving force in the growth of the midfacial area. Scott's hypothesis has been supported by Baume (1961), Wexler and Sarnat (1961, 1965), and Sarnat and Wexler (1966, 1969).

The role of the nasal septum is considered of lesser importance by Moss, Bromberg, Song, and Eisenman (1968) and Stenström and Thilander (1970). According to Moss, facial growth is controlled by a "functional matrix" which comprises the nonskeletal elements of the face, including spaces, muscles, and soft tissues.

Ross and Johnston (1972) concluded that the maxilla drifts forward as part of an overall genetic and environmental pattern of growth, bone being laid down in the sutures and on the maxillary tuberosity. The maxilla is more easily influenced in its growth than the mandible (see Chapter 42).

The role of trauma in interfering with growth and development of the midfacial area seems to be difficult to determine. In making a comparison with another facial area, namely the mandibular, one finds a considerable disparity between the extent of damage suffered by the condylar area and the extent of the ensuing maldevelopment. In some cases of fracture of the condylar area in children, complete restoration of anatomical form occurs without interference with growth and development; in other cases, what seems to be minor damage results in mandibular hypoplasia. Much depends, apparently, upon the extent of damage to the condylar cartilage (Walker, 1957). Reconstructive surgery for nasomaxillary deformities is discussed in Chapter 30.

REFERENCES

Baume, L. J.: The postnatal growth activity of the nasal cartilage septum. Helv. Odont. Acta, *5*:9, 1961.

Baume, L. J.: Patterns of cephalofacial growth and development. A comparative study of the basicranial growth centers in rat and man. Int. Dent. J., *18*:489, 1968.

Beard, C.: Repair of traumatic defects of the lacrimal system (acute). *In* Proceedings of the Second International Symposium on Plastic and Reconstructive Surgery of the Eye and Adnexa. St. Louis, Mo., C. V. Mosby Company, 1967.

Belchier, J.: An account of the bone of animals being changed to a red colour by aliment only. Philos. Trans. *39*:287, 1738.

Björk, A.: Facial growth in man, studied with the aid of metallic implants. Acta Odont. Scand., *13*:9, 1955.

Blackwood, H. J.: Vascularization of the condylar cartilage of the human mandible. J. Anat., *99*:551, 1965.

Blevins, C., and Gores, R. J.: Fractures of the mandibular condyloid process: Results of conservative treatment in 140 patients. J. Oral Surg., *19*:392, 1961.

Broadbent, B. H.: A new x-ray technique and its application to orthodontia. Angle Orthod., *1*:45, 1931.

Broadbent, B. H.: The face of the normal child. Angle Orthod., *7*:183, 1937.

Brodie, A. G.: On the growth pattern of the human head. Am. J. Anat., *68*:209, 1941.

Burdi, A. R., Huelke, F., Snyder, R. G., and Lowry, A. H.: Infants and children in the adult world of automobile safety design: Pediatric and anatomical considerations for design of child restraints. J. Biomech., *2*:267, 1969.

Charles, S. W.: The temporomandibular joint and its influence on the growth of the mandible. J. Br. Dent. Assoc., *46*:845, 1925.

Converse, J. M., and Goodgold, J.: *In* Kazanjian, V. H., and Converse, J. M. (Eds.): The Surgical Treatment of Facial Injuries. 2nd Ed. Baltimore, The Williams & Wilkins Company, 1959, p. 961.

Converse, J. M., and Hogan, V. M.: Open-sky approach for reduction of naso-orbital fractures. Case report. Plast. Reconstr. Surg., *46*:396, 1970.

Disse, J.: Die Ausbildung der Nasenhohlen nach der Geburt. Arch. Anat. Physiol., *29*(Suppl.):54, 1889.

Dufourmentel, L.: Chirurgie de l'Articulation Temporomaxillaire. vol. 1. Paris, Masson et Cie, 1929, p. 228.

Duhamel, H. L.: Quatrième mémoire sur les os. Dans lequel on se propose de rapporter de nouvelles preuves qui établissent que les os croissant en grosseur par l'addition de couches osseuses qui tirent leur origine du périoste. Communication à l'Acad. Roy. des Sciences, *56*:87, 1734.

Enlow, D. H.: The Human Face. New York, Hoeber Medical Division, Harper & Row, 1968.

Ford, F. R., and Woodhall, B.: Phenomena due to misdirection of regenerating fibers of cranial, spinal and autonomic nerves. Arch. Surg., *36*:480, 1938.

Gans, B. J., and Sarnat, B. G.: Sutural facial growth of the Macaca rhesus monkey: A gross and serial roentgenographic study by means of metallic implants. Am. J. Orthod., *37*:827, 1951.

Gregory, T. G.: Personal communication, 1957.

Hamilton, W. J., Boyd, J. D., and Mossman, H. W.: Human Embryology. Baltimore, The Williams & Wilkins Company, 1945.

Hanna, D. C., and Gaisford, J. C.: Facial nerve management in tumors and trauma. Plast. Reconstr. Surg., *35*:445, 1965.

Hellman, M.: A preliminary study in development as it affects the human face. Dent. Cosmos, *69*:250, 1927.

Hellman, M.: The face in its developmental career. *In* The Human Face: A Symposium. Philadelphia, The Dental Cosmos, 1935.

Higley, L. B.: A head positioner for scientific radiographic and photographic purposes. Int. J. Orthod., *22*:699, 1936.

Hollingshead, W. H.: Anatomy for Surgeons. Vol. 1. The Head and Neck. New York, Paul B. Hoeber, Inc., 1958.

Hunter, J.: Works of John Hunter (with notes by James F. Palmer). London, Longman, Rees, Orme, Brown, Breen and Longman, 1835–1837.

Johnson, H. A.: A modification of the Gillies' temporalis transfer for the surgical treatment of lagophthalmos of leprosy. Plast. Reconstr. Surg., *30*:378, 1962.

Kaplan, S. L., and Mark, H. I.: Bilateral fractures of the mandibular condyle and fractures of the symphysis menti in an 18-month-old child. Oral Surg., *15*:136, 1962.

Kazanjian, V. H., and Converse, J. M.: The Surgical Treatment of Facial Injuries. 3rd Ed. Baltimore, The Williams & Wilkins Company, 1974.

Keith, A.: Menders of the Maimed. London, Oxford University Press, 1919.

Keith, A., and Campion, C.: A contribution to the mechanism of growth of the human face. Int. J. Orthod., *8*:607, 1922.

Kostecki, R. J., Casson, P. R., Zallen, R. D., and Converse, J. A.: A case of severe facial trauma in a five-year old child. Unpublished paper, 1969.

Kravits, H., Driessen, G., Gomberg, R., and Korach, A.: Accidental falls from elevated surfaces in infants from birth to one year of age. Pediatrics, *44*(Suppl.):869, 1969.

Krogman, W. M.: The problem of growth changes in the face and skull as viewed from the comparative study of anthropoids and man. Dent. Cosmos, *72*:624, 1930.

Krogman, W. M., and Sassouni, V.: A syllabus in roentgenographic cephalometry. Philadelphia Center for Research in Child Growth, 1957.

Leake, D., Doykos, J., Habal, M. B., and Murray, J. E.: Long-term follow-up of fractures of the mandibular condyle in children. Plast. Reconstr. Surg., *47*:127, 1971.

Lewin, M. L.: Total rhinoplasty in infants. Report of a case of Waterhouse-Friderichsen syndrome. Plast. Reconstr. Surg., *15*:131, 1955.

McCoy, F. J., Chandler, R. A., and Crow, M. L.: Facial fractures in children. Plast. Reconstr. Surg., *37*:209, 1966.

MacLennan, W. D., and Simpson, W.: Treatment of fractured mandibular condylar processes in children. Br. J. Plast. Surg., *18*:423, 1965.

Margolis, H. I.: Standardized x-ray cephalograms. Am. J. Orthod., *26*:725, 1940.

Margolis, H. I.: A basic facial pattern and its application in clinical orthodontics. Am. J. Orthod., *33*:631, 1947.

Maxwell, J. H.: Repair of the facial nerve after facial laceration. Trans. Am. Acad. Ophthalmol. Otolaryngol., *58*:733, 1954.

Moss, M. L., Bromberg, B. E., Song, I. C., and Eisenman, G.: The passive role of nasal septal cartilage in midfacial growth. Plast. Reconstr. Surg., *41*:536, 1968.

Moyers, R. E.: Handbook of Orthodontics. Chicago, Year Book Medical Publishers, 1963.

Negus, V. E.: The Comparative Anatomy and Physiology of the Nose and Paranasal Sinuses. Baltimore, The Williams & Wilkins Company, 1958.

Oliver, P., Richardson, J. R., Clubb, R. W., and Flake, C. A.: Tracheotomy in children. New Engl. J. Med., *267*:631, 1962.

Önne, L.: Recovery of sensibility and sudomotor activity in the hand after nerve suture. Acta Chir. Scand., *300*(Suppl.):1, 1962.

Orban, B.: Oral Histology and Embryology. St. Louis, Mo., C. V. Mosby Company, 1944.

Panagopoulos, A. P.: Management of fractures of the jaws in children. J. Int. Coll. Surg., *28*:806, 1957.

Peter, K.: Atlas der Entwicklung der Nase und des Gaumens beim Menschen. Jena, Gustav Fisher, 1913.

Pfeifer, G.: Kieferbruche im Kindesalter und ihre Auswirkungen auf das Wachstum. Fortschr. Kiefer. Gesichtschir., *11*:43, 1966.

Rakower, W., Protzell, A., and Rosencrans, M.: Treatment of displaced condylar fractures in children: Report of cases. J. Oral Surg., *19*:517, 1961.

Ross, R. B., and Johnston, M. C.: Cleft Lip and Palate. Baltimore, The Williams & Wilkins Company, 1972.

Rowe, N. L.: Fractures of the facial skeleton in children. J. Oral Surg., *26*:505, 1968.

Rowe, N. L.: Fractures of the jaws in children. J. Oral Surg., *27*:497, 1969.

Rowe, N. L., and Killey, G. C.: Fractures of the Facial Skeleton. 2nd Ed. Baltimore, The Williams & Wilkins Company, 1968.

Rushton, M. A.: Unilateral hyperplasia of the mandibular condyle. Proc. R. Soc. Med., *39*:431, 1946.

Salzman, J. A. (Ed.): Roentgenographic Cephalometrics. Proceedings of the Second Research Workshop. Philadelphia, J. B. Lippincott Company, 1961.

Sarnat, B. G., and Wexler, M. R.: Growth of the face and jaws after resection of the septal cartilage in the rabbit. Am. J. Anat., *118*:755, 1966.

Sarnat, B. G., and Wexler, M. R.: Longitudinal development of upper facial deformity after septal resection in growing rabbits. Br. J. Plast. Surg., *22*:313, 1969.

Schour, I., Hoffman, M. M., Sarnat, B. G., and Engel, M. B.: Vital staining of growing bones and teeth with alizarine red S. J. Dent. Res., *20*:411, 1941.

Scott, J. H.: The cartilage of the nasal septum. Br. Dent. J., *95*:37, 1953.

Scott, J. H.: Growth at facial sutures. Am. J. Orthod., *42*:381, 1956.

Scott, J. H.: Studies in facial growth. Dental Practitioner, *7*:344, 1957.

Scott, J. H.: The growth of the human skull. J. Dent. Assoc. South Afr., *13*:133, 1958.

Scott, J. H.: Further studies on the growth of the human face. Proc. R. Soc. Med., *52*:263, 1959.

Scott, J. H.: The analysis of the facial growth from fetal life to adult hood. Angle Orthod., *33*:110, 1963.

Shapiro, H. H.: Maxillofacial Anatomy. Philadelphia, J. B. Lippincott Company, 1954.

Stenström, S. J., and Thilander, B. L.: Effects of nasal septal cartilage resections on young guinea pigs. Plast. Reconstr. Surg., *45*:160, 1970.

Stupka, W.: Die Missbildungen und Anomalien der Nase und des Nasenrachentaumes. Vienna. Julius Springer, 1938. pp. 1–319.

Tessier, P., Guiot, G., Rougerie, J., Delbet, J. P., and Pastoriza, J.: Ostéotomies cranio-naso-orbito-faciales hypertélorisme. Ann. Chir. Plast., *12*:103, 1967.

Topazian, R. G.: Etiology of ankyloses of the tempormandibular joint. J. Oral Surg., *22*:227, 1964.

Walker, D. G.: The mandibular condyle: 50 cases demonstrating arrest in development. Dental Practitioner, *7*:16, 1957.

Wexler, M. R., and Sarnat, B. G.: Rabbit snout growth. Effect of injury to septovomeral region. Arch. Otolaryngol., *74*:305, 1961.

Wexler, M R., and Sarnat, B. G.: Rabbit snout growth after dislocation of the nasal septum. Arch. Otolaryngol., *81*:68, 1965.

CHAPTER 27

DEFORMITIES OF THE FOREHEAD, SCALP, AND CALVARIUM

J. J. LONGACRE, M.D., PH.D., AND JOHN MARQUIS CONVERSE, M.D.

ANATOMY OF THE SCALP

The soft tissue over the cranium consists of five layers (Fig. 27–1): skin; subcutaneous tissue; the occipitofrontalis muscle (epicranius); the galea aponeurotica (a lax layer of subaponeurotic fibroareolar tissue); and the pericranium. From a surgical standpoint the first three strata are considered as forming the scalp proper, since they are intimately connected and are not easily separated.

The *skin* of the scalp is very thick and is attached by tough, fibrous septa to the underlying galea. It has an abundant blood and lymphatic supply and numerous sweat and sebaceous glands.

The *subcutaneous tissue*, because of its fibrous septa, forms an inelastic but firm layer containing the blood vessels. The blood vessels embedded in the unyielding tissue bleed freely when divided because they cannot contract. Because of the abundant anastomoses of the temporal, supraorbital, supratrochlear, posterior auricular, and occipital vessels, scalp flaps with only a small pedicle usually survive and large flaps heal uneventfully. Infection is prone to remain localized because of the fi-

brous septa, but purulent collections are painful because the nerves are compresssed within enclosed compartments.

The paired *occipitofrontalis muscles* (epicranius) and their galeal aponeuroses, which join them across the vertex of the cranium, are attached posteriorly to the external occipital protuberance and the superior nuchal line of the occipital bone. They fuse laterally with the temporal fascia and attach through the substance of the frontalis muscle to the supraorbital ridges and adjacent soft tissues.

The *subepicranial space* lies between the epicranius muscle and the pericranium. This potential space is traversed by small arteries

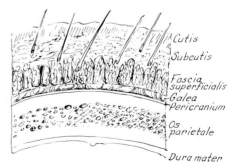

FIGURE 27–1. Diagram of the five layers of the scalp.

822

which supply the pericranium and by the emissary veins connecting the intracranial venous sinuses with the superficial veins of the scalp. This space is considered the danger zone of the scalp because hematoma and infection can spread easily through it, and thrombosis of the emissary veins may extend to the dural sinuses. Pus trapped in this space may destroy the pericranium and cause necrosis of the skull, and can even spread intracranially.

The periosteum overlying the cranium is known as the *pericranium*. In the neonatal skull, the fontanels are bridged by pericranium externally and dura mater internally. When the fontanels are obliterated, the dura mater and pericranium are bound closely to the suture line. Spreading infection and hematoma are thus usually limited to the confines of a single bone. The blood vessels that traverse the pericranium and the small vessels in the outer table of the cranium may afford pathways along which infection extends to the diploë and causes osteomyelitis. When the sutures are obliterated, the pericranium extends from one bone to another without deep sutural attachment.

PHYLOGENY

In describing the development of the cranium it is well to consider first its basic neural and visceral (branchial) components. The neural portion supports and protects the brain and sense organs. Phylogenetically, this part of the skull is a composite consisting of an old cranial base with which are associated the capsular investments of the sense organs. To this has been added more recently the facial skeleton plus a vaulted cranial roof. Thus the skull eventually consists of two components: cranial and facial. Phylogenetically, man inherited only two of the original five bones that protect the eye. They are the lacrimal and the malar bones. The decrease in the number of bones accompanying the movement forward of the orbits from their more lateral position allows for binocular vision. The progressive decrease in the number of bones in the skull as one passes from fish to man is known as "Williston's law." In general the older basal portion is preformed in cartilage, whereas the new facial and roofing bones are formed in membrane. There is, however, so much fusion and overlapping that it is unwise to try to draw too sharp a line of distinction.

The visceral (branchial) portion of the skull consists of reduced and modified remains of the gill arches, which played such an important role in food seizure (jaws) and respiration (gill arches) in our aquatic ancestors. It is of interest that most of the parts retained are still concerned with the same functions, although they have been utilized under different conditions since lung respiration replaced the gill mechanism.

Under air living conditions, the sound receiving mechanism evolves into a more elaborate form with the conversion of the obsolescent proximal ends of the first two visceral arches into the auditory ossicles. The inner aspect of the first branchial pouch becomes the eustachian tube, while the external portion forms the external auditory canal. Around the external auditory orifice, budlike proliferations form as the anlagen of the external ear. The remaining portion of the first branchial arch (Meckel's cartilage) continues forward and becomes the anlage around which two membrane bones are later laid down to form the mandible. The second branchial arch is represented by the stylohyoid ligament and the upper portion of the hyoid bone. The third arch is represented by the lower portion of the hyoid bone, and the thyroid cartilage is formed by the fourth. In the developing embryo the muscles of the face and neck are formed by mesenchymal migration carrying along the original nerve innervation and blood supply from each visceral arch. Deficiency of the mesenchyma results in various hypoplastic syndromes involving the middle and lower third of the face with deformities of the ear and rarely of the eye.

GROWTH OF THE CRANIAL BONES AND FACIAL SKELETON

Congenital deformities of the cranial and facial bones are best understood by studying normal growth. The cranial base is first laid down in cartilage, and this model is gradually replaced with chondral bone in the developing infant. In contrast, the calvaria is formed by the ossification of the preexisting condensed mesenchyma (desmocranium) and by the periosteum, respectively. The preexisting fibrous structures are incorporated with a large number of newly formed fibers in the new bone matrix. Likewise with the maxilla and mandible, the first bone appears in an area of mesenchyma in which definitive collagen fibers are not present until immediately before ossification. In a third type of formation, bone appears among the dense fibers of preexisting fascia, aponeurosis, ten-

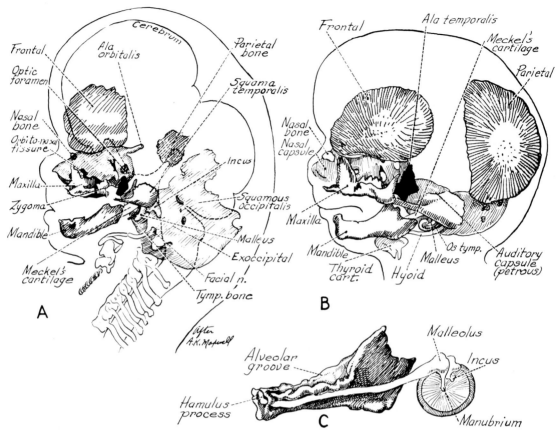

FIGURE 27–2. *A,* Lateral aspect of a model of the skull of a human embryo of about 40 mm (based on Macklin, 1914 and 1921). *B,* Lateral aspect of the skull of an 80-mm human embryo (based on Hartwig's model from Kollman's Handatlas, 1907). (*A* and *B* redrawn from Hamilton, W. J., Boyd, J. D., and Mossman, H. W.: Human Embryology. 3rd Ed. Baltimore, Williams & Wilkins Company, 1962.) *C,* Meckel's cartilage, malleus, and incus of a human fetus 80 mm long. (Redrawn from Kollmann, J., Kiebel, F., and Mall, F. R.: Human Embryology. Philadelphia, J. B. Lippincott Company.) These illustrations appear in color as Figures 26–18 to 26–20.

don, ligament, or cartilage, e.g., Meckel's cartilage (Fig. 27–2, *A, B, C*).

As is well known, the brain grows rapidly; consequently, the cranium triples in volume in the first two years of life, except in premature cranial synostosis (craniostenosis). Growth of the cranium continues but at a slower rate until the seventh year, at which time it has attained 90 per cent of its adult size. Thereafter, the annual increment in growth is almost negligible.

The facial bones do not keep up with the rapid pace of the cranium. After the first year the facial skeleton grows faster and continues to grow over a much longer period.

CONGENITAL DEFECTS OF THE CRANIUM AND SCALP

Congenital defects of the cranium and scalp are rare, only 76 cases having been reported up to 1930. The first patient reported by Campbell (1826) died of hemorrhage from the exposed superior sagittal sinus. This occurred also in patients whose histories were reported by Heidler (1924), Pincherle (1938), and Peer and Van Duyn (1948). According to Ingalls (1933) there were associated defects in other areas of the body in 8 per cent of the cases. Ingalls found an overall mortality of 20 per cent due to hemorrhage and infection. He also found thin-walled blebs in the midline of the head of several embryos as early as the tenth week; he thought that these blebs later ulcerated and produced the defect in the full term infant. The defect has also been attributed to failure of closure of the midline structures; 20 per cent of scalp defects, however, do not occur in the midline. It is now generally accepted that the growth and differentiation of the bones of the vault of the skull are dependent on the growth of the underlying brain. According to Snell (1961) an abnormality in the formation of the underlying brain could be connected with the development of the overlying skin, as both are derived from the adjacent ectoderm.

In the newborn the treatment is conservative, and the patient is placed under continued observation. The indications for operation in the larger lesions overlying the superior sagittal sinus have been stressed by Peer and Van Duyn (1948) and Kahn and Olmedo (1950). These authors point out that if the lesion is more than 1 to 2 cm in width it may become necrotic. Reconstruction with a scalp flap is recommended. In the larger lesions, the skull defect does not close spontaneously, and grafting with bone (split rib grafts) or cartilage is necessary at a later stage to provide adequate protection for the brain. O'Brien and Drake (1961) have surveyed the literature and reported five cases.

Craniopagus. Symmetrical conjoined twins are unusual (one case in 60,000 births) in spite of the fact that the intrinsic conditions capable of giving rise to double monsters exist in all fertilized eggs. According to Stockard (1920–21), if differentiation is interrupted just before the differentiation of the embryonic axis, the resumption of growth may be followed by the establishment of two centers of growth, neither of which is capable of growing at a rate sufficient to inhibit development of the other. When the duplicated parts are of equal size, they are as strongly inclined to be as normal as they are in single individuals.

The treatment of craniopagus twins was reported by Grossman and coworkers (1953), Jayes (1964) and Laskowski and Baldwin (1962).

In the case of the craniopagus twins reported by Grossman, Sugar, Greeley, and Sadove in 1953 (Fig. 27–3), the problem was whether a surgical separation could be attempted. Unfortunately there was little information in the literature that was of any pertinent value; the few previous attempts at separation of other craniopagus twins had failed. Pneumoencephalography disclosed two separated arachnoid spaces and indicated a dural septum between the two brains. Attempts to obtain contrast visualization of the dural venous sinuses failed.

If separation was to be accomplished, an adequate covering for the exposed intracranial structures would be required. Greeley delayed two scalp flaps (Fig. 27–4) 35 cm long and 7.5 cm wide. After three stages, the scalp flaps were completely divided around their periphery. During the first attempt at separation, at 14 months of age, the flaps were elevated from their beds. The final separation was made three weeks later (Fig. 27–5). Since there was a common dural sinus, all of the veins from the one twin had to be clipped and divided. The one twin devoid of a dural sinus never regained consciousness and died 34 days later. The other twin, with the complete dural sinus, cried immediately and moved all extremities. Repair was later done in stages as indicated in Figure 27–4. Figure 27–6 shows the patient as he was nine years after the separation. It was impossible to place bone grafts into the defect because of a residual cyst that collected fluid and required repeated aspiration.

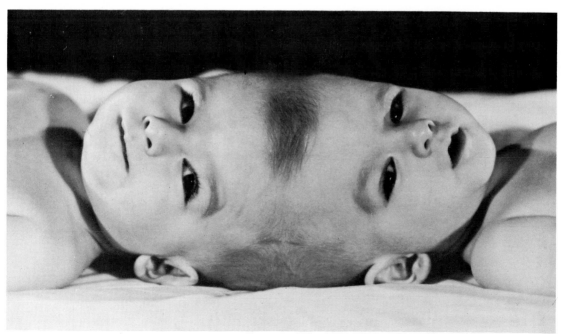

FIGURE 27–3.   Craniopagus twins (R. L. B. and R. D. B.) 11 months of age prior to delaying of flaps and attempt at separation.

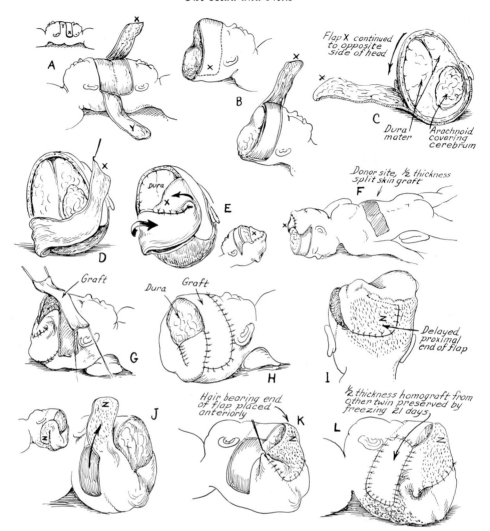

FIGURE 27–4. Origin of circumferential scalp flaps of both infants and stages in covering the exposed intracranial contents by skin flaps in R. D. B. *A*, The flaps, which were replaced after the first attempt at separation on November 26, 1952. *B* to *E*, Re-elevation of skin flaps and transfer to cover the posterior half of the exposed intracranial structures of R. D. B. (December 30, 1952). The arrows in *B* indicate the severance site of the terminal end of the flap. *F* to *H*, Covering of the exposed donor site of the flap with a split-thickness graft from the back of the patient (January 6, 1953). *I*, Extension of the proximal end of the full-thickness flap by delay of the circulation to the base (January 17, 1953). *J*, *K*, *L*, Completion of the rotation of the full-thickness graft to cover the remaining exposed intracranial structures (February 10, 1953). The donor site was covered by a split-thickness graft (March 1, 1953).

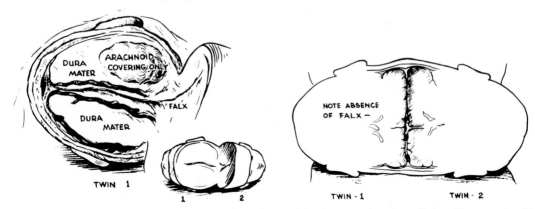

FIGURE 27–5. *A*, Diagram of the arrangement of the abnormal dural venous sinuses, as disclosed by operation. Note the dural defect over the right hemisphere of R. D. B. *B*, Reconstruction of the arrangement of the dural venous sinuses, seen in coronal section. Note the apparent absence of the falx in R. D. B.

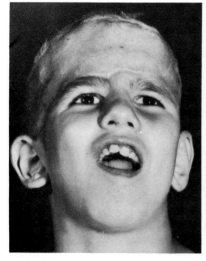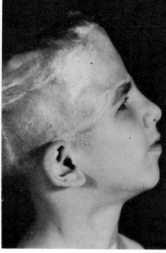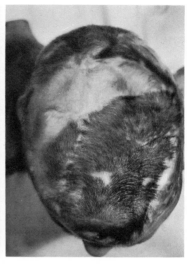

FIGURE 27–6. Surviving twin (R. D. B.) nine years following separation and reconstruction. Since the child had a recurring cyst which enlarged and had to be repeatedly aspirated, no attempt was made to replace the missing bone of the calvarium. R. D. B. died suddenly at the age of 11½ years.

Jayes (1964) has successfully repaired the soft tissue defects in three surviving twins who had been separated from their counterparts (who later died). He has reported that all three are alive; one twin has developed epilepsy, is mentally retarded, and has hemiplegia. Another is physically normal but mentally retarded. The third child is making excellent progress and shows every sign of undergoing normal development. Jayes planned to utilize split rib grafts at a later date to fill the cranial defects. Laskowski and Baldwin (1962) reported the successful separation of craniopagus twins joined at the forehead with their separate brains fused for 2 cm. There was only one artery and not the single venous sinus which had been found in the previously reported cases. Today both girls are bright, alert, and active individuals (Fig. 27–7).

Congenital Aplasia of the Scalp (Aplasia Cutis Congenita). This congenital anomaly, which was described by Campbell in 1826, varies in its extent. It may involve the scalp only, or the scalp and the underlying bone, as in the patient whose case history follows. The malformation may be so extensive as to involve the scalp, cranial vault, and dura.

Aplasia cutis congenita defects are usually less than 2 cm in diameter and often heal spontaneously. Larger defects require surgical closure. The literature has been extensively reviewed by Dingman, Weintraub and Wilensky (1976).

Aplasia cutis congenita is a rare anomaly with little known of the etiology. There have been scattered reports of sequential cases in

the same family, leading to the conclusion that there is a recessive genetic factor involved (Greig, 1931; Kahn and Olmedo, 1950; Savage, 1956; Farmer and Maxmen, 1960; Rauschkolb and Enriquez, 1962; Hodgman, Mathres and Levan, 1965).

Other theories postulated to explain this defect include vascular accidents, direct trauma or pressure, syphilis, and amniotic adhesions as well as chromosomal abnormalities. None of these can fully explain the condition. The

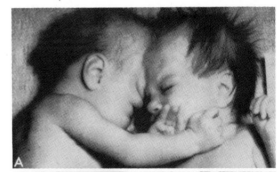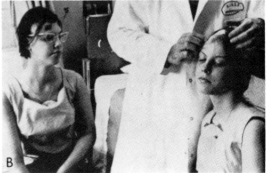

FIGURE 27–7. *A,* Craniopagus twins in the neonatal period. *B,* Appearance of twins in adult life.

scalp or skull defects occur most frequently in the first-born female children. The defects are generally less than 2 cm in diameter and may be symmetrical or stellate in configuration. Most often they are in the midline in the region of the posterior fontanelle. Two or more lesions have been reported in 25 per cent of the cases, and this same group often exhibits symmetrical linear trunk defects. There is never any hair over the defects.

The defect is generally irregular, involving only the epidermis, and heals spontaneously. Absence of the underlying cranial bone is seen in only 20 per cent of the cases (Lynch and Kahn, 1970). Associated anomalies include hydrocephalus, myelomeningoceles, cheiloschisis and palatoschisis, cleft lip, cleft palate, and deformities of the fingers.

Biopsies of the edges of the lesions show no inflammatory reaction. The epidermis is thinned or absent with an atrophic corium. The collagen is compact, with little adipose tissue present. Sweat and sebaceous glands as well as the elastic fibers are absent. The membrane covering the brain consists of a very thin, flattened layer of cuboidal nucleated cells set in a regular manner in a single layer (Montgomery, 1967).

CONGENITAL ABSENCE OF THE SCALP AND CRANIAL VAULT. A full term infant, S.H. (Fig. 27–8, *A, B*), was born with two large defects of the scalp, 2 × 3 cm. on either side of the sagittal sinus in the posterior fontanel area. On radiologic examination there was an underlying defect of the cranium measuring 4 × 5 cm. Over a period of 24 hours, the exposed dura became necrotic, and the child was transferred to the hospital.

Under local anesthesia excision of the necrotic area was performed, sparing the inner layer of the dura and the pia arachnoid. There was no leakage of spinal fluid, but, as debridement was performed on the right side, there was sudden bleeding from one of the emissary veins into the sagittal sinus. This was controlled by Gelfoam, topical thrombin, and digital pressure. The defects were then closed by large rotation flaps (Fig. 27–9). One flap was rotated anteriorly and the other posteriorly. A collodion splint dressing was applied.

The head of the infant was elevated in order to reduce the pressure in the sagittal sinus, and the wound healed uneventfully. Subsequent studies showed that the child had hyperthyroidism and a moderate degree of gargoylism.

CONGENITAL ABSENCE OF THE SCALP, CRANIAL VAULT, AND DURA. Congenital absence of scalp, skull, and dura in a neurologically intact newborn is rare. It has been termed a variant of aplasia cutis congenita, which is usually defined as congenital absence of skin but which occasionally may involve simultaneous loss of scalp, skin, and dura. The surgical treatment of a newborn with a ruptured omphalocele and an extensive area of exposed brain provides a dilemma of priorities and management and is the basis of the following report (Dingman, Weintraub and Wilensky, 1976).

A female infant was transferred to the Pediatric Surgical Service at the University of Michigan Medical Center at six hours of age with a ruptured omphalocele and a large cranial defect. The child was the product of a precipitous delivery following an uncomplicated 36 weeks of gestation. Birth weight was 2.6 kg. The parents were both 26 years of age and were in good health. The mother took vitamins and iron throughout her pregnancy and denied

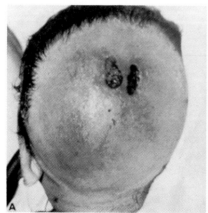 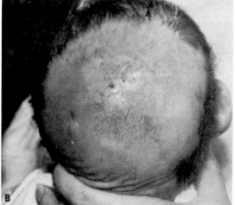

FIGURE 27–8. *A*, A congenital absence of an area of the scalp with beginning necrosis of the dura in newborn infant. *B*, One month following excision of the necrotic areas and reconstruction by means of double rotation flaps.

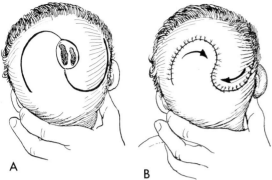

A   B

FIGURE 27-9. *A,* Outline of the proposed rotation flaps for the closure of an occipital defect of the scalp and skull in the infant shown in Figure 27-8. *B,* The rotation flaps have been interpolated, providing adequate coverage of the cranial defect.

any other drug ingestion. The mother had previously delivered a four-month hydatidiform mole and a full-term healthy male. There was no family history of a similar skull or cutaneous defect, syphilis, tuberculosis, or exposure to communicable diseases. At birth the Apgar scores were 2 and 2, the blood pres-

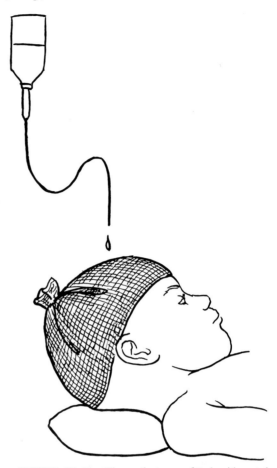

FIGURE 27-11. The patient was fitted with a tube gauze headdress kept moist by a continuous drip of normal saline solution.

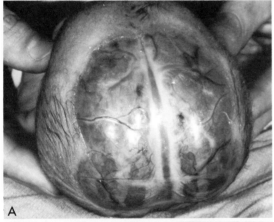

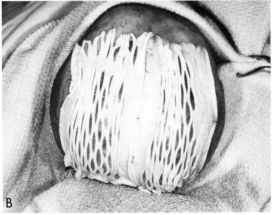

FIGURE 27-10. *A,* Appearance of the congenital defect of the scalp, cranium and dura 11 days after birth. *B,* Skin allografts placed over the defect. (Figs. 27-10 through 27-13 courtesy of Dr. Reed O. Dingman.)

sure 56/34, pulse 156, and temperature 96.8. The child appeared dehydrated and lethargic.

The child had a 7.5 × 5 cm defect involving the skull, scalp, and dura (Fig. 27-10, *A*). This formed a clean, punched-out midline defect over the junction of the sagittal and arachnoid sinuses so that the brain, in fact, was covered by only the thin, transparent pia. The white blood cell count was 21,000, platelet count 123,000, and mixed capillary pH 7.18. Chest roentgenograms showed a pneumomediastinum without an accompanying pneumothorax. The child voided spontaneously. The child was resuscitated and started on antibiotics prior to transfer to the operating room.

The patient's clinical problems required priority decisions. There was only pia covering the child's brain, and thus the risk of hemorrhage, thrombosis, or meningitis was high. On the other hand, the ruptured omphalocele had to be dealt with, despite the fact that most authors advocated the mandatory nature of early scalp closure. It was elected to repair the

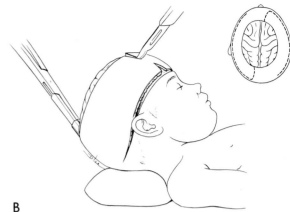

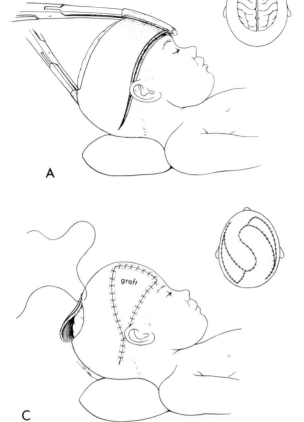

FIGURE 27–12. *A*, Delay of the scalp flap on the right side. The inset shows the extent of the defect. *B*, Division and further delay of the flap. *C*, Transfer of the scalp flaps. The inset illustrates the method of transposition of the flaps over the defect. Split-thickness skin grafts covered the donor areas of the flaps.

omphalocele first and place cadaver skin allografts over the cranial defect (Fig. 27–10, *B*). Autografted skin would offer the advantage of permanent survival, but such a graft would be almost impossible to remove safely when more definitive bony coverage would be necessary.

The omphalocele was repaired primarily without undue abdominal tension. The patient was returned to the neonatal intensive care ward, where the pneumomediastinum resolved. Six hours later the baby had a grand mal seizure. At this time the sodium was 125, potassium 4.6, chloride 86, and CO_2 20; arterial blood gases were normal. Glucose was 40 mg per 100 ml, and calcium was 7.1. Simultaneously the child developed apneic spells and was intubated, placed on a respirator, and given phenobarbital and diphenylhydantoin. Sodium, calcium, and dextrose were administered, and the child's condition was rapidly stabilized. Over the ensuing 18 hours, the child was weaned from the respirator and extubated. The following morning oral feedings were started and she was stooling within 24 hours. The allograft skin did not take well and by the third day was removed.

The child was fitted with a tube gauze headdress (Fig. 27–11), which was kept moist by a continuous drip of normal saline solution. By day four, the child was gaining weight on oral feedings and the serum electrolytes had returned to the normal range. Her head circumference, which was 31 cm at birth (less than the third percentile), grew 1.5 cm at the end of 7 days, and concomitantly the defect increased in size to 9.5 × 7.5 cm. On the eleventh day of life she was returned to the operating room, where bilateral scalp flaps were outlined and delayed (Fig. 27–12, *A*) after intravenous fluorescein testing demonstrated nonperfusion of the distal 4 to 5 cm of the flaps. Allograft skin was again used to cover the defect, and the tube gauze cap with constant irrigation was replaced. Eight days later the flaps were divided and again delayed after fluorescein demonstrated adequate perfusion of all but the distal 2-mm margin of the right scalp flap (Fig. 27–12, *B*). The flaps were then transposed two days later and split-thickness skin autografts were applied to the resulting donor defects (Fig. 27–12, *C*). An additional application of a small split-thickness skin graft to the flap donor

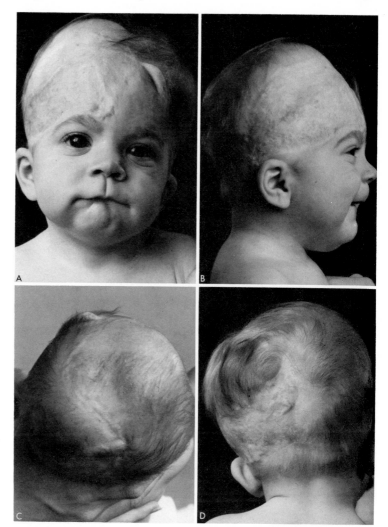

FIGURE 27–13. Appearance of the patient at the age of 10 months. *A, B,* The skin-grafted area of the donor site of the right scalp flap, which covers half of the original defect. *C,* The left scalp flap covers the other half of the defect. *D,* View of the vertex.

area was necessary ten days later. The child did well postoperatively except for one period of seizures; these were felt to be secondary to a tight-fitting head dressing. Treatment included phenobarbital and diphenylhydantoin and replacement of the dressing. No seizure activity has been noted since that time. The patient is currently 12 months old and, although she continues to grow and develop normally, there is no evidence of spontaneous closing of the bony defect as has been reported (Matson, 1957).

Full-thickness flap coverage of the defect was critical, and skin allograft application allowed adequate time to plan and delay the flaps. Fluorescein was used to evaluate flap viability and was definitely helpful, since it predicted loss of the flap in a location that would have recreated the original lesion. At the third scalp flap delay procedure, fluorescein demonstrated full viability and the flaps were successfully rotated (Fig. 27–13).

In the future, consideration will be given to the insertion of split-rib grafts for cranial coverage. It is hoped that some skull growth might occur prior to this. She wears a specially designed plastic helmet, and to date the child is passing growth and mental milestones normally.

Premature Synostosis of the Cranial Sutures. The shape of the head may be severely altered by premature closure of one or more of the cranial sutures (see Chapter 56). Though the synostosis may be present before birth, the abnormality of shape may not be noticed at birth, or may not be appreciated until some time after birth. Whether the brain is involved depends on the extent of the premature closure of the suture lines. When closure of the sutures prevents enlargement of the brain, mental retardation and blindness result. The shape of the head depends upon the sutures involved, the limitation of growth being at right angles to the line of the involved sutures.

Symmetrical premature closure of the

coronal sutures leads to a condition called *acrocephaly, oxycephaly,* or *turret skull.* Björk (1959) inserted pins into various bones of the skull and observed growth to maturity with roentgen cephalometry and presented evidence that premature closure and fusion of the cranial base likewise plays a role. The head is flattened posteriorly and protrudes anteriorly. The facial expression becomes adenoid, and the eyes protrude from widely separated eyelids which tilt downward and outward. The base of the skull is diminished and the cranium bulges in the place where the frontal bossae normally appear. The absence of the occipital bulge is partly responsible for the characteristic appearance. When associated with syndactyly of the hands and occasional polydactyly of the feet, the condition is known as *acrocephalosyndactyly* or *syndrome of Apert.* The appearance of the afflicted patients being similar, it appears as if they all belonged to one family (see Chapter 56).

Craniofacial dysostosis, as first described by Crouzon (1912), is a hereditary synostosis. It consists of acrocephaly, a beaklike nose, a triangular mouth with a short upper lip and protruding lower lip, proptosis of the eyes, and exotropia. The syndromes and their treatment are discussed extensively in Chapter 56.

TRAUMATIC DEFECTS OF THE CRANIUM AND SCALP

Scalp Avulsion

The seriousness of avulsion of the integument over the calvarium and the need to provide cover for the exposed bone were noted by the Egyptians as early as 3000 B.C. Later the famous surgeon Ambroise Paré noted the difficulty in trephining the eburnated exposed calvarium and utilized the cautery to aid in sequestration of the dead outer table.

One of the earliest references in the American literature has been contributed by Douglas (1962), as follows:

The orderly book of "Camp Lady Ambler," October 20, 1776, states "Patrick Vance appointed third surgeon with pay of assistant."

Surgery and surgical instruments were of the most primitive kind on the early frontier. During the Christmas campaign, while the men were quartered at Long Island, the above-mentioned Dr. Vance discovered a treatment for scalped persons. He bored holes in the skull in order to create a new flesh covering for the exposed bone. On being called away he taught James Robertson how to perform the operation.

Frederick Caloit, a scalped patient, was brought in and Robertson had a chance to practice upon him. "He (Vance) bored a few holes himself, to show the manner of

doing it." [Vance] further declared, "I have found that a flat pointed straight awl is the best instrument to bore with as the skull is thick and somewhat difficult to penetrate. When the awl is nearly through, the instrument should be borne more lightly upon. The time to quit boring is when a reddish fluid appears on the point of the awl. I bore at first about one inch apart and as the flesh appears to rise in these holes, I bore a number more. . . . The scalped head cures slowly. It skins remarkably slow, generally taking two years."

With the advent of the industrial revolution there were many victims of scalping as the long hair of the women workers was caught in the unprotected belts and gears of the machines driven by water and steam power. Review of the early literature indicates that many of these unfortunate patients were doomed to die from prolonged infection or intracranial complications. Sequestration of denuded bone and resultant extensive defects surrounded by dense scar were the sequelae in those who survived. Subsequent recurrent breakdown with repeated ulceration frequently terminated in carcinoma.

As early as 1911, Davis reported 81 cases of industrial scalping. In 21 cases the scalp had been replaced only to mummify. In 1924, McWilliams stated that 173 cases had been reported and the scalp replaced in 40, again with no success. During World War I, Cushing (1918) again pointed out the importance of early scalp closure. This was also reemphasized and illustrated by Gillies (1944) during World War II.

Treatment. The immediate surgical care is similar to the supportive care given to any patient who has suffered from trauma, hemorrhage, and shock accompanying an extensive wound. Blood transfusion is frequently indicated to correct the blood loss and secondary hypovolemia. After the patient is prepared under general anesthesia, the wounds are thoroughly cleansed and lightly debrided. The denuded areas should then be converted into closed ones as soon as possible. The therapy applied depends on whether or not the periosteum is present.

TREATMENT WHEN PERIOSTEUM IS PRESENT. The early conversion of the extensive open wound to a closed one with autogenous skin grafting remains the method of choice. The ability of the intact periosteum to support and nourish a skin graft has been well established (Kazanjian and Webster, 1946; Converse, 1955; Kazanjian and Converse, 1959). Thick split-thickness skin grafts provide a much more stable covering than the thin Thiersch graft but require careful suturing and adequate fixation (Fig. 27–14).

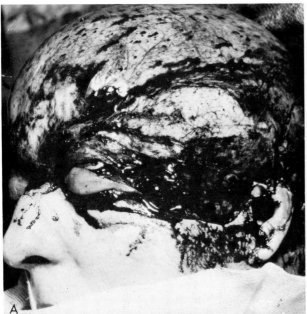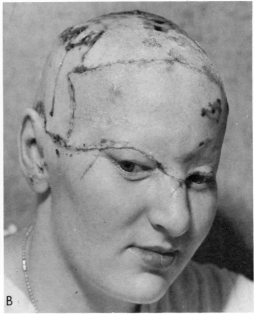

FIGURE 27–14. Traumatic avulsion of the scalp. *A*, Appearance of the patient 24 hours after avulsion of the scalp as a result of hair being entangled in machinery. The pericranium is intact. *B*, After successful split-thickness skin grafting.

Repeated attempts to utilize the full-thickness scalp have generally met with failure. Kazanjian and Webster (1946) pointed out that, even though the subcutaneous fat is removed, including most of the hair follicles, the skin of the scalp is so thick that it is far less likely to survive than are the split-thickness grafts.

Osborne (1950) reported a case in which thick split-thickness grafts from the avulsed scalp were applied to the pericranium with success. Meister (1955) used "deep" scalp grafts in two cases but obtained no hair growth, even though epithelization was attained. Delak (1955) reported one successful take of a thinned scalp graft with some fuzz three months later. According to Robinson (1952) replacement even after laborious thinning down to a full-thickness skin graft is not to be recommended. Robinson further suggested that, until further research has been undertaken on the split scalp graft, immediate coverage with split-thickness skin grafts of the areas with a pericranial base remains the method of choice.

A notable exception is a case reported by Lu (1969), in which he reported an unexpectedly successful result in a 7 year old patient with a subtotal avulsion of the scalp. The avulsed scalp was replaced in toto and was revascularized.

Miller, Anstee and Snell (1976) were successful in replanting a totally avulsed scalp by microvascular anastomoses. The procedure was successful because the detached scalp was not unduly damaged and suitable recipient vessels were available in the superficial temporal region.

TREATMENT WHEN PERIOSTEUM IS DESTROYED. The outer table of the calvarium receives its blood supply from the scalp through the periosteum. Hence, when the bone is exposed by avulsion, it must be immediately covered, either by a local flap in moderate and even large sized defects or by a flap from a distance. A description of the closure of these defects is given by Converse (1954b, 1955). In the scalp all the arteries extend to the vertex, anastomose freely, and form a rich network. The mobility and abundant blood supply of the scalp permit the closure of large areas with hair-bearing scalp by transposing large and long flaps on a narrow pedicle (Fig. 27–15). The closure of defects by mobilization, rotation, and advancement of local flaps is the method of choice (Fig. 27–16). The nonstretchable scalp can be made to cover a large area by multiple incisions through the galea according to the technique of Kazanjian and Converse. The surrounding tissues are stretched after undermining the plane between the galea and pericranium, raising the flaps, and making a number of vertical incisions through the nonstretchable galea. These may be crisscrossed with similar horizontal incisions (see Fig. 27–16, *F*) to relieve the tension and permit return of the flaps to their original position without compromising the blood supply.

Orticochea (1971) has devised an ingenious three-flap technique for the closure of moder-

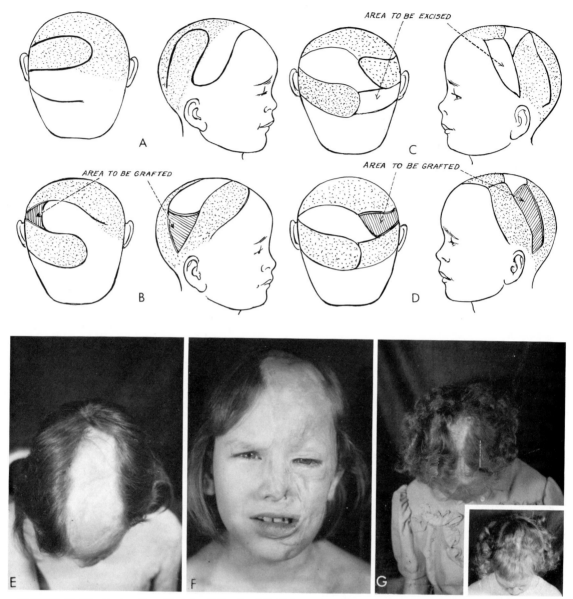

FIGURE 27–15. Restoration of hairline (following full-thickness burn) by transposed scalp flaps. *A,* Design of flaps. *B,* The hair-bearing flap has been transposed forward and the non–hair-bearing backward. The remaining donor defect is covered with a split-thickness skin graft applied over the pericranium. *C,* On the contralateral side, the scarred tissue will be excised; the hair-bearing flap is outlined. *D,* The hair-bearing flap has been transposed and the remaining donor defect is grafted. *E, F,* Large skin-grafted area of scalp. *G,* After transposition of flaps (inset), the patient is able to cover the remaining skin-grafted area with a luxuriant growth of hair.

ate sized and large defects with variations (Figs. 27–17 and 27–18). A four-flap technique is also feasible (Orticochea, 1967) (Fig. 27–19). Because of the vascularity of scalp flaps, they remain viable when the base of the flap is at the periphery, where it receives the nutrient vessels of the scalp.

If soft tissue coverage is not provided, the outer table of the cranial bone undergoes necrosis and is eventually extruded. Exfoliation may be accelerated by drilling a series of burr holes through the outer table of the cranium. Granulations growing up from the diploë eventually join and provide a base of granulation tissue which will accept a skin graft. A more rapid method is to remove the eburnated dead bone with an osteotome down to bleeding bone. In a week to ten days, granulations

Text continued on page 837.

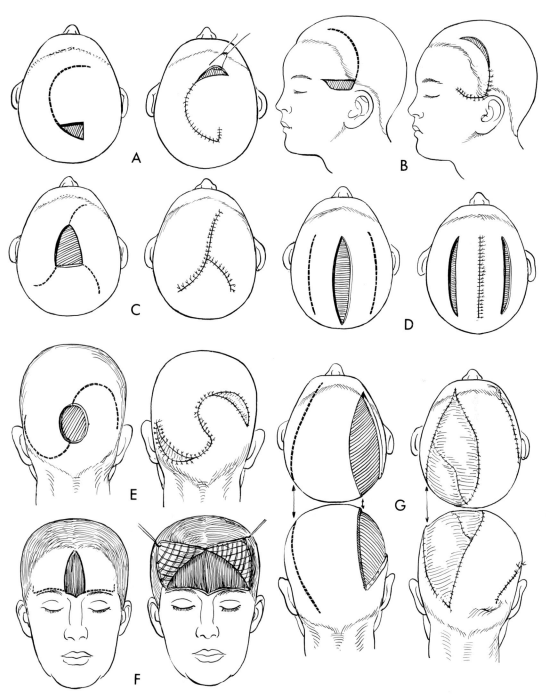

FIGURE 27–16.　Some techniques for the closure of scalp defects. *A, B,* Rotation flaps. *C,* Gillies' tripod technique (1944). *D,* Bipedicle flaps. *E,* Double opposing rotation flaps. If complete closure cannot be obtained, split-thickness skin grafts are applied over the pericranium to cover the remaining exposed areas. *F,* Kazanjian and Converse's crisscross incisions through the frontalis muscle and/or the galea aponeurotica to distend the flaps and achieve closure of the defect. *G,* A large flap transposed over a lateral scalp defect. The residual defect is skin-grafted (over the pericranium).

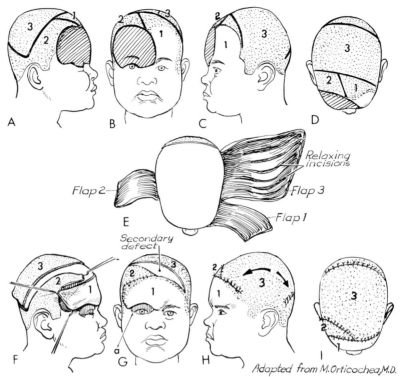

FIGURE 27–17. Development of the surgical technique. It is preferable to cut flaps 1 and 2 at an angle as shown. The secondary defect that results after juxtaposing flaps 1 and 2 is smaller than the primary one. (Modified from Orticochea, M.: New three-flap scalp reconstruction technique. Br. J. Plast. Surg., *24*:184, 1971.)

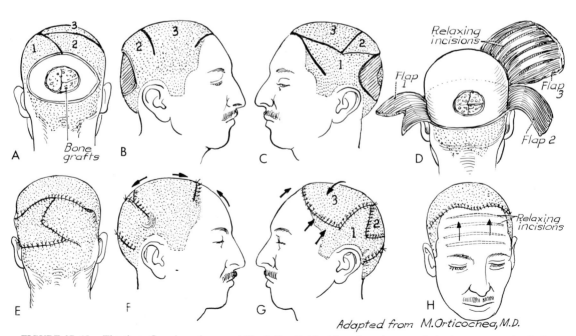

FIGURE 27–18. The three flaps have been mobilized. Parallel incisions have been made in the aponeurosis of a large flap (3) transverse to the longitudinal axis of the skull. Flaps 1 and 2 are sutured in juxtaposition but without tension because their pedicles are narrow. (Modified from Orticochea, M.: New three-flap scalp reconstruction technique. Br. J. Plast. Surg., *24*:184, 1971.)

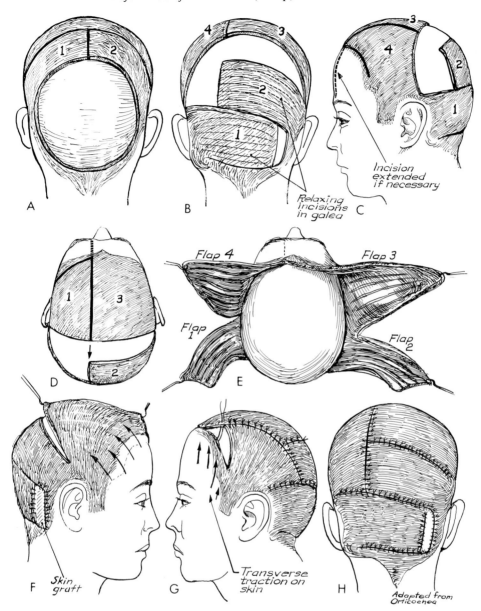

FIGURE 27–19. Four-flap technique. This technique is particularly applicable in the child. (Modified from Orticochea, M.: Four-flap scalp reconstruction technique. Br. J. Plast. Surg., *20*:159, 1967.)

cover the area and will accept a thick split-thickness skin graft.

For smaller scalp defects which are not amenable to coverage by means of local flaps, the outer table can be burred down until pin-point bleeding is noted. A split-thickness skin graft can be successfully applied on such a bed without any delay.

Large losses of the scalp and cranium secondary to burns cannot be repaired with local scalp flaps if the surrounding tissue is subject to circulatory and dystrophic alterations. Such a condition is often seen in recurrent carcinoma treated by irradiation. These defects are best repaired with an abdominal jump flap (Figs. 27–20 and 27–21) or a tube flap (Fig. 27–22) transferred to the arm as an intermediate carrier. It is necessary to remove all the necrotic bone, repair the defect with a flap transferred from a distance, and at a later date provide bony protection to the underlying brain with split-rib bone grafts inserted under the flap.

McLean and Buncke (1972), employing microsurgical revascularization techniques (see Chapter 14), covered a bare cranial defect with a free omental transplant anastomosed to the superficial temporal artery and vein; the omentum, in turn, was covered with a skin graft (Fig. 27–23).

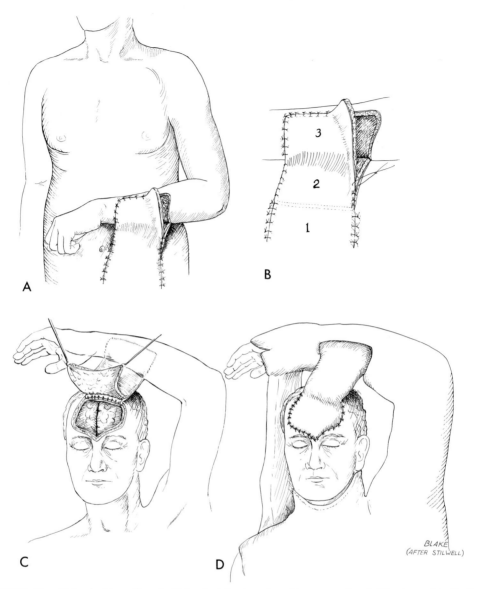

FIGURE 27–20. Abdominal jump flap. *A,* Abdominal flap transferred to arm carrier. *B,* Flap is graphically divided into three sectors. Part 1 will cover the cranial defect. The underside of part 2 is covered with a "hinge flap" raised from the forearm. Part 3 is transferred to the arm carrier. *C, D,* At a later stage the flap is transferred on the arm carrier to the scalp defect. (From Converse, J. M., Campbell, R. M., and Watson, W. L.: Repair of large radiation ulcers situated over the heart and brain. Ann. Surg., *133*:95, 1951.)

Baudet, Molenaar and Montandon (1976) have successfully closed a full-thickness defect of the scalp and cranium in a 35 year old female by a combined procedure consisting of bone grafting the defect by split-rib grafts and providing soft tissue coverage, in the same stage, with a microvascular free groin flap. The circular defect was 11.25 cm in diameter and resulted from the resection of a recurrent irradiated sarcoma.

Defects of the Cranium

Historical Review. In 1889, Seydel, in repairing a defect of the skull, grafted an osteo- periosteal graft from the tibia, which he reduced to small pieces, to repair a cranial defect. Müller (1890) and König (1890) used a flap of scalp with a portion of the outer table attached. Von Hacker (1903) transplanted a single osteoperiosteal graft from the tibia as a cranial graft. Keen (1909) filled defects from chips removed by drilling the outer table of the skull, anticipating the chip-bone grafting technique of Mowlem (1944) during World War II. During a six-year period Delagenière and Lewin (1920) reported 104 cases of tibial osteoperiosteal grafts with only two failures. Kazanjian and Converse (1940) reported 18 successful

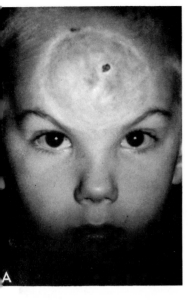
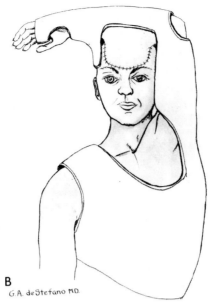
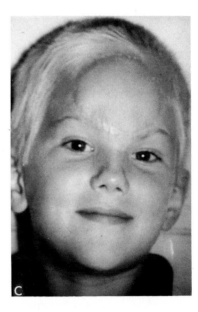

G.A. deStefano MD.

FIGURE 27–21. *A,* A malignant lesion had been resected four years previously and the area immediately covered with a split-thickness skin graft. Repeated trauma resulted in chronic ulceration and a continuous breakdown. *B,* The exostosis and the ulcerated grafted area were excised and covered with a flap from the hairless portion of the forearm. *C,* Two years following reconstruction.

cranioplasties using osteoperiosteal grafts removed from the tibia.

In 1915, Kappis employed the full thickness of the twelfth rib with periosteum to cover a dural and skull defect. Weber (1916) and

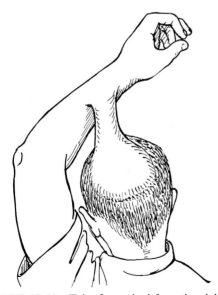

FIGURE 27–22. Tube flap, raised from the abdomen, transferred via the forearm, to provide integumental cover of exposed bone after resection of a radiated recurrent basal cell carcinoma. The patient's arm was immobilized by a plaster cast similar to that illustrated in Figure 27–21.

Schmidt (1916) reported the use of rib grafts. In 1917 R. C. Brown of Australia suggested splitting the rib, leaving the inner half as protection for the thoracic cavity. In 1921, Ballin suggested repairing a dural defect with fascia and laying the split ribs "cut" face down on the fascia. Fagarasanu (1937) split the rib in order to gain more substance.

Morestin in 1915 advocated costal cartilage. Westermann in 1916 transplanted a graft from the sternum, and in 1920 MacLennan used scapula. Mauclaire (1908) and Phemister (1914) employed iliac bone for the repair of cranial defects, and Phemister (1914) used the outer iliac crest. Pickerill in 1931 employed the inner table of the ilium for cranial defects and later in 1947, in a long-range follow-up, concluded there was no doubt that surgically, anatomically, and psychologically the patient's own tissues provide the best means of reconstruction.

In 1928, Brown presented a ten-year postal card follow-up of his split-rib cases. Mowlem (1944) advocated the merits of cancellous bone. Macomber (1949) used cancellous iliac bone for defects of the forehead, nose, and chin. Sodeberg and Mulvey (1947) also claimed that cancellous bone had superior osteogenic properties. McClintock and Dingman (1951) reported the successful use of autogenous iliac bone in 14 cranioplasties. Kiehn and Grino (1953) reported the relief of symptoms follow-

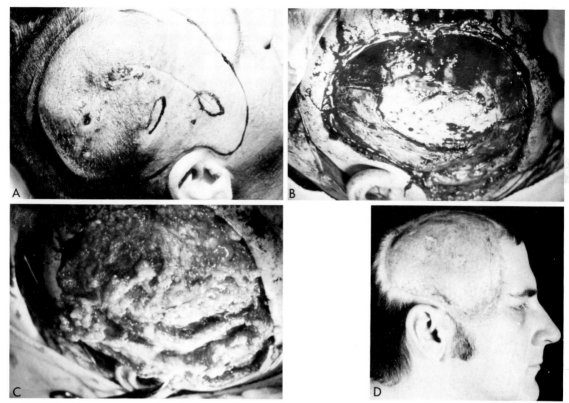

FIGURE 27–23. Reconstruction of a scalp defect with autotransplant of omentum revascularized by microsurgical techniques. *A,* Neurofibroma involvement of scalp. *B,* Resulting defect following excision. *C,* Omental autotransplant in scalp defect. *D,* Omental autograft with overlying skin graft. An arteriogram three weeks after surgery showed a patent omental arcade in the temporal area. (From McLean, D. H., and Buncke, H. J., Jr.: Autotransplant of omentum to a large scalp defect, with microsurgical revascularization. Plast. Reconstr. Surg., 49:268, 1972. Copyright 1972. The Williams & Wilkins Company, Baltimore.)

ing removal of a tantalum plate in three cases and reconstruction with flaps and iliac bone.

In a monograph on cranioplasty, Wolff and Walker (1945) stated that for defects up to 8 cm, autogenous bone was the choice; but for larger defects inorganic materials should be used.

It is of interest that a hammered gold plate was used, before the dawn of history, to repair a frontal defect of the skull in a Neolithic Peruvian chieftain. The same type of gold plate was suggested by Fallopio, but later decried by Paré. Gold was utilized by the French (Estor, 1917) during World War I, but it was found to be too soft and expensive. Lead plates were used by Mauclaire (1908) but produced acute lead poisoning, and silver was utilized by Savariaud (1912), resulting in localized argyria.

Subsequently tantalum (Pudenz and Odom, 1942), vitallium (Geib, 1941), and stainless steel (Scott and Wycis, 1946) have been extensively utilized but have the following disadvantages. They are radiopaque, conduct heat and cold, and produce varying degrees of local reaction at the time of implantation. The incidence of infection and subsequent extrusion is fairly high. White (1948), in an extensive follow-up of patients operated upon during the period between 1943 and 1946, found that the complications amounted to 10.6 per cent in 66 cranioplasties performed with lucite and 12.3 per cent in 130 after plating with tantalum. He found that the scarred scalp is likely to break down under a plate and that plates over the mastoid, frontal, and supraorbital areas tend to loosen and perforate the soft tissues. The danger with short wave diathermy in patients with metals embedded in their tissues must be seriously considered.

Small and Graham (1945–46) pointed out the high incidence of epilepsy resulting from the intense fibrosis set up by the foreign body reaction. Newer inorganic materials have been employed more recently for large frontal bone defects. These have been cast from impressions taken of the defect; complications, including fluid collection, infection, and eventual extrusion, have occurred. It must be further borne in mind that inorganic substances have no growth potential and hence should not be utilized in the growing child. Grotesque malformations of the skull and skeleton have followed the early repair of cranial defects with fixed metallic plates and mesh. These complications contrast with the relatively uncomplicated postoperative course following the use of autogenous bone grafts for the repair of frontal bone defects.

Conditions for Success in Bone Grafting. As previously emphasized in Chapter 13, a covering of well-vascularized soft tissue is an essential condition for success. Local or distant flaps must resurface the area to be bone-grafted if soft tissue over the cranial defect has been destroyed or is inadequately vascularized. Bone to bone contact between the graft and host bone is essential. Absence of infection is self-evident.

SPLIT-RIB GRAFTS. Much has been written about cartilage, skin, and bone banks. The bank of autogenous bone (the ribs) within each individual possesses the ability to redeposit itself repeatedly, if care is taken not to destroy the periosteum of the rib bed (Longacre, 1955; Longacre and de Stefano, 1957a, b, c; Longacre and coworkers, 1959; Holmstrand

and coworkers, 1960). The supply of bone is almost unlimited and can be removed without producing respiratory distress or ensuing deformity if it is done at intervals. It is a well-known fact that rib fractures in the aged and cachectic heal. It has been pointed out by Albright and Forbes (1957) that, when multiple pathologic fractures occur in certain syndromes, the only ones that heal are rib fractures. The ribs possess an inherent ability for osteogenesis. Within a few weeks after total removal of a rib, there is evidence of calcification, and within a short time a complete new rib has re-formed. Roentgenograms taken years later show no deformity of the thoracic cage. Only very careful examination will indicate which ribs have been utilized (Fig. 27–24). In a patient with Romberg's hemifacial atrophy, we have used a rib regenerated from the same rib bed as often as five times.

Clinical experience shows the low morbidity after rib resection, as compared to that after the resection of a similar amount of bone from the ilium or tibia. In addition, the ilium should not be utilized in a growing patient because of the danger of disturbing the growth center of the cartilaginous crest. However, Crockford and Converse (1972) have reported a technique of harvesting bone grafts from the ilium without disturbing the secondary centers of os-

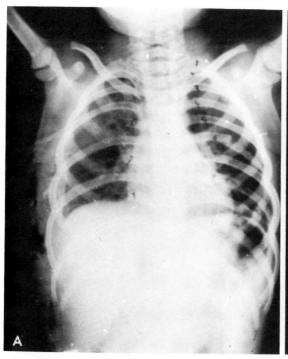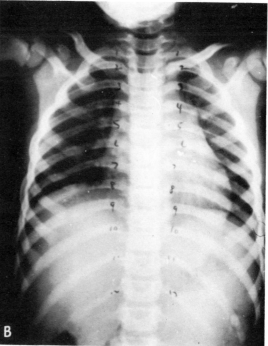

FIGURE 27–24. *A,* Roentgenogram shows regeneration of the left sixth, eighth, and tenth ribs, removed three weeks before resection of the right fifth, seventh, ninth, and eleventh ribs. *B,* Completed regeneration and growth one year after resection.

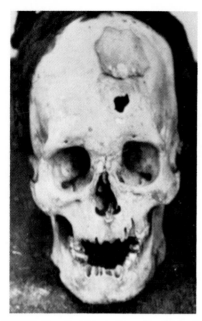

FIGURE 27-25. Prehistoric Peruvian skull with frontal defect repaired with hammered gold plate.

care are surviving severe and mutilating trauma to the skull and facial skeleton. The resection of tumors and osteomyelitic areas produces extensive defects. As the result of intensive irradiation therapy and radical ablation of recurrent carcinoma, large defects of the cranium are produced. The radical unroofing of the calvarium as a life-saving measure in the treatment of acute lead encephalitis (McLaurin and Nichols, 1957) accounted for extensive defects (75 to 90 per cent of the calvarium).

Defects of the cranium have presented a problem since the earliest records of man (e.g., the Edwin Smith Papyrus) and are seen in the remains of the trephined skulls of Peruvian Neolithic man (Fig. 27-25). Rarely does the calvarium regenerate, and then only in very young children after a portion of it has been removed for craniosynostosis or osteomyelitis. It is well known that the ossification of a linear fracture of the skull requires months in children, while in an adult it will require years. In contrast, a fracture through the base ossifies after a relatively short time. This difference in healing may be explained by the fact that the calvarium originates from membranous bone, while the base originates from cartilage (chondocranium).

An 18 month old child (Fig. 27-26, *A*) had survived 40 per cent total destruction of the skull and its coverings with the exposure of the anterior, middle, and posterior cranial fossae. After the infection had been cleared up, the area was covered with postage stamp skin grafts. Since the area still remained soft, it was decided to prepare a delayed flap of the remaining scalp and rotate it over the defect,

sification (see Chapter 13). This technique is indicated only in small cranial defects. With regard to the amount of bone obtainable, we have resected eight full length ribs (four alternate ribs from each side of the thoracic cage) in a child within a period of two weeks without producing any cardiorespiratory embarrassment.

TECHNIQUE. In this age of speed and power with its associated increase in head injuries, more patients as the result of improved

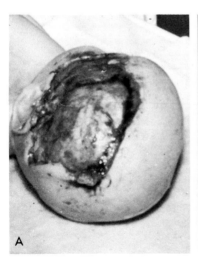
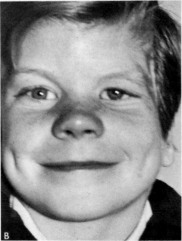
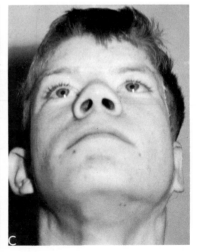

FIGURE 27-26. *A,* Photograph of an 18 month old child who had survived 40 per cent total destruction of the cranium and its coverings with exposure of the anterior, middle, and posterior cranial fossae. *B,* Photograph 6½ years following completion of reconstruction with split-rib grafts. *C,* Note symmetrical development of the skull 16 years after reconstruction.

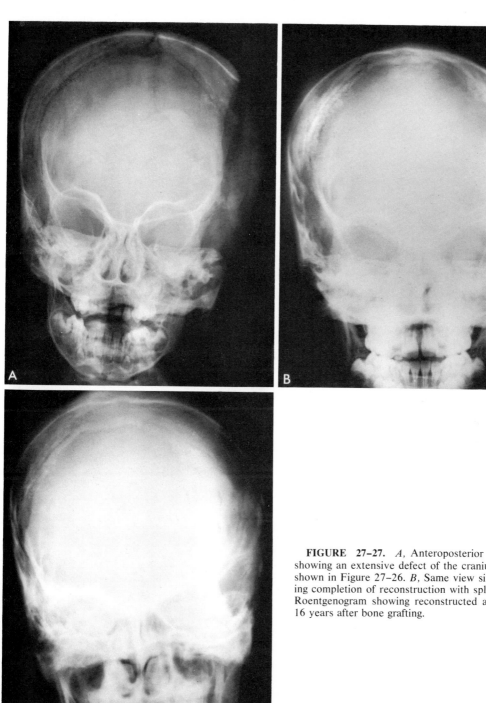

FIGURE 27–27. *A*, Anteroposterior roentgenogram showing an extensive defect of the cranium in the child shown in Figure 27–26. *B*, Same view six years following completion of reconstruction with split-rib grafts. *C*, Roentgenogram showing reconstructed area unchanged 16 years after bone grafting.

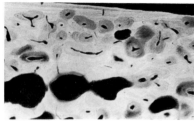
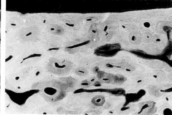
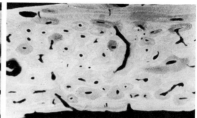

FIGURE 27–28. A six-year biopsy of the patient shown in Figure 27–26 shows complete restoration of the cranial defect with formation of an outer and inner table.

after having excised the previously grafted area. Despite the improvement in the blood supply, there was still no evidence of regeneration of the bone one year after the original injury. The diameter of the defect had increased from 13.5 cm to 15 cm during the interval (Fig. 27–27, *A*). It was felt that four full length rib grafts (if taken singly in four separate operations) would not disturb the cardiorespiratory mechanism of the child and still would provide sufficient autogenous bone. The bone grafting was done in stages; after two operations there was some purulent drainage due to reactivation of infection. The wounds healed, however, without the extrusion of a single fragment. Within one year there was osteogenesis extending from the edge of the skull to the split-rib grafts and between the widely separated grafts themselves. It has now been 17 years since the reconstruction was completed. The long-term result is shown in Figure 27–26, *B* and *C*, and in Figure 27–27, *B* and *C*. The defect is now reconstructed with a plaque of solid bone, except in the posterior fossa where no split-rib grafts were placed. In these plaques are to be found vestiges of the original rib grafts (Fig. 27–27, *B*). It is of interest that the circumference of the skull measured 53 cm at the age of nine years. The boy was active and alert and led a normal life. A six-year biopsy (Fig. 27–28) was taken which showed complete restoration of the defect, with the formation of an inner and outer table. At age 18 years, the patient is fully grown. Note the symmetry of skull (Fig. 27–27, *C*).

Another example is that of a 4 year old child (Fig. 27–29, *A*) with extensive defects measuring 14 × 16 cm on either side of his skull. Two years previously he had been admitted in a moribund state with acute lead encephalitis. As the result of an extensive unroofing of the skull with radical incision of the dura, the child survived, and two years later he had a residual I.Q. of 90. One of the resected cranial segments, which had been removed and kept under sterile conditions in the bone bank, had

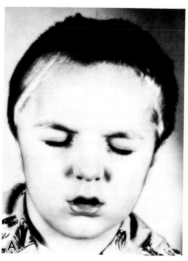
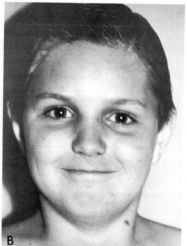
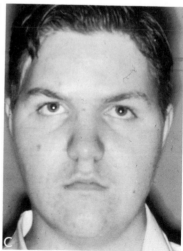

FIGURE 27–29. Cranial defect. *A*, A 4 year old child with extensive defects of the cranium secondary to an extensive bilateral cerebral decompression performed two years previously for acute cerebral edema associated with acute lead encephalopathy. *B*, Six years following completion of reconstruction of the 75 per cent defect of the cranium. Note the symmetry and good contour. *C*, Symmetrical skull 16 years after reconstruction.

later been used to reconstruct one side of this "satchel handle" defect. Osteomyelitis ensued, and the refrigerated autogenous graft was removed. Two years later there was very little evidence of bone regeneration (Fig. 27–30, *A*), and he was forced to wear a special helmet to protect the brain. The eighth and tenth ribs were resected at one procedure, and part of the defect on the left side was reconstructed. After an interval of 24 days the sixth, eighth, and tenth ribs were removed from the right side and the costal beds closed carefully with a running suture of 3–0 chromic catgut. The ribs were then split lengthwise to provide sufficient bone to reconstruct the entire defect on the right side of the skull. Ten days later the seventh rib was removed from the left side of the thorax and split lengthwise in three separate grafts. There was evidence of almost complete regeneration of the eighth and tenth ribs at this time. The split-rib grafts transplanted 34 days before were found to be solidly incorporated between the dura and the scalp and appeared on gross examination to be well vascularized. Figure 27–30, *C* and *D*, shows the progressive thickening of the reconstructed skull, with the formation of an inner and outer table.

Clinically it has been noted that the skulls of these children develop at a normal rate, even in a child of 18 months in whom all the growth centers on one side of the skull had been destroyed. Over a period of 16 years of observation following repair, there has been no apparent difference in growth between the unaffected and the reconstructed sides (even though 90 per cent of the growth of the calvarium is completed by the age of eight) (Fig. 27–30, *E*, *F*). In other children in whom a growth center was destroyed and the defect bridged with an inorganic implant, growth failed to occur, resulting in an asymmetry between the two sides of the cranium.

LONGITUDINAL STUDIES

Upon analysis of our results (Longacre and deStefano, 1957b) with 146 autogenous bone and cartilage grafts to the head and face, we were impressed with the permanence of the autogenous osseous transplant and the manner in which it would stand up under reactivated infection. In addition, there was direct evidence in measurements and moulages of the continuous growth of these grafts in young patients observed over a period of six to 18 years.

The literature is filled with preliminary and so-called long-term follow-up of a mere two or three years. Results which first appeared as excellent during this short time may not be as good when followed over a more extended period. This is particularly true when the factor of growth and development is considered in the reconstruction of extensive defects of the cranial bones and facial skeleton in the developing child.

Longacre has performed more than 700 operations on humans utilizing split-rib grafts during the past 20 years. In addition, long-range experimental observations have been made in several large series of macaque rhesus monkeys. Our clinical findings in humans have closely paralleled the more detailed experimental observations in the monkeys (for details see Chapter 13).

Iliac Bone Grafts. Iliac bone may be utilized in frontal and other cranial defects measuring up to 10 cm in diameter. Iliac bone grafts are particularly indicated in frontal defects, as they provide a smooth contour.

REPAIR OF FULL-THICKNESS DEFECTS OF THE FRONTAL BONE

A preferred technique for wide exposure of the frontal bone is the raising of a bifrontal or coronal scalp flap (Fig. 27–31, *A*). This type of exposure is preferable to exposure through residual scars, unless they are conspicuous and require repair; usually the scars are not conspicuous by the time bone repair is being considered.

The incision through the scalp extends downwards on each side between both preauricular areas. The flap is raised through the fibroareolar tissue between the galea aponeurotica and the pericranium, and, as the dissection is continued downward, it reaches the frontalis muscle, which is raised from the periosteum of the frontal bone to the level of the supraorbital arches. In defects involving the lower portion of the frontal bone, the periosteum is incised, the supraorbital nerve is liberated from its canal (see Chapter 56) and the periorbita is raised from the anterior portion of the roof of the orbit when the defect involves the supraorbital rim.

As the raising of the flap reaches the bony defect, careful dissection is required because of the adherence of the dura to the periosteum and the flap; in many cases the tissues may be adherent and dense scar tissue present.

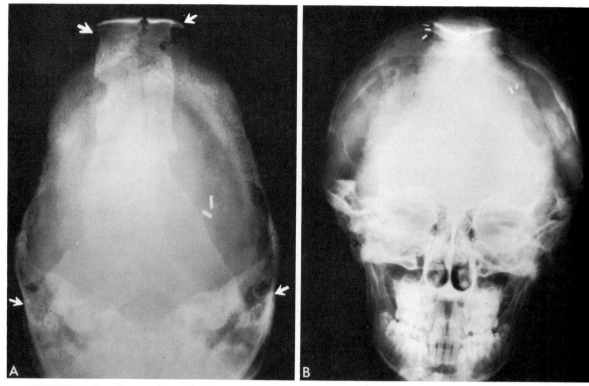

FIGURE 27–30. Same patient as in Figure 27–29. *A*, Extensive satchel handle defect two years after radical decompression for acute lead encephalopathy. *B*, Six years after reconstruction of the skull defects. Note formation of large bone plaques.

Illustration continued on opposite page

The extent of the bony defect is outlined. The periosteum is incised around the periphery of the defect, a periosteal elevator raises the periosteal cuff thus formed around the defect, and the cuff is folded into the defect (Fig. 27–31, *B*).

The periosteum around the periphery of the defect is elevated, as the iliac bone graft will be placed under it after bridging the bony defect (Fig. 27–31, *B*). The iliac bone taken from the inner table of the ilium has a curvature favorable to the restoration of contour of most cranial and lateral frontal defects. The shape of the graft and size of the graft are determined by a template of malleable Asche metal (Fig. 27–31, *C*). The cortex of the graft from the inner table of the ilium is placed toward the dura and the cancellous portion under the soft tissues (Fig. 27–31, *D*). A central frontal defect may require a graft without the curvature. The curvature of the graft can be modified by bending the graft after weakening the cortex by a number of parallel cuts through the partial thickness of the cortex; in young patients the bone is malleable, and adequate curvature can be obtained by bending it into the suitable contour. In small and moderate sized defects, a single onlay graft is adequate (Fig. 27–31, *D*). The overlapping edges of the graft, which are placed between the surrounding bone and the periosteum, are thinned and beveled by means of an air-turbine drill activating a large oval-shaped or Lindemann spiral burr. This precaution is essential to prevent the edge of the graft from forming a conspicuous peripheral ridge. A mosaic of corticocancellous and cancellous grafts is then built up to complete the coverage of the defect and to provide adequate contour when necessary (Fig. 27–31, *E, F*).

Usually the dura is covered with scar tissue, but under the bone overlay a dead space, which will fill with blood and serum, should be obliterated with cancellous bone chips packed into the cavity.

Fixation of the bone graft is optional (Fig. 27–31, *F*). The flap is replaced, sutured, and a pressure dressing applied for seven days.

Patients who have undergone reconstruction of frontal bone defects by this technique are shown in Figures 27–32 and 27–33.

In large cranial and frontal bone defects, the problem of obtaining sufficient bone becomes more complex. It is in these large defects that sequential split-rib grafting is indicated. The

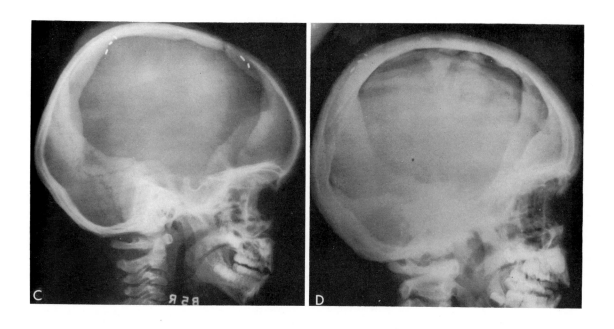

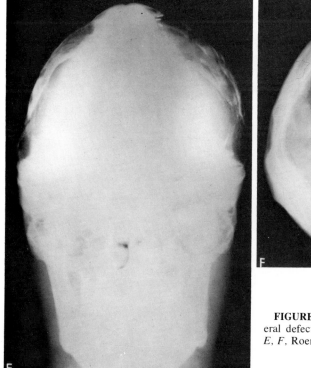

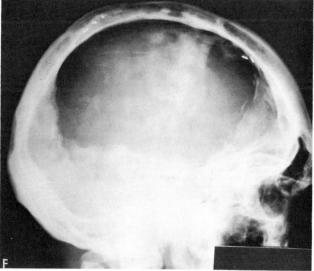

FIGURE 27–30 *Continued.* *C*, Lateral view of extensive bilateral defect. 14 × 16 cm. *D*, Lateral view after reconstruction. *E, F*, Roentgenograms 16 years following reconstruction.

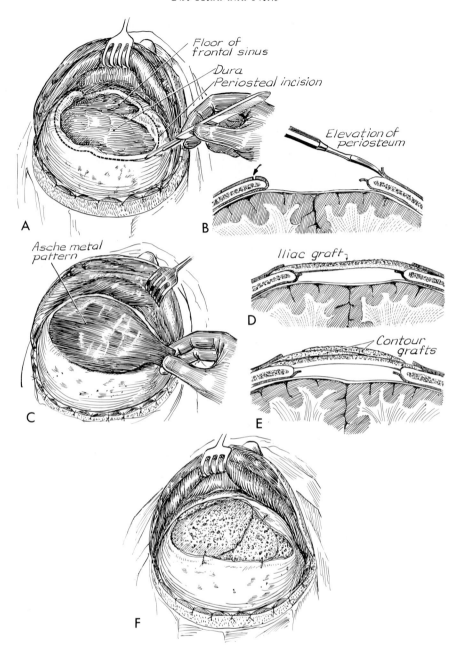

FIGURE 27–31. Technique of repair of a frontal bone defect with iliac bone graft. *A*, A bifrontal (coronal) flap has been raised, leaving the periosteum attached to the frontal bone. The dotted line indicates the incision through the periosteum around the defect. *B*, After incision, the periosteum is raised; the periosteum surrounding the defect is reflected into the defect. *C*, A pattern is made (Asche metal) which will be used to outline the size of the graft to be resected from the medial aspect of the ilium. *D*, Bone graft in position. *E*, *F*, When necessary, to improve the contour, additional cancellous bone grafts are placed over the main graft.

contour can be improved in large frontal bone defects by the addition of flat pieces of iliac bone, consisting mostly of cancellous bone, which straddle the split rib grafts.

The Frontal Sinus in Frontal Bone Defects. Radical operations for frontal sinusitis, compli-

cated by spreading osteomyelitis, may necessitate the resection of the full thickness of the frontal bone, the anterior and posterior walls of the frontal sinuses, and adjacent supraorbital and nasal bone. Reconstruction is then required after a suitable time interval. The advent of antibiotics has made possible the con-

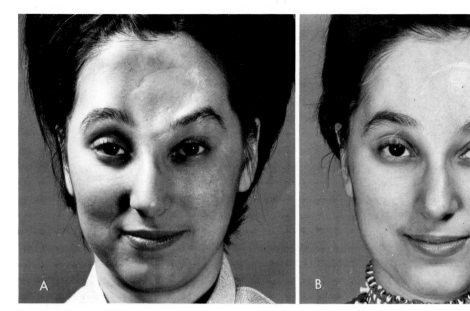

FIGURE 27–32. *A,* Large midfrontal defect resulting from an automobile accident. Two successive metallic implants had been placed by the patient's neurosurgeon to restore contour. Both implants were rejected. *B,* Patient three years after iliac bone grafting according to the technique illustrated in Figure 27–31. (From Kazanjian and Converse.)

trol of spreading osteomyelitis and obviated the need for radical surgery.

Less radical operations are still performed for the cure of frontal sinusitis, leaving in their wake a deformity resulting from the resection of the anterior wall of the frontal sinus. Reconstruction by bone grafting is indicated (Fig. 27–34).

Glabellar fractures may result in the loss of bone of the anterior wall of the frontal sinus or a depressed, malunited fracture (Figs. 27–35 and 27–36). The treatment is similar to that illustrated in Figure 27–34.

Complications caused by repeated inflammatory episodes and suppuration have been observed because of the failure to eliminate the mucous membrane–lined cavities of the frontal sinuses. Large frontal sinuses extend far laterally, and the remainder of the sinus may be overlooked. The roentgenogram usually shows the size and position of the frontal sinus. In unusual cases, it will show the presence of the frontoethmoidal cell between the frontal sinus and the roof of the orbit. The bony defect involving the anterior wall of the frontal sinuses may not extend over the entire height and width of the frontal sinuses. The lateral portions of each sinus should be identified. All of the mucous membrane should be removed with a large size curette. "Nature abhors a vacuum,"

and the sinus cavity must be eliminated. The cavity is filled with corticocancellous bone chips. The frontal duct is curetted, thus removing the lining mucous membrane, and a bone chip is plugged into the duct. A bone graft overlay is then placed over the defect (see Fig. 27–34).

Respective Indications and Variations in Technique. The iliac bone graft, whether wired into the defect or employed as an overlay in conjunction with smaller grafts, has the advantage of smoothness, an important consideration in a conspicuous area of the body. Large defects can be repaired by this technique, the limit in size being the surface of bone that can be removed from the medial aspect of the ilium.

In large defects of the calvarium too extensive for iliac bone grafting, the split-rib technique performed in stages is the only feasible technique and is of particular value in the child. A disadvantage of the split-rib technique is the slightly irregular surface provided by the juxtaposed grafts. While this inconvenience is of minor importance over the hair-bearing portion of the cranium, it has an esthetic disadvantage in the repair of defects of the frontal bone. Körloff, Nylén, and Rietz (1973) have achieved good results in a series of frontal bone de-

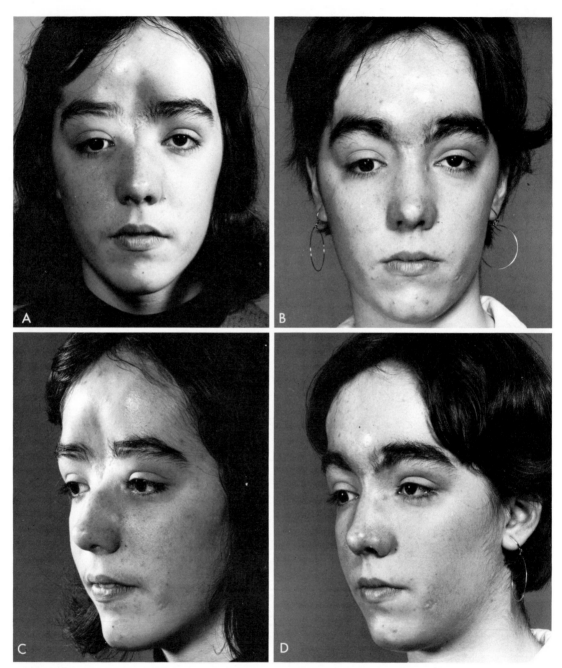

FIGURE 27–33. *A, C,* Bony defect involving the frontal bone, the skeletal structures forming the glabella and the root of the nose, and the medial part of the supraorbital arches. The frontal sinuses were of enormous size, and a large cavity communicating with the nose had become relined with mucous membrane. The problem was to achieve a line of separation between the cutaneous covering and the lining mucous membrane and to place a bone graft between these two layers. *B, D,* This was achieved, and iliac bone graft reconstruction was done according to the technique illustrated in Figure 27–31. Additional bone grafts restored contour to the root of the nose and the supraorbital arches. (From Kazanjian and Converse.)

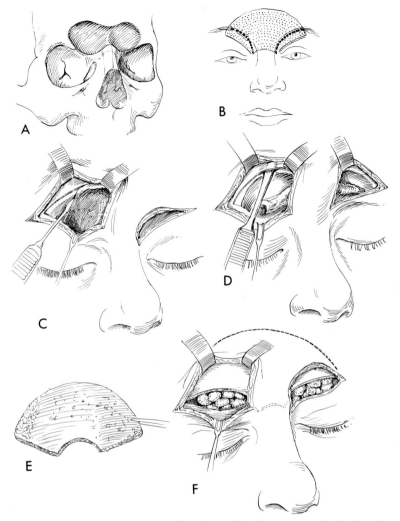

FIGURE 27–34. Reconstruction of a frontal bone deformity resulting from an operation for frontal sinusitis complicated by osteomyelitis. The operation required resection of the anterior wall of the frontal sinuses and the medial portion of each supraorbital arch. *A*, The area diagonally lined represents the defect in the frontal bone. Incisions for exposure are made in the eyebrows, the site of previous operative scars. *B*, The defect in the frontal bone. *C*, Exposure of the area. An incision has been made through the periosteum above the defect, and the periosteum is reflected into the defect and removed with the mucous membrane. *D*, The periosteum is raised around the defect for a distance of 2 to 3 cm. *E*, The shape of the graft removed from the inner table of the ilium. The graft consists of the inner table with cancellous bone. *F*, The bone graft placed over the defect has subperiosteal contact with the bone surrounding the edges of the defect. The lower margin of the bone graft has been suitably shaped to restore the contour of the supraorbital arches. Note the underlying bone chips. (From Converse, J. M.: Technique of bone grafting for contour restoration of face. Plast. Reconstr. Surg., *14*:332, 1954.)

fects by split-rib bone grafting in two stages: a first layer of split-rib grafts is placed under the edges of the defect over the dura (Fig. 27–37, *A, B*); ten months later, a second layer of grafts is wedged into the defect at right angles to the first layer of grafts (Fig. 27–37, *C, D, E*).

Another technique (Marchac, 1974) splices a single layer of split-ribs into the diploë of the bone surrounding the defect for better fixation (Fig. 27–38).

In order to avoid the irregular surface that may result from reconstruction of a frontal bone defect by split-rib grafting, slabs of cancellous iliac bone grafts may be laid, mosaic fashion, over the split-ribs (Fig. 27–39).

Contour Restoration of the Frontal Bone. With a depressed fracture of the anterior wall of the frontal sinus or a sloped forehead, as occurs in patients with craniofacial dysostosis (see Chapter 56), the full thickness of the bone is not involved.

Exposure by raising the bifrontal scalp flap,

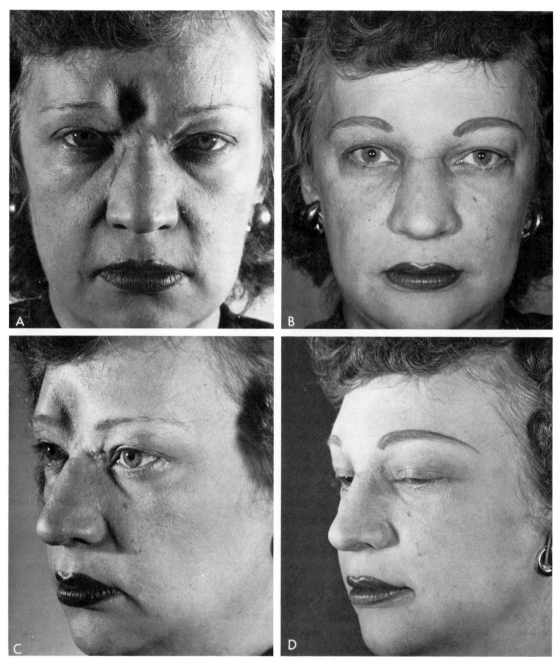

FIGURE 27–35. Reconstruction of the frontal bone. Before (*A* and *C*) and after (*B* and *D*) bone grafting according to the technique illustrated in Figure 27–34. (From Converse, J. M., and Campbell, R. M.: Bone grafts in surgery of face. Surg. Clin. North Am., *34*:375, 1954.)

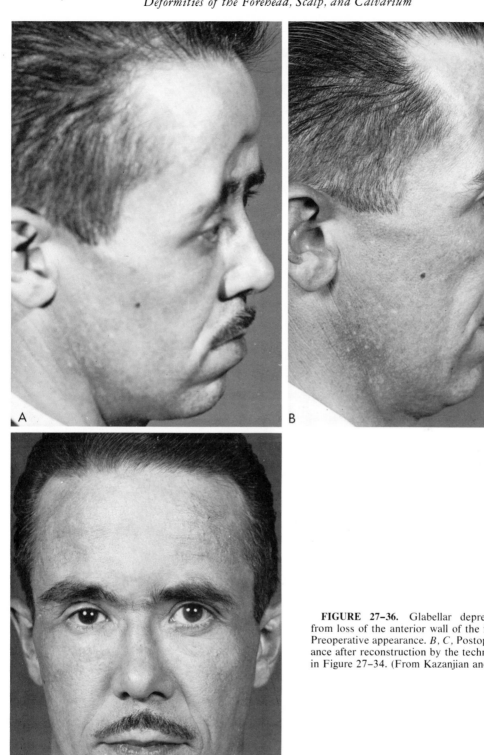

FIGURE 27–36. Glabellar depression resulting from loss of the anterior wall of the frontal sinus. *A*, Preoperative appearance. *B*, *C*, Postoperative appearance after reconstruction by the technique illustrated in Figure 27–34. (From Kazanjian and Converse.)

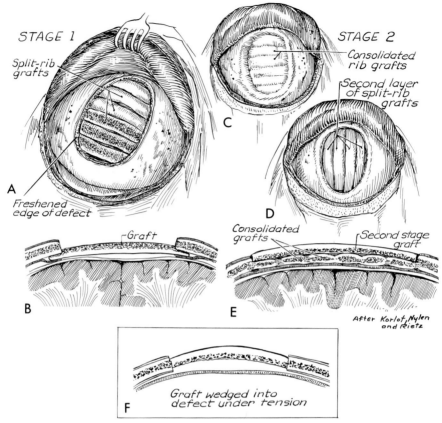

FIGURE 27-37. Repair of the frontal bone by staged, double-layer split-rib grafts (Körlof, Nylén, and Rietz). *A, B,* The first layer of split-rib grafts is placed under the edges of the defect. *C, D, E,* After consolidation of the first layer, a second layer of split-rib grafts is wedged into the defect at right angles to the first layer (After Körlof, Nylén, and Rietz, 1973). *F,* Using another technique, a single layer is wedged between the edges of the defect.

described in the preceding pages, exposes the depressed area. Onlay bone grafts contoured to shape must be placed under the periosteum of the frontal bone in close contact with the bone. Iliac bone grafts and split-rib grafts will restore contour. When split-ribs are employed, they are placed side by side, split surface and cortical surface alternating. Slivers of the bone

may be placed in the intervals between the surface of the grafts to obtain a smooth contour.

Costal cartilage grafts have provided a satisfactory means of restoring supraorbital arch depression and are an alternative source of grafting material. As stated earlier in this chapter, autografts are preferred to all other transplants or implants.

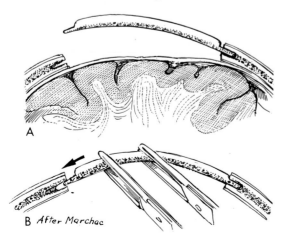

FIGURE 27-38. The split-rib grafts are spliced into the diploë of the bone at the edge of the defect for better fixation (Marchac, 1974).

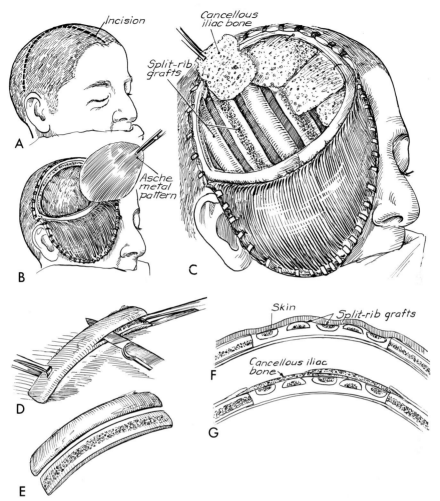

FIGURE 27–39. Split-rib grafts combined with cancellous iliac bone grafts. *A*, Incision for exposure of a large parietal defect. *B*, Pattern taken for size. *C*, The split-rib grafts (*D, E*) to be wedged in position. *F*, Irregular contour if the split-rib grafts are not covered by cancellous iliac bone grafts as in *G*.

REFERENCES

Albright, F., and Forbes, A. P.: Personal communication, 1957.

Ballin, M.: A method of cranioplasty. Surg. Gynecol. Obstet., *33*:79, 1921.

Baudet, J., Molenaar, A., and Montandon, D.: Personal communication, 1976.

Björk, A.: Roentgencephalometric Growth Analysis. Transactions of International Symposium on Congenital Anomalies of the Face and Associated Structures. December, 1959.

Brown, R. C.: The repair of skull defects. Med. J. Aust., *11*:409, 1917.

Brown, R. C.: Cranioplasty by split-rib method. J. Coll. Surg. Aust., 1928.

Campbell, W.: Case of congenital ulcer on the cranium of a fetus. Edinburgh J. Med. Sci., *2*:82, 1826.

Converse, J. M.: Techniques of bone grafting for contour restoration of the face. Plast. Reconstr. Surg., *14*:332, 1954.

Converse, J. M.: Surgical closure of scalp defects. *In* Kahn, E. A., Bassett, R. C. Schneider, R. C., and Crosby,

E. C. (Eds.): Correlative Neurosurgery. Springfield, Ill., Charles C Thomas, Publisher, 1955.

Converse, J. M., Campbell, R. M., and Watson, W. L.: Repair of large radiation ulcers situated over the heart and the brain. Ann. Surg., *133*:95, 1951.

Crockford, D. A., and Converse, J. M.: The ilium as a source of bone grafts in children. Plast. Reconstr. Surg., *50*:270, 1972.

Crouzon, O.: Etudes des maladies familiales nerveuses et dystrophiques. Bull. Mém. Soc. Méd. Hôp. Paris, 1912.

Cushing, H.: A study of a series of wounds involving the brain and its enveloping structures. Br. J. Plast. Surg., *5*:558, 1918.

Davis, J. S.: Scalping accidents. Johns Hopkins Hosp. Rep., *16*:257, 1911.

Delagenière, H., and Lewin, P.: A general method of repairing loss of bony substance and of reconstructing bones by osteoperiosteal grafts taken from the tibia. Surg. Gynecol. Obstet., *30*:441, 1920.

Delak, Z.: Successful replacement of the completely avulsed scalp. Br. J. Plast. Surg., *8*:55, 1955.

Dingman, R. O., Weintraub, W. H., and Wilensky, R. J.: Personal communication, 1976.

Douglas, B.: Personal communication, 1962.

Estor, E.: Cent cas de prosthèse cranienne par plaque d'or. Bull. Mém. Soc. Chir. Paris, 48:463. 1917.

Fagarasanu, I.: Procédé de cranioplastie par des greffons costaux redoublés; procédé due "grillage protecteur." Tech. Chir., 29:57, 1937.

Farmer, W. W., and Maxmen, M.: Congenital absence of skin. Plast. Reconstr. Surg., 25:291, 1960.

Geib, F. W.: Vitallium skull plates. J.A.M.A., 117:8, 306, 1941.

Gillies, H.: Note on scalp closure. Lancet, 2:310, 1944.

Greig, D. M.: Localized congenital defects of the scalp, Edinburgh Med. J., 38:341, 1931.

Grossman, H. J., Sugar, O., Greeley, P. W., and Sadove, M. S.: Surgical separation in craniopagus. J.A.M.A., 153:201, 1953.

Heidler, H.: Kongenitaler Hautdefekt am Kopfe. Wien., Klin. Wochenschr., 37:114, 1924.

Hodgman, J. E., Mathres, A. W., and Levan, N. E.: Congenital scalp defects in twin sisters. Am. J. Dis. Child., 110:293, 1965.

Holmstrand, K., Longacre, J. J., and de Stefano, G. A.: Biophysical studies of split-rib grafts in the repair of the cranium. Plast. Reconstr. Surg., 26:286, 1960.

Ingalls, N. W.: Congenital defects of the scalp. Studies in the pathology of development III. Am. J. Obstet. Gynecol., 25:861, 1933.

Jayes, P. H.: Plastic repair after separation of craniopagus twins. Br. Med. J., 1:1340, 1964.

Kahn, E. A., and Olmedo, L.: Congenital defect of the scalp. Plast. Reconstr. Surg., 6:435, 1950.

Kappis, A.: Zur Deckung von Schadeldefekten. Zentralbl. Chir., 42:897, 1915.

Kazanjian, V. H., and Converse, J. M.: Reconstruction after radical operation for osteomyelitis of frontal bone. Arch. Otolaryngol., 31:94, 1940.

Kazanjian, V. H., and Converse, J. M.: The Surgical Treatment of Facial Injuries. 2nd Ed. Baltimore, Williams & Wilkins Company, 1959.

Kazanjian, V. H., and Webster, R. C.: The treatment of extensive losses of the scalp. Plast. Reconstr. Surg., 1:360, 1946.

Keen, W. W.: Surgery, Its Principles and Practice. Philadelphia, W. B. Saunders Company, 1909.

Kiehn, C. L., and Grino, A.: Iliac bone grafts replacing tantalum plates for gunshot wounds of the skull. Am. J. Surg., 85:395, 1953.

König, F.: Der knöcherne Ersatz Grosser Schädeldefekte. Zentralbl. Chir., 17:467, 1890.

Körlof, B., Nylén, B., and Rietz, K.: Bone grafting of skull defects. Plast. Reconstr. Surg., 52:378, 1973.

Laskowski, E. J., and Baldwin, M.: The repair of scalp, skull and dural defects in a case of craniopagus. Plast. Reconstr. Surg., 29:597, 1962.

Longacre, J. J.: Surgical correction of extensive defects of scalp and skull with autogenous tissues. Transactions of 1st International Congress of Plastic Surgeons, Stockholm, 1955, p. 346.

Longacre, J. J., and de Stefano, G. S.: Reconstruction of extensive defects of the skull with split-rib grafts. Plast. Reconstr. Surg., 19:186, 1957a.

Longacre, J. J., and de Stefano, G. A.: Further observations of the behavior of autogenous split-rib grafts in reconstruction of extensive defects of the cranium and face. Plast. Reconstr. Surg., 20:281, 1957b.

Longacre, J. J., and de Stefano, G. A.: Repair of extensive defects of the scalp and skull with autogenous tissues. J. Int. Coll. Surg., 27:324, 1957c.

Longacre, J. J., de Stefano, G. A., Davidson, D. A., and Holmstrand, K.: Observations on the behavior of split-

rib grafts in the reconstruction of extensive defects of the calvarium and facial skeleton. Transactions of 2nd International Congress of Plastic Surgeons, London, 1959, pp. 290.

Lu, M. M.: Successful replacement of avulsed scalp. Plast. Reconstr. Surg., 43:231, 1969.

Lynch, P. J., and Kahn, E. A.: Congenital defects of the scalp. A surgical approach to aplasia cutis congenita. J. Neurosurg., 33:198, 1970.

MacLennan, A.: The repair by bone graft of gaps in the skull due to congenital deficiency, injury, or operation. Glasgow Med. J., 93:251, 1920.

Macomber, D. W.: Cancellous iliac bone in depression of forehead, nose and chin. Plast. Reconstr. Surg., 4:157, 1949.

McClintock, H. G., and Dingman, R. O.: The repair of cranial defects with iliac bone. Surgery, 30:955, 1951.

McLaurin, R. L., and Nichols, J. B.: Extensive cranial decompression in the treatment of severe lead encephalopathy. Pediatrics, 20:4, 1957.

McLean, D. H., and Buncke, H. J.: Autotransplant of omentum to a large scalp defect, with microsurgical revascularization. Plast. Reconstr. Surg., 49:268, 1972.

McWilliams, C. A.: Principles of the four types of skin grafting. J.A.M.A., 83:183, 1924.

Marchac, D.: Personal communication, 1974.

Matson, D. D.: Congenital defects of the scalp and skull. In Neurosurgery of Infancy and Childhood. 2nd Ed. Springfield, Ill., Charles C Thomas, 1957.

Mauclaire, H.: Bréche cranienne restaurée par la prosthèse metallique. Comments on article by Rouvillois: Bull. Mém. Soc. Chir. Paris, 34:232, 1908.

Meister, C.: Attempts to restore hair growth. Br. J. Plast. Surg., 8:44, 1955.

Miller, G. D. H., Anstee, E. J., and Snell, J. A.: Successful replantation of an avulsed scalp by microvascular anastomoses. Plast. Reconstr. Surg., 58:133, 1976.

Montgomery, H.: Congenital aplasia. In Dermatopathology. Vol. 1. New York, Harper & Row, 1967, p. 75.

Morestin, H.: Les transplantations cartilagineuses dans la chirurgie réparatrice. Bull. Mém. Soc. Chir. Paris, 41:1994, 1915.

Mowlem, R.: Cancellous chip bone grafts; report on 75 cases. Lancet, 2:746, 1944.

Müller, W.: Zur Frage der temporären Schädelresektion an Stelle der Trepanation. Zentralbl. Chir., 17:65, 1890.

O'Brien, B., and Drake, J.: Congenital defects of the skull and scalp. Br. J. Plast. Surg., 13:102, 1961.

Orticochea, M.: Four flap scalp reconstruction technique. Br. J. Plast. Surg., 20:172, 1967.

Orticochea, M.: New three-flap scalp reconstruction technique. Br. J. Plast. Surg., 24:184, 1971.

Osborne, M. P.: Complete scalp avulsion. Ann. Surg., 132:198, 1950.

Paré, A.: Of wounds made by gunshot, other fierie engeines, and all sorts of weapons. In the Workes of that Famous Chirurgion Ambrois Parey, translated from the Latin and compared with the French by T. Johnson, T. Cotes and R. Young, London, 1634.

Peer, L. A., and Van Duyn, J.: Congenital defects of the scalp; report of a case with fatal termination. Plast. Reconstr. Surg., 3:722, 1948.

Phemister, D. B.: The fate of transplanted bone and regeneration of its various constituents. Surg. Gynecol. Obstet., 19:303, 1914.

Pickerill, H. P.: New method of osteoplastic restoration of the skull. Med. J. Aust., 2:228, 1931.

Pickerill, H. P.: Note on cranial autoplasty. Br. J. Surg., 35:204, 1947.

Pincherle, B.: Nouveau-née avec ulcération congénitale du

cuir chevelu, mutilations multiples des phalanges et syndactylie partielle. Arch. Méd. Enf., *41*:96, 1938.

Pudenz, R. H., and Odom, G. L.: Meningocerebral adhesions: Experimental study of effect of human amniotic membrane, amnioplastin, beef allantonic membrane, Cargile membrane, tantalum foil and polyvinyl alcohol films. Surgery, *12*:318, 1942.

Rauschkolb, R. R., and Enriquez, S. I.: Aplasia cutis congenita. Arch. Dermatol., *86*:54, 1962.

Robinson, F.: Complete avulsion of the scalp. Br. J. Plast. Surg., *5*:37, 1952.

Savage, D.: Localized congenital defects of the scalp. J. Obstet. Gynec. (Br.), *63*:351, 1956.

Savariaud, M.: Prosthèse du crane avec plaque d'argent extensible. Bull. Mém. Soc. Chir. Paris, *38*:238, 1912.

Schmidt, G. B.: Schádelplastik: Besprechung. Beitr. Klin. Chir., *98*:604, 1916.

Scott, M., and Wycis, H. T.: Experimental observations on the use of stainless steel for cranioplasty. J. Neurosurg., *3*:310, 1946.

Seydel, H.: Eine neue Methode, grosse Knochendefekten des Schädels zu keckung. Zentralbl. Chir., *16*:209, 1889.

Small, J. M., and Graham, M. P.: Acrylic resin for the closure of skull defects. Br. J. Surg., *33*:106, 1945–46.

Snell, R. S., quoted by O'Brien, B., and Drake, J.: Congenital defects of the skull and scalp. Br. J. Plast. Surg., *13*:102, 1961.

Sodeberg, B. N., and Mulvey, J. M.: Mandibular reconstruction in jaw deformities. Plast. Reconstr. Surg., *2*:191, 1947.

Stockard, C. R.: Structural expression: An experimental study of twins, "double monsters" and single deformities. Am. J. Anat., *28*:115, 1920–21.

Von Hacker, H.: Ersatz von Schädeldefekten durch unter der Kopfschwartz verschobener oder ein gelappte Periostknocken. Beitr. Klin. Chir., *37*:499, 1903.

Weber, H.: Schädelplastik. Berl. Klin. Wochenschr., *53*:1115, 1916.

Westermann, C. W. T.: Zur Methodik der Deckung von Schädeldefekten. Zentralbl. Chir., *43*:113, 1916.

White, J. C.: Late complications following cranioplasty with alloplastic plates. Ann. Surg., *128*:743, 1948.

Wolff, J. L., and Walker, A. D.: Cranioplasty, a collective review. Int. Abstr. Surg., *81*:1, 1945.

CHAPTER 28

DEFORMITIES OF THE EYELIDS AND ADNEXA, ORBIT, AND THE ZYGOMA

John Marquis Converse, M.D.,
Byron Smith, M.D.,
Mark K. H. Wang, M.D.,
W. Brandon Macomber, M.D.,
John Clarke Mustardé, F.R.C.S.,
Burgos T. Sayoc, M.D.,
Ray A. Elliott, Jr., M.D.,
Augustus J. Valauri, D.D.S.,
Serge Krupp, M.D.,
and Donald Wood-Smith, F.R.C.S.E.

The Eyelids and Their Adnexa

John Marquis Converse, M.D.,
and Byron Smith, M.D.

The eyelids are essential for the protection of the cornea. The upper lid protects the cornea and aids in visual function. Lacerations through the eyelids and defects of the eyelid tissue must be repaired for the protection of the cornea.

The extraocular musculature governs ocular function and binocular vision. Restoration of

858

adequate extraocular muscle function is essential.

Malunited fractures of the orbit result in malformation and deformity; the architecture of the orbit must be restored if functional disturbances of the ocular globe are to be eliminated.

The lacrimal apparatus may be lacerated, obstructed, or destroyed. The flow of tears through the nasolacrimal duct, although not essential in all cases, must often be restored by short circuiting the flow of lacrimal secretions into the nasal cavity.

In performing operations in the orbital region, the primary considerations should always be the protection of the eye and the maintenance of vision.

GENERAL ANATOMICAL CONSIDERATIONS

The structures under study in this chapter rest on the upper portion of the midface skeleton. The area may be divided into three portions: a central or nasomaxillary area and two lateral orbitozygomatic (or maxillozygomatic) areas. The nasomaxillary area is composed of the nasal structures which rest upon the maxilla in front of the interorbital space (see Chapter 25, Fig. 25–1). The lateral or orbitozygomatic areas discussed in this chapter are formed in large part by the orbital cavities.

The anatomy of the orbits has been described in Chapter 25. The orbital contents consist of the ocular globe and the cushion of

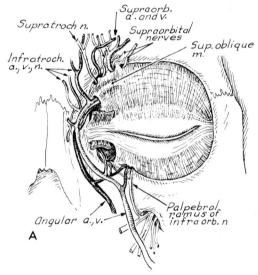

FIGURE 28–1. The medial and lateral canthal tendons, nerves, and arteries which traverse the septum orbitale. *A*, The septum orbitale (orbital septum). *B*, The septum orbitale and the orbicularis muscle have been removed.

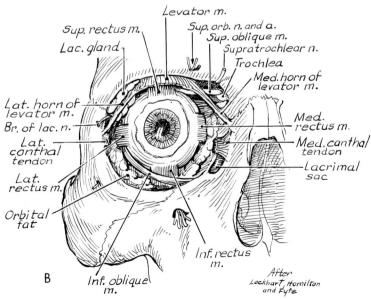

fat which surrounds it. The ocular globe occupies the anterior half of the orbital cavity, and its movements are controlled by the extraocular muscles; the posterior half of the orbital cavity contains the optic nerve, orbital fat, vessels, muscles, and the nerves supplying the extraocular musculature. Tenon's capsule divides the orbital cavity into anterior (precapsular) and posterior (retrocapsular) portions.

As stated in Chapter 25, the septum orbitale (orbital septum) maintains the orbital contents in position. The septum orbitale is a fascial structure, inserted on the inner aspect of the rim of the orbit (Figs. 28-1 and 28-2). The septum orbitale attaches to and blends with the levator aponeurosis in the upper eyelid for a distance of a few millimeters above the upper border of the tarsus; in the lower eyelid, the septum orbitale is attached to the lower border of the tarsus. The eyeball is protected by the orbital rims, which are exposed to trauma because of their prominence. Serious functional disturbances may arise from the displacement of these bones, because of the close relationship of the orbital rims to structures within the orbital cavity.

The supratrochlear and supraorbital nerves and, more medially, the trochlea of the superior oblique muscle are located along the superior rim of the orbit (see Fig. 28-1, *A*). The

tendon of the superior oblique muscle functions in a cartilaginous pulley, the trochlea, which is fixed by ligamentous fibers immediately behind the superomedial angle of the orbital margin. Fractures involving the superior rim of the orbit may result in compression of the supraorbital nerve, with consequent anesthesia in its area of distribution. Diplopia may also result from injury to the pulley of the superior oblique muscle, thus affecting the balance of the extraocular muscles. The lacrimal gland is lodged in the lacrimal fossa behind the lateral portion of the superior rim of the orbit.

The frontal process of the maxilla and the lacrimal bone share in the formation of the groove for the lacrimal sac. Displaced fragments of bone in this area may injure the lacrimal sac and other portions of the lacrimal apparatus.

The lower rim of the orbit is formed by the anterior limits of the zygomatic and maxillary components of the orbital floor. When the floor of the orbit is fractured and displaced downward, the lowered level of the eyeball may produce ocular dysfunction. Diplopia is usually the consequence of entrapment of the orbital contents in the area of a blowout fracture in the floor of the orbit. Escape of orbital fat through the fractured orbital floor into the subjacent maxillary sinus is the most frequent cause of traumatic enophthalmos.

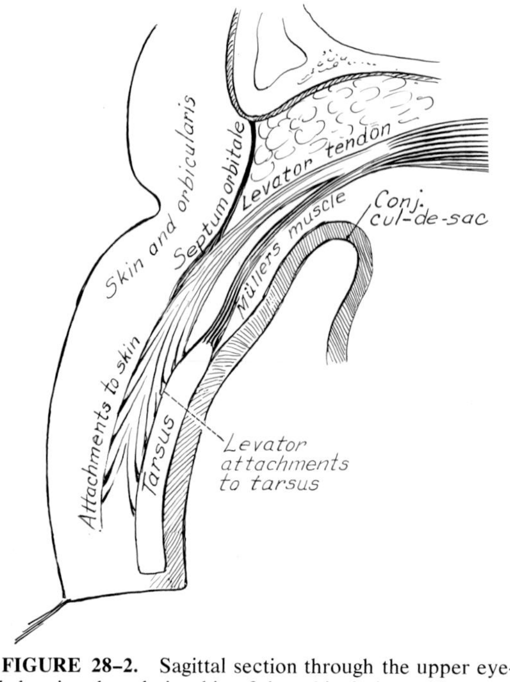

ANATOMY OF THE EYELIDS

Familiarity with the anatomy of the eyelids is a prerequisite for any operative procedure in this area. The anatomy of the orbital region has been studied and defined by Jones (1967) in a number of publications. The eyelids are composed of thin skin, areolar tissue, orbicularis oculi muscle, tarsus, septum orbitale (orbital septum), tarsal (meibomian) glands, and conjunctiva.

The tarsal plates are thin, elongated plates of connective tissue (Fig. 28-3) which contribute to the form and support of the eyelids. The superior tarsus is semilunar in form, approximately 10 mm in width at its center; the inferior tarsus is smaller, thinner, and elliptical in form, and has a vertical dimension of approximately 5 mm.

The anatomy of the margin of the eyelid is important from a surgical viewpoint, as an understanding of its structure is helpful when suturing wounds or incisions extending through it. The eyelid margins are thick. Upon the

FIGURE 28–2. Sagittal section through the upper eyelid showing the relationship of the orbicularis oculi muscle, septum orbitale, levator palpebrae superioris, and Müller's muscle.

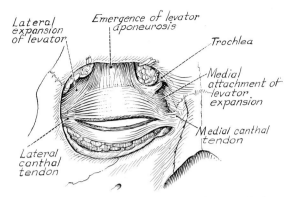

FIGURE 28–3. The tarsal plates, the levator palpebrae superioris, and their relationship to the medial canthal and lateral canthal tendons.

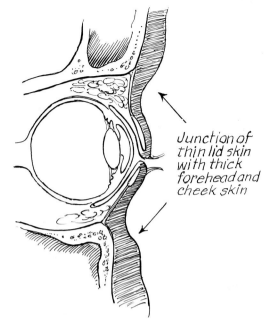

FIGURE 28–4. Difference in thickness of the cutaneous tissues at the orbital margin where the eyelid skin meets the surrounding facial skin.

inner portion of each eyelid margin, between the tarsus and the conjunctiva, are situated the tarsal (meibomian) glands. When the eyelid is everted, they appear as a string of tiny pearls (the white line). The tarsal glands are imbedded in grooves in the inner surfaces of the tarsus.

It is important to keep in mind that the eyelid margin has an anterior and a posterior border which must be realigned when suturing a full-thickness laceration or an operative incision which extends through it.

Skin and Subcutaneous Fascia. The skin of the eyelids is thin and elastic; it is moderately adherent to the orbicularis muscle over the tarsus and is more mobile and loose as the orbital rim is approached. The eyelid skin becomes thicker at the junction with the skin of the cheek and the other areas surrounding the orbit (Fig. 28–4), the area of transition corresponding roughly to the bony orbital margins.

The Orbicularis Oculi Muscle. The orbicularis muscle surrounding the palpebral fissure is responsible for lid closure. Although in appearance it is one continuous muscle, it has been divided arbitrarily into three subdivisions (Fig. 28–5) (Jones, 1967):

1. The orbital portion which forms a muscular ring extending over the orbital margin.
2. The pretarsal portion (pretarsal muscle) overlying the tarsus.
3. The preseptal portion (preseptal muscle) overlying the septum orbitale.

The anatomical arrangement is similar in both the upper and lower eyelids, with some variations resulting from functional differences between the lids.

1. The orbital portion of the orbicularis muscle extends in a circular fashion widely around the orbit, interdigitating with fibers of

the frontalis muscle (Figs. 28–5 and 28–6), and it is adherent to the skin lateral to the lateral canthus; the orbital portion arises from the medial canthal tendon.

2. The pretarsal muscle divides medially into a superficial head and a deep head (Fig. 28–6, *A, B, C*). The superficial head joins its counterpart in the opposing lid to form the medial canthal tendon, which inserts above and anterior to the anterior lacrimal crest. The deep head, after joining its counterpart, ex-

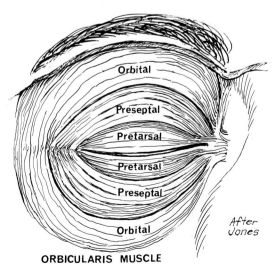

ORBICULARIS MUSCLE

FIGURE 28–5. The three subdivisions of the orbicularis oculi muscle. (After Jones.)

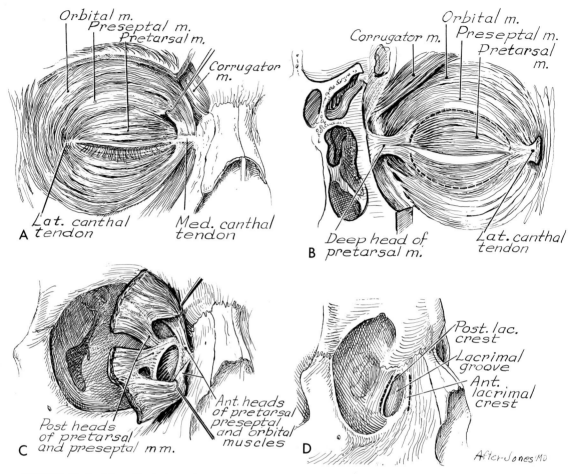

FIGURE 28–6. The orbicularis oculi muscle. *A,* The medial and lateral canthal tendons showing the superficial head of the pretarsal muscle which joins its counterpart from the opposing lid to form the medial canthal tendon. The hook raises the preseptal muscle whose fibers insert on the orbital margin below the medial canthal tendon. *B,* The orbicularis oculi muscle seen from behind. The deep head of the pretarsal muscle after joining its counterpart extends posterior to the lacrimal sac, blending with the lacrimal sac diaphragm to insert behind the posterior lacrimal crest (Horner's muscle). *C,* Anterior view illustrating the anterior heads of the pretarsal and preseptal muscles, as well as the posterior heads. *D,* The skeletal anatomy of the medial canthus. (After Jones.)

tends posteriorly to the lacrimal sac, blending with the lacrimal sac diaphragm to insert immediately behind the posterior lacrimal crest (Figs. 28–6, *C, D* and 28–7). The deep head of the tarsal portion of the orbicularis has also been known as Horner's muscle or the tensor tarsi muscle.

3. The preseptal muscle has superficial and deep fibers (Figs. 28–6, *A, B* and 28–7). The superficial fibers of each preseptal muscle (upper and lower) insert on the orbital margin below the medial canthal tendon (Fig. 28–8, *A*). Deeper fibers insert on the lacrimal diaphragm. The deepest fibers insert on the posterior lacrimal crest just above the deep heads of the pretarsals (Fig. 28–6, *C*). The lacrimal pump mechanism is explained by the medial movements of the lids, emptying the ampullae,

shortening the canaliculi, thus forcing fluid into the lacrimal sac. The preseptal muscles through their intimate connection with the lacrimal diaphragm produce a negative pressure in the lacrimal sac. The elasticity of the diaphragm returns it to a position of rest, and fluid is forced into the nasolacrimal duct.

In the lateral canthus, both preseptal muscles form a "raphé" (see Fig. 28–8, *B*), a convenient term to designate the loops of muscle bundles which are firmly attached to the skin of the lateral canthus (Jones, 1974a). The pretarsal muscles of the upper and lower lids are inserted into the orbital tubercle, situated behind the orbital rim on the lateral orbital wall, through the intermediary of the lateral canthal tendon (Figs. 28–8, *C* and 28–9). There is space between the tendon and the raphé which

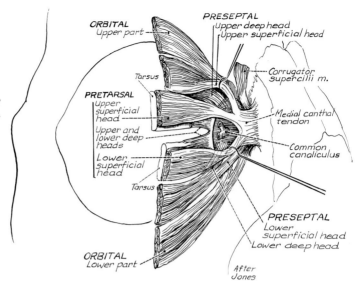

FIGURE 28–7. Details of the anatomy in the right medial canthal area (front view).

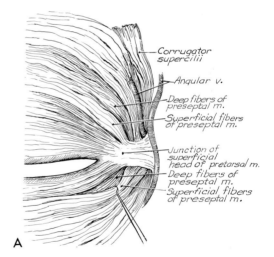

FIGURE 28–8. *A*, The anatomy of the orbicularis oculi muscle at the right medial canthus. *B*, The lateral palpebral raphé. *C*, The lateral canthal tendon and the anatomy of the structures of the lateral canthus. (After Jones.)

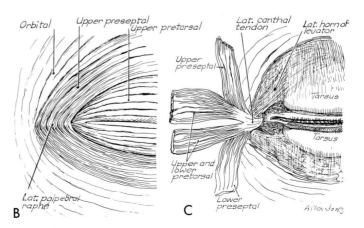

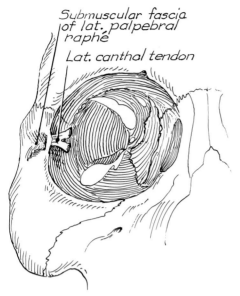

Submuscular fascia of lat. palpebral raphé

Lat. canthal tendon

FIGURE 28–9. The respective attachments of the lateral palpebral raphé and the lateral canthal tendon. (After Jones.)

deepens laterally. A lateral palpebral artery passes through this space, supplying both eyelids.

The heads of the pretarsal and preseptal muscles inserted on the posterior lacrimal crest have a particular surgical importance, for they not only aid in maintaining the eyelids against the ocular globe but also maintain the depth of the naso-orbital valley. When anatomical disorganization of the medial canthal region occurs in naso-orbital fractures, reattachment of the canthal tendon posteriorly to the lacrimal groove is essential to reestablish the depth of the naso-orbital valley.

An intricate fascial system, known as Lockwood's suspensory ligament, supports the orbital contents and is attached to the orbital walls, medially to the posterior lacrimal crest and laterally below the lateral orbital tubercle.

The Levator Palpebrae Superioris and Müller's Muscles and Their Relationships. The levator palpebrae superioris is a thin, flat, triangular muscle which arises from the undersurface of the lesser wing of the sphenoid above and in front of the optic foramen. At its origin, it is narrow and tenuous, but soon it broadens, ending in a wide aponeurosis (see Fig. 28–3; Fig. 28–10). The levator aponeurosis fans out medially and laterally into two extensions. The lateral extension is quite strong and presses into the lacrimal gland, dividing it into orbital and palpebral lobes. It attaches to the lateral canthal tendon. The me-

dial extension attaches to the posterior lacrimal crest. The levator aponeurosis has a firm attachment to the anterior surface of the tarsus and to the skin of the eyelid, forming the superior tarsal fold of the upper eyelid. The levator aponeurosis is attached to and blends with the orbital septum for a distance of about 3 to 5 mm above the upper border of the tarsus. Above this level, the levator aponeurosis is separated from the septum orbitale by preaponeurotic fat, which lies between the septum orbitale and the levator aponeurosis and has different characteristics from the orbital fat which is situated posterior to the septum orbitale.

Müller's muscle (Fig. 28–10) extends from the junction of the muscular portion of the levator muscle and its aponeurosis to the superior border of the tarsus and overlies the underlying conjunctiva. Whereas the levator muscle is a striated muscle innervated by the third cranial nerve, Müller's muscle is a smooth muscle and receives its innervation from the sympathetic nervous system.

CLOSURE OF THE PALPEBRAL FISSURE. Closure of the palpebral fissure is produced by contraction of the orbicularis oculi muscle. Opening of the palpebral fissure is the result of relaxation of the orbicularis oculi and contraction of the levator palpebrae superioris and Müller's muscles.

In paralysis of the seventh nerve, closure of the upper eyelid can be produced only by relaxation of the levator palpebrae superioris muscle, which is innervated by the third cra-

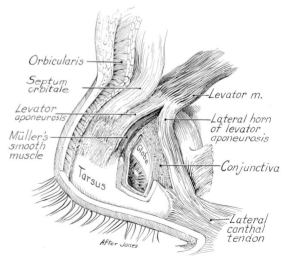

Orbicularis

Septum orbitale

Levator aponeurosis

Müller's smooth muscle

Tarsus

Levator m.

Lateral horn of levator aponeurosis

Conjunctiva

Globe

Lateral canthal tendon

After Jones

FIGURE 28–10. Diagrammatic sagittal section illustrating the structures of the upper eyelid, including the levator muscle, its aponeurosis, and its relationship with Müller's muscle and the septum orbitale. (After Jones.)

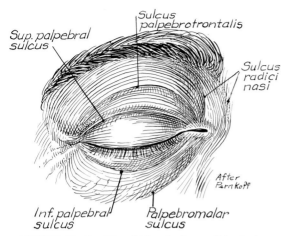

FIGURE 28–11. The folds of the eyelids (redrawn after Pernkopf). Pernkopf designated the folds using Latin terminology (superior palpebral sulcus = supratarsal fold, and so on).

nial nerve; the eyelid descends by gravity. It is not possible for the patient to squeeze the eyelids together because of the paralysis of the orbicularis oculi muscle.

The skin of the eyelids is folded upon itself, the excess of skin permitting closure of the palpebral fissure. The upper limit of the tarsus of the upper lid is demarcated by a crease, the supratarsal fold (Fig. 28–11). The tarsus disappears under an overlapping fold of the upper part of the lid when the eyelid is raised. The tarsus of the lower lid is much smaller, and the skin covering the tarsus lacks such definite demarcation. Closure of the palpebral fissure is produced mainly by the downward displacement of the upper eyelid (Fig. 28–12). Blinking movements of the lids, produced by contraction of the orbicularis oculi muscle (which acts as an antagonist to the levator palpebrae superioris muscle), have an important role in activating the lacrimal pump, providing periodic compression of the lacrimal sac for the evacuation of tears.

The Conjunctiva. The conjunctiva lines the inner aspect of the eyelid and is reflected onto the globe. The tarsal conjunctiva is densely adherent to the tarsal plates; the remainder of the conjunctiva is loosely bound to the underlying epibulbar and fornix tissues. The depth of the conjunctival cul-de-sac varies; Figure 28–13 outlines the depth of the cul-de-sac.

The eyelids have unusual mobility and are therefore vulnerable to the effects of scar contracture, whether within themselves or in the adjacent tissue.

Sensory Innervation. An awareness of the

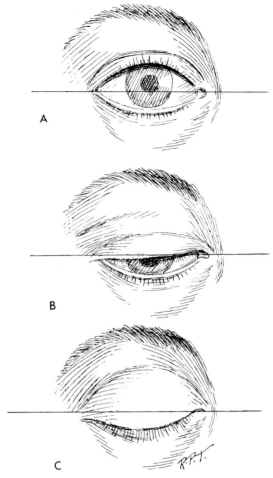

FIGURE 28–12. *A,* In the forward gaze, the medial and lateral canthi are situated along the same horizontal plane. *B, C,* As the upper eyelid descends, it extends below the horizontal plane. Closure of the palpebral fissure is produced mainly by the downward displacement of the upper eyelid.

sensory innervation is important, local anesthesia being frequently employed for operations in the orbital region. The eyelids are in-

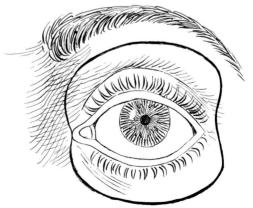

FIGURE 28–13. The depth of the conjunctival fornix is outlined.

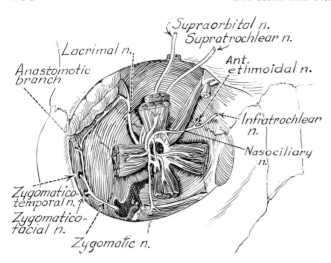

FIGURE 28–14. The sensory nerves of the orbit.

nervated by the ophthalmic and maxillary nerves, which are distributed from the trigeminal ganglion in Meckel's trigeminal cave, a space in the floor of the middle cranial fossa immediately near the apex of the petrous portion of the temporal bone.

The ophthalmic nerve, first division of the trigeminal, enters the orbital cavity through the superior orbital fissure, distributing lacrimal, frontal, and nasociliary branches (Figs. 28–14 and 28–15). The lacrimal nerve contributes afferent filaments to the lacrimal gland and to the upper eyelid and skin in the region of the lateral orbital border. The frontal nerve (Fig. 28–16), bifurcating in the orbital cavity into supraorbital and supratrochlear branches, transmits sensation from the skin of the forehead and scalp, the frontal sinus, and the major portion of the upper eyelid. The nasociliary nerve is distributed mainly to the internal and external nose.

The maxillary nerve, second division of the trigeminal, leaves the cranium through the foramen rotundum, traverses the pterygopalatine fossa, supplies short sphenopalatine nerves to the sphenopalatine ganglion, zygomatic nerve, and posterior-superior alveolar nerves, and continues through the infraorbital canal or groove in the floor of the orbit. The portion of the maxillary nerve in the orbital floor is referred to as the infraorbital nerve. The zygomatic nerve is the orbital branch of the maxillary nerve, branching from the latter in the pterygopalatine fossa and extending

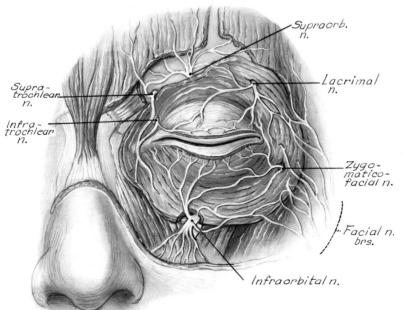

FIGURE 28–15. The peripheral distribution of the sensory nerves of the orbit.

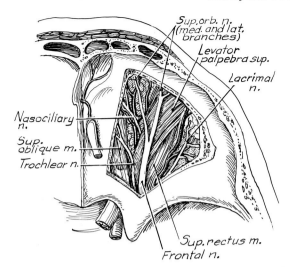

FIGURE 28–16. Transverse section after removal of the roof of the orbit, illustrating the position of the frontal nerve and the other nerves of the orbit.

through the inferior orbital fossa into the orbit, where it bifurcates into zygomaticotemporal and zygomaticofacial branches. The zygomatico-temporal nerve joins the lacrimal nerve in the orbit, reaches the temporal fossa by way of the zygomaticotemporal foramen in the zygoma, penetrates the temporal fascia, and transmits sensation from the skin of the anterior temporal region, where it has connections with the neighboring filaments of the facial nerve. The zygomaticofacial nerve, passing through the zygomaticofacial foramen on the outer region of the face, connects with terminal filaments of the facial nerve.

The infraorbital nerve (see Fig. 28–15), after giving off middle and anterior superior alveolar branches from the floor of the orbit, emerges upon the face through the infraorbital foramen and subdivides into terminal branches, which include the inferior palpebral, external nasal, and superior labial nerves, which transmit sensation from the upper lip and cheek and adjacent areas.

GENERAL OPERATIVE CONSIDERATIONS

Regional Anesthesia of the Eyelids. Regional block anesthesia of the eyelids may be achieved by injecting at various points along the superior rim of the orbit to produce block anesthesia of the lacrimal, frontal, supraorbital, and supratrochlear nerves. Additional injec-

tions in or near the infraorbital foramen and in the region of the zygomaticofacial foramen on the lateral surface of the zygoma result in block anesthesia of both upper and lower lids.

A convenient technique of obtaining regional anesthesia of the upper lid is to inject a local anesthetic solution below the midportion of the supraorbital arch, extending the needle 4 cm backward in order to block the frontal nerve (see Fig. 28–16). This permits the patient to open and close his lids during the operation, a useful maneuver during operations for ptosis or lid retraction.

Care of the Cornea. Protection of the cornea from desiccation, irritation, and trauma during and after the operation is an essential consideration in all surgery of the eyelids and orbital region. Desiccation can be prevented by the administration of a few drops of saline in the conjunctival sac periodically during an operation when the lids cannot be closed. During operations in the orbital area, the use of a plastic contact protective shell should be routine, when possible (Fig. 28–17). The contact shell prevents desiccation and injury of the cornea by an instrument or abrasion by gauze during the surgical procedure.

A carefully applied dressing is essential to avoid corneal irritation during the postoperative period. It is distressing for the surgeon to be obliged to remove a pressure dressing over

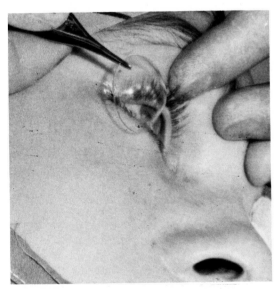

FIGURE 28–17. Protective lens being inserted into the conjunctival sac. A transparent lens is shown in the photograph in order to allow the sclera and the cornea to be seen through the lens. Colored lenses are preferable, as there is less risk of forgetting to remove them postoperatively and thus risking corneal abrasion.

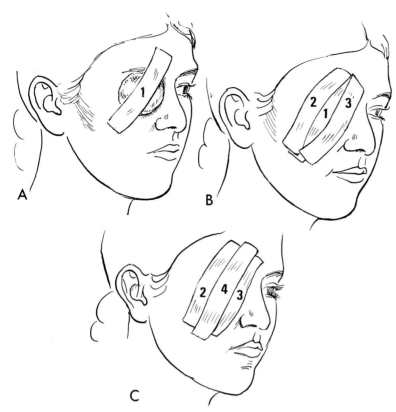

FIGURE 28–18. The eye dressing. *A,* An eye pad has been placed over the orbital region and is maintained in place with a strip of paper tape. *B, C,* The dressing is reinforced with additional tape. A moderately compressive pressure dressing may be placed over the eye dressing and maintained by a head bandage when required.

a reconstructed lid, particularly if a skin graft has been used, because the patient is complaining of symptoms of corneal irritation—a grating sensation in the eye or recurring shooting pain. At the end of the operation, the conjunctival sac should be washed carefully with normal saline solution to free it of any loose particles of gauze, eyelash, cotton, or other foreign body. An occlusive suture should always be used if a pressure dressing is applied over the eye in order to avoid opening of the eyelids and exposure of the cornea to the dressing (see Fig. 28–19). The dressing itself should be applied carefully so that it is not displaced during the postoperative period. Figure 28–18 illustrates the application of adhesive tape over the dressing to ensure its proper immobilization. A figure-of-eight bandage can be employed to reinforce this dressing, when indicated.

In order to avoid postoperative corneal abrasion, deep sutures should be placed in such a manner that the knots are buried in the tissue or placed externally when the lid is being reconstructed. A continuous buried suture, which may be pulled out after healing, is particularly useful in ensuring the approximation of tissue over the corneal region. Skin grafts should not be placed in the conjunctival sac if

they are to be in contact with the cornea; only conjunctiva or other mucosal tissue is tolerated by the cornea.

OCCLUSIVE LID SUTURE. Temporary lid closure may be achieved by inserting one or two horizontal mattress sutures (Fig. 28–19). A double-armed suture (4–0 silk), with a needle at each end, is used for this procedure. The sutures are placed from below upward in order that the knot may be tied in the upper lid; this precaution facilitates removal of the suture.

Another method of occlusive suture is a continuous to-and-fro suture between the upper and lower eyelid margins (Fig. 28–20). This type of suture may be left in position for many weeks and is as effective as a tarsorrhaphy.

TARSORRHAPHY. Tarsorrhaphy, or the formation of a lid adhesion, has been extensively used in the past to ensure occlusion of the eyelids. It is contraindicated in the protection of the cornea in burn ectropion of the eyelids, as the lids pull apart (see Chapter 33) and the lid margins are deformed. It is, however, a useful emergency measure if occlusion of the eyelids must be ensured in ocular pathology.

After local anesthesia has been obtained by infiltration, two fixation forceps are placed 1 cm apart on the lid (Fig. 28–21, *A*). The lid is

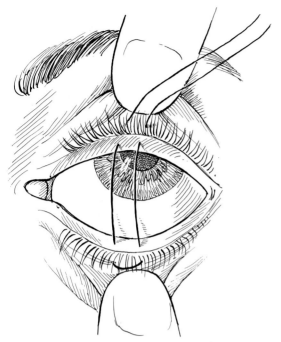

FIGURE 28–19. Occlusive suture used to prevent opening of the palpebral fissure and corneal abrasion when a pressure dressing is placed over the eye.

lid (Fig. 28–21, *D*). This procedure increases the surface contact between the raw areas of the lid and improves the chance of successful adhesion (Fig. 28–21, *E*). The procedure is repeated in another portion of the eyelid and also in two areas of the opposing eyelid. Mattress sutures of 4–0 silk are placed through protective soft rubber dam plates, which are not essential if the occlusive sutures are not tied under excessive tension, which would cause them to cut through the skin. The sutures penetrate the skin 5 mm from the lid margin, entering the wound first through one lid, then the other, and finally emerging to be tied (Fig. 28–21, *F*). In certain ophthalmologic cases, it may be necessary to do a complete tarsorrhaphy, denuding the entire length of both eyelid margins (Fig. 28–22). Procedures such as the one illustrated in Figure 28–22 should be used only if they are definitive, as the eyelid margin is inalterably damaged. Occlusive sutures (see Figs. 28–19 and 28–20) are usually sufficient.

LACERATIONS OF THE EYELIDS

A distinction must be made between the laceration which extends through the eyelid skin only and the laceration which extends through the tarsus and eyelid margin.

Laceration Through Skin Only. If there is no loss of tissue, approximation of the wound

punctured and counterpunctured along its free margin with the tip of a sharp knife. A 1.5 × 4 mm strip of lid margin tissue is undermined with the knife and removed (Fig. 28–21, *B*). The tip of the knife is stabbed through the middle portion of the denuded area thus formed for a depth of 3 mm (Fig. 28–21, *C*). The incision splits the

FIGURE 28–20. Continuous to-and-fro suture between the upper and lower eyelid margins to occlude the lids. *A*, Placing of the continuous suture. *B*, The suture is tightened, occluding the lids. Such a suture can be left for many weeks or even months without causing irritation. A suture of 4–0 or 5–0 monofilament nylon is employed.

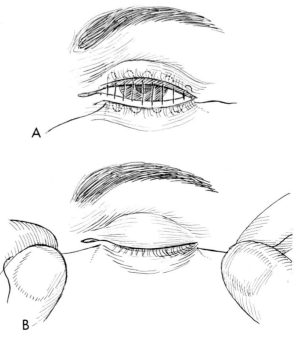

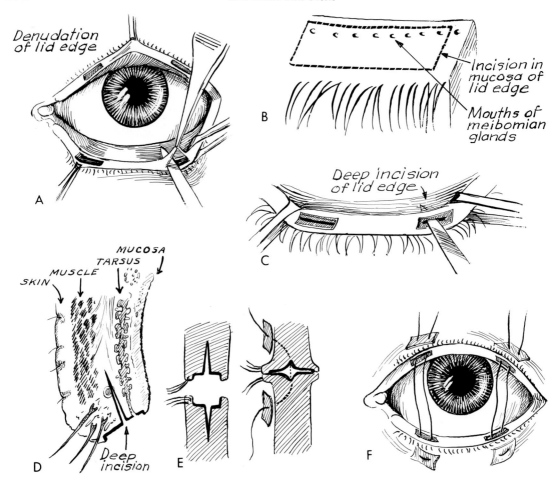

FIGURE 28–21.   Technique of partial tarsorrhaphy. *A*, Excision of two small rectangles along the margin of each eyelid. *B*, Outline of the excised area. *C*, An incision 3 mm in depth is made into the tarsal plate. *D*, Sagittal section showing the depth of the incision in the denuded portion of the lid margin. *E*, The incision allows spreading of the denuded areas and a wider surface of contact. *F*, Sutures are placed through the denuded areas and through small pieces of rubber dam.

edges usually leaves an inconspicuous scar. Sutures should be removed in 48 to 72 hours, as epithelization along the suture tract will result in cystlike nests of sebaceous material that require subsequent removal. If the laceration is horizontal, parallel to the lid folds, and does not extend through the levator apo-

FIGURE 28–22.   Complete tarsorrhaphy. *A*, The greater portion of the margin of each lid is denuded. *B*, The lids are held occluded by a continuous suture.

neurosis resulting in ptosis, simple approximation is adequate. Vertical scars also frequently heal without being conspicuous, but occasionally they result in a linear contracture, causing an upward pull on the lid margin. This is particularly serious if the laceration lies near a lacrimal punctum, as the punctum may be pulled away from the lacrimal lake. In such a case, a Z-plasty procedure done at the initial suture of the wound would obviate this inconvenience.

Little debridement is required, as the blood supply of the area is abundant. Interrupted sutures or continuous subcuticular sutures are used.

Lacerations Involving the Lid Margins. Lacerations of the lid margins may be approximated without undue tension. In the past, many various forms of overlapping dissections and complicated repairs were utilized. These included Wheeler's halving technique (1936)

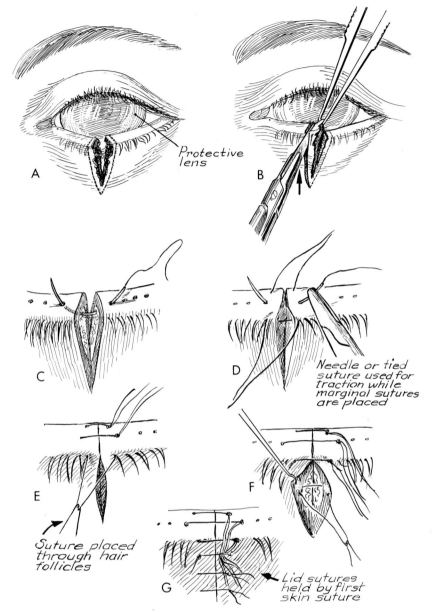

FIGURE 28–23. Repair of lacerations through the lid. *A*, A scleral lens has been placed in the conjunctival sac. *B*, The wound edges are freshened using a razor-blade knife. *C*, The first suture placed through the line of the ducts of the tarsal glands aligns the margins. *D, E*, Additional sutures are placed through the posterior and anterior edges of the lid margin and tied. *F*, Pretarsal and muscle sutures are placed and tied. *G*, Wound suture completed.

and Hughes' tongue and groove technique (1955). The technique most generally employed is that of Mustardé (1966). The simplest possible method is often the best. To ensure precise alignment of the lid margin, the needle is placed along the line of the ducts of the tarsal glands in the midmarginal area (Fig. 28–23, *A, B, C*), downward into the wound in the tarsal gland area, and across the wound, up the opposite side, and out through the line of the tarsal glands of the opposite side of the defect

(Fig. 28–23, *C*). The needle puncture should be approximately 1.5 mm from the cut edge. Traction upon this suture approximates the wound edges and aligns the anterior and posterior lid margins. Additional sutures are placed at the posterior and anterior lid margins and are tied, leaving the suture ends long (Fig. 28–23, *D, E, F*). The needles of the sutures should be atraumatic and the suture material 6–0 in size.

After the three marginal sutures have been

tied, moderate upward traction ensures good positioning of the wound edges. Pretarsal and muscle sutures are then placed, tied, and trimmed closely (Fig. 28–23, *F*). The skin is sutured with a continuous suture or several interrupted sutures. The skin suture, 2 mm from the lashes, is tied over the ends of the three marginal sutures (Fig. 28–23, *G*). This prevents the sutures from irritating the cornea during the postoperative period. An eye patch is placed over the eye but is not essential. After 24 hours, the dressing is removed. The skin sutures are removed within three or four days. The marginal sutures should be left in position a week or longer, depending upon the amount of tension upon the wound. After the skin sutures have been removed, it is advisable to place a strip of paper tape across the wound horizontally to assure its protection during the following three or four days. Ordinarily it is not necessary to place an occlusive suture or perform a tarsorrhaphy in the treatment of lid lacerations.

Visual magnification using loupes or the microscope permits precise approximation of the edges of the transected layers.

Closure of Moderate Sized Defects by Direct Approximation. In the event of tissue loss in the middle section of either the upper or lower lid, direct closure may exert undue tension upon the horizontal dimension of the lid. Should it be determined that tension is excessive, release of the structures at the lateral canthus provides additional substance for closure.

Lateral canthotomy is done with scissors (Fig. 28–24, *A*). The skin and conjunctiva are dissected from the lateral canthal tendon and raphé. The vertical incision across the lower half or upper half of the raphé may then be done (Fig. 28–24, *B*). As the vertical incision is made, a release in the horizontal tension is immediately noticeable (Fig. 28–24, *C*). If the release is not achieved, this indicates that all of the structures between the skin and the conjunctiva have not been sufficiently dissected. Ordinarily 5 to 10 mm in the horizontal dimension of the lid may be gained by this method (Fig. 28–24, *D*). This technique is applicable to the upper as well as the lower lid.

Repair of Injuries to the Levator Palpebrae Superioris. Lacerations extending through the levator muscle or its aponeurosis must be repaired. The diagnosis and repair of the resulting traumatic ptosis are described in a later section of the chapter (see page 921).

Avulsion of the Eyelid. Dog bites, human bites, and accidents of varying types have been the cause of partial or complete avulsion of an eyelid. If the eyelid is partially avulsed, the ex-

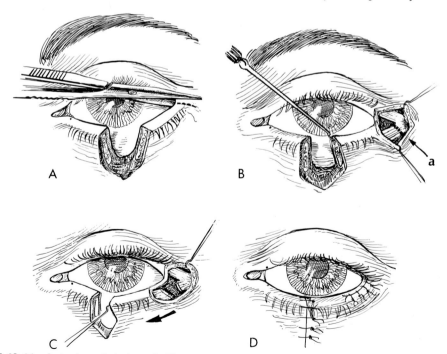

FIGURE 28–24. Lateral cantholysis to facilitate the closure of a moderate sized defect. *A,* Lateral canthotomy. *B,* The conjunctiva is dissected from the lateral canthal tendon, and the lower crus of the tendon is severed (a). *C, D,* Closure of the defect is thus facilitated.

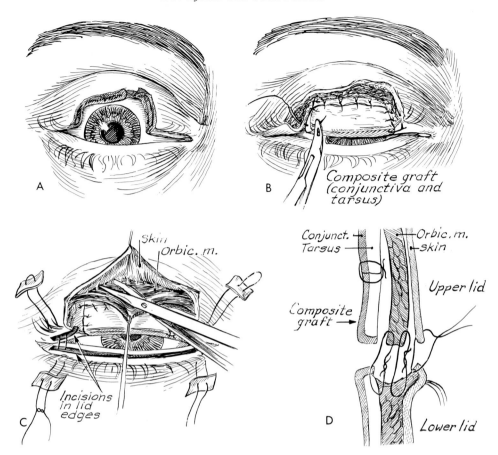

FIGURE 28–25. Immediate reconstruction of an avulsed upper eyelid. *A, B,* The skin and orbicularis oculi muscle fibers are dissected and will be advanced over the tarsus. Intermarginal adhesion is prepared. *C,* Mobilization of the orbicularis oculi muscle fibers and the skin. *D,* Sagittal section showing method of placing sutures. (After A. Callahan.)

cellent blood supply allows careful replacement, suture of all the structures, and usually anatomical and functional restoration. In dog bites, abundant irrigation is required to remove the necrotizing effect of the canine saliva. One of the most unusual cases of total avulsion of the upper lid and its replantation has been reported by Callahan (1956).

A woman, aged 22, experienced a bite of her right upper lid. When she was brought into the hospital shortly after injury at 3 A.M. on Sunday morning, she did not bring the detached portion of the lid with her. Her friends were dispatched to the scene of the injury for it.

Examination showed a large central coloboma of the right upper lid. The defect in the lid tarsus measured 5 mm vertically by 15 mm horizontally; the defect in the skin and orbicularis was about 10 mm vertically by 15 mm horizontally. The rigidity of the tarsus and the angle of bite caused less tarsus to be lost than skin. Tooth marks were evidenced by the V-shaped notch torn in the tarsus at each end of the coloboma. The right eye was uninjured.

The detached portion of the lid was found on the floor with some trash and brought back to the hospital. A night attendant placed it in an envelope on the patient's chart. At 8 A.M. it was recovered by a resident who placed it in a medicine glass filled with penicillin solution (50,000 units per cc). This detached portion was a single piece the size of the defect, and it had been bitten off squarely.

The plan for repair [Fig. 28–25] was to use the tarsus and lid margin of the detached portion, to discard the skin and orbicularis, to use sliding flaps of muscle and skin to form the anterior lamina, and to prevent damage from postoperative contracture (vertical tension) by uniting the upper lid with the lower along a wide intermarginal adhesion.

The patient's inebriation had subsided sufficiently by 9 A.M. for the repair to begin.

When replantation of the eyelid tissue is not possible because of destruction or loss, the eyeball remains exposed. When the upper eyelid is lost, desiccation of the cornea from lack of corneal protection initiates a keratolytic process which terminates in destruction of the eye.

Protection of the eye is imperative if the avulsed eyelid tissues cannot be replaced. When the lower eyelid is destroyed, closure of the upper lid protects the cornea. Protection of the cornea cannot be assured when the upper lid is destroyed. The lower lid is separated into cutaneous, muscular, and tarsoconjunctival layers. The inner tarsoconjunctival layer is advanced to cover the globe; the musculocutaneous layer is advanced as far as possible; and the remaining raw area over the tarsoconjunctival layer is covered with a skin graft.

The eye is in serious danger when both upper and lower eyelids are avulsed. Sectioning the inferior rectus muscle permits upper rotation of the eyeball and protection of the cornea until later reconstructive procedures can be considered. The use of soft lens and moisture chambers provides protection until adequate surgical measures can be taken.

The repair of other full-thickness defects is discussed on page 881.

TUMORS OF THE EYELIDS AND ORBIT

MARK K. H. WANG, M.D.,
AND W. BRANDON MACOMBER, M.D.

Benign Tumors of the Eyelids

CONGENITAL BENIGN LESIONS

Benign tumors of the eyelid in children are usually congenital. They are frequently classified according to their developmental origin from single or multiple germ layers. The relatively common hemangioma, nevus, and neurofibroma arise from a single germ layer, while the dermoid cyst and teratoma have origin in more than one germ layer. Benign tumors rarely interfere with lid function, but their early rapid growth is often alarming.

Hemangiomas and Lymphangiomas. The majority of hemangiomas are present at birth or appear shortly thereafter. Approximately 85 per cent are evident within the first year of life. More than half of them occur on the head, and the eyelid is commonly involved. Hemangiomas and lymphangiomas are also discussed in Chapter 65. The pathology of hemangiomas and lymphangiomas of the lids is similar to that of other areas.

Surgical excision is indicated when spontaneous recession does not occur rapidly or when the tumor is of such size that it interferes with the function of the eyelid. Excision is effective if the wound can be closed without causing ectropion of the involved lid (Fig. 28–26). If a large skin defect results from the excision, a full-thickness skin graft is advisable. Split-thickness grafts or grafts from the contralateral upper lid are desirable in the defect of the upper lid; grafts from the postauricular or supraclavicular area give the best color match and texture in the lower lid.

Fortunately, the tarsal plate is rarely involved by the tumor; thus, resection of the whole thickness of the eyelid is not indicated. Secondary hypertrophy and enlargement of the tarsus is occasionally encountered, and a partial resection of the tarsus may be needed to restore the involved eyelid to proper size. The musculature of the lids should be preserved whenever possible. Preservation of the levator palpebrae superioris muscle of the upper eyelid is of prime importance.

COMPLICATIONS

Hemorrhage. The main complication in hemangiomas is hemorrhage. A large cavernous hemangioma has a very rich blood supply. Surgical excision requires tedious and meticulous dissection, with isolation and ligation of individual vessels. A blood transfusion may be indicated for moderately large lesions; the patient should be crossmatched, and blood should always be available.

Ptosis and loss of the supratarsal fold. The large mass of the tumor may cause elongation of the levator aponeurosis and resulting ptosis of the eyelid, as well as loss of the supratarsal fold. Levator shortening and restoration of the fold remedy this complication (Fig. 28–26).

Neurofibroma. This is a congenital tumor which appears to have a genetic component. Its presence in the eyelid is often associated with neurofibromas of the cornea, iris, ciliary body, retina, choroid plexus, or orbit. The neurofibroma is frequently accompanied by patches of cutaneous pigmentation (café au lait spots); multiple tumors arising from the sheaths of cranial, spinal, peripheral, and sympathetic nerves; or developmental defects in the orbital or temporal bones.

The tumors are usually first observed in early childhood or about the age of puberty, and growth is characteristically slow. Unilateral involvement of an upper lid is the usual picture, and the temporal portion of the lid is often affected first. The involved lid is diffusely

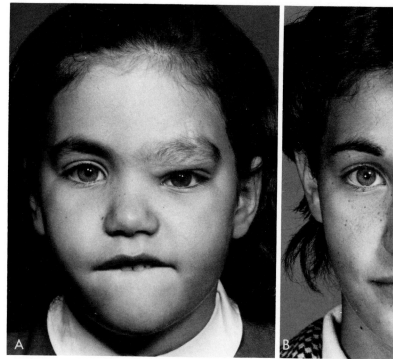
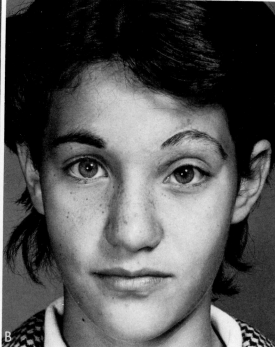

FIGURE 28–26. Lymphangioma of the left upper eyelid. *A*, Seven year old girl with lymphangioma of the upper lid. *B*, Six years following resection of the tumor, shortening of the levator aponeurosis, and formation of a new supratarsal fold (case of Dr. John M. Converse and Dr. Byron Smith).

thickened, and the overlying skin is frequently pigmented (Fig. 28–27). Partial ptosis of the upper lid is common, and in large tumors the entire eyelid is enormously enlarged, and the thickened skin hangs in folds. Palpation of cordlike structures in the lax folds of skin gives the feeling of a "bag of worms."

Microscopically, the neurofibroma is chiefly composed of long, slender cells, the elongated nuclei of which may show palisading, whorls, and eddies—the true perineural fibroblastoma. These cells are intermingled in a background of loose, tangled, or reticular tissue and sheath of Schwann reaction. Mucocystic degeneration is common.

TREATMENT. Treatment is rarely sought until the lesion begins to affect the appearance and function of the involved eyelid. In early cases, complete excision of the tumor and the involved skin should be attempted. This is often difficult because of the diffuse nature and lack of clear demarcation of the tumor. Repair of the surgical defect may require a skin graft.

When extensive involvement of the eyelid results in thickened and pendulous skin and subcutaneous layer, the underlying tarsus may also be stretched and hypertrophic. Because of the benign nature of the lesion, radical whole

thickness excision of the involved lid is rarely indicated. The goals of surgical treatment should be reduction of the bulk of the eyelid to nearly normal, correction of the ptosis if present, and maintenance of adequate movement of the lids.

The skin and subcutaneous tissue. If the skin is not thick and hypertrophic, excision of the redundant portion with complete removal of the subcutaneous tumor usually is sufficient. A transverse incision is made, with the lower incision about 1 mm above the eyelashes, extending from the medial to the lateral canthus. The upper incision of the ellipse is made after carefully estimating the amount of redundant skin to be excised. The skin above the excised area is undermined as thinly as is compatible with its viability, and the main bulk of the tumor is excised in toto down to the tarsal plate. Care must be taken to preserve the levator muscle and aponeurosis during the dissection. Primary closure of the wound is then done.

When the eyelid skin is thick and hypertrophic, its complete excision along with the subcutaneous tumor down to the tarsus is indicated. The levator palpebrae aponeurosis must be preserved. A strip of skin 1 mm in width is

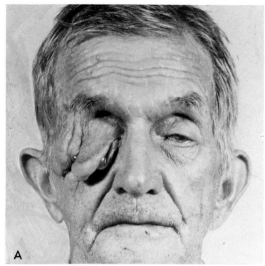

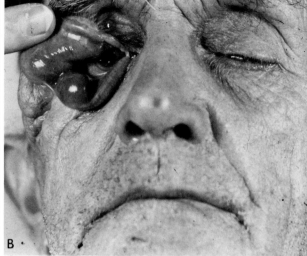

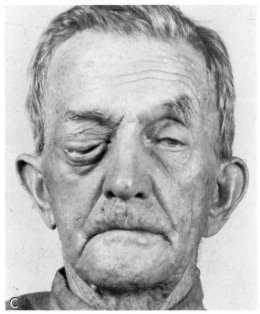

FIGURE 28-27. Neurofibroma of the upper and lower eyelids, severe type. *A, B,* Preoperative appearance. Note the full-thickness enlargement of the involved eyelids. *C,* Three months after fractional full-thickness resection of the involved eyelids.

preserved above the eyelashes to avoid their destruction. The defect is repaired with a split-thickness skin graft.

The tarsus and conjunctiva. When the tarsal plate is enlarged and hypertrophic, reduction of its mass is beneficial. A transverse excision of tarsus and conjunctiva between the lid margin and the insertions of the levator palpebrae muscle will reduce excess in the vertical dimension, and a vertical wedge resection is used to reduce excessive width. Following partial resection, the tarsus is reapproximated with a continuous running suture of No. 36 stainless steel wire or other type of nonabsorbable suture. Both ends of the wire are left long to facilitate its later removal. The loose

areolar tissue superficial to the tarsus is approximated with a layer of interrupted 5-0 plain catgut sutures, and skin closure is completed either by direct closure with a running 6-0 black silk suture or by skin grafting.

Ptosis. A degree of ptosis is invariably present in all severe cases of neurofibromatosis of the upper eyelid. The deformity may result from simple hypertrophy of the lid or weakness of the overstretched levator palpebrae aponeurosis. If ptosis persists after a satisfactory reduction in size of the involved lid, it should be corrected.

When the levator palpebrae muscle is functional and does not appear to be thin and atrophic, shortening the aponeurosis will achieve the desired effect. If there is no detectable levator function, the suspension technique is employed. Both of these techniques are described later in this chapter (see Ptosis of the Upper Eyelid).

COMPLICATIONS

Necrosis of the skin. This occurs when excessive thinning of the skin is performed during excision of the main bulk of the subcutaneous tumor. It can be avoided if the skin is excised and the defect is covered with a skin graft.

Lack of symmetry. If the involvement of the eyelid is extensive, symmetry with the unaffected eyelid may not be obtainable, even after maximal removal of the bulk of the tumor and restoration of the levator muscle function by shortening the aponeurosis or by suspension by a fascia lata graft.

Dermoid Cyst. The dermoid cyst is a congenital cystic tumor composed of at least 90 per cent dermal elements. The dermoid cyst is to be distinguished from the teratoma, which contains elements of all three germ layers and less than 90 per cent dermal elements. Dermoid cysts are common lesions in the region of the orbit. The most common site is above the lateral third of the eyebrow. Rarely does a dermoid cyst occur within the orbit or on the lower eyelid.

A typical dermoid cyst appears during the first year of life as a lump above the eyebrow. The cyst is smooth and firm and often seems firmly adherent to the underlying bone. It is occasionally tender but rarely painful. The overlying skin is unaffected and nonadherent, and sinus tracts are rare. The tumor is situated under the muscle and periosteum, and a craterlike depression is often produced on the surface of the underlying bone. Growth is slow, and function of the eyelid is unaffected.

In this region the dermoid cyst develops along the line of embryonic fusion of the nasooptic groove, from infolding of the ectoderm during embryonic development. Such cysts are simple in structure. The wall is relatively thick and is lined by squamous epithelium resembling skin with hair follicles and sweat and sebaceous glands. The content is a greasy, cheesy material which is often mixed with hair. Rarely, a mesodermic structure such as bone or cartilage is found.

TREATMENT. Complete surgical removal is the only effective treatment for a dermoid cyst. The cyst is exposed through a muscle-splitting incision and removed in toto, preferably intact. When the cyst is adherent to the bone, the overlying periosteum is removed with the tumor. If cordlike extensions are present, as the aftermath of a previous rupture of the cyst, they should also be removed. Careful and thorough hemostasis is important to avoid ecchymosis of the eyelid. Closure is accomplished by meticulous layer approximation using 5–0 plain catgut for subcutaneous sutures and 6–0 silk sutures for the skin.

COMPLICATIONS

Recurrence. This happens when part of the cyst wall is left behind. It is therefore important not to rupture the cyst during dissection, so that complete removal can be ensured. Local scarring, a sequel to previous infection, may trap islands of epithelial cells and cause recurrence. Such scarred areas, therefore, must be completely excised.

Injury to the facial nerve. The temporal branch of the facial nerve courses upward laterally to the eyebrow to supply the frontalis muscle. A dermoid cyst is most often situated underneath the lateral portion of the eyebrow. During dissection one must be careful not to injure the nerve. This can be extremely difficult if there is extensive scarring from previous infection.

Teratoma. This is the second type of congenital cyst encountered in the eyelid region, though it is seen much more rarely than those discussed above. The teratoma is thought to originate in a developing blastomere, some cells of which become separated or displaced and, after a dormant period, become activated and evolve into a teratoma. The structure is complex. Its wall is thick and characteristically contains elements derived from all three germinal layers. The teratoma may contain well-developed structures, such as skin, hair, nails, and teeth, as well as brain, glandular tissue, and a variety of other tissues. Unlike the dermoid cyst, the teratoma may be malignant in character.

TREATMENT. Complete excision is the only method of cure. The involved bone surrounding the tumor must be removed. If the defect is large enough to produce deformity, immediate reconstruction with a bone graft should be performed, assuming the lesion is benign.

ACQUIRED BENIGN LESIONS

Most of the benign tumors of the eyelid in adults are of epithelial origin from the skin or its appendages. Kwitko, Boniuk, and Zimmerman (1963), in reviewing 1176 eyelid lesions, found 50 per cent of them to be benign in nature.

Keratoacanthoma. This is a well-localized, elevated, hemispherical, rapidly growing tumor, with a central keratin crater. The name was first introduced by Helsham and Buchanan in 1950. There are three clinical varieties: (1) the verrugoma type, covered by a firmly attached scale; (2) the molluscum sebaceum type, with a central crater containing soft, greasy, bony material; and (3) the nodular-vegetating type, with a small, lobulated surface. Histologically the lesion has a conical configuration with a central, keratin-filled crater lined by epithelium. Numerous papillary projections extend into the crater from the epithelium. The entire lesion extends into the dermis with an inflammatory infiltration at its base. Although virus particles have been found in 40 to 60 per cent of tumor cells, attempts to culture the virus have been unsuccessful.

Boniuk and Zimmerman (1967), in reviewing 44 cases of keratoacanthoma of the eyelid, found that half were of less than one month's duration, and none had been present more than four months. The size varies from 0.4 to 1.0 cm in diameter. Most keratoacanthomas present no symptoms, though occasionally the lesion may be itchy, or even painful.

TREATMENT. Although spontaneous recession of the lesion has been reported, surgical excision is still the treatment of choice. In light of its rapid growth and the difficulty of differential diagnosis from squamous cell epithelium, watchful waiting is seldom justified.

The lesion should be excised through a transverse incision, and closure can be achieved with or without a skin graft. Recurrence is rare.

Inverted Follicular Keratosis. Boniuk and Zimmerman (1963) described this lesion of the eyelid as one often confused with squamous cell epithelioma. The lesion usually appears as a warty or verrucous growth. Sometimes it may be nodular or papillary. Some lesions are heavily pigmented. About 40 per cent appear at the lid margin. Most of them are less than 0.5 cm in diameter. Occasionally the lesion causes itching or burning or may ooze blood. On microscopic examination, the tumor lies in the junctional areas between epidermis and dermis and is composed of cells simulating the basal layer of epidermis or squamoid cells arranged concentrically in small nests, with keratin formation in the center of the nests. Some of the lesions have an inverted, cup-shaped appearance, with the normal adjacent epidermis

extending upward to partially cover the side of the tumor mass.

Melanotic Freckle. A lesion situated on the eyelid and conjunctiva was first described by Hutchinson in 1894. It often starts as a small brown or black flat spot on the skin of the eyelid of a middle-aged adult. It gradually and irregularly enlarges in size and increases in pigmentation. The course is uneven, waxing and waning with time. About 20 to 30 per cent of these freckles become malignant. The lesion is differentiated from the junctional nevus, which usually appears before adolescence, has a stable course, and rarely becomes malignant. The lesion is also discussed in Chapter 65.

Histologically, it is composed of melanocytes situated in the basal layer of the epidermis. Malignant changes are characterized by thickening and elevation of a segment of the lesion. It may ulcerate or bleed. Microscopically, the melanocytes invade the dermis. Beneath the tumor, there is chronic inflammatory cell accumulation.

TREATMENT. Because of the high incidence of malignant change, melanotic freckles should be excised. Local wide excision is adequate. No regional node dissection is indicated when there is no clinical involvement.

Pyogenic Granuloma. This lesion was first described in 1897 by Poncept and Dor. It is bluish red or brownish red, has a smooth surface, and is pedunculated or mushroom-shaped. It varies in size from a pinhead to a cherry, bleeds easily, and grows rapidly. The lower eyelid and canthal region are most often involved. It is claimed to be viral in origin and shows no predilection as to age or sex. Recurrence after excision sometimes occurs.

Inclusion Cyst. There is a great variety of cysts which occur in the eyelid. The dermoid cyst has been previously described. There is also the common type of sebaceous cyst originating from eyelid skin. Opening into the eyelid margin, there are three types of glands. The glands of Moll, modified apocrine sweat glands, open into the eyelash follicles or separately between the lashes. Cysts from these glands are skin-colored or pinkish and semi-translucent. They arise from the lid margin and can grow as large as 1 cm in diameter. The glands of Zeis are small sebaceous glands connected with the lash follicle. Cysts of this origin are also marginally situated. The meibomian glands are situated on the orbital side of the lid margin. Cysts of this origin protrude toward the orbit, causing early eye irritation. Protrusion and irritation are also characteristic of cysts of the glands of Krause and Wolfring, two sets of accessory lacrimal glands located in the subconjunctival connective tissue of the eyelids.

Xanthoma. The eyelid is the commonest site of cutaneous xanthomas. They usually occur in older women and are slow growing and often multiple. Eyelid xanthomas are symmetrical, soft, yellow-brown, slightly elevated, and velvety. They occur in the upper and lower eyelids near the inner canthus and are symptomless. Composed of foam cells containing lipid and found in the upper dermis, they are associated with hyperlipemia and hypercholesterolemia in approximately 35 per cent of the cases. Surgical removal is performed for esthetic reasons.

Trichoepithelioma. The lesions are benign, nonulcerative, and frequently multiple. They appear as small, slightly elevated, flat, pale or translucent, circular or slightly irregular, hard tumors with a few projecting hairs of a very fine texture. Microscopically, they are characterized by many immature hair follicles, some containing hair. Excision is the method of choice.

Syringomas or Clear Cell Hidradenoma. This is a benign tumor developed from a sweat gland or its ducts. The areas most frequently affected are the eyelid and chest wall. They are round, small, multiple, firm, and slightly raised lesions, yellowish or brownish red in color and waxy in appearance. As a syringoma grows, the center becomes cystic or puckered after the rupture of the cyst. They occur in women at puberty and are found most often bilaterally in the lower eyelids. Microscopically, the tumors retain the structure of typical sweat glands. When dilatation of ducts occurs, hypoplasia of the epithelial lining is dominant. Malignant transformation of this tumor is rare, but when it occurs, the tumor is locally invasive and may give rise to distant metastases to bone or lymph nodes.

Malignant Tumors of the Eyelids

Most malignant lesions of the eyelid are epithelial in origin. They are superficial, slow-growing, and easily diagnosed. Approximately 90 per cent of all skin cancers are located in the region of the head and neck. The incidence of epithelioma of the eyelid is estimated by various authorities to be from 2.5 to 16.8 per cent of all skin cancers. In a review of 853 skin cancers, Macomber, Wang, and Sullivan (1959) found the incidence of eyelid involvement to be 9.4 per cent.

There is no significant difference in the incidence between sexes. The frequency of involvement increases with the age of the patient, with the highest incidence occurring in sixth and seventh decades (Holmström, Bartholdson and Johanson, 1975). The lower eyelid and the medial canthus are the regions most commonly involved. This distribution has been similarly reported by Birge (1938), Driver and Cole (1939), Stetson and Schultz (1949), Hunt (1947), del Regato (1949), Zimmerman (1962), and Smith (1975). It is quite possible that the wearing of improperly fitted eyeglasses, producing constant pressure and irritation on the medial canthus, may be a significant extrinsic factor in the etiology of medial canthus lesions, and irritation by chronic eye discharges on the lower eyelid may be reponsible for the frequency of lesions there. Various authors have also implicated sunlight, chemical irritation, old scars, and precursory keratosis as etiologic factors.

Pathology. The basal cell epithelioma is the most common malignant lesion of the eyelid, and the squamous cell epithelioma ranks next. The ratio of basal cell to squamous cell epithelioma varies from 4.4:1 as reported by Birge (1938) to 38.6:1 as reported by Kwitko, Boniuk, and Zimmerman (1963). Holmström, Bartholdson and Johanson (1975) reported an incidence of basal cell carcinoma of nearly 90 per cent in the Swedish study. Malignant melanoma of the skin of the eyelid is uncommon (less than 1 per cent of all the malignant lesions), and melanomas originating from the palpebral conjunctiva are also extremely rare.

The typical *basal cell epithelioma* appears first as a small, firm, waxy nodule with a few telangiectatic vessels on its surface. The nodule slowly increases in size and undergoes central ulceration. At this stage, it appears as a slowly progressive ulcer surrounded by a pearly, firm, rolled border. Occasionally it is pigmented. At other times it may be raised and cystic in appearance.

A basal cell epithelioma is a localized neoplasm which invades tissue by direct extension. Regional metastasis is extremely rare. In the eyelids it may invade the tarsal plate and conjunctiva. In advanced cases, local permeation along the adjacent lymphatics may cause paramarginal subcutaneous extension or intraorbital involvement when the affected lymphatics reach the bulbar conjunctiva or penetrate the orbital fascia. Birge (1938) reported the incidence of bulbar involvement to be 25.9 per cent, while in the authors' series of 42 cases (Macomber, Wang, and Gottlieb, 1954), 7 per cent had intraorbital extension. When the primary lesion is on the medial canthus, it tends to extend over the side of the nose rather than to the tarsal plate of the eyelid (Hollander and Krugh, 1944). Occasionally the lacrimal duct and ethmoid sac are involved (Stetson and Schulz, 1949).

Lacassagne (1933) pointed out that eyelid skin has an extremely thin epidermis. It was his opinion that outside irritations such as sunlight, pressure, or trauma may easily disturb the basal cell layer through this thin epidermis and favor the development of a lesion. Morax (1926) was of the opinion that a basal cell epithelioma of the eyelid arises primarily from the meibomian sebaceous glands and more rarely from the glands of Zeis or sweat gland of Moll. Traube (1954), however, held that basal cell lesions originated chiefly from the lid skin near its margin and only rarely from the accessory glands.

Basal cell epitheliomas or adenocarcinomas originating in the meibomian glands appear as ulcerated nodules near the lid margin. Ginsberg (1965) collected 142 cases reported in the literature up to 1963. According to him these tumors represent 1 per cent of eyelid cancer. They are more common in the upper than the lower lid. About 17 per cent of the adenocarcinomas showed regional metastasis. Microscopically, one observes definite lobular formation with occasional groups of typical sebaceous cells. The tumor is composed of two types of cells. The cells in the central portion are vacuolated, while those at the periphery are elongated, with deeply eosinophilic cytoplasm, arranged perpendicularly to the septa. Basal cell epitheliomas originating in the glands of Moll are usually found on the lid margin near the inner canthus of the lower eyelid. A cyst of the gland is the usual precursor. Microscopically, there is no connection between the tumor cells and the surface epithelium or the adnexal structures near it.

The *squamous cell epithelioma* is characterized as a firm, raised, ulcerated skin lesion. It grows more rapidly and infiltrates neighboring structures earlier than a basal cell epithelioma. Not infrequently, it metastasizes to the regional lymph nodes. The upper and outer lid lesions tend to metastasize to preauricular nodes (Stetson and Schulz, 1949), whereas lesions of the lower eyelid and inner canthus spread to cervical nodes (Hardin and Robinson, 1951). Ackerman and del Regato (1947) estimated that not more than 5 per cent of squamous cell epitheliomas spread to the regional lymph nodes.

Malignant melanoma of the eyelid may derive from a preexisting nevus or melanotic freckle. Reese (1953) stated that junctional activity is present in 90 per cent of the nevi of the eyelid skin and lid margin. Thus nevi at locations subject to chronic irritation, such as the caruncle, margin of the eyelids, and semilunar folds, are more predisposed to malignant change. Such malignant change from a nevus is relatively rare, as compared with that from melanotic freckles (20 to 30 per cent).

Malignant melanomas of the conjunctiva are rare. They are most commonly seen in the fifth, sixth, and seventh decades. They are usually oval and polypoid when appearing at the fornix or the caruncle, and flat when in the scleral triangle near the limbus. Their surface is either smooth or rough with rich vascularity; their color is frequently dark brown. Growth can be slow or rapid. Metastasis to distant organs is unfortunately characteristic of this disease.

The above malignant skin lesions are also discussed in Chapter 65.

Treatment

SURGERY VERSUS IRRADIATION. The primary aim of treatment is complete extirpation of the neoplasm in the shortest possible time, with the least possible structural deformity and functional impairment of the eyelids.

In the selection of a form of therapy for the early lesion, the physician may be guided by the availability of experienced radiotherapists, since satisfactory results have been reported by both qualified surgeons and radiotherapists. The authors favor surgical excision for the following reasons:

1. Side effects such as cataracts, extensive and deforming cicatrization of the eyelid, persistent conjunctivitis, and stenosis of the tear ducts are still of sufficiently high incidence to present a problem after a curative dose of radiation.

2. If irradiation is performed without benefit of biopsy, the physician is deprived of microscopic confirmation of a clinical diagnosis. A radioresistant lesion may therefore be treated for extended periods of time without effect, fol-

lowing which permanent cure may be accomplished only with considerable difficulty or may be completely impossible.

3. Advanced lesions are not satisfactorily controlled by irradiation if they have already invaded deep structures, such as the orbit or facial bones.

4. Granted a satisfactory response to radiation therapy checked by gross examination of the treated area, there is still no confirmation of complete destruction of the lesion. A sectional examination of the surgical specimen, on the other hand, provides microscopic evidence of the completeness of the surgical excision and provides the soundest basis for accurate prognosis.

5. When a previously irradiated lesion shows a recurrence, the lesion is invariably radioresistant and requires surgery. Surgical excision of such a lesion requires eradication not only of the recurrent lesion but also of the entire irradiated area, transforming what originally might have been a simple reconstructive problem into one of major complexity.

6. In conclusion, roentgen irradiation of tumors tends to cause epidermization of the lid margin and the adjacent palpebral conjunctiva, which in turn causes corneal irritation, an intolerable complication for the patient. A conjunctival or mucosal graft, taken from the oral mucosa, is required to replace the troublesome area of epidermization. Depigmentation, scarring, and telangiectasis are additional disfiguring sequelae of X-ray therapy. More serious complications such as cataract, persistent conjunctivitis, and stenosis of the lacrimal puncta are less frequent because the ocular globe is adequately shielded but are observed when high doses of X-irradiation are administered. The present availability of many varied reconstructive procedures makes possible a radical, extensive excision, rarely followed by severe deformity or impaired function, even in advanced cases.

As Holmström, Bartholdson and Johanson (1975) have remarked, eyelid cancer provides two hazards: loss of vision and loss of life. Whether treated by irradiation or surgery, the cure rate has been reported to exceed 90 per cent (Driver and Cole, 1939; Stetson and Schulz, 1949). The goal of permanent eradication of the cancer and the preservation of eyelid function without ancillary complications can best be attained by surgery (Reeh, 1963; Wang, Macomber and Elliott, 1964; Huffstadt and Heybroek, 1966; Wynn-Williams, 1967; Beare, 1973).

RECONSTRUCTION OF DEFECTS OF THE EYELIDS

As in other parts of the body, defects either are congenital in origin or result from trauma or from the resection of lid tissue for the eradication of a tumor, benign or malignant. The principles of eyelid reconstruction apply to all defects irrespective of their etiology.

Development of Reconstructive Surgery of the Eyelids. Von Graefe in 1818 constructed a lower lid with a cheek flap. His method was improved upon by Fricke (1829), who introduced a procedure for both upper and lower lid reconstruction using zygomatic and temporal flaps. The use of an arm flap to reconstruct the eyelid was a common practice among the surgeons of the nineteenth century.

Such large flaps, though generally successful, had several disadvantages: (1) the reconstructive procedures frequently caused considerable discomfort to the patient; (2) the skin transplanted was frequently a poor match for the adjacent skin in color, texture, and thickness; (3) scars, some extremely deforming in themselves, were produced at the donor site; (4) lid function was frequently poor because the reconstructed lid was thick and nonpliable.

Following Reverdin's report (1869) introducing the concept of the skin graft, many attempts were made by the surgeons of the period to utilize the new technique in eyelid reconstruction. Lawson (1871) is credited with the first successful skin graft in a case of ectropion in 1870. In the same year, Le Fort (1872) in France and Wolfe (1876) in England succeeded in transplanting full-thickness skin grafts. It was not until the principles of grafting full-thickness skin were well understood and widely employed that the percentage of good results with skin grafts exceeded those obtained with flaps.

With these early successes in eyelid reconstruction came an awareness of the need for a conjunctival lining of the new lid. Teale in 1860 reported the correction of a symblepharon by using a conjunctival flap. In 1884 Bock used mucous membrane as a graft for the repair and replacement of a conjunctival defect. Stellwag (1889) reported the use of vaginal mucosa for such a purpose.

The poor cosmetic results with skin from various donor areas, such as the arm and leg, led Gradenigo in 1904 to graft eyelid skin for an eyelid defect. He was the first to introduce one of the principles of eyelid reconstruction: the use of eyelid tissue to replace eyelid defects. Eyelid skin in the form of both flaps and grafts was used by him as well as other surgeons with success.

Landolt in 1881 was the first to employ the tarsoconjunctival flap. This concept was further expanded and developed by Cirincione in 1901. In 1912 Ischreyt reversed the procedure and reconstructed an upper lid defect in a similar manner. This marked the beginning of full-thickness eyelid reconstruction.

Esser (1919) first reported a full-thickness rotation flap from the lower eyelid to repair a defect of the upper eyelid. Cutler and Beard (1955) used a bridge full-thickness flap from the lower eyelid advancing upward for the same purpose. In addition to the use of skin and mucosal grafts for eyelid reconstruction, de Blaskovics (1918) reported the first free tarsal graft; Yonens, Westphal, Barfield, and Yonens (1967) reported composite full-thickness lower eyelid grafts for upper eyelid reconstruction.

The contributions of such surgeons as Dupuy-Dutemps (1927), Wheeler (1939), and Hughes (1943) and the more recent contributions of Mustardé and Smith, to mention only a few, have served to refine the technique of eyelid reconstruction to the high point of effectiveness that it has now reached.

Exenteration of the orbit was first described in 1583 by Bartisch. The resulting cavity was left uncovered and allowed to granulate and heal over slowly by peripheral epithelization. The contracting scar resulted in severe deformity and often great discomfort. Davis in 1919 mentioned the application of a Thiersch graft for the immediate coverage of the orbital cavity but expressed dissatisfaction with the technique. Wheeler in 1922 pointed out the feasibility of applying an immediate skin graft directly over bone, muscle, tendon, fascia, or periosteum without waiting for granulation tissue to appear in the orbital cavity. This principle continues to be practiced by most surgeons today, when indicated.

The lateral advancement of an island flap, described by Kazanjian in 1949 (Fig. 28–28), was probably one of the first island flaps with a subcutaneous pedicle used for eyelid reconstruction in our era.

In more extensive defects, the tarsoconjunctival flap, first described by Landolt (1881), modified by Köllner (1911) (see Fig. 28–39) and by Hughes (1937), and further modified and utilized in a variety of ways, has been popular. It is interesting to note that Köllner spared the lower portion of the tarsus, thus preventing entropion, trichiasis, and up-

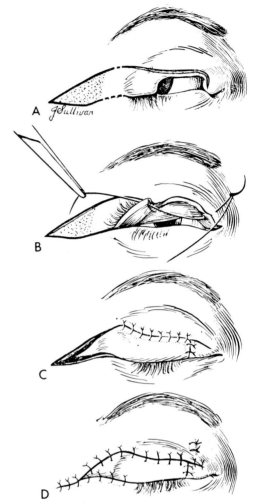

FIGURE 28–28. Full-thickness loss of eyelid tissue. Kazanjian's (1949) repair by island flap. *A,* Incision of flap, permitting advancement of the lateral portion of the upper lid. *B,* The edges of the defect are approximated by sutures. *C,* Lid reconstructed after advancement of the lateral portion. *D,* Operation completed.

ward bowing of the upper lid, a complication of the procedure advocated by Landolt and Hughes and subsequently modified to avoid such complications.

A radical departure has been the development of the Mustardé technique (1959) utilizing a composite chondromucosal graft from the nasal septum and a rotation flap from the cheek. There are thus two schools of thought in direct opposition. Each of these techniques and some of their applications are now described.

Eyelid Reconstruction

JOHN C. MUSTARDÉ, F.R.C.S.

Repair of a Defect by a Skin Graft. Resection of tumors of the eyelids involves resection of an adequate amount of normal tissue so as to avoid the possibility of local recurrence. The amount of normal tissue to be resected around the apparent limit of the tumor will vary from 3 mm in a cystic basal cell tumor to 5 or 6 mm around a sclerosing basal cell lesion or a squamous cell epithelioma. Resection in depth need not be as extensive as the lateral resection, because the constantly moving layer of orbicularis muscle tends to prevent deep spread of the tumor until fairly late in the course of the disease. It therefore follows that, provided there is sufficient normal skin between the clinical limits of the tumor and the lash line, it will usually be possible to excise the tumor along with some or all of the underlying orbicularis muscle and cover the defect by means of a skin graft. A full-thickness skin graft, taken from the sulcus behind the ear, will obviate any likelihood of contraction and subsequent deformity of the lid. In addition, the postauricular skin provides an excellent color and texture match in the lower lid and in the region of the medial or lateral canthus. It is not suitable in the upper lid, where its thickness may cause some interference with the free movement of the lid.

Tumors which have penetrated deeper than the orbicularis muscle but are not yet extending closer to the lid margin than the distance given above may still be resected adequately, at least in the lower lid and at the canthus, unless there is some indication that the tumor has invaded close to the conjunctival layer. Such defects can be filled by a local flap from the skin of the nose, the cheek, or if necessary the forehead. Small, deep lesions at the medial canthus can readily be resurfaced by a V-Y glabellar flap, but more extensive lesions may require a two-stage transfer of midline forehead skin.

Full-Thickness Defects. In patients in whom the tumor extends closer to the lid margin than the limits given above, resection in the manner described must always leave a possibility of local recurrence, and in such instances the safest procedure is to perform a full-thickness resection of all layers of the eyelid, including the lid margin and the conjunctiva in the affected zone. Such a drastic approach when dealing with eyelid tumors may seem to be extending the surgical resection unnecessarily far, but in a personal series of 162 lid tumors treated by full-thickness lid resection, there has not been a single recurrence.

The problem of reconstructing the defect in an eyelid after resection of a tumor must take into account the fact that the eyelid requires, as a minimum, a mucus-secreting layer for lining and a skin layer to form a cover. Apart from this, however, there are basic differences between the requirements for a reconstructed lower lid and for a reconstructed upper lid. These stem mainly from the effects of gravity and age on the eyelid tissues and from the fact that the reconstructed lower eyelid will no longer have the support of a normal orbicularis muscle to impart an uplifting sling action. It is well known that, even in a normal eyelid, once the orbicularis muscle action has been interfered with, the tissues of the eyelid will gradually stretch, and this includes the lid margin and the tarsal plate. The same stretching and sagging process will take place in a reconstructed lower lid over the course of years, and as many of these patients are in the later decades of life, the stretching process may happen quite rapidly after surgery — within a year or 18 months in some cases.

A permanent means of support for the reconstructed part of the lower lid must be provided in all except minor repairs, and a suitable material must be introduced which will not in itself sag in the process of time and lose its supportive action. This rules out the tarsal plate from the upper lid, auricular cartilage, and fascia lata, because, being basically connective tissue structures, they will gradually stretch with time and aging. The most satisfactory material is true cartilage, and although rib cartilage could be used, it has a tendency to curl if cut in thin slices and in any event necessitates a comparatively major procedure for the removal of suitable costal cartilage. Cartilage from the nasal septum is ideal for the procedure and has the considerable additional merit of having a mucosal surface attached to it, so that a composite graft of mucosa and cartilage can be used to provide not only the supportive skeleton of the new part of the lid but also a secreting mucous membrane lining.

Paufique and Tessier (1962) advocated a composite graft consisting of the lateral cartilage of the nose and underlying nasal mucoperichondrium over the septal composite graft favored by Mustardé. They did not describe possible complications, such as obstruction of the nasal airway, resulting from this procedure.

If the alternative type of reconstruction is used, i.e., providing a flap of *skin* lined with a composite graft of cartilage and mucosa, almost all of the above defects are obviated.

Lower Lid Reconstruction

Of the two basic layers of a reconstructed eyelid, the skin layer and the lining layer, one can be a graft, but one must of necessity be a flap with a continuously intact blood supply. If a flap is used for the *lining* layer, this means bringing down conjunctiva, possibly with some of the tarsal plate in its lower part, from the upper fornix and swinging it across over the cornea to form the lining of the reconstructed portion.

There are difficulties in utilizing such a conjunctival flap, with or without a portion of the tarsal plate attached to it, because the amount of conjunctiva and tarsus available for anything except a minor reconstructive procedure of the lower lid will be insufficient to line the lower lid and at the same time continue to provide adequate lining for the upper fornix and the posterior surface of the upper lid. As a result, there is always the risk that the upper lid will have a tendency toward entropion and

even trichiasis, the lashes rubbing on the cornea.

Moreover, the tarsal plate which has been brought down with the conjunctival flap will lie toward the fornix of the lower lid, and the margin, which is that part requiring the stiffening effect of a skeleton, will remain comparatively unsupported. Finally, in all except marginal lower lid reconstructions, the transposed tarsal plate, although perhaps providing an apparent supportive skeletal action at the time of surgery, will certainly stretch with the course of time, and the lid margin will eventually sag.

The technique is illustrated in Figure 28–29. The area of excision and the rotation flap are shown in *A*. The flap, having been raised, is sutured to the tissues near the lateral canthus (*B*); a portion of the flap will serve as the skin of the lower lid. A measured septal composite graft (g) of cartilage and mucosa (chondromucosal graft) is sutured to the edges of the defect (*C*); the portion of the rotation flap which will serve as the skin layer is indicated by the two

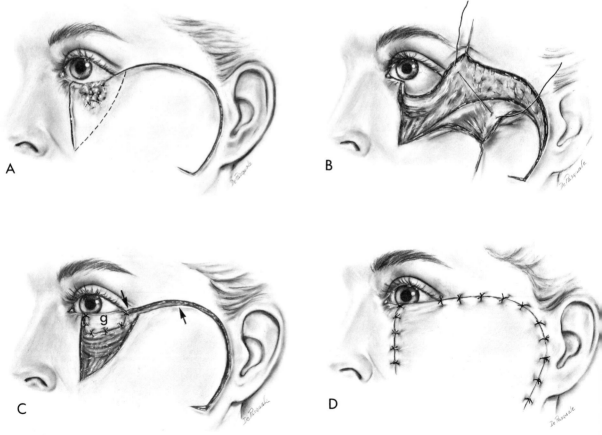

FIGURE 28–29. Lower eyelid reconstruction. *A*, The area of excision and the rotation flap are outlined. *B*, The flap is raised, rotated, and sutured to the tissues near the lateral canthus. *C*, A measured septal composite graft (g) of cartilage and attached mucous membrane is sutured to the edges of the defect. *D*, The rotation flap is in position. The operation is completed (Mustardé).

arrows. The skin flap has been rotated, and the operation is completed (*D*). In moderate sized defects of the lower lid, a lateral advancement flap (Fig. 28–30, *A*) or a lateral advancement flap facilitated by a relaxing incision to release tension may be employed (Fig. 28–30, *B, C*).

In V-shaped defects of moderate size Mc-Gregor (1973) suggested adding a Z-plasty to the lateral end of the flap (Fig. 28–31). When reconstructing a lower eyelid defect, he also suggested that the flap be designed by means of an incision continuing the upward curve of the lower lid margin as far as the temporal hairline (Figs. 28–31 and 28–32). In this technique for the repair of V-shaped defects — which could also readily be repaired by the Cutler-Beard technique (1955) (see Fig. 28–42) — the tarsus is advanced, and additional chondromucosal septal graft is provided.

Marginal Defects. Where excision of the lesion results in a defect of the marginal zone

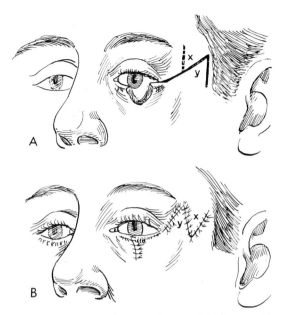

FIGURE 28–31. The upward curve of the flap provides adequate vertical length and avoids dragging down of the reconstructed eyelid; the Z-plasty releases excessive tension. (After McGregor.)

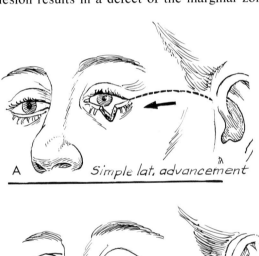

A *Simple lat. advancement*

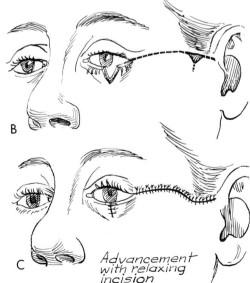

C *Advancement with relaxing incision*

FIGURE 28–30. *A*, Repair by a lateral advancement flap. *B, C*, Advancement facilitated by a relaxing incision. (After McGregor.)

only, the skin flap of which the reconstructed portion of the lid is to be built can be brought down as a bipedicle flap from the area of redundant skin above the upper lid supratarsal fold (Fig. 28–33, *A*). The bipedicle (Tripier) flap should be lifted, along with the underlying orbicularis muscle, in order to ensure an adequate blood supply to the skin (Fig. 28–33, *B*), and it should be lined by a composite nasal graft of cartilage and mucosa (Fig. 28–33, *C, D*). It may be felt that, to repair such a shallow defect, it is unnecessary to include the cartilaginous skeletal element, but a mucosal graft alone will tend to contract to some extent and will pull the skin layer backward, so that there is risk of the epithelium, and possibly even small hairs, rubbing on the cornea. The cartilage incorporated in the flap will also ensure that the maximum height of the reconstructed margin will be maintained permanently (Fig. 28–33, *E*). The two pedicles are divided after two weeks and returned to the upper lid (Fig. 28–33, *F*). It is considered unnecessary, and indeed unwise, to insert a layer of lashes into a reconstructed lid because of the risk of distortion of the hairs and possible trichiasis at a later date. From a purely cosmetic point of view, an intact upper lash line will disguise the lack of lashes in the reconstructed lower lid (Fig. 28–33, *F, G*).

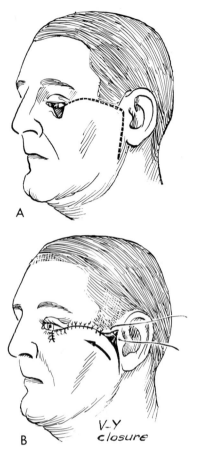

A

B

V-Y closure

FIGURE 28–32. McGregor's incision continues the upward curve of the lower eyelid margin into the temporal area to the hairline, similar to Dieffenbach's technique.

Reconstruction of Defects Other than Marginal. For the reconstruction of lid defects in which the loss of tissue extends in a vertical direction beyond 4 or 5 mm, a more adequate source of skin is to be found by advancing the peripheral orbital tissue lateral to the lateral canthus (Smith and Cherubini, 1970) (see Fig. 28–35) . This can be brought in most readily by raising the cheek skin, along with this thin orbital skin, as a flap and transferring it medially in order to provide a skin layer on which to build up a new sector of the lower lid. Whether the cheek skin is rotated in the manner of an Imre flap, or whether it is allowed to slide medially by a modified Dieffenbach technique, which depends on closing the secondary preauricular defect by a V-Y procedure or a Z-plasty along the horizontal line, will depend on the individual preference and experience of the surgeon (see Fig. 28–32). The author's own preference is for a rotation flap utilizing a backcut when a large rotation is

required to reconstruct an extensive defect (Figs. 28–34, 28–35).

Small defects of up to a quarter of a lid can be closed by direct apposition of the cut edges. A three-layer type of closure which allows the tarsal plate to be accurately splinted by means of a pull-out suture will ensure good healing with a minimum of scar on the skin surface and without any notching of the lid margin (see Fig. 28–23).

When a defect slightly larger than a quarter of the lid length is being reconstructed, a division of the lower crus of the lateral canthal tendon (cantholysis) will permit the defect to be closed in the manner described above without tension on the wound (see Fig. 28–24). For the closure of defects beyond one-third of the lid length, additional tissue must be brought in from the lateral side, and the degree of rotation and transposition of the cheek flap must be judged in accordance with the amount of tissue which is required for the new lid sector (see Figs. 28–34 and 28–35). When the reconstructed sector of the lid is not more than a quarter of the lid length, it may be lined by conjunctiva brought up from the lower fornix, but in more extensive reconstructions, the new lid sector should be lined with a composite graft of nasal septal cartilage and mucosa. If this is not done, there may be a gradual sinking down in the course of time of the reconstructed margin of the lower lid.

It should be noted that the septal cartilage must be thinned to about 1.5 mm in thickness to avoid producing an excessively bulky lower lid. The thinning of the cartilage has an important secondary function in that it will permit the cartilage to curl in the direction of the perichondrium, and thus the composite graft will become curved concavely to fit snugly onto the contour of the eye.

On rare occasions the cheek skin may not be available, and in such a case the skin of the forehead may have to be utilized. Such a skin flap may be brought down from the midline of the forehead; this is preferable to lifting the flap from the region above the eyebrow, as the latter procedure tends to raise the eyebrow unnaturally. Forehead flap skin is rather thick, however, and, in addition, will require a two-stage procedure to bring it down to reconstruct the lower lid.

Reconstruction of the Upper Lid

The problems to be faced in the reconstruction of the upper lid are quite different from those

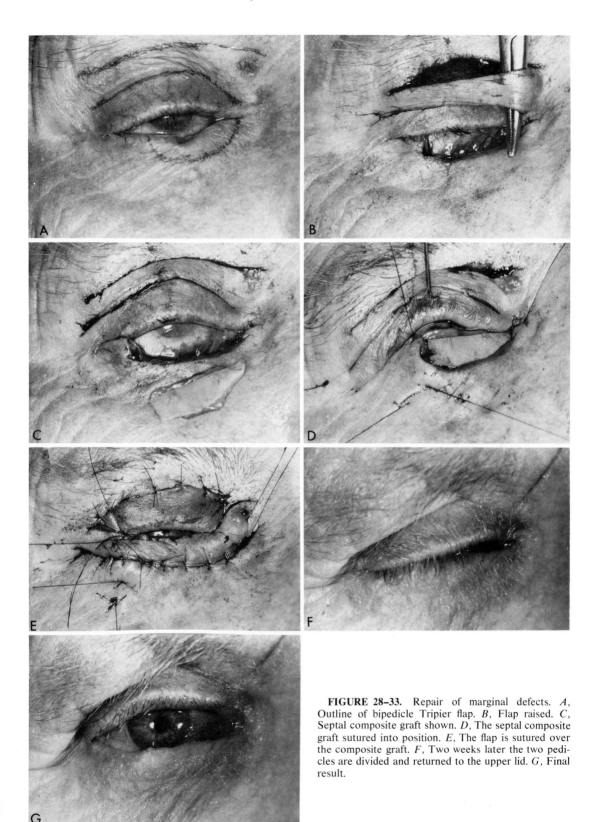

FIGURE 28–33. Repair of marginal defects. *A*, Outline of bipedicle Tripier flap. *B*, Flap raised. *C*, Septal composite graft shown. *D*, The septal composite graft sutured into position. *E*, The flap is sutured over the composite graft. *F*, Two weeks later the two pedicles are divided and returned to the upper lid. *G*, Final result.

which one encounters in the reconstruction of the lower lid. Whereas in the lower lid one seeks to fashion a structure which will, by its inherent rigidity, withstand the effects of gravity and time, in the upper lid gravity and time are, if anything, working on the side of the surgeon. What is required is a structure with a basic skin covering and mucus-secreting lining, yet one which will be sufficiently flexible to alter its shape from convex on looking downward to concave on looking upward; at the same time, however, it must cling closely to the contour of the eyeball and have a reasonably firm margin.

No tissue or combination of tissues, other than another eyelid, can reproduce an upper lid which can in any way satisfy all of these specifications; it is well worth sacrificing a part of the lower lid in order to be certain of an adequately functioning upper lid. This is the basis of the Abbé type of full-thickness flap, which has been adapted from Esser's (1940) original transposition of an upper lid flap in order to reconstruct defects in the lower lid.

Marginal Defects.   Marginal defects in the upper lid may be treated in the same way as

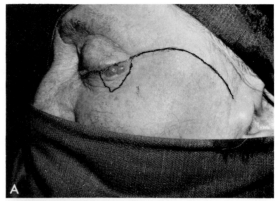
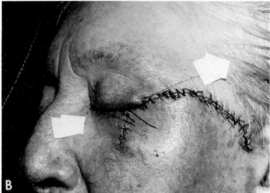

FIGURE 28–35.   Reconstruction of a lower lid defect. *A,* Outline of the subtotal excision of the lower eyelid. Note the variation in the outline of the rotation flap from Figure 28–34, *A. B,* Result obtained according to the technique illustrated in Figure 28–29.

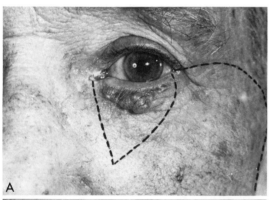
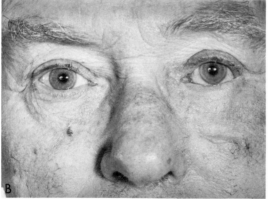

FIGURE 28–34.   Reconstruction of a lower lid defect. *A,* Outline of the area of excision and rotation flap. *B,* Operation completed according to the technique illustrated in Figure 28–29.

are marginal defects in the lower lid by using a bipedicle Tripier flap from the loose peripheral skin of the upper lid and bringing this down along with some of the orbicularis muscle (see Fig. 28–33). If the defect is a very wide one, the pedicles of the skin flap may be set in position at the first operation without the need to divide and transpose the pedicles at a second stage. Smaller defects, however, will best be reconstructed by division of the pedicles in two weeks, as was described for the lower lid. In young patients the defect left by the Tripier flap must be grafted. The lining of the small skin flap should consist of nasal mucosa alone with no cartilage attached, as this would interfere with the change of shape of the lid margin. Buccal mucosa should not be used, as it contracts so much that it inevitably causes entropion of the lid margin.

Defects Affecting the Vertical Dimension of the Lid

SMALL DEFECTS OF THE UPPER EYELID. Small defects of the upper lid up to one quarter of the length of the lid may be closed by direct approximation, and a division of the upper crus of the lateral canthal tendon may be done to relax the lid when closure of a defect of up to one-third the width of the lid is required.

MODERATE DEFECTS OF THE UPPER EYE-LID. Defects of up to half of the lid may be closed by rotating a small full-thickness flap of the lower lid, which is based on the marginal vessels. These vessels run about 3 or 4 mm from the margin of the lid, and the pedicle should be at least 5 or 6 mm in width to avoid damaging them.

The fact that one can resect about a quarter of an eyelid and still close the defect because the tissues of the lid stretch quite considerably means that, when considering the size of flaps to be used to fill a specific defect in the upper lid, one can reduce the width of the flap by as much as a quarter of the original lid length, and it will be quite possible to fill the defect with a smaller flap. In practice it is not wise to outline the full-thickness flap from the lower lid any smaller than a quarter of the lid length, as it then becomes rather too small to handle adequately.

The position of the flap can be determined by marking out on the lower lid an outline of the defect in the upper lid and making the central point between the marks the site of the hinge of the lower lid flap. The flap can be designed on either the lateral or medial side of the hinge, and the defect in the lower lid is closed to within a few millimeters of the margin, taking care to avoid damaging the small vessels in the pedicle itself.

The conjunctiva and the tarsal plate are sutured using one or more continuous, fine, pull-out nylon sutures (6–0) so as to avoid any knots rubbing on the cornea. These sutures can be pulled out in a week, or about ten days if they show any resistance to withdrawal. The orbicularis muscle is closed with 6–0 catgut, and the skin is approximated with 5–0 or 6–0 silk sutures.

After two weeks the small pedicle is divided, and the lid margins are revised. This may entail splitting the edges of the lower marginal wound to a depth of several millimeters in order to equalize the edges of the wound. If the lower lid is at all tight, relaxation may be obtained by dividing the lower crus of the lateral canthal tendon through a small horizontal stab wound at the lateral canthus.

During the first stage of the procedure, if the defect in the upper lid lies near the center, the cut end of the levator muscle should be identified and sutured to the connective tissue in the center of the small lid flap, just distal to the tarsal plate. This will ensure satisfactory levator

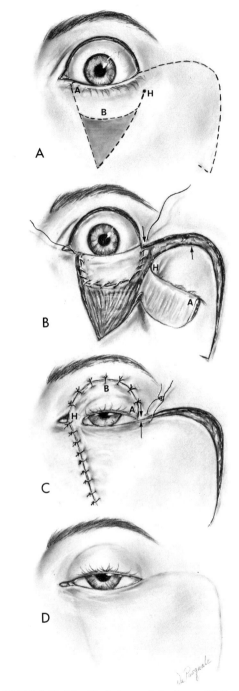

FIGURE 28–36. Technique of the lower lid "switch" flap to reconstruct a large defect of the upper lid. *A,* The dotted lines outline the portion of the *lower* lid which will serve to reconstruct the *upper* lid. The rotation flap and its "cut-back" to reconstruct the *lower* lid is also outlined. The point H indicates the hinge of the pedicle. The shaded area indicates the triangle of skin to be excised. *B,* The septal composite graft has been sutured to the edges of the lower lid defect. The arrow indicates the nylon suture supporting the graft. The lower lid and the rotation flap have been elevated. *C,* The lower eyelid flap has been rotated on its pedicle hinge H and sutured in position in the upper eyelid. The rotation flap (note supporting suture lateral to lateral canthus) covers the raw area over the composite graft and cheek. *D,* Final appearance.

function, and the remaining peripheral part of the orbicularis muscle will, along with gravity, produce adequate closure of the lid.

Techniques for closing these moderate defects of the upper lid have been described in which a procedure similar to that described for reconstruction of the lower lid is employed — i.e., the orbital skin lateral to the lateral canthus is moved toward the midline and lined with conjunctiva. Such techniques may present a simpler means of reconstructing a moderate sector of the upper lid for those not familiar with the Abbé "switch" flap operation, but they involve more scarring of the cheek and tend to bring toward the midline some of the bulk of the tail of the eyebrow. Sectioning of the conjunctiva of the upper fornix on the lateral side may occlude some of the ductules from the lacrimal gland, with resultant cyst formation. If the defect in the upper lid lies on the medial half, one must remember that the mobile central part of the levator aponeurosis is being brought across to be tethered to the medial canthus. This may result in a mechanical ptosis which is extremely difficult, if not impossible, to correct.

LARGE DEFECTS OF THE UPPER EYELID.

Large defects of the upper lid will require larger lower lid "switch" flaps to reconstruct them (Fig. 28–36), but it is worth remembering that because the lid tissues will stretch to such an extent as to permit closure of a defect of about a quarter of the lid, the size of the "switch" flap to be used can be reduced by a quarter of the lid length. If this quarter is marked out on the lateral side of the upper lid defect when it is extrapolated onto the lower lid, the point H in Figure 28–36, *A, B* will represent the site of the pedicle hinge; the remainder of the defect width represents the size of the "switch" flap required to fill the defect.

The reconstructed segment of the lower lid should be lined with a composite graft of nasal septal mucosa and cartilage, as described in lower lid reconstruction (Fig. 28–36, *B*). The flap can lie on either side of the hinge, depending upon which side presents the greater amount of tissue (Fig. 28–36, *C*); the flap should be designed on the lateral side of the hinge if it is going to encroach on the punctum of the lower lid. Because a larger secondary defect is produced in the lower lid, it is usually necessary to rotate the cheek to allow a small new segment of the lower lid to be con-

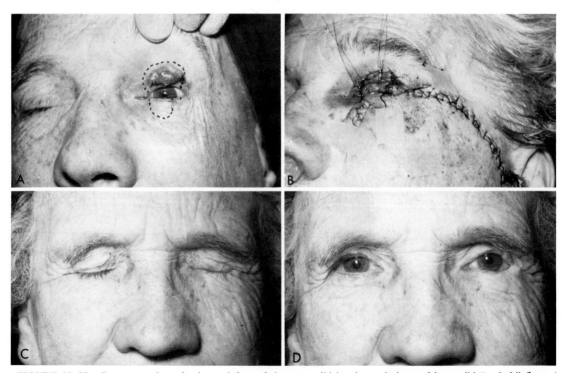

FIGURE 28–37. Reconstruction of a large defect of the upper lid by the technique of lower lid "switch" flap. *A,* Outline of the upper lid defect and of the portion of the lower lid to serve as the "switch" flap. *B,* After completion of the operative procedure illustrated in Figure 28–36. *C,* Closure of the palpebral fissure after completion of the reconstruction. *D,* Appearance in the forward gaze.

structed; as the size of the "switch" flap increases, the lower lid reconstruction becomes more extensive. The marginal vessels must be preserved in the flap, which is divided after two weeks (Fig. 28–36, *D* and 28–37).

Total Reconstruction of the Upper Lid. A total replacement of the upper lid may be achieved in the same manner, but no design or formula for placing the hinge is required, and the "switch" flap from the lower lid should be confined to the lateral three-quarters of the lid, thus preserving the lower lacrimal drainage apparatus (Fig. 28–38, *A* to *D*). The new lower lid segment is lined with a composite graft (Fig. 28–38, *E*), and the pedicle should be at least 6 mm in width in order to preserve the marginal vessels. The "switch" flap is carried nasally on the cheek flap and then rotated 180 degrees (Fig. 28–38, *F, G*). Care must be taken to avoid damage to the vascular supply by keeping the dissection deep to the orbicularis muscle, as far at least as the margin of the orbit. The stump of the levator muscle must be attached by sutures to the connective tissue of the "switch" flap. The pedicle is divided 2 1/2 weeks following large reconstructions, and the lid margins are then revised (Fig. 28–38, *H, I*).

Total Reconstruction of the Upper and Lower Lids. Mustardé (1974) advised a wide dissection of the conjunctiva of both lids; the conjunctiva is sutured over the cornea. A forehead flap is used to cover the conjunctiva. At a later date, the forehead flap, after the return of the pedicle to the forehead, is split into upper and lower eyelids to allow vision. Although the result is far from satisfactory from an esthetic viewpoint, the cornea is saved.

Eyelid Reconstruction

Byron Smith, M.D.

Indications. Eyelid repair and reconstruction are indicated following trauma, in congenital malformations, and for defects resulting from neoplastic disease and numerous other conditions in which the lids have been damaged or destroyed. Considerable progress has been achieved with the development of more refined instruments, sharper needles, improved suture materials, more efficient anesthesia, improved surgical techniques, and greater precision in operative technique aided by the use of visual magnification by operating loupes and microscopes.

The Three Sections of the Eyelids. For the convenience of description, the eyelids may be divided into three sections along a horizontal plane: the central (or middle), the medial (or nasal), and the lateral (or temporal).

1. The central section is made up of the entire substance of the upper and lower lids and their opposing margins.

2. The lateral section is composed of the lateral canthus, lateral fornix, lid margins, conjunctiva, and secreting lacrimal structures.

3. The medial section encompasses the structures of the medial canthus, such as the caruncle, puncta, lacrimal ducts, medial canthal tendon, lid margins, and surrounding bone.

The medial canthus is somewhat more complicated in its anatomy than the lateral canthus; the upper lid is more complicated in its anatomy and function than the lower lid. Knowledge of the intricate structures and functions of these anatomical units is necessary before engaging in reconstructive surgery of the eyelids.

Development of the Tarsoconjunctival Flap Technique. The development of the tarsoconjunctival flap technique has been reviewed earlier in this chapter (see p. 882). Hughes (1937) described a tarsoconjunctival flap technique for reconstruction of the lower lid similar to that of Landolt (1881) and popularized the technique. Cutler and Beard (1955) employed a bridge flap from the lower lid for partial and total upper eyelid reconstruction similar to the technique of Köllner (1911). The popularity of the Hughes technique waned when entropion and trichiasis occurred, which was attributed to the incision at the white line. Since that time the technique has been modified—the horizontal incision, parallel to the lid margin, which determines the advancing edge of the tarsoconjunctival flap, is placed at least 4 to 5 mm away from the edge of the lid margin—and these complications have not occurred.

Large Defects in the Central Section of the Lower Eyelid

In large defects in the central section of the lower lid, replacement of the lid tissue by lid tissue is usually possible. If borrowing techniques from the same, opposing, or contralateral lids are utilized, only minimal structural, functional, and cosmetic damage should be

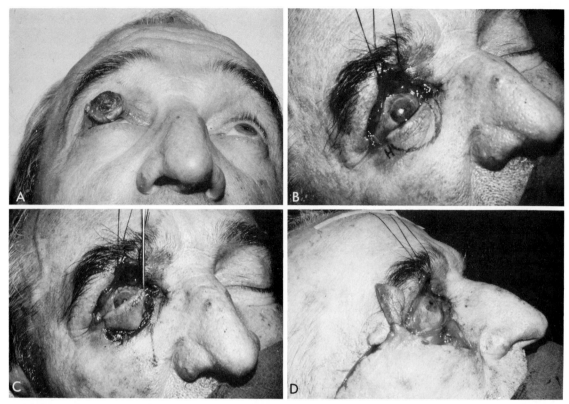

FIGURE 28–38. *A*, Large tumor of the upper eyelid. *B*, After resection of the upper lid. Note outline of donor lower lid tissue and pedicle hinge (H). *C*, The lower lid flap is prepared for rotation. *D*, The lower lid flap is raised on its pedicle at point H. The triangle of skin has been excised (see Fig. 28–36, *A*), and the rotation flap incised.

Illustration continued on opposite page

inflicted upon the donor lid. If such damage is predictable, the advisability of using other methods—advancement or transposition flaps from the forehead, temporal region, or cheek—should be considered. Usually these techniques require more surgical skill and extensive dissection, cause more scars, and involve more postsurgical complications than may be expected from simpler techniques.

For the restoration of large horizontal defects in the central area of the lower lid, the technique of Köllner (1911), the modified technique of Hughes (1937, 1945), and the technique of Cutler and Beard (1955) provide the best functional and cosmetic results. In order to utilize these techniques, a normal opposing upper lid is mandatory.

The First Stage. The horizontal dimension of the defect in the lower lid is measured (Fig. 28–39, *A*). It is essential to maintain a well-supported upper lid margin, despite the fact that some of the upper tarsus has been transposed. The horizontal incision parallel to the lid margin which establishes the advancing edge of the tarsoconjunctival flap *should be at least 4 to 5 mm above the internal surface of the*

upper lid margin (Fig. 28–39, *B*, *C*). With the scissors hugging the tarsus, the flap should be dissected high beneath the surface of the levator muscle (Fig. 28–39, *C*). In the event that the dissection is not carried far enough backward and superiorly, a late residual retraction and increased arching of the upper lid may be the consequence of this error in technique.

The portion of the tarsoconjunctival flap that is used for the repair should be approximately 25 per cent narrower in width than the defect. Older patients have lax eyelids, and a wider tarsoconjunctival flap would result in a reconstructed lower lid which has a tendency to be ectropic because of excessive horizontal length.

After the tarsoconjunctival flap has been dissected and advanced into the defect, the leading margin of the advanced tarsus is attached to the recipient site and conjunctival base by interrupted sutures of 6–0 chromic catgut (Fig. 28–39, *B*). The knots are tied externally so that they do not irritate the ocular globe. The margins of the tarsal flap are then securely attached to adjacent margins of the lower lid defect by a tongue and groove technique (Fig. 28–39, *D*, *E*).

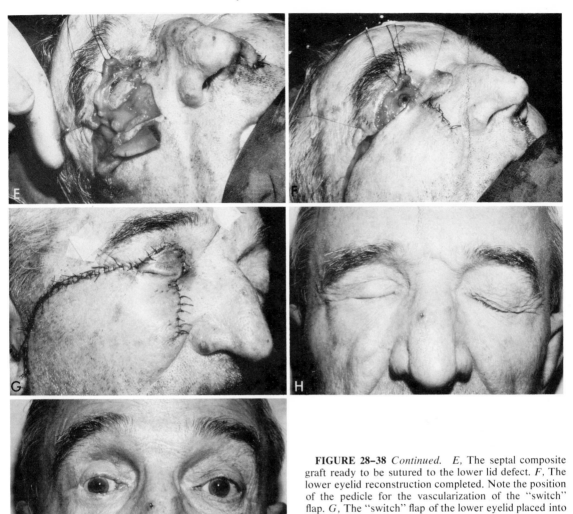

FIGURE 28–38 *Continued.* *E,* The septal composite graft ready to be sutured to the lower lid defect. *F,* The lower eyelid reconstruction completed. Note the position of the pedicle for the vascularization of the "switch" flap. *G,* The "switch" flap of the lower eyelid placed into the upper lid defect. *H,* Closure of the palpebral fissure of the reconstructed lids. *I,* Appearance in the forward gaze.

Once in place, the tarsoconjunctival flap furnishes the posterior layers of the lid. This leaves a rectangular raw area over the tarsus (Fig. 28–39, *E*), which is resurfaced by a full-thickness skin graft (Fig. 28–39, *F*) or an advancement flap from the cheek. The choice of a graft or an advancement flap is determined by the laxity in the surrounding skin. In the aged patient, the skin is redundant and lax and readily available. If there is any vertical tension on a proposed advancement flap from below, it is contraindicated; postoperative retraction in such a flap invites late postoperative ectropion. If the advancement flap from below is feasible and selected as the method of closure, the flap is sutured to the anterior surface of the advanced

tarsoconjunctival flap with interrupted 6–0 silk sutures. The margins are likewise closed with interrupted sutures. If there is any puckering at the base of the advancement flap, the excess tissue is removed by excision of a triangle of skin on each side.

A full-thickness skin graft is usually the preferable technique in any but the aged patient with loose skin. Available donor skin for grafting is removed from behind the ear or from the supraclavicular area. In large defects of the lower lid, a skin graft should not be taken from the contralateral upper lid, because it is not sufficiently thick. The graft is neatly fitted into the defect and sutured on all sides with 6–0 silk sutures. The remainder of the upper lid margin

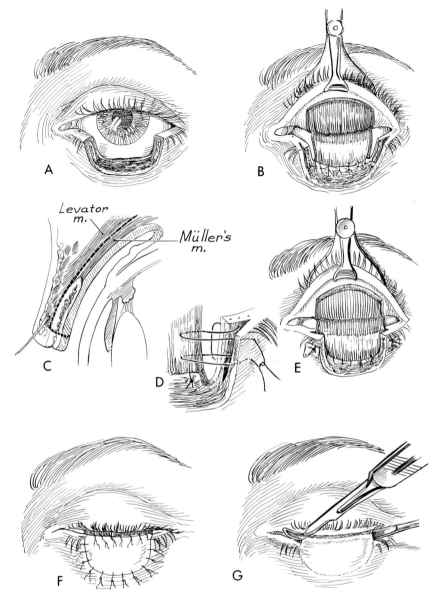

FIGURE 28–39. Reconstruction of a large central defect of the lower eyelid. *A*, Large lower eyelid defect. *B*, Tarsoconjunctival flap from the upper eyelid is sutured into the lower lid defect. Erhardt clamp was used to evert the upper lid. Note that the incision through the tarsus is made parallel to the lid margin and no closer than 4 mm. The remaining tarsal border ensures stability of the lid margin and avoids entropion. *C*, In sagittal section, the incision through the conjunctiva and tarsus and the plane of dissection extending upward between the levator and Müller's muscles are outlined. Note the margin of tarsus left undisturbed, an essential precaution to prevent postoperative entropion of the upper lid. *D*, Technique of imbricating the tarsoconjunctival flap into the edge of the defect. *E*, The tarsoconjunctival flap is in position, each edge being imbricated into the wound edges of the defect. *F*, A full-thickness retroauricular or supraclavicular graft has been sutured over the tarsoconjunctival flap. *G*, Four weeks later a grooved probe is passed under the tarsoconjunctival flap, which is sectioned. (After B. Smith and T. D. Cherubini, 1970.)

is then slid over the surface of the tarsoconjunctival flap into the position it normally occupies. It is not necessary to suture the upper lid to the tarsoconjunctival flap. A moderately compressive pressure dressing is then applied with a few strips of adhesive tape. The dressing is changed in 48 hours. The sutures are removed at the end of one week. A dressing of

a protective nature is kept in place for approximately ten days. The patient is advised to avoid attempting to open the eye until the second stage of the reconstructive procedure.

EYELASH GRAFTING.   The eyelashes in the lower lid are fine and sparse, and their restoration is not essential. If one chooses to do a lash graft from the brow, surgery is done six weeks

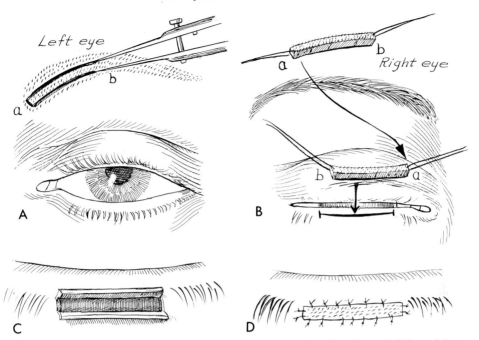

FIGURE 28-40. Eyelash grafting. *A*, Outline of cilia graft from contralateral eyebrow. *B*, Cilia graft is transplanted to the defect in the lower eyelid; it is rotated, its medial end becoming its lateral end. *C*, Two flaps raised to receive the graft. *D*, Graft has been sutured into position. The direction of the lashes is more satisfactory when removed from the opposite brow and then reversed.

following the first stage. A horizontal incision is made at the upper edge of the flap, and the margins are undermined to prepare the recipient site. A strip of eyebrow, approximately four hairs in breadth, is resected (Fig. 28–40, *A*, *B*), reversed, and sutured into the recipient site with interrupted 6–0 sutures (Fig. 28–40, *C*, *D*). The base of the graft should be freed of excessive fat, but damage to the root bulbs must be avoided. During the postoperative period, the transplanted cilia have a tendency to fall out, but they usually grow back in about two months. The transplanted lashes grow to an excessive length, and the patient must be advised to keep them trimmed appropriately.

The Second Stage. Three weeks after the cilia graft has been done, the palpebral fissure may be opened (Fig. 28–39, *G*). Excess tissue along the lid margins should be leveled off with a pair of spring-handled scissors. The upper lid is everted, and excessive irregularities are resected. Any irregular tissue or residual epidermis beneath the upper lid causes irritation of the cornea. If the operation has been correctly executed, the upper lid falls back into its usual position, and the lower lid has an adequate contour and function within the next few weeks (Fig. 28–41).

Large Defects in the Central Area of the Upper Eyelid

The upper lid is involved by malignant tumors less frequently than the lower lid. Large central defects of sufficient magnitude to require the addition of tissue borrowed from the lower lid require a technique somewhat different from the procedure described for borrowing tissue from the upper to restore the lower lid. The Cutler-Beard technique is preferred in repairing large central defects of the upper lid.

The First Stage. The defect in the upper lid should be trimmed so that the edges are smooth and straight. The horizontal dimension of the defect in the upper lid is measured. The donor flap is then designed on the external surface of the lower lid (Fig. 28–42, *A*). In this technique the margin of the lower lid is retained (Fig. 28–42, *B*). Within this small bridge, the marginal artery traverses the substance of the lid and ensures the blood supply. It is essential to avoid injuring the bridge flap or the marginal artery. The horizontal incision delineating the advancing upper margin of the composite flap should be situated approximately 4 mm below and parallel to the lid margin (Fig. 28–42, *B*). Vertical incisions are

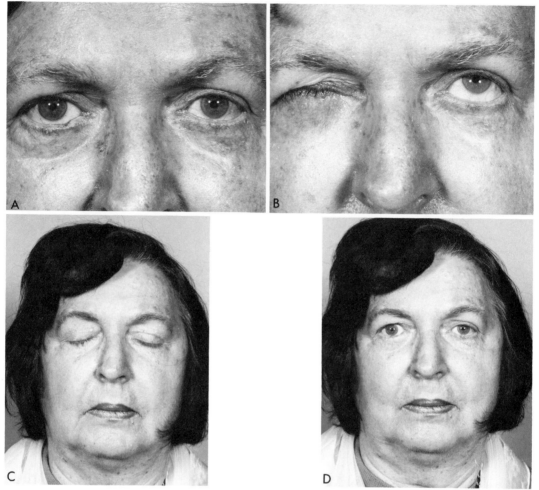

FIGURE 28–41. Reconstruction of a large central segment of the right lower lid. *A*, Malignant lesion of the right lower lid will require extensive resection. *B*, The large segment of the lower lid has been resected, and a tarsoconjunctival flap has been freed from the upper lid, forming the inner portion of the lower lid, as illustrated in Figure 28–39, *E*. The tarsoconjunctival flap is covered by a full-thickness retroauricular graft, as shown in Figure 28–39, *F*. *C*, After separation of the lids (see Fig. 28–39, *G*). The patient shown occluding the lids. *D*, Appearance of the patient in the forward gaze. Note excellent contour of the lower eyelid. There is excess skin in the upper eyelid which could have been removed. The patient, however, was satisfied with the result.

made on either side of the designed flap (Fig. 28–42, *B*).

The lower lid is then everted, exposing its tarsal surface. A horizontal incision is made through the tarsus approximately 4 mm below the lid margin, at the level of the previously made horizontal skin incision. The horizontal and vertical incisions through the soft tissues and the tarsus are then connected. Finally, vertical incisions downward through the conjunctiva are made, following the lines of the previous skin and tarsal incisions.

The bridge is gently elevated as the skin-muscle tarsoconjunctival flap is advanced into the defect of the upper lid (Fig. 28–42, *C*). Interrupted sutures of 6–0 chromic catgut attach the conjunctiva of the flap from the lower lid to that of the upper lid (Fig. 28–42, *C*). These sutures usually pick up the conjunctiva, the levator aponeurosis, and the attached structures. The margins of the flap are also approximated to the tarsus and conjunctiva of the recipient bed (Fig. 28–42, *C, D*). Lastly, the skin of the advanced flap from the lower lid is sutured to the skin of the recipient bed of the upper lid with 6–0 silk on atraumatic needles (Fig. 28–42, *C*).

It is undesirable and unnecessary to close the tissues along the inferior margin of the bridge containing the marginal artery. During the first two postoperative weeks, the skin spontaneously becomes adherent to

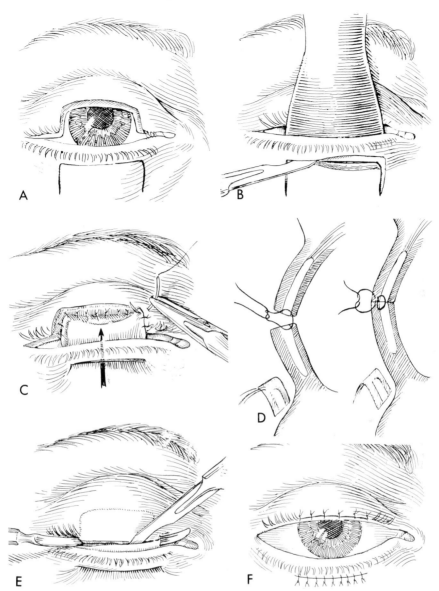

FIGURE 28–42. Reconstruction of a large central segment of the upper lid by the Cutler-Beard bridge flap technique. *A*, Defect of upper eyelid and outline of flap from the lower eyelid. *B*, Bridge flap is incised. Lid plate is in position to maintain stretch on tissues of the lower lid during incision. *C*, Flap has been advanced, being passed under bridge consisting of intact full-thickness lower lid margin. Interrupted sutures of 5–0 plain catgut have been used to approximate the conjunctiva of the flap and the edges of the lid defect. Suturing of skin is begun. *D*, In sagittal section, buried sutures approximating edges of the tarsus are shown. *E*, After six weeks, the flap is divided over a grooved probe. *F*, The donor flap has been released and returned to its original position.

the conjunctiva. Attempts at closure by sutures invite excessive compression and the possibility of injury to the marginal artery and sloughing of the bridge. The bridge is protected by a dressing, so that pressure is not applied to the margin of the lower lid during the postoperative period. The skin sutures are removed in seven days. It is sometimes desirable to leave the marginal sutures of the upper lid in place for approximately ten days.

During the postoperative period, the advancement flap from the lower lid stretches and elongates. In some patients this flap elongates to as much as double its original length in a period of eight weeks.

If it is felt desirable to do a cilia graft, the procedure is done in a similar fashion to that described for the lower lid. The lashes should be placed at the suitable level in alignment with the residual lashes on either side of the flap.

The Second Stage. Six weeks after the first stage, the flap may be released, restoring the margin of the upper lid. As recommended by Reeh (1967), it is advisable to leave approximately a millimeter of excess to allow for ultimate contraction during healing (Fig. 28–42, *E, F*). The flap from the lower lid is then freshened and replaced into its original position. Ordinarily very little or no deformity is obvious in the lower lid after the early postoperative reaction has subsided. The fact that the advancement flap elongated during the early postoperative period is a factor in avoiding retraction of the lower lid margin in the final stage (Fig. 28–43). A reverse procedure is employed to reconstruct a defect of the lower lid (Fig. 28–44).

Defects of the Lateral Segment of the Eyelid

Small defects in the lateral canthus may be closed by direct approximation. Should the tissues heal with a defective angle or shortened palpebral fissure, subsequent lateral canthoplasty may rectify the residual defect.

If the defect in the lateral canthus is of significant dimensions, involving the upper lid, the lower lid, and the lateral canthus, a more involved technique becomes necessary. A carcinoma of the lateral canthus ordinarily leaves a large defect. Carcinomas involving the lateral as well as the medial canthus are potentially dangerous and have a propensity toward recurrence unless widely excised.

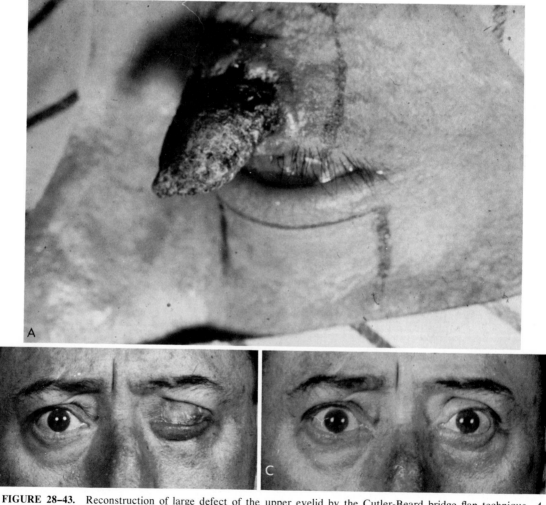

FIGURE 28–43. Reconstruction of large defect of the upper eyelid by the Cutler-Beard bridge flap technique. *A,* Large malignant lesion of the upper lid. Note the outline of the bridge flap from the lower eyelid. *B,* Appearance of the patient during the intermediary period when the tarsoconjunctival flap from the lower lid has been advanced into the defect of the upper lid, as shown in Figure 28–42, *C. C,* Appearance of the patient at completion of the reconstruction.

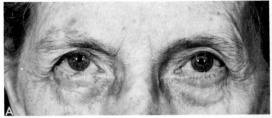
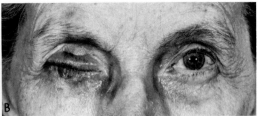
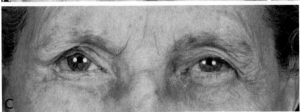

FIGURE 28-44. The bridge flap technique for the reconstruction of a defect of the lower lid. *A*, Patient with malignant lesion of the right lower lid. *B*, Appearance of the patient after the bridge flap has been inserted from the upper lid into the lower lid. *C*, Final appearance of the patient after the completion of the reconstruction.

In determining the lines of transmarginal incision for the excision of the lateral canthal tumor, the operating microscope is a most useful aid. The tarsal glands in the area of the cancer, as well as along its advancing edge, tend to be obliterated. The incision through the lid margin should be well beyond the evidence of microscopic involvement. If in doubt, it is preferable to err on the radical rather than on the conservative side. Additional biopsies may be taken from the wound edges after the block containing the carcinoma has been excised. The initial incisions for the resection of the lateral canthus carcinoma should be vertical through the lid margins, upward toward the upper cul-de-sac, and downward toward the lower cul-de-sac. This maneuver releases the lateral canthus so that the internal surface may be inspected and dissected under direct vision. After the lateral canthus and its adjacent tissues have been resected, it is desirable to pin the tissue to a piece of cardboard, so that the pathology laboratory may retain proper orientation in the sectioning of the tissue.

Of the various means of closure of a large lateral canthal defect, the tarsoconjunctival flap from the upper lid is the preferred technique (Fig. 28-45). The flap is prepared according to the technique employed in the large central lower lid defects. After the flap has been sufficiently dissected and released, it is displaced downward and outward into the canthal defect. The advanced margin of the tarsoconjunctival flap is sutured to the recipient bed with 6–0 chromic catgut sutures (Fig. 28-45, *A, B*). The nasal extremity of the flap is interdigitated into the recipient lower lid margin. The temporal (lateral) edge of the flap should be well fixed to the orbital margin or tissues adjacent to it. If one chooses, an ar-

tificial lateral canthal support may be designed using a turnover flap from the periosteum and superficial tissues over the lateral orbital margin (Fig. 28-45, *C*). This fabricated tendon is then sutured to the anterior surface of the tarsoconjunctival flap (Fig. 28-45, *D*).

After the tendon has been sutured into position, the external raw surface is exposed. In the older patient, the defect may be covered by undermining and advancing skin from the adjacent area or by rotating lateral tissue, as advocated by Mustardé (1966) and McGregor (1973). If the skin in the area is scarred or is under tension, as in the younger patient, a full-thickness retroauricular skin graft can be employed. Another technique is the transposition of a temporal flap (Fig. 28-45, *E, F*). The interpalpebral bridge is divided six to eight weeks following the first stage. Ordinarily, lash grafting at the lateral canthus is not necessary.

Defects in the Medial Segment of the Eyelid

Cancers involving the medial canthus are frequently insidious, recognized late, and inadequately treated. They are particularly resistant to any type of treatment other than early radical resection. Since the anatomy of the medial canthus is more complicated than that of the lateral canthus, surgical excision and restoration are more involved than similar surgery in the lateral canthal area. The lacrimal excretory ducts, the medial canthal tendon, and the caruncle are in close proximity. The resection may include all of these structures, including the lacrimal sac, if necessary. The initial incisions are similar in outline to those described

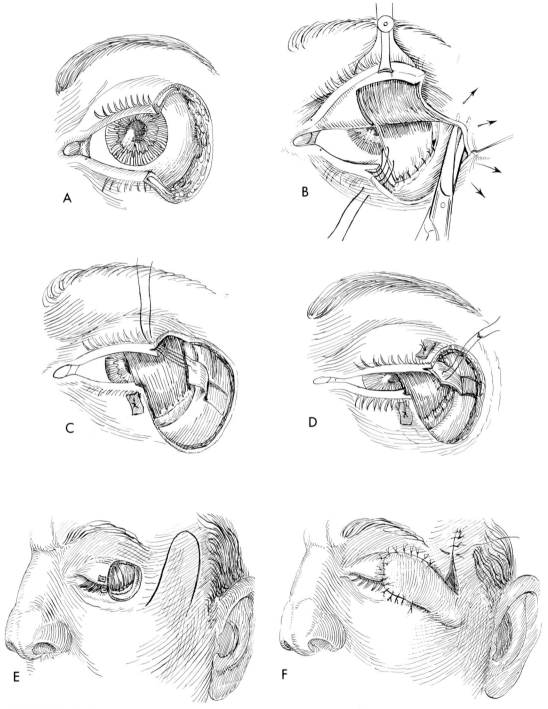

FIGURE 28–45. Reconstruction of the lateral portions of the upper and lower eyelids. *A*, Outline of defect. *B*, The flap of tarsoconjunctiva has been raised from the undersurface of the upper eyelid and is advanced to form the tarsoconjunctival layer of the new lateral canthus. Medially, eyelid tissue is split to allow more intimate junction with the tarsoconjunctival flap. *C, D*, New lateral canthal raphé is fashioned from periosteum and sutured to the lateral portion of the tarsoconjunctival flap. *E, F*, Temporal transposition flap sutured in position over the tarsoconjunctival flap.

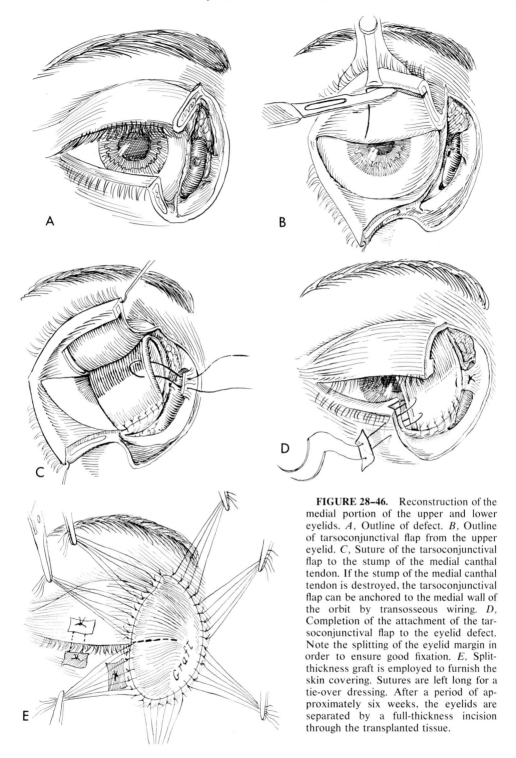

FIGURE 28–46. Reconstruction of the medial portion of the upper and lower eyelids. *A,* Outline of defect. *B,* Outline of tarsoconjunctival flap from the upper eyelid. *C,* Suture of the tarsoconjunctival flap to the stump of the medial canthal tendon. If the stump of the medial canthal tendon is destroyed, the tarsoconjunctival flap can be anchored to the medial wall of the orbit by transosseous wiring. *D,* Completion of the attachment of the tarsoconjunctival flap to the eyelid defect. Note the splitting of the eyelid margin in order to ensure good fixation. *E,* Split-thickness graft is employed to furnish the skin covering. Sutures are left long for a tie-over dressing. After a period of approximately six weeks, the eyelids are separated by a full-thickness incision through the transplanted tissue.

for the lateral canthus. Vertical incisions are made temporal (lateral) to the involved area, upward to the cul-de-sac in the upper lid, and downward to the lower cul-de-sac in the lower lid.

One may expect considerable bleeding from the angular vein. After the transmarginal incisions have been extended into the fornices, it is advisable to make the encircling incisions around the nasal (medial) aspect of the mass.

The tissues are dissected down to the periosteum, and the entire medial canthal area is resected. The resection is delineated by the bony contour. If the conjunctiva in the caruncular area is involved, the dissection is extended toward the medial rectus muscle, so that all of the diseased tissue is removed (Fig. 28–46, *A*). Closure is started by outlining and freeing a tarsoconjunctival flap from the upper lid, as was described for the reconstruction of lateral canthal defects (Fig. 28–46, *B*). The flap is advanced into the defect (Fig. 28–46, *C*). It is attached nasally by transnasal wires and sutured to the edges of the defect (Fig. 28–46, *D*). Since the skin overlying the lateral aspect of the nose is difficult to advance, the raw area is best closed by a split-thickness or a full-thickness skin graft, taken from the upper lid of the contralateral eye or from the postauricular or the supraclavicular areas (Fig. 28–46, *E*). The graft is patterned to fit the defect accurately. The skin graft usually heals well and attaches itself to the underlying bone. After the graft has been sutured into its recipient bed with interrupted 6–0 silk sutures, a small pressure dressing is tied down to the surface to maintain the graft in its recipient bed. A moderately compressive pressure dressing is applied for approximately three days. When the dressing is removed, the pack on top of the graft may be carefully raised and the graft inspected. The dressing may then be left in position for one week.

When the lacrimal excretory system is deformed or eradicated, postoperative epiphora is not unusual. If this becomes a complication of sufficient significance, various means of management are available. Excessive secretion is verified by lacrimal function tests; relief may be obtained by resection of the palpebral lobe of the lacrimal gland. If this treatment is undesirable, the only alternative is a conjunctivorhinostomy (see Fig. 28–126). Conjunctivonasal intubation is more complicated and difficult in these cases than it is when the medial canthus has a normal contour. With careful adjustment of the tube, however, it is possible to obtain satisfactory lacrimal drainage (see p. 988).

It is needless to reiterate that the surgeon should study the pathology of the tumor. After the initial healing, the scarred area should be observed periodically for years, every three months for the first 18 months, and then every six months for three years. From that time on the patient should be examined carefully each year.

RECONSTRUCTION OF THE EYELIDS: A DIVERGENCE OF OPINION

JOHN MARQUIS CONVERSE, M.D.

Two schools of thought have thus developed concerning the technique of reconstructing major defects of the eyelids. Smith (1959) is of the opinion that the best result can be obtained from utilizing lid tissue for repair of a lid defect, similar to the concept of repairing a defect of the lip with tissue from the opposing lip. Poor results had been previously obtained with the tarsoconjunctival flap technique because a rim of tarsus of 4 to 5 mm was not preserved. The result was notching, entropion, and trichiasis. This technique presupposes that tissue from the opposing lid is available. It is obvious that experience in ophthalmic plastic surgery and a thorough knowledge of eyelid anatomy are required to obtain good results by the tarsoconjunctival flap technique. Consequently the technique of Mustardé has appealed to surgeons with little experience in ophthalmic plastic surgery.

Failures have been observed following reconstruction by both techniques; these can be attributed to inexperience. Holmström, Bartholdson and Johanson (1975) stated that in a series of 203 cancers of the eyelid, composite chondromucosal flaps were used in a number of cases. Conspicuous scars and a bulky distorted lid margin contrasted with the superior results obtained by the tarsoconjunctival flap technique.

The Mustardé technique is indicated in patients in whom tissue from the opposing lid is unavailable and in those with advanced cancers which require more tissue for satisfactory reconstruction than can be obtained from the opposing lid, particularly in patients of advanced age.

COMPOSITE GRAFTS

Horizontal defects of the lids may be closed by means of composite grafts from one of the other unaffected lids, provided that the tissues are available without causing a permanent defect in the donor lid (Jones, 1966). The composite graft is taken as a block of tissue from the donor lid and transplanted into the recipient bed in the defective lid (Fig. 28–47). The technique is more difficult and requires more

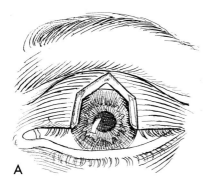

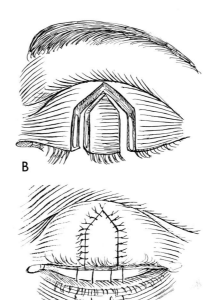

FIGURE 28–47. Composite graft in eyelid defects. *A*, Moderate defect of upper eyelid. *B*, Composite graft, smaller in width than defect, has been removed from the donor eyelid and is placed in the defect. *C*, Sutures have been placed in the pretarsal fascia to approximate the edges of the tarsus to orient the graft. Suturing of the graft has been completed by interrupted sutures approximating the skin margins. Two occlusive mattress sutures are placed to join the eyelids and immobilize the area during the healing of the graft.

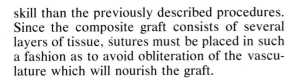

skill than the previously described procedures. Since the composite graft consists of several layers of tissue, sutures must be placed in such a fashion as to avoid obliteration of the vasculature which will nourish the graft.

EXCISION OF CANTHAL DEFECTS AND HEALING BY SECOND INTENTION: CHEMOSURGERY

This type of treatment may appear to be heresy to the plastic surgeon. The technique of restoration by granulation tissue proliferation of medial canthal defects was described by Beard and Fox (1964). It consists of resecting all of the necessary tissue in the medial canthal area and packing the wound open (Fig. 28–48, *A*). The nasal (medial) extremities of the upper and lower lids are maintained in apposition by a temporary interpalpebral suture. Relatively large medial canthal defects fill in very rapidly. As scar tissue forms, the nasal extremities of the upper and lower lids are pulled into position by gradual contraction (Fig. 28–48, *B*). In some situations, the residual canthus may be pulled somewhat upward or downward and require late surgical revision. Similar observation was made in the treatment of recurrent basal cell carcinomas of the medial canthal area treated by chemosurgery (see Chapter 65). After progressive healing, only minor corrective procedures were needed.

This technique has also been employed for the treatment of large lateral canthal defects and has been found as advantageous as in medial canthal defects. The technique is probably an excellent one for the inexperienced surgeon. More sophisticated surgery in the hands of the experienced surgeon is described and preferable. However, a radical resection followed by healing by contraction is preferable to an inadequate excision if the surgeon is not qualified to perform the reconstruction.

It is in the eradication of malignant tumors of the canthi—of the medial canthus, in particular—that chemosurgery (see Chapter 65) finds its most valuable application. The histologic control provided by this technique guards against inadequate excision and recurrence.

FAR ADVANCED LESIONS INVOLVING THE ORBITAL CONTENTS

W. Brandon Macomber, M.D.,
and Mark K. H. Wang, M.D.

Exenteration of the Orbit

Exenteration of the orbit is a radical operation reserved for treatment of malignant tumors

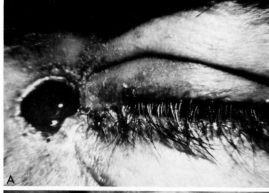

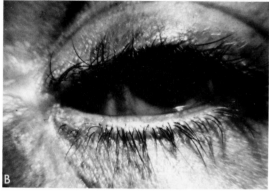

FIGURE 28–48. Excision of a canthal defect and healing by second intention. *A*, Defect resulting from resection of a malignancy of the medial canthus. *B*, After healing by second intention, the canthus is maintained in the depth of the naso-orbital valley.

which have invaded the orbit. It is a disfiguring and psychologically traumatic operation, although a life-saving procedure that should be undertaken without delay when it is indicated following histologic confirmation of the indication for orbital exenteration.

Wadsworth (1974) has reviewed the types of exenteration: (1) complete exenteration with excision of the eyelids and orbital contents; the cavity is allowed to granulate; (2) complete exenteration with excision of the lids and the orbital contents; a split-thickness skin graft is applied over the bone; (3) complete exenteration with preservation of the eyelids and occasionally of the conjunctiva; (4) complete exenteration with preservation of the eyelids and transfer of a temporalis muscle flap; (5) complete exenteration and repair of the orbital defect by a skin flap.

Complete Exenteration Without Primary Skin Grafting. This technique allows spontaneous re-epithelization after the granulation tissue has filled a portion of the cavity. Spontaneous epithelization results in considerable distortion of the adjacent structures, which are drawn into the orbital cavity. This technique is principally indicated in cases in which recurrences are deemed possible and when radiotherapy may be required as an adjuvant method of treatment.

Complete Exenteration and Skin Grafting. Skin grafting of the orbital cavity avoids a long period of granulation, suppuration, and progressively slow healing. The open skin-grafted orbital cavity still allows inspection if recurrence of the tumor is feared.

Complete Exenteration with Preservation of the Eyelids. In rare instances, the orbital contents can be exenterated and the lids preserved. Permanent occlusion of the eyelids is obtained by a complete tarsorrhaphy. The procedure can be done as a primary procedure after filling the orbital cavity with Gelfoam. It can also be done as a secondary procedure after having allowed the orbital cavity to granulate. If the eyelids tend to sink into the orbit long after the healing process has been completed, a sphere can be implanted in the orbit to correct the sunken appearance (Wadsworth, 1974). It is obvious that this type of procedure can be employed only in cases in which the risk of recurrence of the tumor has been eliminated.

Complete Exenteration with Preservation of the Lids and Transfer of a Temporalis Muscle Flap. In this technique, a temporalis muscle flap is introduced into the orbital cavity and is covered with a split-thickness skin graft.

Complete Exenteration and Repair of the Orbital Defect by a Skin Flap. The advantage of this technique, as well as the technique in which the eyelids can be preserved, is that the patient is relieved of an unsightly cavity that requires constant cleansing of secretions and desquamation from a skin graft.

Indications for Exenteration. Exenteration is indicated for various malignant orbital tumors, including the sarcomas (except lymphosarcoma), malignant melanoma and malignant melanosis of the conjunctiva, and the more malignant mixed tumors or primary carcinomas of the lacrimal gland. Malignant melanoma of the choroid requires exenteration only when there is nonencapsulated extension into the extraocular orbit (Reese, 1953).

Malignant tumors arising in the eyelids, accessory sinuses, or other periorbital structures may invade the orbit. In such cases, exenteration in continuity with the primary tumor resection may offer the best opportunity for a cure.

Exenteration is not indicated for benign tumors and pseudotumors of the orbit, meningiomas, malignant melanomas confined to the globe, or retinoblastomas, nor can it be used with hope of cure in tumors metastatic to the orbit, except in the rare instance when the primary tumor and other metastases have been eliminated (Pack and Ariel, 1959).

Preoperative Evaluation. A preliminary surgical biopsy is recommended for the identification of all extraorbital neoplasms, lesions of the conjunctiva, and accessible extraocular tumors of the orbit for which exenteration is being considered. If frozen section diagnosis is doubtful, delay until permanent sections can be obtained is far better than risking an unwarranted radical operation. There is little evidence to suggest that this brief delay will affect prognosis.

Preoperative definition of the extent of tumor invasion is required to plan the extent of the surgery. Radiologic examination, including tomography, of the orbit, adjacent facial bones, and accessory sinuses should be routine when exenteration is being considered, and orbital venography may also be helpful (Dayton and Hanafee, 1969). Since an exact definition of the total lesion may not be possible before the operation, the surgeon must be prepared to extend the procedure, as indicated by the operative findings.

Preparation for such a deforming operation necessitates a frank discussion with the patient. Only when he understands the gravity of the situation and the goal of the surgeon will he be likely to accept the consequent deformity. A plan for early rehabilitation should be offered whenever possible.

Technique. General endotracheal anesthesia is required. For simple exenteration, a 10- × 10-cm split-thickness skin graft (0.012 to 0.015 inch in thickness) is obtained from a hairless donor site, usually on the lateral aspect of the buttock. The graft is wrapped in gauze moistened with normal saline and set aside.

The exenteration is begun with an incision around the rim of the orbit, which is extended through eyelid skin, subcutaneous tissue, and muscle to expose the periosteum. The canthal tendons are raised from the bone after the periosteum is incised around the orbital rim.

Separation of the periorbita is begun on the lateral wall, using a blunt elevator. Sharp dis-section may be needed to free the periobita and neurovascular structures in the region of the inferior and superior fissures, and as the plane of dissection is developed medially, the ligamentous part of the trochlea must be severed from the frontal bone along the anterosuperior portion of the nasal quadrant. Care must be taken to avoid perforation of the thin roof of the orbit and the paper-thin lamina papyracea of the ethmoid bone.

When subperiosteal dissection has been completed to the apex of the orbit, curved enucleation scissors are introduced along the lateral wall, the neurovascular bundle traversing the optic foramen is severed close to bone, and the specimen is removed en bloc. The orbit is packed with gentle pressure for several minutes. The larger vessels are ligated with absorbable suture material, and meticulous hemostasis is completed with pinpoint electrocoagulation. The defect is then ready for repair.

When the tumor invades the bony orbit or involves periorbital tissues, the operative plan is extended to afford adequate margins of resection. In no instance, however, is a less radical exenteration performed.

The previously obtained skin graft is placed in the orbit without tension, and all folds and wrinkles are smoothed to assure accurate approximation over the bone. Any excess is trimmed as the graft is sutured to the borders of the defect with a continuous suture. Interrupted sutures are placed around the periphery of the graft at 1- to 2-cm intervals, and the ends are left long to tie over the dressing.

The graft is covered with a single layer of xeroform gauze, and the orbital cavity is packed firmly with fluffed gauze or with a bolus of ordinary steel wool wrapped in gauze. The latter technique is favored whenever a skin graft is placed on a firm bed, as dried blood does not affect its resilience. The dressing is secured in the orbit with tie-over sutures, and any exposed suture lines are covered with xeroform gauze. The outer dressing is completed with fluffed gauze tapered away from the orbit and a roller gauze head bandage. It is important to maintain general anesthesia until the dressing is completed and manual support over the dressing during extubation in order to lessen the risk of bleeding beneath the graft.

All but the very elderly are kept in bed with an elevated backrest until the first dressing change on the fifth or sixth postoperative day. Antibiotics are used only when an extended resection uncovers dura, or an opening into the nose, mouth, or accessory sinus has occurred.

Controversy Concerning Closure of the Orbital Cavity. After exenteration for a rapidly growing malignant tumor which may require additional treatment by irradiation, skin grafting is contraindicated. Skin grafting is indi-

cated, however, if the radical procedure has eradicated the tumor.

Considerable controversy exists over whether or not to cover the open orbital cavity, because such a procedure hides the area to

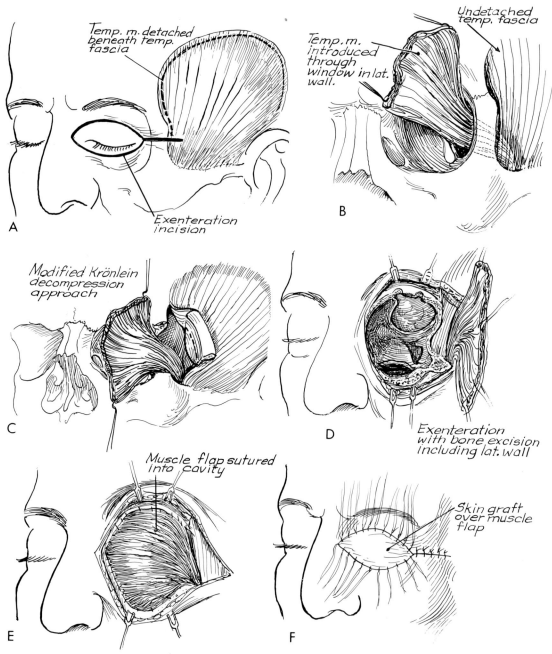

FIGURE 28–49. Closure of exenterated orbit by a temporalis muscle flap covered by a skin graft (after Webster). *A,* Outline of incisions for the orbital exenteration. The broken line indicates the temporalis muscle flap. *B,* One technique: the temporalis muscle flap, devoid of fascia, is introduced through the lateral orbital wall. *C,* Another technique: the orbital rim is detached to facilitate the procedure, then replaced. *D,* In this technique the entire lateral wall has been resected. A portion of the roof and floor of the orbit has also been resected to ensure complete eradication of the tumor. *E,* The temporalis muscle is sutured to the soft tissues around the exenterated orbital cavity. *F,* A split-thickness skin graft is sutured over the muscle. (From Webster, J. P.: Temporalis muscle transplants for defects following orbital exenteration. Trans. Internatl. Soc. Plast. Surg. © 1957, The Williams & Wilkins Company, Baltimore.)

be observed for a possible recurrence. This decision will also depend upon the type and size of the tumor.

Preservation of the eyelids to act as flaps for the repair (Spaeth, 1948) will decrease the size of the area to be grafted, but this technique offers no significant cosmetic benefit and introduces some technical difficulties, because the suture line for the graft falls within the orbit rather than at the rim.

Forehead and scalp flaps can be used to decrease the depth of the defect and afford a stable cover. Thomson (1970) reviewed the literature on repair techniques while introducing an ipsilateral forehead-scalp flap. Campbell (1948, 1954) reported the use of the temporalis muscle to reconstruct orbital and maxillary defects after resection for cancer. Naquin (1956) and Webster (1957) suggested the use of a temporalis muscle flap resurfaced by a skin graft (Fig. 28–49). Bakamjian and Souther (1975) have described a technique for the transfer of the muscle into the orbital cavity. A wide scalp flap is raised from the temporal fascia. After exposing the temporal region, the temporal fascia is incised along the entire temporal ridge down to the bone. The muscle is freed subperiosteally, and the attachments of the temporal fascia to the lateral and medial edges of the zygomatic arch are divided. If care is taken to avoid injuring the deep temporal branches of the internal maxillary artery, the coronary process may also be severed in order to provide additional mobility to the muscle flap.

The objections common to all of these flap techniques are (1) potential masking of tumor recurrence and (2) additional deformity in the donor area.

When an extended operation unroofs structures such as dura, the base of the skull, or an accessory sinus, a skin flap will afford the safest cover for the additional defect. A local flap of forehead or scalp is preferred, as the excellent blood supply affords the opportunity for immediate transfer. The flap is returned to the donor area in a second operation, leaving behind sufficient subcutaneous tissue to accept a split-thickness skin graft. With this technique, the deformity of the exposed donor site is minimized, and the grafted area lies under the prosthesis.

Flap reconstruction of the eyelids and orbit to accommodate a standard type of enucleation prosthesis has not been satisfactory, and the cosmetic results certainly do not justify the procedure, even if one could be certain that the tumor were completely eradicated. Modern prosthetic techniques afford cosmetic results far superior to those obtainable with present methods of surgical reconstruction, and a prosthesis is readily removed for early detection of recurrent tumor (see Chapter 67).

Recurrence. Careful preoperative evaluation for resectability and wide removal of the initial tumor offer the best opportunity for local cure, but when radical surgery is performed for highly malignant tumors, a significant recurrence rate is unavoidable. Radiation offers little benefit to patients with persistent tumor. Local recurrence of the tumor requires prompt surgical excision if any chance for cure can still be hoped for.

Complications. Hematoma and bone infection must be prevented. Immediate repair of the defect has greatly reduced the feared complication of osteomyelitis. When wound infection is encountered, prompt drainage and vigorous antibiotic therapy are required. Careful hemostasis and an effective dressing should prevent significant hematoma formation.

Large losses of graft tissue, from any cause, will require secondary grafting once the wound is covered by healthy granulation tissue. Small residual defects, however, can be expected to heal without further grafting. Frequent change of normal saline compresses helps keep the wound clean in preparation for regrafting or while final healing is taking place.

The deformity produced by exenteration is severe. Psychologic preparation of the patient is both necessary and rewarding. Naquin (1956), in reviewing 48 cases of exenteration, reported one case in which postoperative depression was severe enough to require psychiatric care. He also reported one case of persistent postoperative trigeminal neuralgia which required surgery.

The Intracranial Approach for Tumors Involving the Anterior Cranial Fossa. The intracranial approach affords the only means of total eradication of a tumor transgressing the orbital roof or involving the cranial fossa (see Chapter 64).

ECTROPION

JOHN MARQUIS CONVERSE, M.D., AND BYRON SMITH, M.D.

The term ectropion denotes an outward turning or eversion of the eyelid margin. It may vary in degree from the mild eversion of a portion of the lid to a total eversion of the entire lid. This latter occurrence is more frequent in the lower lid because of the smaller size of the tarsal plate; in the upper lid, the eyelid is turned inside out only when a considerable amount of skin has been destroyed.

Congenital ectropion is a rare condition. It results from a deficiency of tissue in the outer layers of the eyelids, causing an outward turning of the lid margin. *Acute spastic ectropion* is seen in exophthalmos. The backward pull of the orbicularis oculi muscle tends to evert the eyelid margin. *Senile ectropion* results from loss of muscle tone in the orbicularis oculi muscle and a resulting elongation of the eyelid; it is usually accompanied by epiphora. The conjunctiva becomes hyperemic and hypertrophic and may become keratinized. *Paralytic ectropion* is the result of loss of function of the orbicularis oculi muscle in facial paralysis. The eyelid tends to fall away from the eye, and epiphora is the frequent accompaniment of this condition. Exposure of the cornea may lead to the serious complication of ulcerations. *Cicatricial ectropion* is caused by loss of tissue in the outer layer of the eyelid as a result of trauma, most frequently thermal burns.

Spastic and Senile Ectropion. Spastic ectropion usually requires no treatment other than the relief of the causative pathologic state—for example, exophthalmos.

The Kuhnt-Szymanowski type of operation has been useful in the past in the treatment of senile ectropion. The lid is split into two layers, a deeper tarsoconjunctival layer and a superficial layer consisting of the skin and orbicularis oculi muscle. The lid is shortened by removing a wedge from the tarsoconjunctival layer, the width of the wedge being that amount that will bring the lid into firm contact with the globe when the tarsal edges are approximated. A skin incision is then made upward and laterally from the lateral canthus for a distance of about 15 to 20 mm. The skin is drawn laterally and a triangle of excessive skin resected. The main complications of this technique are entropion and trichiasis caused by splitting of the lid along its margin.

In extreme cases of senile ectropion, it may be necessary to perform a similar operation and also to excise a wedge from the orbicularis oculi muscle in order to remove the excess of distended muscle and thus tighten it.

Several methods are available for the correction of ectropion of the medial half of the lower lid. The degree of the deformity and the expe-

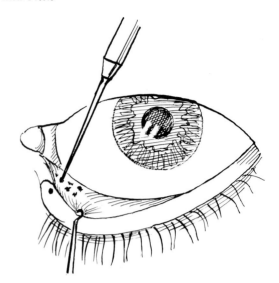

FIGURE 28–50. Technique of punctate cauterization of the inner layers of the medial portion of the lower lid for the correction of senile ectropion.

rience of the surgeon dictate the selection of the most desirable means of management.

Minimal ectropion of the punctum of the lower lid may be tolerated without sufficient symptoms to justify surgical correction. Cauterization of the internal layers of the lower lid is an uncontrolled method which has been employed for several decades (Fig. 28–50). It has met with some success in the hands of experienced surgeons. Likewise, horizontal resection of tissues inferior to the lower canaliculus has limited indications. In more severe deformities in which there is a need for both horizontal and vertical shortening of the lid, neither of the above methods provides sufficient countermeasures to produce the desired result.

The "Lazy T" Method of Treatment (Smith, 1975). The "lazy-T" method of vertical and horizontal correction has been employed by Smith for a number of years for the treatment of moderately severe ectropion. As the term "lazy-T" implies, the incision for this procedure takes the shape of a "T," with the horizontal bar lying inside the lower lid (Fig. 28–51).

The procedure may be done under local or general anesthesia. If local anesthesia is employed, the tissues should be distorted as little as possible by the injection. A lapse of 15 or 20 minutes between the injection and the start of surgery also allows time for some of the distortion from the local anesthetic solution to dissipate. If general anesthesia is used, this complication is eliminated.

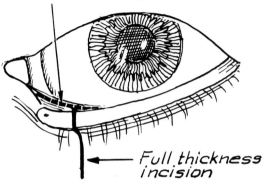

Incision through tarsus and conj.

Full thickness incision

FIGURE 28–51. The "lazy T" method. The incision is made in the form of a "T" with the horizontal bar inside the lower lid.

Technique. As indicated in Figure 28–52, *A*, fixation of the lid margin is maintained with forceps, and gentle traction pulls the lid into an accentuated position of ectropion. Using a razor knife, a horizontal incision is made below the level of the lower canaliculus. A lacrimal probe may be inserted into the lower canaliculus to identify the level of its location. The incision is made sufficiently deep to section the tarsoconjunctival layer of the lower lid and sufficiently long to allow for correction of the ectropion.

The inferior margin of the incision is undermined (Fig. 28–52, *B*, *C*) sufficiently to allow for adequate overlap of the incision when the margins are crisscrossed by two-forceps manipulation (Fig. 28–52, *D*, *E*). The amount of tissue to resect from the lower flap is calculated by this means. Only the amount of tissue to be resected is undermined, as the lower, undetached tissues assist in maintaining the correction.

When the horizontal resection of tissue has been achieved (Fig. 28–52, *F*), apposition of the wound edges corrects the vertical component of the deformity. The horizontal component remains. In Figure 28–52, *G*, a vertical incision lateral to the punctum is extended through all layers of the lower lid from the lid margin down into the depth of the lower fornix. This incision may be made with a sharp knife or with scissors. As shown in Figure 28–52, *H*, the two sections of the lower lid are then crisscrossed by means of two-forceps manipulation. Sufficient horizontal traction is applied to give an estimate of the dimensions of the marginal resection necessary to correct the horizontal component of the deformity. After

resection of the wedge of lower lid tissue, apposition of the wound margins should place the lower lid margin in an optimal position and establish contact of the lid with the globe.

Figure 28–52, *I*, *J* shows the closure of the initial, horizontal tarsoconjunctival incision with fine caliber, interrupted, absorbable sutures, such as plain catgut or Dexon. The vertical transmarginal incision is then closed as a lid laceration or wound (Fig. 28–52, *K*). This is usually done with 6–0 silk sutures. The initial suture is placed through the mouths of the meibomian glands. Traction upon this suture, or merely placing a needle in this area, aligns the lid margin in correct position to enable accurate placement of an anterior and a posterior marginal suture (Fig. 28–52, *L*). The anterior marginal suture is placed through ciliary exits.

Two buried muscle sutures are placed and tied (Fig. 28–52, *M*). The long ends of the middle and posterior marginal sutures are brought forward and held beneath the marginal suture at the eyelash (Fig. 28–52, *M*, *N*). This maneuver prevents the suture ends from floating into the palpebral fissure.

The remainder of the skin incision is closed with interrupted silk sutures (Fig. 28–52, *N*). Ointment is not applied, because it may seep into the wound and delay healing. A moderately compressive Telfa dressing is applied. The silk sutures may be removed in one week. After wound reaction subsides, the lid margin assumes a normal position, and the punctum is in contact with the lacrimal lake.

Paralytic Ectropion. In lagophthalmos due to facial paralysis, it is necessary to protect the cornea by means of a moist chamber, a patch at night, and adhesive tape support of the lower lid laterally. If the cornea needs additional protection, a number of surgical procedures can be employed. These are discussed in the chapter on facial paralysis (see Chapter 36).

Cicatricial Ectropion. Cicatricial ectropion is the result of the destruction of the skin of the eyelid and of the surrounding facial area. Cicatricial ectropion most frequently results from burns but also results from lacerations that have been improperly treated, from the excessive removal of skin in the excision of tumors, or following the removal of the skin in cosmetic operations on the eyelids (see Chapter 37). The treatment of cicatricial ectropion consists of readjustment of the displaced tissue or application of a skin graft to replace the destroyed skin.

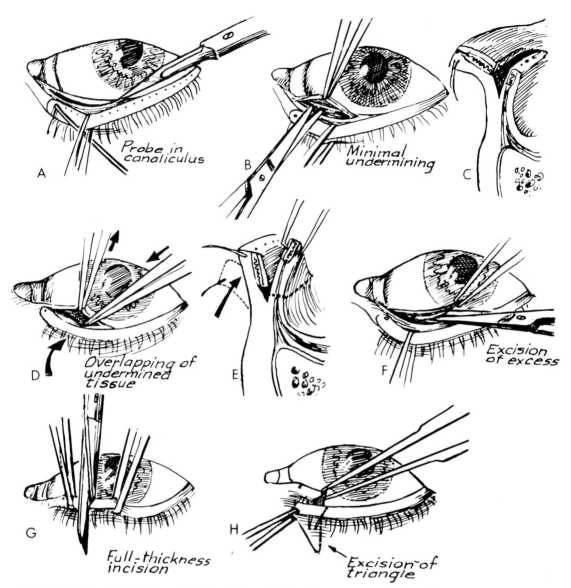

FIGURE 28–52. The technique of the "lazy T" method. *A*, A forceps everts the lower lid. A razor knife incises horizontally below the canaliculus. *B*, The inferior margin of the incision is undermined. *C*, Sagittal section demonstrating the depth of the undermining. *D*, The lower margin of the incision is overlapped over the anterior margin. *E*, Sagittal section illustrating the overlap. The dotted line indicates the line of resection. *F*, The excess tissue is resected. *G*, A vertical incision lateral to the punctum extends through all the layers of the lid down to the lower fornix. *H*, The two sections of the lid are criss-crossed and overlapped. As indicated by the dotted line, a triangle of excess tissue is resected.

The Z-plasty procedure will correct linear contractures causing ectropion. *Skin grafting is required to replace loss of skin.* Skin from the opposing or the contralateral upper lid is adequate for small defects—eversion of the lower punctum, for example. When more extensive skin loss occurs, especially following thermal burns, skin grafts from other donor areas are required. Split-thickness skin grafts are favored to correct ectropion of the upper lid, as the thinner skin allows the formation of the folds of the upper lid; the graft is removed from the medial aspect of the arm, the supraclavicular area (in the male patient), and any other suitable area. The lower lid requires a full-thickness graft to provide adequate support; the graft is removed, preferably from the retroauricular area or the supraclavicular area (in males).

Tarsorrhaphy is unnecessary and contrain-

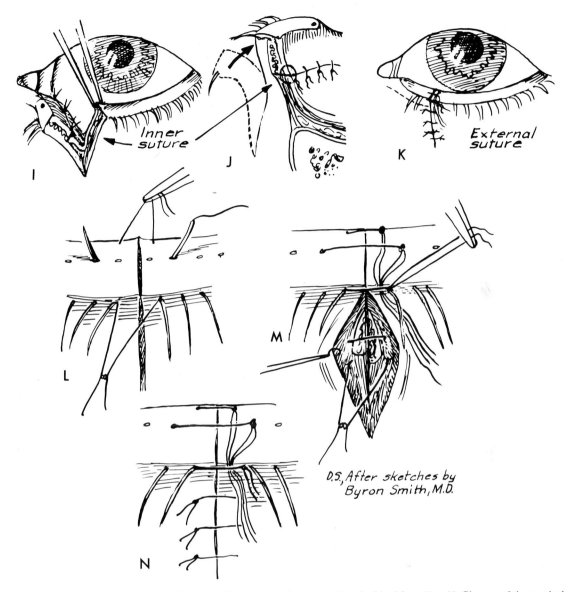

FIGURE 28–52 *Continued.* *I, J,* Closure of the horizontal tarsoconjunctival incision. *K* to *N,* Closure of the vertical transmarginal incision in the same fashion as a full-thickness transmarginal laceration (see Fig. 28–23).

dicated, as it deforms the eyelid margin and may lead to troublesome epithelization and corneal irritation.

Details concerning skin grafting of the eyelids for the correction of ectropion are described in Chapter 33.

Temporal Flap for Ectropion of the Lower Eyelid. In the repair of lower lid ectropion of long duration, particularly when tissue loss has occurred over the infraorbital margin, a skin graft may not be adequate. Bone may be exposed as a result of the destructive process

(Fig. 28–53, *A, B*) or after release of the lid from its ectropic position. A skin flap from the temporal area can be employed. A temporal flap transposition is shown in Figure 28–54. In ectropion of the lower lid uncorrected for a long period of time, the lid margin has become elongated; the conjunctiva has hypertrophied and is occasionally ulcerated. It is necessary to excise a section of the lid margin and tarsus in such cases to restore adequate horizontal lid dimension (Fig. 28–54, *C*). The secondary defect in the temporal region is closed by direct approximation.

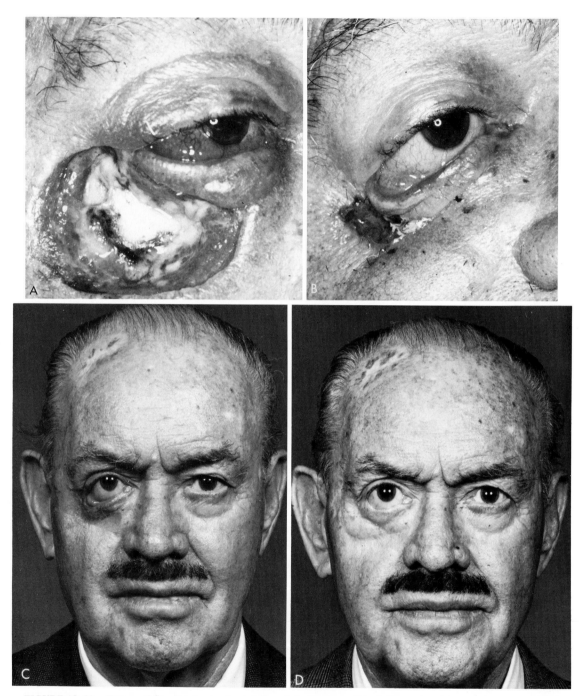

FIGURE 28–53.   Temporal flap for repair of ectropion of the lower eyelid. *A*, Extensive defect of the lower eyelid involving the rim of the orbit and a portion of the zygoma, as well as the cheek skin. *B*, After spontaneous healing of the wound. Note the severe contraction and downward displacement of the lateral canthus. *C*, A full-thickness skin graft was employed to relieve the ectropion of the lower lid but was not adequate to correct the deformity. *D*, The temporal flap illustrated in Figure 28–54 was employed to complete reconstruction.

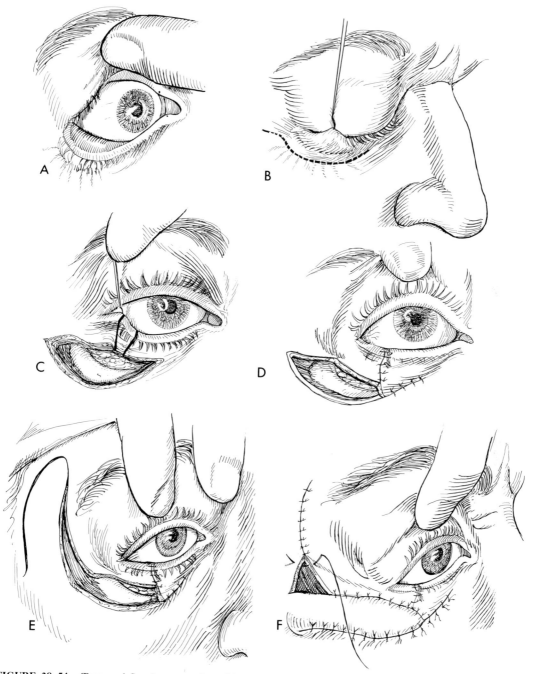

FIGURE 28–54. Temporal flap for correction of lower eyelid ectropion. *A*, Ectropion of the lower eyelid resulting from the defect shown in Figure 28–53. As a result of longstanding ectropion, the lid was elongated in its horizontal dimension. *B*, Outline of the incision. *C*, Excision of a full-thickness section of the lid to diminish the horizontal dimension. *D*, After suture of the eyelid margin. *E*, Outline of the temporal flap. *F*, The temporal flap is in position, and the temporal defect is closed by direct approximation.

ENTROPION

Entropion is an inward turning of the lid margin and the lashes against the cornea; the friction of the lashes against the cornea causes irritation. In contrast, in trichiasis the lashes only are turned in, and the lid margins are in normal position.

Primary or congenital entropion of the lower lid is rare and is due either to lack of a normal tarsal plate or to hypertrophy of the marginal fibers of the orbicularis oculi muscle. The condition is progressive and involves the whole of the lower lid margin. Surgical correction is almost always necessary. Eversion of the lid may be accomplished by excision of skin and hypertrophied orbicularis muscle fibers (Fox, 1956).

Secondary entropion results from the lack of lid support, from a small or absent ocular globe, or from backward pressure on the ciliary margin by an excess fold of skin, as in epiblepharon. A frequent cause of secondary entropion is scarring of the conjunctiva or the subconjunctiva, which pulls on the lid margin and causes a bowing of the tarsus. Correction of this condition is achieved by a number of methods using either the skin or the conjunctival approach. The tarsoconjunctival wedge operation and its modifications (see Fig. 28–55) have been successful.

Cicatricial entropion or inversion of the lid differs from the spasmodic or degenerative type; although traumatic entropion may involve both the upper and lower eyelids, the noncicatricial type is usually limited to the lower eyelid.

Two types of cicatricial entropion occur. The lid margin may be uninjured in the first type; owing to the loss of conjunctiva, however, adhesions of the lid to the globe cause the inversion, and the entropion is thus secondary to symblepharon. Inversion and distortion of the lid margin are due to scarring in the second type. In this condition, some of the eyelashes are turned in, and trichiasis, contact of the eyelashes with the globe and cornea, results. The eyelashes are normally inserted into the outer portion of the lid margin and sweep outward and upward. Entropion is a turning in of the lid margin; the eyelashes in this process may or may not contact the eyelid. Trichiasis may be present without true entropion, whereas entropion and trichiasis may be present together. The direction of the base of the hair follicle and the shaft of the hair may be changed owing to injury; thus the eyelash, instead of being directed outward, may be directed inward, resulting in trichiasis. Trichiasis may also result from scarring of the inner aspect of the eyelid margin and is not an infrequent complication after reconstructive operations on the eyelids.

The treatment of entropion due to symblepharon requires the correction of the symblepharon in a first stage by releasing the adhesions between the globe and the lid. The treatment of symblepharon is considered later in this chapter. Correction of entropion is nec-

essary in a second stage if entropion persists after the relief of symblepharon.

The Wedge Operation. This operation (Fig. 28–55) utilizes the principle of introducing a composite wedge of tarsus and conjunctiva into an incision made along the inner margin of the lid in order to produce an eversion of the lid margin and correct the entropion (Fig. 28–55).

The tarsoconjunctival graft is removed from the inner aspect of the lid near the upper portion of the tarsus, the lid being everted by an Erhardt clamp (Fig. 28–55, *B*, *C*). The donor area of the graft may be left to epithelize spontaneously. An incision is made at the inner aspect of the upper lid margin immediately behind the inverted eyelashes (Fig. 28–55, *D*). The incision is extended upward at an angle of 45 degrees to avoid injuring the base of the eyelash hair follicles (Fig. 28–55, *E*). The oblique incision also permits rotation of the eyelid margin. The wedge, consisting of the composite graft of conjunctiva and tarsus, is inserted into the incision near the lid margin to maintain the corrected position (Fig. 28–55, *F* to *I*).

Epilation for Trichiasis. Isolated eyelashes in contact with the bulbar conjunctiva often resist conservative treatment. In such cases, the hair follicles of the offending eyelashes are destroyed by either electrolysis or excision of the tissue containing the eyelashes.

When only a few eyelashes deviate from the normal direction and contact the cornea, electrolysis or diathermy may suffice to destroy the hair follicles of the misdirected lashes. The needle is inserted along the shaft of the eyelash, and a very weak current is employed for one or two seconds. The eyelash is then pulled out with a cilia forceps without removing the needle. If the eyelash is not loosened, the electric current is again applied for a longer time with more intensity. Failure to loosen the eyelash may be due to misdirection of the needle. Reinsertion of the needle may be necessary. The lash can be removed by simple brushing with a cotton-tipped applicator if the hair root is properly coagulated. This treatment has limitations, because it is impossible to remove a number of eyelashes in close proximity to each other without risking necrosis of the eyelid margin. In such cases, it is advisable to complete electrolysis in multiple stages.

Surgery is often the simplest method for the removal of misdirected eyelashes and is particularly applicable in the lower lid.

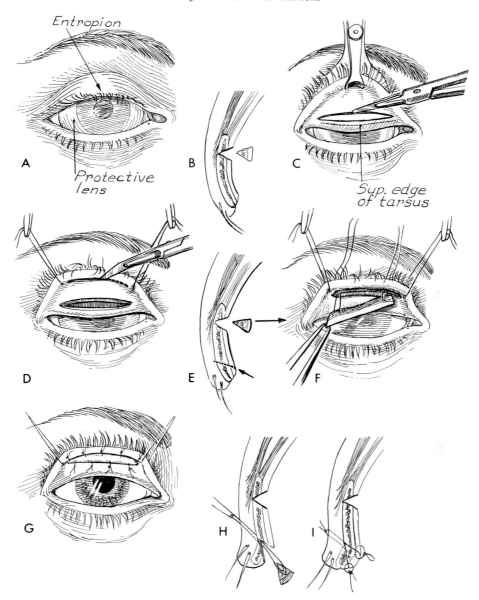

FIGURE 28–55. Tarsal wedge technique for the correction of entropion. *A,* Protective lens is placed in the conjunctival sac. *B,* A wedge of tarsus is excised from the donor site. *C,* The lid is everted on an Erhardt clamp. A wedge of tarsus and conjunctiva approximately 2 mm in width is excised. *D,* The incision is made parallel to the posterior marginal edge directly behind the area of the offending lashes. *E,* The dotted line indicates the direction of the incision. *F,* The tarsal wedge is placed into the recipient site. *G,* The tarsal wedge has been sutured into position with fine catgut sutures. *H, I,* Sagittal section depicting the position of the graft of tarsoconjunctiva wedged into the recipient bed. (After B. Smith and Cherubini, 1970.)

SYMBLEPHARON

Chemical burns are a frequent cause of symblepharon, a rare condition in flash and fire burns. Lacerations extending through the lid, conjunctival cul-de-sac, and sclera, if inadequately repaired, also result in symblepharon. The raw areas of the globe and the inner surface of the lid, when healed, are fused by a cicatricial band. The entire inner surface of the lid may adhere to the globe in extensive symblepharon, whereas in less extensive cases the adhesions may involve only a portion of the lid joined to the globe by a cicatricial band. In the latter type, correction of symblepharon may frequently be accomplished by a Z-plasty (Fig. 28–56). When the adhesion between the eyelid and the globe extends over a wider surface, after the adhesion is freed, the adjacent conjunctiva may be raised and advanced over the raw area, covering the scleral defect with a conjunctival graft (Fig. 28–57). Preserved scleral allografts have been used successfully to repair defects in this area.

Conjunctival Flap from the Opposing Eyelid. The conjunctiva of the upper lid is a source of supply for extensive cases of symblepharon of the lower lid. The technique consists of freeing the lower lid from the globe (Fig. 28–58, *A*). After this procedure, a horizontal incision is made through the conjunctiva 4 mm above the upper lid margin. The conjunctiva of the upper lid is undermined freely, advanced, and maintained in position in the depth of the fornix by a mattress suture with the ends brought out through the skin (Fig. 28–58, *B*); the lids are held in apposition by a continuous to and fro suture. After healing is completed, the lids and flap are separated (Fig. 28–58, *C*).

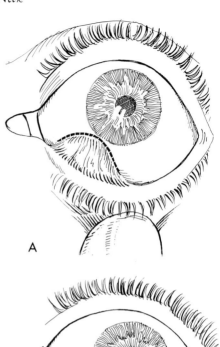

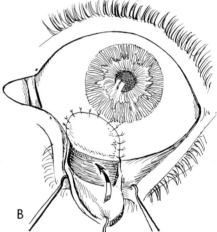

FIGURE 28–57. Correction of symblepharon. *A*, Freeing of an adhesion between the eyelid and the ocular globe. The scarred tissue over the sclera is employed to provide lining for the lower lid. *B*, The scleral defect is covered by a conjunctival graft.

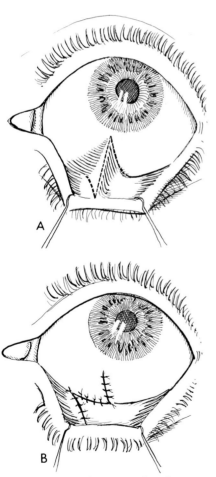

FIGURE 28–56. Z-plasty procedure for correction of symblepharon.

Conjunctival or Mucosal Grafts. A small conjunctival defect can be repaired by a graft of conjunctiva removed from the opposing eyelid of the same eye or from an eyelid of the other eye (Fig. 28–59). Mucosa is obtained from the buccal wall of the oral cavity when a larger surface is required.

Transplantation of a thin split-thickness skin graft, although a simpler method, should not be employed because friction of the dermoepidermal graft against the eyeball and cornea causes irritation, leading to keratoconjunctivitis or even more serious sequelae.

Sections of mucosa as large as 1.5 × 5 cm are removed from the buccal wall (Fig. 28–60). The tissue is preferably taken from the vicinity

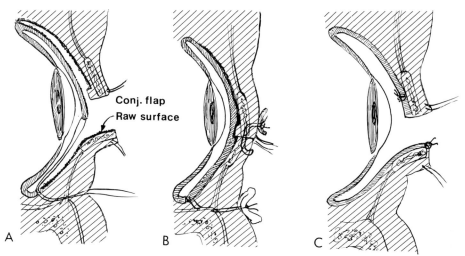

FIGURE 28–58. Conjunctival flap for the correction of symblepharon. *A*, The conjunctiva is outlined in sagittal section on the upper lid; the defect in the lower lid is also outlined. *B*, The upper lid flap has been advanced into the lid defect, and the lids are held together by occlusive sutures. *C*, After healing, the occlusive sutures are removed, the flap is cut, and the palpebral fissure is opened.

of the lower portion of the cheek wall below the parotid duct; the looseness and elasticity of the mucosa in this region permit the direct approximation of the donor area. The graft is spread over a wet-gloved finger, and the submucosal tissue is removed with scissors. A split-thickness mucosal graft may also be removed by means of the Castroviejo electric mucotome (Fig. 28–61).

In extensive symblepharon, a wide area of the conjunctival surface of the eyelid and of the sclera must be covered, and the conjunctival cul-de-sac must be reestablished. After obtaining the graft of oral mucosa, the scar tissue is resected and the fornix is extended to the periosteum of the infraorbital margin. The graft is then sutured to the edges of the conjunctival and scleral defect (Fig. 28–62).

The lower margin of the graft is anchored with through-and-through sutures to assure the depth of the conjunctival fornix (Fig. 28–62). The infraorbital margin should be exposed and the graft applied against it in order to assure further the depth of the conjunctival cul-de-sac. If more positive fixation is needed in the fornix, silicone tubing is used to maintain the graft in the depth of the fornix (Fig. 28–62, *A*). A doughnut type of scleral lens can also be

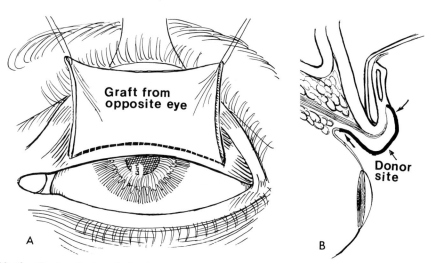

FIGURE 28–59. Conjunctival graft for the correction of symblepharon. *A*, Outline of graft from the upper lid. *B*, Sagittal view illustrating the position of the donor site on the upper lid.

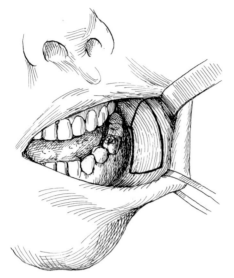

FIGURE 28–60. Area of the buccal mucosa from which a full-thickness mucous membrane graft may be removed. The graft is usually made thinner by trimming the undersurface with scissors.

placed in the cul-de-sac (Fig. 28–62, *B*). This type of lens is an ordinary scleral lens from which the corneal part has been removed (see Fig. 28–64).

PTOSIS OF THE UPPER EYELID

Ptosis of the upper eyelid, or blepharoptosis, refers to the abnormally low level of the upper eyelid during fixation with the involved eye. During normal downward gaze, the upper eyelid follows the excursion of the eye downward. When this fails to occur, the condition is referred to as lagophthalmos (lid lag).

According to Rycroft (1962), until 1811 ptosis of the upper eyelid was treated by the excision of skin alone, after the fashion of the ancient Arabian surgeons. Even Scarpa at that time used this time-honored technique. Von Graefe, however, no doubt influenced by the teachings of his father and Dieffenbach, felt that a strip of orbicularis oculi muscle should also be excised. There is no doubt that on his trips to London and Ireland von Graefe must have spoken of this technique. Bowman (1859), who was his friend, used the technique on several occasions but clearly was not completely satisfied with it.

Methods for the correction of ptosis, a drooping of the upper eyelid as a result of insufficient levator muscle action or stretching of the levator aponeurosis (in congenital exophthalmos, such as in craniofacial dysostosis), or of absence of muscle function, differ.

If levator muscle function is present, various operations have been devised, originating from de Blaskovics' operation (1923), to shorten the levator and the tarsus through a conjunctival approach. If levator muscle function is absent, suspension of the upper eyelid to the active frontalis muscle is the most commonly employed procedure. The authors have abandoned the technique of using the superior rectus muscle in the treatment of ptosis, be-

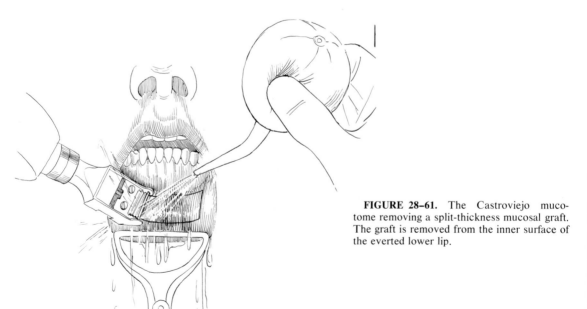

FIGURE 28–61. The Castroviejo mucotome removing a split-thickness mucosal graft. The graft is removed from the inner surface of the everted lower lip.

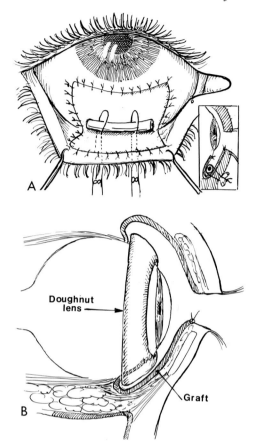

FIGURE 28–62. Relief of symblepharon by a mucosal graft. *A,* The graft has been sutured over the raw surface of the sclera and lower eyelid. Position of mucosal graft and polyethylene tubing maintaining the depth of the cul-de-sac (sagittal section). *B,* The cul-de-sac can also be maintained by a fenestrated scleral lens.

cause the other means of treatment are more effective and accompanied by fewer complications. The best results are obtained by suturing or shortening the levator muscle.

Principles of Operative Treatment of Congenital and Acquired Ptosis. The results of surgery for ptosis depend on three factors: the nature of the ptosis, the type of operation selected, and the skill with which the operation is done (Berke, 1949, 1952, 1957, 1959, 1962). The best cosmetic and functional results in congenital or acquired ptosis are achieved by resection of the levator, provided the levator muscle action is adequate.

Before deciding what type of operation is indicated, one must make three important observations: measurement of the amount of levator action; a notation of the position of the normal lid with respect to its cornea in the primary position; and an appraisal of the position of the normal upper lid fold.

1. MEASURING LEVATOR ACTION. Measuring the levator action of the ptotic lid is best done by placing a millimeter ruler over the lid with one hand and then noting the amount of elevation of the lid, from a position of looking down to a position of looking up, while immobilizing the brow with the thumb of the other hand. This maneuver should be repeated several times until the excursion of the lid is the same on two or more tests while the head is held stationary.

Smith (1974) uses the retinoscope as a means of studying the relationship of the upper lid margin to the pupil. He also requests eating or gum chewing as part of the examination to detect the presence of the jaw-winking phenomenon. The position of the cornea is examined during forced closure of the lids by opening the lids passively during voluntary forced closure of the eyes. The position of the cornea during this act helps to disclose the position of the eye during sleep. It is encouraging to find that the eyes drift upward because the position affords better coverage of the cornea during sleep in the presence of various degrees of lagophthalmos commonly seen in postoperative ptosis cases. Hypotropia may influence the position of the cornea during this test.

Isaksson and Johanson (1962) considered that, among the methods for studying levator muscle function, electromyography was the best. The amount of levator action will determine whether resection of the levator is indicated and, if so, where the ptotic lid should be placed at the time of operation. Thus, if the levator action is only 3 mm or less, 50 to 90 per cent of these lids will be undercorrected following resection of the levator, even though the ptosis is intentionally overcorrected at the time of operation. If, however, the levator action measures over 4 mm, resection of the levator should give a satisfactory result in over 60 per cent of the cases, that is, not more than 1 mm of overcorrection or undercorrection.

2. POSITION OF THE NORMAL LID. The position of the normal lid before operation and that of the ptotic lid at the end of operation must be estimated with the cornea in the primary position. The estimated placement of the ptotic lid at the end of operation, as shown in Table 28–1, is designed to produce 1 mm or less of overcorrection. This is advisable because it is easier to remedy overcorrection than undercorrection. Overcorrection can be cured by a partial tenotomy or a recession of the levator, whereas undercorrection requires a second resection of the levator (provided the

TABLE 28–1. *Placement of Ptotic Lid for Various Amounts of Levator Action in*
Congenital Monocular Ptosis When Normal Lid Covers Cornea 2 to 3 mm
and the External Approach Is Used

AMOUNT OF LEVATOR ACTION	PTOTIC LID SHOULD COVER CORNEA	EXPECTED POSTOPERATIVE LIFT	FALL	EXPECTED OVERCORRECTION OR UNDERCORRECTION
2–3 mm	0 mm	0 mm	2–3 mm	Under 1–2 mm
4–5 mm	1–2 mm	0 mm	0–1 mm	Over 0–1 mm
6–7 mm	2–3 mm	0–1 mm	0 mm	Over 0–1 mm
8–9 mm	3–4 mm	2–3 mm	0 mm	Over 0–1 mm
10–11 mm	6 mm	4–5 mm	0 mm	Over 0–2 mm

From Berke, R. A.: Plastic and Reconstructive Surgery of the Eye and Adnexa. Washington, Butterworth & Company, 1962.

levator action is adequate) under less favorable conditions, namely abnormal tissue planes and scar tissue induced by the first operation. The dangers of overcorrection are keratopathy, corneal opacity, ulceration, and possible eventual perforation.

The position of the normal lid with respect to the cornea must be noted before operation, because this position represents the point at which the ptotic lid should rest after operation when healing is complete. The position of the normal lid also serves as a useful guide as to where the ptotic lid should rest at the conclusion of the operation. If the cornea on the ptotic side is turned up (as it usually is under general anesthesia), the globe must be rotated downward to the primary position manually in order to place the lid at the correct position decided on before operation. Thus, an accurate determination of the normal position of the nonptotic lid is a necessary preoperative observation in avoiding postoperative overcorrection or undercorrection.

3. THE UPPER LID SUPRATARSAL FOLD. The position and contour of the normal upper lid fold are also important preoperative observations, because they indicate where the skin incision should be made in the ptotic lid in order to cause the ptotic upper lid fold to match that of the normal side after operation.

In most children the normal upper lid fold is 4 or 5 mm above the lashes in the midline, being 1 or 2 mm closer to the lashes in its temporal and nasal extremities. Therefore, the skin incision should be made to conform to this curve—that is, the two ends of the skin incision should usually be closer to the lashes at the extremities than in the midline of the lid. In a few patients the normal lid fold may blend with the palpebro-orbital fold, which usually is 10 to 18 mm above the lashes, to create a high upper fold matching that on the normal side.

In bilateral ptosis, the upper lid fold can be placed anywhere above the lashes, provided both folds are placed at the same distance from the lashes.

When the levator action is 2 mm or less in congenital ptosis, undercorrection is the rule, because in such cases the levator tissue will usually be found to be too thin and delicate to support the lid. In this situation one must resort to suspending the ptotic lid from the brow.

SURGICAL TREATMENT OF ACQUIRED BLEPHAROPTOSIS

The surgical treatment of acquired ptosis is a more complex matter because this type of ptosis has so many different causes. Nevertheless, experience has demonstrated that resection of the levator is the operation of choice in acquired ptosis when levator activity is more than 2 mm. Therefore, this operation is indicated in incomplete paralysis of the third nerve, in ptosis secondary to blepharochalasis, in chronic progressive external ophthalmoplegia, in Horner's syndrome, in ptosis following enucleation, in ptosis associated with hemangioma or neurofibromatosis of the lid, in juvenile or senile hereditary ptosis, and in ptosis following trauma to the levator.

In most of the acquired ptoses, postoperative overcorrection is the rule, unless the ptosis is adequately corrected at the time of operation. In some of these patients, exposure keratitis occurs after operation, especially in adults with paralysis of the superior rectus muscle or absence of Bell's phenomenon. However, exposure keratitis is seldom a serious complication if the lower lid is pulled up to cover the cornea during sleep.

Primary and Late Primary Repair of Traumatic Ptosis

It is essential to determine the cause of ptosis of the upper eyelid. Is it due to transection, actual destruction or fibrosis of the levator palpebrae superioris muscle, or paralysis of the levator muscle secondary to third nerve injury? In compound fractures involving the roof of the orbit and the supraorbital region, detached fragments of bone may extend downward, pressing on the levator mechanism and interfering with the raising of the lid. Some severe injuries with loss of bone in the region of the orbital rim may result in ptosis by herniation of the brain down over the eyeball. In other injuries, a loss of bone in the region of the floor of the frontal sinus with infection and hypertrophic granulations in the frontal sinus may cause a tumorlike mass to press downward on the upper eyelid, also causing ptosis.

True ptosis of the upper eyelid must be distinguished from pseudoptosis, which is seen in blowout fractures when the downward position of the eyeball increases the supratarsal fold and gives an illusion of ptosis (see Chapter 25).

In some levator injuries, no levator function can be demonstrated in the period immediately after the injury, but over a period of weeks and months the function improves rapidly. These patients still require levator repair, but such repair can be performed with better results once the nerve has recovered its conduction. Furthermore, the delay allows the healed tissues to soften, so that it is easier to identify the levator.

In all deep transverse lacerations of the upper eyelid, it is essential to verify the integrity of the levator palpebrae superioris muscle. If the patient cannot raise his upper lid for reasons other than edema, primary suture of the severed levator aponeurosis should be considered. In the early stages after injury, this may be difficult to determine because of edema.

The levator is frequently involved in injuries to the lid, especially in automobile accidents in which glass cuts are frequent, and also in injuries from various types of machinery. In addition, the opportunity for primary repair of the levator is frequently missed by the surgeon at the time of injury. In many instances, this is because the lid injury may be minimal in comparison to other injuries that the patient has sustained and is therefore given secondary consideration. Furthermore, the repair is often made by a general surgeon who frequently forgets that the levator aponeurosis lies directly superficial to the conjunctiva, and this is the region in which the most care must be taken. He tends to suture the skin, and perhaps even repair lacerations of the tarsus, but may neglect the levator itself. In many instances, the surgeon who undertakes the primary repair must be forgiven, because the lid may frequently be so severely damaged that it is almost impossible to achieve adequate repair. Extensive swelling of the lids occurs even after very trivial injury and contributes to the difficulty of diagnosis and repair.

Suturing of a torn, lacerated, or avulsed levator muscle shortly after injury is difficult. Since the levator is a thin, broad muscle and its aponeurosis is fragile, the surgeon faces the difficult task of locating and identifying it in the presence of acute tissue injury, ecchymosis, and edema. When the lid is so severely injured that it is not possible to achieve adequate repair or when the ptosis is discovered weeks after the injury, it is advantageous to delay the surgery for a period of six months (Smith and Obear, 1967).

Local anesthesia is indicated when locating the proximal portion of the levator, as voluntary contractions by the patient during upward gaze are very helpful; regional anesthesia by blocking the frontal nerve is also helpful (see p. 923).

The operating microscope is useful in detecting remnants of the supratarsal fold. The external approach is the best method to expose the anterior surface of the levator. Careful dissection is necessary in lacerated lids, since the anatomy is distorted. The anterior surface of the tarsal plate is identified first by dissecting the lower skin flap and pretarsal orbicularis oculi muscle. The upper skin flap is dissected superficial to the unaffected levator aponeurosis and the closely associated septum orbitale. Posterior to the septum orbitale, orbital fat lies superficial to the levator muscle. The superior rectus muscle lies deep to the levator. Should it become impossible to identify the levator in the wound, the surgeon must then proceed with dissection and identification of the levator and its nasal or temporal anterior attachments. After this identification is accomplished, the dissection is extended superiorly and posteriorly until the levator is identified at the apex of the wound. The dissection is then continued on both sides of the laceration. When the anterior surface of the levator is exposed, the extent of the laceration is visible. The repair is done with 6–0 chromic catgut. Under ideal circumstances, the severed ends of the muscle are approximated into their normal anatomical relationships (Fig. 28–63). If tissue has been lost, surgical judgment dictates the positioning of sutures. The lid fold is closed with double-armed 6–0 silk sutures passed from the conjunctival surface through opposing skin edges and tied to restore the supratarsal fold.

The complication of a shortened superior conjunctival fornix sometimes necessitates use of a 0.2-mm split-thickness graft of oral mucous membrane. Postoperatively, the contour of the fornix is retained by a centrally perforated scleral contact transparent contact shell (Fig. 28–64). The shell is retained for approximately two weeks. The shells are available through most contact lens laboratories. Failure to use the shell in indicated cases may mean the difference between the failure and success of the operation.

Under no circumstances should the tarsus be resected as a means of ptosis correction. The tarsus is the main supporting structure of the upper lid; it is responsible for marginal contour and lash direction and acts as an an-

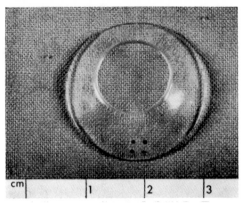

FIGURE 28–64. Contact fenestrated scleral shell for the fornix retention. The corneal portion of the shell has been removed to prevent corneal abrasion and encourage adequate drainage. The shell is inserted after the graft has been sutured in position.

chorage for muscular action. Ptosis correction in the presence of a resected tarsus is a difficult undertaking.

It should be noted that some lacerations of the levator muscle are complicated by retained foreign bodies, scleral injury, and superior rectus muscle trauma. If the laceration extends through the tarsus and the lid margin, the wound is firmly closed, as is done in a lid laceration. If the surgeon employs binocular loupes or an operating microscope and fine interrupted sutures, healing without deformity is assured.

The skin sutures are removed within three or four days. The marginal sutures should be left in position a week or longer, depending upon the amount of tension upon the wound. After the skin sutures have been removed, it is advisable to place a strip of paper tape across the wound horizontally to assure its protection during the following three or four days. Ordinarily it is not necessary to place an occlusive suture or to perform a tarsorrhaphy in the treatment of lid lacerations.

Levator Resection Operation for Ptosis

The Conjunctival Approach. In 1859, Bowman described the first resection of the levator aponeurosis through the conjunctiva. He everted the lid, excised the upper edge of the tarsus with slightly more than 1 cm of the levator, and sewed the two edges together. In 1923 de Blaskovics described another method for resection of the levator, in which the upper lid was everted on a lid retractor, the conjunctiva

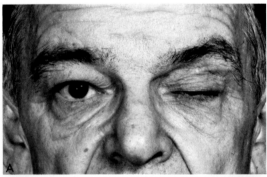

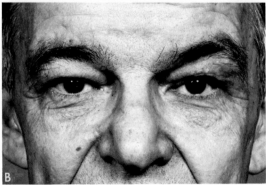

FIGURE 28–63. Late primary repair of traumatic blepharoptosis. *A,* A 50 year old man with traumatic laceration of the upper lid involving the levator palpebrae superioris muscle. *B,* The surgery was performed six months after the injury, utilizing an external approach with a 15-mm levator resection. The postoperative lid symmetry is excellent (Figs. 28–63 and 28–64 from Smith, B., and Obear, M. F.: Traumatic blepharoptosis. Surg. Clin. N. Am., *47*:515, 1967.)

was reflected upward, and 10 to 20 mm of the levator was excised, correcting to 4 to 8 mm of the ptosis. In 1952, Berke modified the Blaskovics procedure by completely freeing the levator attachment to gain additional correction. Later, Iliff (1954) simplified the operation further by excising the conjunctiva of the upper fornix along with the levator. These operations through the conjunctiva usually give excellent results only when the levator action is good.

The Cutaneous Approach. The first operation for resection of the levator through a skin incision was described by Eversbusch (1883). Many modifications of this original operation have been made. More levator tissue can be excised through the external route, and better results can be achieved when the levator action is poor. Berke (1959) attributed the better results obtained by the skin approach to greater exposure and to firmer anchorage of the transplanted levator to the tissues of the upper lid. Thus he concluded that the external approach is the method of choice when the levator action is poor but that either approach may be used when the levator action is good.

The Fasanella-Servat Operation and Its Modifications. The Fasanella-Servat operation was described in 1961. According to Fasanella (1973), the procedure is indicated only in instances of mild ptosis (1.5 to 2 mm) in which levator function is good and a satisfactory lid fold is present. Two exceptions to this rule are post-enucleation cases, in which 3 mm of ptosis can be corrected, and myogenic acquired ptosis, in which as much as 4 mm can be corrected. In *all* instances, levator function must be good or the operation will fail.

Present indications according to Fasanella are as follows: (1) bilateral congenital ptosis; (2) unilateral congenital ptosis; (3) ptosis following disease processes; (4) ptosis associated with Horner's muscle syndrome; (5) myogenic acquired senile ptosis; (6) ptosis following enucleation; (7) ptosis following orbital surgery; (8) ptosis following scar cicatrization; (9) ptosis following chronic conjunctivitis; (10) ptosis following incomplete ptosis repair; (11) ptosis following cataract extraction; (12) ptosis following repeated corneal transplantation; (13) ptosis following glaucoma procedures; (14) special situations.

ANESTHESIA. In most instances for adults and always for children, general anesthesia is preferred. If local anesthesia is decided upon, any of the usual solutions may be used, and one has a choice of three approaches:

1. A 4-cm needle (No. 22 or 23) is introduced precisely at the midpoint of the upper lid just below the bony orbital margin at some distance from the frontal nerve, reducing the chance of striking the vessels accompanying the nerve. The needle is gently passed directly posteriorly until it touches the curving roof of the orbit, is withdrawn slightly, and is advanced further until it again touches the roof. This is repeated until the entire length of the 4-cm needle has been inserted. Only a few milliliters of the solution is injected. The resulting anesthesia encompasses the entire upper lid except for a minimal area at the temporal or nasal extremities where sensory overlap may occur from adjacent nerves. The frontal region of the forehead is also blocked. Because of the sensory overlay, 0.5 ml of anesthetic solution is injected in the area of the supraorbital nerve and the same amount in the area of the lacrimal nerve.

2. A second choice is to inject under the skin just above the tarsal plate; approximately 1 ml can be used. To minimize bleeding, another 0.5 ml with norepinephrine is injected, using a No. 30 needle, through the conjunctiva of the everted lid just above the tarsal plate. The lid is returned to its normal position and massaged to help spread the solution. This is also an aid in permitting the forceps to grasp the tissues firmly and precisely without pain.

3. A third choice, advocated by Beard (1969), is to inject 1 ml of anesthetic solution with norepinephrine under the conjunctiva of the everted lid. Both Fasanella and Beard agree that this amount causes difficulty in applying the clamps. Beard adds 0.25 ml of the solution under the skin of the temporal area where the suture is to be buried.

TECHNIQUE. The eyelid is everted without the use of a Desmarre retractor or similar instrument, which will push the skin and subcutaneous tissues inward where they can be picked up in the bite of the hemostatic forceps. This avoids postoperative unwanted skin folds and "peaked" lids.

A selection of two thin, curved, hemostatic forceps and two straight forceps to match the variations of the tarsal plate should be available. Most tarsal plates have a "D" shape with an upward convexity, but a few are almost straight.

The height of the midportion of the adult tarsus is approximately 11 mm. The forceps are placed on the lower edge of the everted lid 3 mm or less from the everted upper border of the tarsus (Fig. 28–65, *A*). The forceps grasp the conjunctiva, tarsus, levator (or some thin ante-

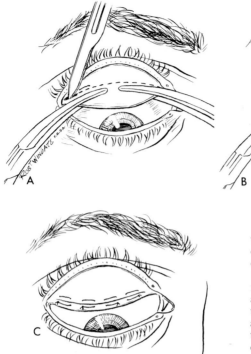

FIGURE 28–65. The Fasanella-Servat operation (1973). *A*, The eyelid is everted. *B*, Two thin, curved hemostatic forceps are placed on the lower edge of the everted lid 3 mm or less from the upper border of the tarsus. The first of the interrupted incisions is made. The interrupted incisions are extended in steps of 4 to 5 mm. A mattress suture is placed after each incision. *C*, The sutures are tied so as to hold the tissues firmly yet allow the lid to be returned to its normal position at the end of the procedure.

rior fibers of the levator 4 or 5 mm below the superior edge of the tarsus), and Müller's muscle. A question arises as to whether any of the fibers of the levator are grasped by the clamp. In any case, all loose tissues are held taut by the clamps.

Incisions are extended in steps of 4 to 5 mm, and a suture is placed after each incision (Fig. 28–65, *B*). These interrupted incisions minimize bleeding and serve as a safety factor in preventing retraction or loss of the levator. The sutures are tied tightly enough to hold the tissues firmly yet allow the lid to be returned to its normal position at the end of the procedure (Fig. 28–65, *C*). One should always avoid dog-ears and raggedness of the tarsal plate, which may cause corneal abrasion.

The sutures must be placed so that, at most, 3 mm of tarsus, 3 mm of levator and Müller's muscle, and 6 mm of conjunctiva can be excised and must be at a safe margin from the cut edge to avoid the risk of the sutures pulling out and causing postoperative bleeding. Reaching *too* high with the sutures may be another cause of the "peaked" lid.

Two 4–0 black silk sutures through the lower lid, the upper lid, and the brow are used with protective pieces of rubber bands or "cotton mosquitos." The sutures are tied just tightly enough to mold and hold the upper lid in a smooth, symmetrical curve matching the other side, if the contralateral side is normal.

Sodium sulfanilamide ointment is used generously. Vaseline gauze, a cotton eye pad slightly moistened on the inside, a second eye pad, and Elastoplast establish a firm monocular bandage. To control edema, ice is placed in a rubber glove, inserted into a stockinette, and affixed to the forehead. Systemic antibiotics may be used if desired. The patient may be discharged on the day of the operation or the next day if there is no pain. The two silk sutures are removed on the third or fourth day.

In the original Fasanella procedure (Fig. 28–65), four or five interrupted 5–0 to 6–0 sutures were placed, but owing to reports of corneal abrasions, especially after use of centrally

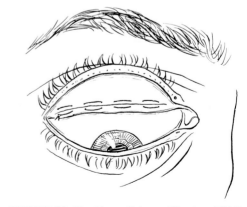

FIGURE 28–66. Fasanella's modification (1966) using a continuous suture, the knot being placed temporally.

placed knots (Fig. 28–65, *C*), Fasanella now recommends that such sutures be used *exclusively* for minimal ptosis following enucleations. In 1961 Fasanella pointed out that the danger of corneal damage could be averted by using a continuous suture with one knot tied temporally (Fig. 28–66) or a running serpentine suture (Fig. 28–67, *A*) followed by return as a continuous suture to the point of origin (Fig. 28–67, *B*).

Beard's modification (1969) is a running serpentine suture of 5–0 to 6–0 plain catgut (Lukens double-armed, gas sterilized). The suture is placed from the temporal to the nasal aspect, passing back and forth between the tarsal conjunctiva and the palpebral conjunctiva about 1 mm from the hemostats (Fig. 28–68, *A*); the tissue included in the hemostats is then excised, and the suture is returned to its point of origin in a running fashion, uniting the palpebral conjunctiva to the upper tarsal edge. A small skin incision is made in the upper eyelid fold over the temporal end of the operative site. Both ends of the suture are brought out

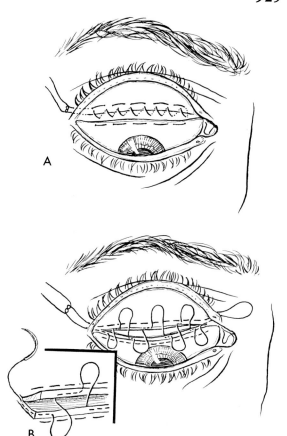

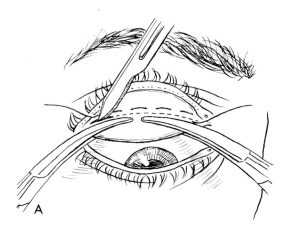

FIGURE 28–68. *A*, Beard's modification (1969). A running "serpentine" suture of 5–0 or 6–0 plain catgut is placed from the temporal to the nasal aspect about 1 mm from the hemostats; the suture passes back and forth between the tarsal conjunctiva and the palpebral conjunctiva. The tissue included in the hemostat is then excised, and the suture is returned to its point of origin as a running continuous suture uniting the palpebral conjunctiva to the upper tarsal edge. The ends of the suture are brought out through the skin in the temporal portion of the supratarsal fold and tied. By this modification, no knots touch the cornea or the sclera. *B*, Tensel's modification (1970) of the Beard suture. The return of the suture from medial to lateral is placed in the "subsubstance."

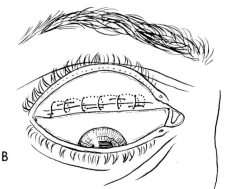

FIGURE 28–67. *A*, Fasanella's other alternate method of suturing in a running continuous or "serpentine" fashion. *B*, The running continuous or "serpentine" suture is returned, and the suture is tied on the temporal side.

through the incision and tied; the knot retracts beneath the skin. By this modification, no knots touch the cornea or sclera.

Tenzel (1970) suggested a modification of the Beard suture in that the return of the suture from medial to lateral be a "subsubstance" suture (Fig. 28–68, *B*).

Fasanella states that he presently uses the Beard suture as the procedure of choice, but he now prefers to make the incision along the crushed tissue held within the clamps, as suggested to him by Simington (1972). The crushing does not appear to devitalize the tissues; in chalazion surgery, the tarsus is crushed without ill effects.

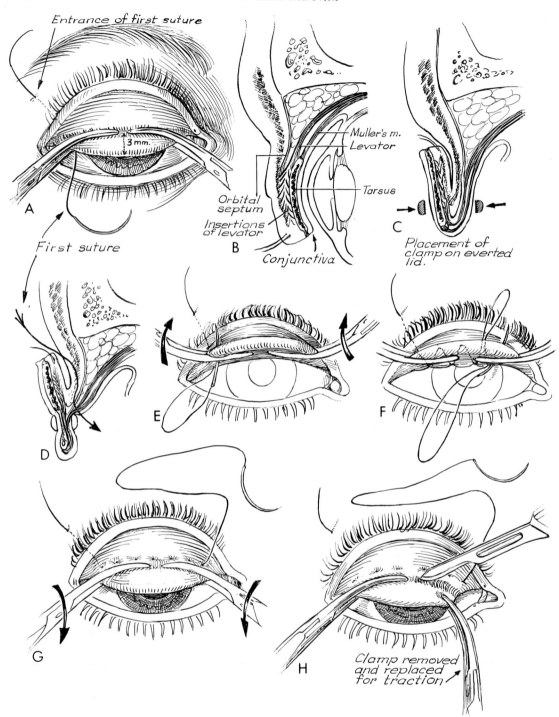

FIGURE 28–69. Smith's modification of the Fasanella-Servat operation. *A,* The lid is everted, and hemostats are placed 3 mm above the everted upper border of the tarsus. A suture is inserted, entering above the lateral canthus and exiting just about the clamp. *B,* Cross section illustrating the anatomy of the upper eyelid. *C,* The arrows indicate the position of the hemostat on the everted lid. *D,* Cross section illustrating the position of the lid after it has been everted and showing the tissues grasped by the hemostat: conjunctiva, tarsus, orbital septum, levator, Müller's muscle, and conjunctiva; the infolded skin and orbicularis muscle are avoided. *E,* The clamped portion of the lid is elevated, and suturing is begun. *F,* The suture is continued across the area held by the clamp. *G,* The suture is brought out through the conjunctiva beyond the clamped area. *H,* The clamp on the nasal side is removed and placed on the edge of the tarsus as a retractor. A scalpel makes a through-and-through incision into the crushed tissue left by the removed hemostat.

Illustration continued on opposite page

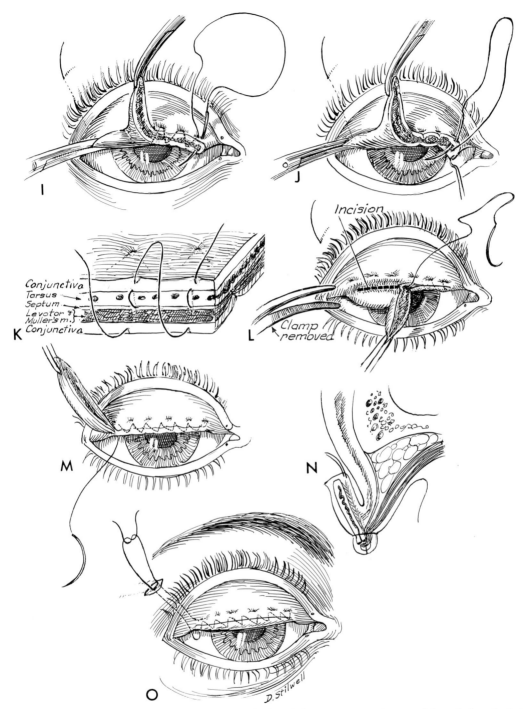

FIGURE 28–69 *Continued.* *I,* The incised tissue is raised, and the suture enters the wound through the subsubstance layer. *J, K,* The subsubstance suture extends laterally, picking up the fibers of the levator, Müller's muscle, and the septum orbitale in the lower bites. *L,* The lateral clamp is now removed, the through-and-through incision and suture continued laterally. *M,* The suture is continued to the lateral edge. *N,* Cross section showing the position of the sutures. *O,* The suture is brought out through an incision at the lateral end of the supratarsal fold and tied beneath the skin.

The Fasanella-Servat procedure using the Beard suture (1969) with the incision made along the crushed tissue, as recommended by Simington, is illustrated in Figure 28–68.

Smith (1974) also prefers the Beard suture but modifies it slightly by placing the through-and-through suture from the tarsal conjunctiva to the palpebral conjunctiva in such a way as to minimize the amount of suture material appearing on the conjunctival surface. For the same purpose he also uses the "subsubstance" sutures to close the raw edges, as suggested by Tenzel.

In the Smith modification, the lid is everted, and hemostats are placed 3 mm above the everted upper border of the tarsus (Fig. 28–69, *A*). Figure 28–69, *B* illustrates the anatomy of the eyelid. Figure 28–69, *C* shows the position of the hemostat on the everted lid. A suture is inserted, entering above the lateral canthus and exiting just above the clamp on the palpebral-conjunctival side (Fig. 28–69, *A, D*). The anatomy of the lid before and after it has been everted is shown in Figure 28–69, *A, D*. The clamp grasps conjunctiva, tarsus, orbital septum, levator, Müller's muscle, and again conjunctiva, avoided the in-folded skin and orbicularis muscle.

The clamped portion of the lid is elevated, and the suture is brought from the palpebral-conjunctival side to the tarsal side, above the clamp (Fig. 28–69, *E*). The suture is continued across the area held by the clamps (Fig. 28–69, *F*). Each entrance of the needle is placed as close to the last exit of the suture as possible, and the suture is angled to form a "V" to the opposite side. In this way, abrasion of the cornea by a large amount of suture material is avoided. Figure 28–69, *G* shows the minimal amount of suture material indented into the conjunctiva on the tarsal side.

The clamp on the nasal side is now removed and placed on the edge of the tarsus to act as a retractor. A through-and-through incision is made into the crushed tissue left after the removal of the hemostat (Fig. 28–69, *H*). The suture is brought out into the wound through the subcuticular layer (Fig. 28–69, *I*). The subcuticular suture is continued laterally, picking up the fibers of the levator, Müller's muscle, and septum in the lower bites (Fig. 28–69, *J, K*).

The lateral clamp is now removed and the through-and-through incision continued laterally along the bed of the clamp; a small area is left attached for traction purposes (Fig. 28–69, *L, M*). The subcuticular suture is continued to the lateral edge (Fig. 28–69, *M*). The

sagittal section (Fig. 28–69, *N*) shows the position of the suture. A stab incision is made at the site of the first entrance of the suture above the lateral canthus; the ends of the subcuticular suture are brought out through an incision at the lateral end of the supratarsal fold and are tied beneath the skin (Fig. 28–69, *O*).

Iliff uses three interrupted 4-0 black silk stay sutures (Fig. 28–70, *A*) instead of the interrupted sutures shown in Figure 28–65. These are temporary sutures which provide hemostasis and secure the tissue firmly. The tissues are excised and the hemostats removed (Fig. 28–70, *B*). A modified, completely buried, 6-0 chromic running suture is applied and knotted (Fig. 28–70, *C*). These bites are firm and buried and approximate raw edge to raw edge. They do not include the conjunctiva and cause no irritation to the cornea. At this stage the interrupted sutures shown in Figure 28–70, *B* are removed (Fig. 28–70, *D*). Iliff has added still another ingenious step; if he wants to achieve a "wee bit" more correction prior to applying the clamps to the tissues, he reaches high with several sutures through conjunctiva and levator, pulls these tissues toward the clamps, applies the clamps, and then proceeds with the operation as outlined by him. Iliff points out that, if one knows the anatomy of the levator palpebrae superioris muscle and its aponeurosis, one can by this maneuver contribute an additional lift.

There are three insertions of the levator (Fig. 28–70, *E*):

1. The main insertion is in the skin through fibers that cross the antagonist, the orbicularis. This insertion is marked by the superior palpebral sulcus. The accentuation of the superior palpebral fold with the eyes looking up is an index of levator function. This is one of the main conditions looked for in selecting cases for this operation.

2. Part of the levator is inserted in the anterior face of the tarsus at 4 or 5 mm below its superior edge, i.e., the superior third to half of the anterior face of the tarsus. The principal attachment to the tarsus is through the unstriped Müller's muscle, which attaches itself to the superior edge of the tarsus.

3. The third attachment of the levator is to the conjunctiva of the upper cul-de-sac via the fascial sheath of the muscle. There may be a similar attachment to the superior rectus.

Beard (1969) is of the opinion that the Fasanella-Servat operation is successful because of the tarsectomy. Putterman (1973) believes that the good results are due to resection and

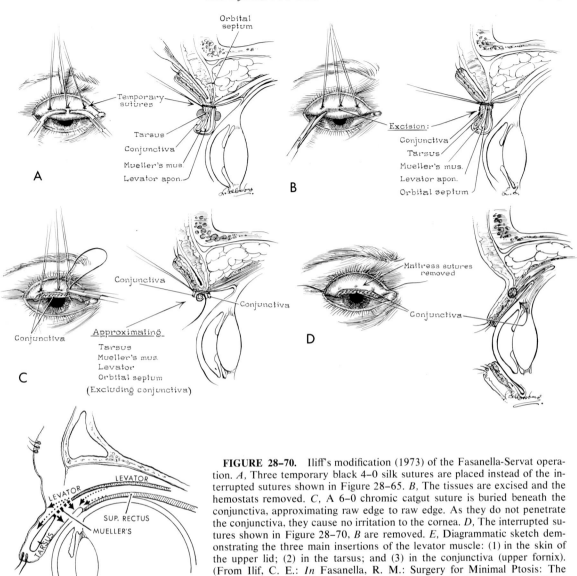

FIGURE 28–70. Iliff's modification (1973) of the Fasanella-Servat operation. *A,* Three temporary black 4–0 silk sutures are placed instead of the interrupted sutures shown in Figure 28–65. *B,* The tissues are excised and the hemostats removed. *C,* A 6–0 chromic catgut suture is buried beneath the conjunctiva, approximating raw edge to raw edge. As they do not penetrate the conjunctiva, they cause no irritation to the cornea. *D,* The interrupted sutures shown in Figure 28–70, *B* are removed. *E,* Diagrammatic sketch demonstrating the three main insertions of the levator muscle: (1) in the skin of the upper lid; (2) in the tarsus; and (3) in the conjunctiva (upper fornix). (From Ilif, C. E.: *In* Fasanella, R. M.: Surgery for Minimal Ptosis: The Fasanella-Servat Operation. Trans. Ophthalmol. Soc. U.K., *93*:425, 1973.)

advancement of Müller's muscle. According to Fasanella (1973), perhaps a combination of both of these—the small block resection and bites of suture into the tarsus and what remains of the conjunctiva and levator—is responsible for the successful results.

Levator Shortening Operation (Jones, 1974a)

A description of an operation devised by Jones (1974a) was included in a chapter written by Callahan (1974). The operation has been employed by Smith (1975) with good results. The operation is performed on the sedated patient under local anesthesia. An incision is made 6 mm above the lashline, extending through the skin and orbicularis oculi muscle but not through the fascia beneath the muscle. An Erhardt clamp is attached near the lid margin, and the skin-muscle layer is retracted upward. Careful blunt dissection extending upward under the muscle layer for a distance of 10 to 12 mm exposes the fat over the levator aponeurosis (preaponeurotic fat). The patient is asked to look upward, and this maneuver identifies the aponeurosis. An opening is made through the septum orbitale; the septum orbitale is incised, and a squint hook is

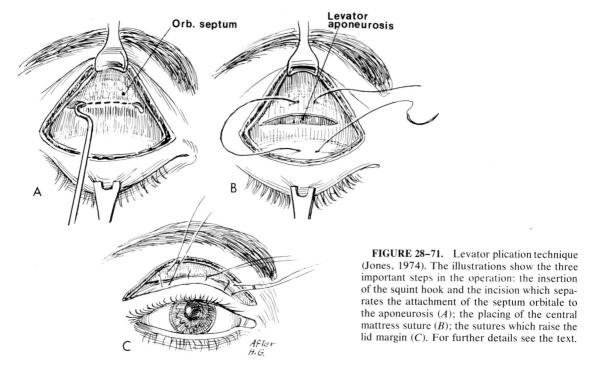

Orb. septum

Levator aponeurosis

A

B

C

After H.G.

FIGURE 28–71. Levator plication technique (Jones, 1974). The illustrations show the three important steps in the operation: the insertion of the squint hook and the incision which separates the attachment of the septum orbitale to the aponeurosis (*A*); the placing of the central mattress suture (*B*); the sutures which raise the lid margin (*C*). For further details see the text.

inserted separating it from its attachment to the aponeurosis (Fig. 28–71, *A*).

A catgut suture picks up a section of the aponeurosis, approximately 7 to 8 mm wide, in the central portion of the aponeurosis (Fig. 28–71, *B*); the mattress suture is inserted below through the tissue along the upper border of the tarsus just medial to the midline of the eyelid (Fig. 28–71, *B*).

The Erhardt clamp is removed. The first tie of a surgeon's knot provides temporary fixation for the evaluation of the position of the lid margin. If sufficient lift has not been obtained, the upper portion of the mattress suture is removed and reinserted into the tissue and the aponeurosis at a higher level. The procedure may have to be repeated until the lid is lifted to a satisfactory level (Fig. 28–71, *C*). Once this is achieved, an additional suture is placed on each side of the central suture to elevate the medial and lateral thirds of the eyelid.

External Levator Resection

When the levator muscle is present and functioning and the ptosis exceeds 4 mm, the levator operation through a transcutaneous approach gives better results than any of the other ptosis procedures. Even when poor levator function is demonstrated, this procedure

frequently produces an acceptable postoperative result.

A scleral contact lens is inserted (Fig. 28–72, *A*). It is essential that the reader refer to Figure 28–2 for the diagrammatic representation of a sagittal section of the upper eyelid. It will be noted that the septum orbitale separates the orbicularis muscle from the underlying orbital fat. The levator aponeurosis is deep to the orbital fat. Near the tarsus the septum orbitale blends with the levator aponeurosis and spreads over the anterior surface of the tarsus. The levator aponeurosis interdigitates with the fibers of the orbicularis muscle. Deep to the levator, between the muscle and the conjunctiva, are the thin fibers of Müller's muscle, which inserts on the upper border of the tarsus.

The first procedure is to identify the upper border of the tarsus, which indicates the supratarsal fold.

The upper eyelid is elevated, puckering the skin at the supratarsal fold. The line is marked with ink and incised after injection of a solution of local anesthetic solution to separate the skin from the underlying orbicularis muscle (Fig. 28–72, *B, C*). The eyelid is stretched horizontally to facilitate the procedure. A razor knife separates the skin from the orbicularis muscle downward to the lower margin of the tarsus remaining deep to the roots of the lashes.

The upper margin of the incision is undermined for a distance of a few millimeters (Fig. 28–72, *D*).

At the lateral end of the incision, scissors undermine the pretarsal portion of the orbicularis muscle, separating it from the pretarsal fascia (Fig. 28–72, *E*). The pretarsal portion of the orbicularis muscle is raised as a flap and excised (Fig. 28–72, *F*). A puncture incision is then made at the superolateral edge of the tarsus, lateral to the levator aponeurosis (Fig. 28–72, *G*), and a straight hemostat is passed through the conjunctiva (Fig. 28–72, *H*). One blade of the hemostat is passed across the conjunctival cul-de-sac just above the tarsus; the other rests over the levator aponeurosis, Müller's muscle, and a few preseptal orbicularis fibers (Fig. 28–72, *H, I*). The tissues incorporated within the blades of the hemostat are freed from the tarsus by an incision (Fig. 28–72, *J*).

The conjunctiva is now separated from Müller's muscle and the levator. Saline solution injected between the layers (Fig. 28–72, *K*) facilitates the dissection, which is extended upward (Fig. 28–72, *L*), separating the conjunctiva from Müller's muscle, care being taken to avoid injuring the superior rectus muscle.

Müller's muscle is then sutured with catgut to the upper margin of the tarsus (Fig. 28–72, *M*). The skin and orbicularis muscle are retracted upward, downward traction is exerted upon the hemostat, and the septum orbitale is incised laterally and medially (Fig. 28–72, *N*); orbital fat prolapses through the openings in the septum orbitale. The levator is freed medially and laterally from the levator expansions upward toward the trochlea and along the lateral orbital wall (Fig. 28–72, *O*). A double-armed suture of 6–0 silk is passed through the central portion of the tarsus but not through the conjunctiva. It is then passed through the structures held by the hemostat at a level situated between 1 and 2 cm above the level of the hemostat (Fig. 28–72, *P, Q*). The level at which the suture is placed depends upon the amount of shortening desired. The suture is tied (Fig. 28–72, *R*); the contact lens is removed; and the operator is guided by the level of the eyelid margin in relation to the upper limbus when the suture is tightened. The central portion of the eyelid margin should rest just below the upper limbus (Fig. 28–72, *S*). Exposure of the cornea is a complication which occurs if the eyelid margin is too high; it should be adjusted, and if necessary the suture

should be removed and replaced at the suitable level. The additional mattress sutures are tied, and the tissue below the hemostat is excised (Fig. 28–72, *T*). Three additional vertical mattress sutures of 6–0 chromic catgut are placed through the upper portion of the tarsus; they traverse the levator and the skin margins to reinforce the attachment of the levator aponeurosis to the tarsus and assure the position and depth of the supratarsal fold (Fig. 28–72, *U, V*). A temporary occlusive suture (Fig. 28–72, *W*) protects the cornea and relieves the tension on the sutures, assuring the fixation of the levator aponeurosis to the tarsus. It is removed after 24 hours.

The cornea should be inspected frequently during subsequent days for evidence of keratopathy. The patient is encouraged to close his eyes forcefully to stimulate activity of the orbicularis muscle. A solution of 0.5 per cent methylcellulose is instilled into the conjunctival sac every hour if there is some corneal exposure, and an ointment is applied at night to protect the cornea. This procedure is the most frequently employed in our series of cases of levator injury and resulting traumatic ptosis of the upper eyelid and in congenital defects such as blepharophimosis (see Fig. 28–84).

When tissue destruction is so marked that the muscle cannot be found or when it is denervated, one must resort to suspension methods. The muscle is rarely denervated by penetrating lacerations, as it is innervated posteriorly, and it is rare that loss of conduction of the superior division of the third (oculomotor) nerve occurs in the orbit. Third nerve paralysis may be a complication of a skull fracture, resulting in loss of function of the levator.

Frontalis Suspension for Blepharoptosis

According to Burian (1962), Hess in 1893 conceived a method of provoking the formation of fibrous bands between the frontalis muscle and the skin on the margin of the lid so that they would work as tendons. He made a long incision in the eyebrow and separated the skin of the lid from the orbicularis muscle down to the tarsus. Two or three mattress sutures were inserted through the skin and then led under the skin in the wound of the eyebrow and through the frontalis muscle to come out 2 cm above the eyebrow. The mattress sutures were then

Text continued on page 936.

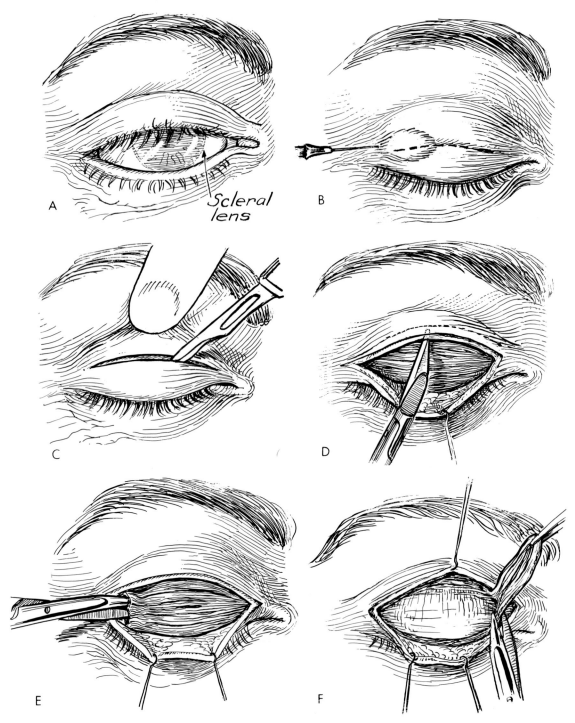

FIGURE 28–72. External levator resection: modified Blaskovics operation. *A*, The protective lens has been inserted. *B*, The upper border of the tarsus has been indicated by an ink line. Injection of a solution of Xylocaine-epinephrine separates the skin from the underlying orbicularis muscle. *C*, An incision is made following the ink line. *D*, The skin is separated from the orbicularis muscle by sharp dissection. *E*, Scissors incise and undermine the pretarsal portion of the orbicularis muscle, separating it from the pretarsal fascia. *F*, The pretarsal portion of the orbicularis muscle is raised as a flap and excised.

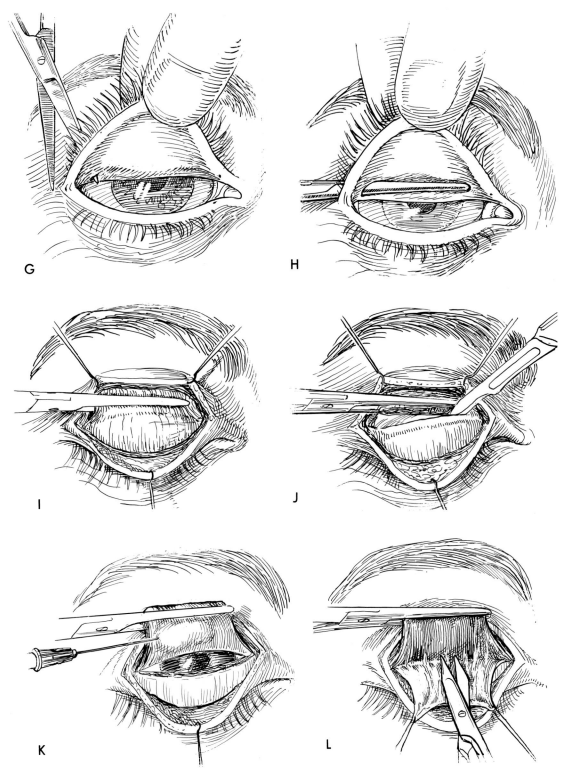

FIGURE 28–72 *Continued.* *G*, A puncture incision is made at the superolateral edge of the tarsus, lateral to the levator aponeurosis. *H*, A straight hemostat is passed through the conjunctiva. *I*, One blade of the hemostat extends across the conjunctiva just about the tarsus. The other blade rests over the levator aponeurosis, Müller's muscle, and a few preseptal orbicularis fibers. *J*, The tissues incorporated within the blades of the hemostat are freed from the tarsus by an incision. *K*, Injection of saline solution separates the conjunctiva from Müller's muscle and the levator. *L*, The plane of dissection is found between Müller's muscle and the conjunctiva.

Illustration continued on following page

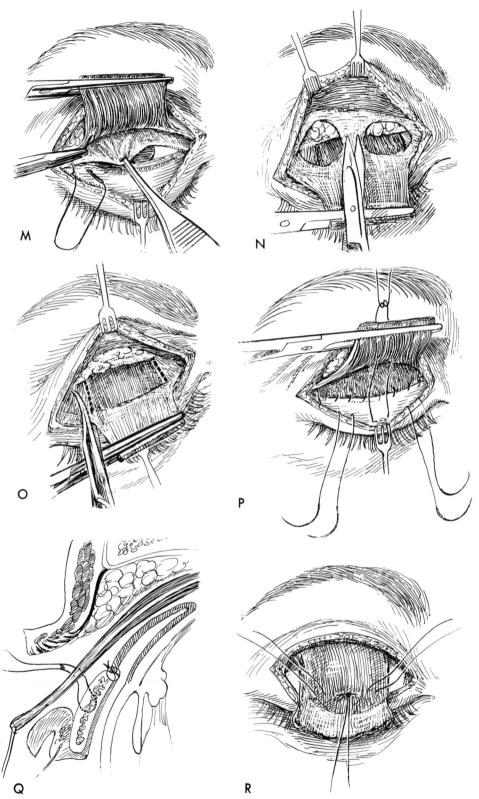

FIGURE 28–72 *Continued.* *M*, Müller's muscle is sutured with catgut to the upper margin of the tarsus. *N*, The skin and orbicularis muscle are retracted upward, and the septum orbitale is incised laterally and medially. *O*, The levator is freed medially and laterally from the levator expansions. *P*, A double-armed suture of 6–0 silk is passed through the central portion of the tarsus but not through the conjunctiva; a suture is then placed through the structures held by the hemostat at a level situated between 1 and 2 cm above the level of the hemostat. *Q*, Sagittal section showing the position of the suture illustrated in Figure 28–72, *P*. *R*, A mattress suture is tied; additional sutures have been placed medially and laterally.

Illustration continued on opposite page

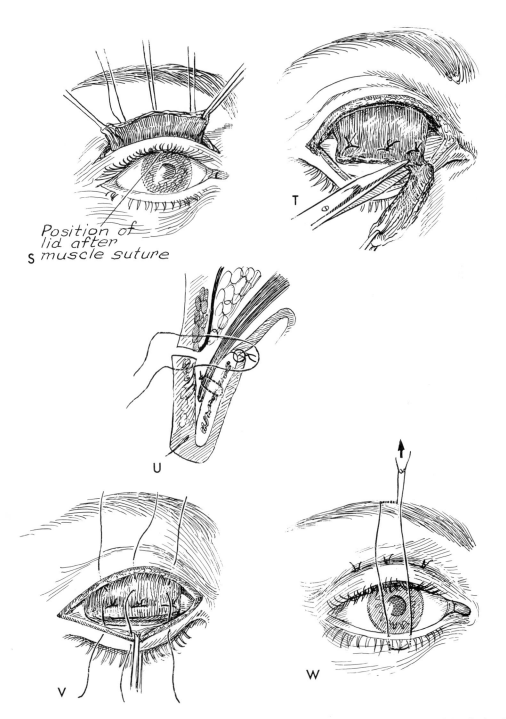

FIGURE 28-72 *Continued.* *S,* The contact lens has been removed, and the operator is guided by the level of the eyelid margin in relation to the upper limbus when the suture is tightened. *T,* Additional mattress sutures have been tied, and tissue below the hemostat is excised. *U,* Sagittal section illustrating the position of a mattress suture of 6-0 chromic catgut placed through the upper portion of the tarsus, traversing the levator and the supratarsal fold. *V,* Position of three sutures placed according to the technique shown in Figure 28-72, *U. W,* At the completion of the operation, an occlusive suture protects the cornea and relieves tension on the sutures, assuring fixation of the levator aponeurosis to the tarsus.

knotted on glass pearls under appropriate tension. These sutures stayed in for two weeks, during which period resistant fibrous bands were supposed to have developed. No doubt, the effect was due to the fibrous contraction of the large wound in the lid, but the results were poor. This led to the use of permanent suspension of the lid by stitches, inserted subcutaneously, connecting the tarsus with the frontalis muscle. From the use of silk sutures, surgeons passed on to physiologically inert suture material, such as silver and stainless steel wire, and finally to alloplastic sutures..

As mentioned in König's (1928) monograph, it was Payr who originated the use of fascia (1928). Payr made three incisions: one along the upper border of the tarsus, another in the eyebrow, and a third higher up on the forehead. After tunneling the skin between the incisions, he introduced a large strip of fascia lata and sutured it to the upper border of the frontalis muscle; the effect was excellent.

Later surgeons made only the tarsal and brow incisions. Lexer (1923) introduced two narrow tapes of fascia through small incisions on the internal and external parts of the brow and on corresponding parts of the tarsus. Elschnig (1913) did an operation similar to that of Payr but sutured the lower end of the strip transcutaneously. He encountered the development of a purulent infection, but the final result was satisfactory.

Many surgeons have used strips of fascia in different ways. Risdon (1945) made a small incision above the eyebrow, tunneled from there to near the canthus, then paralleled one-half of the upper lid margin and cut upward to the incised area, thus making a tunnel in the form of a triangle. Two or three such triangles were made, and fascial strips were threaded through the tunnels and sutured to the fibers of the occipitofrontalis muscle. The authors have favored a modification of the Friedenwald-Guyton (1948) suture technique, employing a double rhomboid suture (Fig. 28–73).

Technique of Frontalis Suspension. The double triangular or rhomboid suture has become popular in recent years (Fig. 28–73). It is performed with fascia lata or one of the in-

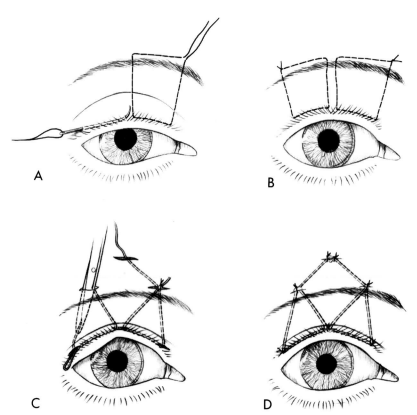

FIGURE 28–73. Frontalis fixation for ptosis when levator function is absent. Prior to location of the incisions above the eyebrow, the frontalis muscle is tested. If the frontalis is paralyzed, the suspension technique cannot be used. One part of the frontalis muscle may contract more than others, and the incisions should be placed to utilize that part. *A, B,* Double rhomboid frontalis fixation technique. Suspension material is threaded from lid margin upward to emerge from the incisions above the brow (see text for details). Note the special needle for introducing the suspension material. *C, D,* Double triangular suture.

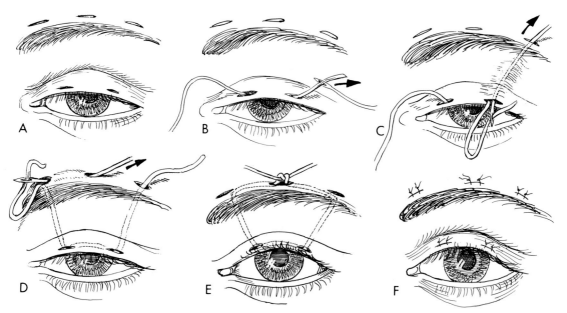

FIGURE 28–74. Frontalis suspension technique of Tillett and Tillett (1966). Modified emplacement of a Silastic strip. *A*, At the juncture of the horizontal thirds of the lid, two linear incisions are made 3 mm from and parallel to the lid margin. Each incision is about 4 mm long. The skin, subcutaneous tissues, and orbicularis muscle are opened to expose the anterior tarsal surface. Three linear incisions are made just above the eyebrow. The first is placed in the midline of the brow directly over the midline of the lid. The medial incision is placed medially to a vertical line extending from the medial margin of the incision, and the lateral incision is made lateral to the lateral marginal incision. These incisions above the brow are opened to the frontalis muscle aponeurosis, but not to the periosteum. *B*, Insertion of the Silastic strip (No. 40). The Wright needle has been inserted from the lateral to the medial incision, the needle point having been pushed behind the orbicularis muscle, picking up some fibers of the epitarsus. When the point emerges through the medial incision, one end of the strip is inserted in the needle's eye. As the needle is drawn back out through the lateral incision, the strip is left in place in the lid near the margin. *C*, The needle has been directed down through the upper lateral incision and brought posterior to the orbicularis muscle in the plane of the orbital septum along the anterior surface of the tarsus to emerge in the lateral lid incision. One end of the strip has been inserted in the needle's eye. *D*, Both ends of the strip have been drawn through the respective brow incisions. The needle has not yet been detached from the strip at the medial end. The needle has been inserted in the midbrow incision and out through the medial incision. One end of the Silastic strip has been inserted through the eye of the needle so that it can be drawn out through the medial incision. *E*, Both ends have now been drawn up through the midbrow incision and through the Watzke sleeve. If desired, a suture may be tied around the ends of the sleeve to prevent slipping; this has been unnecessary in our experience. *F*, The skin incisions have been closed. (After Callahan, 1974.)

organic materials. Autogenous fascia lata is removed by means of a fascial stripper (see Chapter 9, Fig. 9–1), or a thin strip of tendon is removed from the extensor of the fifth toe (more difficult to use in the thin tissues of the lid). Autogenous grafts have the advantage of not being rejected in the midst of an inflammatory reaction, a not infrequent complication with inorganic materials. When this complication occurs, the suspension material is removed. After a quiescent period, fascia lata suspension can then be employed. Callahan (1974) has reported success with the technique of Tillett and Tillett (1966), which uses a Silastic band for the frontalis suspension of the upper lids in cases of blepharophimosis (Fig. 28–74). Mustardé (1974) has returned to the use of autogenous fascia lata.

For the double rhomboid suspension (Fig. 28–73, *A, B*), three incisions are made above the eyebrow extending through the temporalis muscle. Two separate rhomboid suspensions are done, the knots being tied laterally and medially.

In performing the double triangular frontalis fixation (Fig. 28–73, *C, D*), two small incisions are made above the eyebrow to the frontalis muscle, one medially and the other laterally. Three incisions are made through the skin and orbicularis oculi muscle immediately above the eyelashes. Another incision is made about 6 cm above the central portion of the eyebrow which extends through the frontalis muscle (Fig. 28–73, *C*). Two strips of fascia, tendon, Supramid, or other inorganic material are threaded upward through the eyelid incisions, emerging through the incisions above the eyebrow, where they are knotted (when fascia is employed they are also sutured) under sufficient tension to form a supratarsal fold, arch, and elevation of the lid. The two long ends are passed subcutaneously to emerge through the central wound above the eyebrow, where they are tied together. The incisions are closed by direct approximation with sutures (Fig. 28–73, *D*).

A pressure dressing is applied for 24 hours. A solution of 0.5 per cent methylcellulose is instilled into the palpebral fissure every hour during the day, and ointment is applied for pro-

tection during sleep. Stippling of the cornea may appear during the early postoperative phase, but usually within a few days the cornea becomes tolerant of the new lid position.

The main disadvantage of the frontalis operations is that ptosis in looking up and

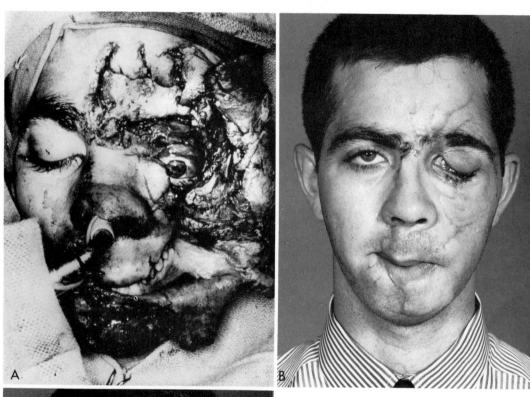

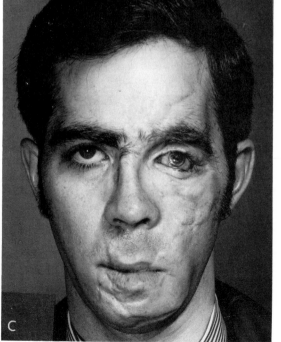

FIGURE 28–75. Scleral lens to protect the cornea in ptosis with paralysis of the orbicularis oculi muscle. *A*, Patient immediately after an automobile accident. Note the complete disorganization of the face and destructive lesions around the orbit. *B*, The patient after primary surgery. *C*, The patient has been improved by a series of operations, which have included levator shortening, reestablishment of continuity of the upper eyelid, and full-thickness graft to the lower lid. Because of paralysis of the orbicularis oculi muscle, caused by the multiple lacerations and avulsion of tissue, and of inability to occlude the lids, the patient wears a lens to protect the cornea.

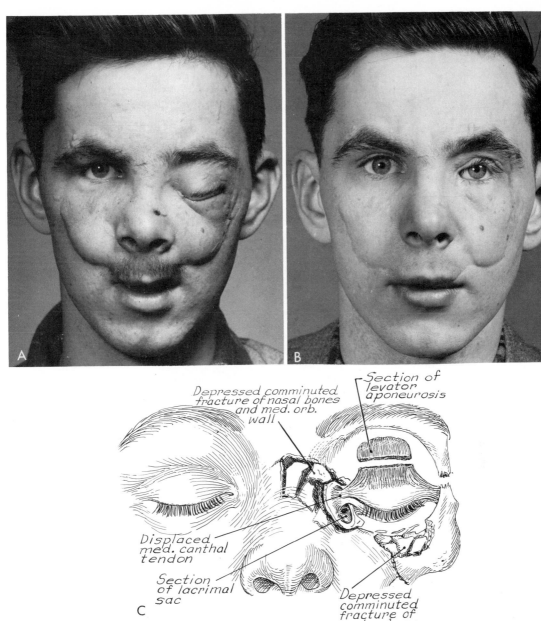

FIGURE 28-76. Multiple facial injuries with section of the levator aponeurosis. *A,* A 20 year old patient who was projected through the windshield suffered a shearing off of soft tissues of the face and a section of the upper eyelid. In a rebound injury, the patient was projected against the dashboard, suffering naso-orbital and orbital fractures. The soft tissues had been avulsed from the facial skeletal framework, and a blowout fracture had occurred in the left orbit. *B,* The patient after reconstructive surgery involving treatment of the blowout and naso-orbital fractures, medial canthoplasty, dacryocystorhinostomy, and repair of the severed levator aponeurosis. Bone grafting was necessary to restore the contour of the nose. *C,* Some of the lesions suffered by the patient, including multiple fractures of the nose, section of the levator aponeurosis, comminuted fracture of the zygoma, and blowout fracture of the left orbit. (From Converse, J. M., and Smith, B.: Naso-orbital fractures. Trans. Am. Acad. Ophthalmol., Otolaryngol., 67:659, 1963.)

lagophthalmos in looking down usually occur. The lid can be raised only by lifting the brow, and the pull exerted by the fascia for elevating the lid tends to pull the lid away from the globe.

In exceptional cases when only remnants of the levator are present and when paralysis of the orbicularis oculi and the frontalis muscles is present, caused by destruction of the temporofacial division of the facial nerve, frontalis suspension cannot be employed. Figure 28-75 shows a physician who suffered severe injuries causing permanent paralysis of the orbicularis oculi and frontalis muscles. A scleral lens was necessary in this case to protect the cornea, as shortening of the lid was required. The newly developed soft plastic lens is better tolerated than the lens formerly employed for this purpose.

Reestablishing the continuity of the levator and levator resection, whether done early or late (Fig. 28–76), are the best methods of correcting ptosis of the upper eyelid when levator function is present.

EPICANTHUS: CONGENITAL AND TRAUMATIC

Congenital Epicanthus. Congenital epicanthus is often bilateral and is transmitted as a dominant trait. It is characterized by a fold of skin which extends from the bridge of the nose, overhanging and partially hiding the medial canthus. The fold may arise from the eyebrow, the tarsal fold, or the skin of the upper lid above the tarsal fold. It occurs with varying frequency in all races but is most common among Orientals. Variations include epicanthus inversus, characterized by a skin fold which originates in the lower lid and swings upward into the upper lid. This is differentiated from (1) epicanthus palpebralis, the most common condition, in which the fold arises from the upper lid above the tarsal region; (2) epicanthus tarsalis, in which the fold arises from the skin over the tarsus; and (3) epicanthus superciliaris, in which the fold runs from the eyebrows toward the normal lower lid.

The correction of congenital epicanthal folds is surgical and can be performed at an early age.

Various techniques have been proposed for the correction of epicanthal folds. The tech-

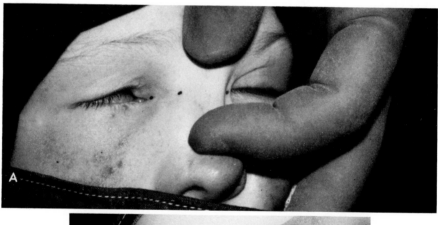

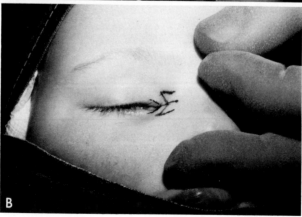

FIGURE 28–77. Mustardé's four-flap technique for the correction of an epicanthal fold. *A,* A point is marked at the proposed site of the new canthus (midway between the center of the pupil and the midline of the nose). The skin of the nose is pulled medially to obliterate any fold present, and a second point is marked at the site of the actual canthus. *B,* A line is drawn between these two points, and from the center two diverging lines are drawn at an angle of 60 degrees and slightly shorter in length (1 to 2 mm) than the original horizontal line. Back cuts of a similar length are now drawn at a 45 degree angle. Paramarginal incisions also of the same length are drawn on the upper and lower eyelids. (Figs. 28–77 to 28–80, courtesy of Mr. J. Mustardé.)

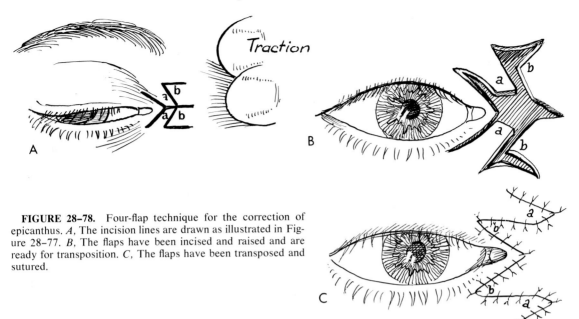

FIGURE 28-78. Four-flap technique for the correction of epicanthus. *A,* The incision lines are drawn as illustrated in Figure 28-77. *B,* The flaps have been incised and raised and are ready for transposition. *C,* The flaps have been transposed and sutured.

nique of Blair, Brown, and Hamm (1932) has been supplanted by that of Mustardé (1963) for the correction of epicanthal folds of congenital origin.

RECTANGULAR FLAP (FOUR-FLAP) TECHNIQUE. Mustardé (1974) described his rectangular flap, or four-flap, technique as follows: epicanthal folds, whether accompanied by telecanthus or not, may be treated by the four-flap technique, irrespective of the position of the folds or their severity.

A point is marked on the skin of the nose (Fig. 28-77, *A*) at the site of the proposed new canthus (halfway between the center of the nose and the center of the pupil). The nasal skin is pulled medially to obliterate the fold, and another mark is made at the actual canthus (Fig. 28-77, *A*). These two points are then joined, and from the midpoint lines are drawn at 60 degrees and only slightly shorter in length than the distance between the two points (Fig. 28-77, *B*). From the top of these vertical lines, back cuts of 45 degrees are drawn, and again the length of these should be the same as that of the vertical lines (Fig. 28-77, *B*). Finally, paramarginal lines of the same length are drawn along each lid margin (Fig. 28-77, *B*). The skin flaps so outlined are incised down to the orbicularis muscle and are raised (Fig. 28-78). If telecanthus is present, the excessive amount of medial canthal tendon is excised, and the medial canthus is sutured to the periosteum of the nose with any nonab-

sorbable material, such as silk or stainless steel wire. In patients with extremely wide telecanthus, the stumps of the two medial canthal tendons should be wired to one another using a permanent transnasal stainless steel wire passed by means of a curved awl. The flaps are now transposed and sutured in place using 4-0 chromic catgut for the first suture to unite the two points originally marked (Fig. 28-79, *A, B*). Any excess tissue of the flaps is trimmed, and the rest of the suturing is done with 6-0 chromic catgut, so that the sutures will not require removal (Fig. 28-79, *C, D*). Ethnic epicanthus may be corrected and may be combined with removal of fat from the upper lid, with formation of an upper lid furrow (Fig. 28-80).

It is essential that the final scar of the operation should run *through* the medial canthus so as to avoid any possibility of a secondary cicatricial fold. The operation is equally suitable for children who have a degree of telecanthus as well as epicanthus, or it may be used for telecanthus alone — for instance, in severe blepharophimosis. It may also be used for simple epicanthal folds without any degree of telecanthus. A similar procedure is used for all types of conditions, and the presence or absence of a fold itself is ignored in making the design.

Traumatic Epicanthus. Double-opposing Z-plasties have been used extensively in the treatment of traumatic epicanthus (Converse

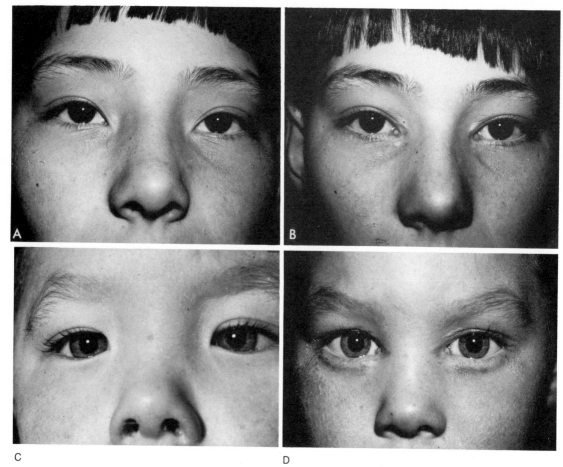

FIGURE 28–79.   Preoperative (*A*) and postoperative (*B*) views of epicanthal folds corrected by the four-flap technique. *C, D,* Preoperative and postoperative views of more accentuated epicanthal folds corrected by the four-flap technique.

and Smith, 1966). The double-opposing Z-plasty technique may be preferable in cicatricial epicanthus, particularly in the repair of naso-orbital fractures. The incisions made through the skin for double-opposing Z-plasties also serve as the point of entry to the medial orbital wall and nasal dorsum in these cases. The medial canthal tendon is then reattached to the medial orbital wall (see section of chapter entitled Malunited Naso-orbital Fractures). The pathology underlying the traumatic epicanthal fold is scar tissue resulting in a contractile linear band or the disruption of the skeletal anatomy of the area.

Whereas the epicanthal fold itself can be disregarded in Mustardé's technique, the incision for the traumatic epicanthal fold must extend through the scar itself (Fig. 28–81). If the scar is wide, it may have to be excised, but in most cases the Z-plasty will redistribute the scar and result in its progressive softening.

DYSTOCIA CANTHORUM

Under this term is classified a whole range of canthal deformities and displacements that will not be discussed in this text. An exception is canthus inversus, usually a downward tilt of the medial canthus resulting from faulty cicatrization of naso-orbital fractures. Medial canthoplasties are required for repair and are discussed in a later section of the chapter (see page 1012).

EPIBLEPHARON

Epiblepharon, as its name of Greek derivation indicates, is a deformity that is characterized by a fold of skin and conjunctiva which covers the caruncle and a variable portion of the sclera. The deformity is frequently associ-

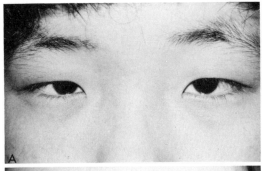
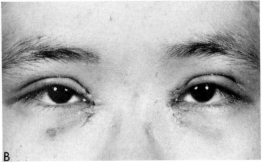
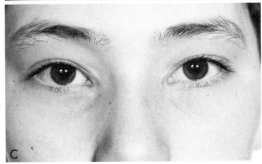

FIGURE 28–80. Example of more severe epicanthus with absence of superior palpebral folds and telecanthus. *A,* Appearance of the patient preoperatively. *B,* After the correction of the epicanthal folds by the four-flap technique and the formation of supratarsal folds. *C,* Appearance after healing of the wounds.

ated with congenital epicanthus and blepharophimosis. Epiblepharon also occurs in traumatic epicanthus, orbital hypertelorism, and post-thermal deformities involving the medial canthal area (the naso-orbital valley). The treatment consists of replacing the medial canthus against the medial orbital wall and restoring its angular shape. The Mustardé "jumping man" incisions, outlining quadrilateral flaps, combined with a shortening of the elon-

FIGURE 28–81. Double-opposing Z-plasties. Two Z-plasties done in opposing directions constitute an excellent technique for relaxing tension and releasing contracture of a linear scar. It is of particular usefulness in areas where only small flaps may be designed. Limited amount of tissue in the confined naso-orbital valley limits the size of the Z-flaps. *A,* Design of the opposing Z-plasties. *B,* Flaps are raised, and deep scar tissue is excised. *C,* Transosseous wires have been placed through the bony skeleton of the nose for fixation of the canthal buttons (see *F* and *G*). *D,* The flaps have been transposed. *E,* Double opposing Z-plasties completed. *F, G,* The canthal buttons are maintained by through-and-through wiring, assuring the coaptation of the flaps to the underlying skeleton and preventing hematoma. (Converse, 1964.)

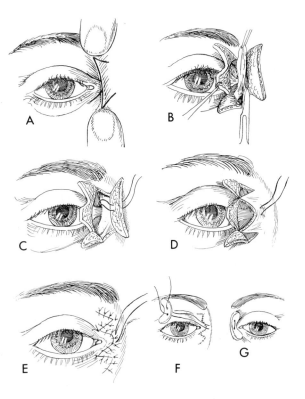

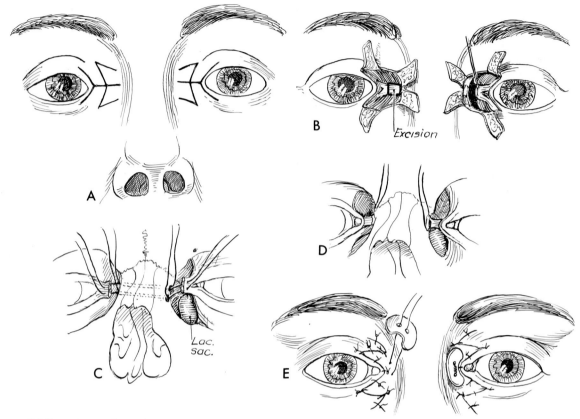

FIGURE 28–82. Correction of epiblepharon. *A,* Design of Mustardé's "jumping man" incisions. *B,* The flaps are raised. The medial canthal tendon is shortened. *C, D,* Transnasal wires are threaded through the stump of the medial canthal tendons. *E,* Operation completed. The buttons are placed to prevent hematoma formation.

gated medial canthal tendon as illustrated in Figure 28–82 may be adequate to correct the deformity.

More complicated cases, particularly following trauma (fractures, burns), may require more extensive procedures. Resection of subcutaneous scar tissue, raising the periorbita, and sectioning the inferior branch of the lateral canthal tendon to release lateral tension may be required. Firm attachment of the medial canthus to the bone is essential (Fig. 28–82, *C*). This technique is indicated in epiblepharon caused by burn contracture and is combined with a medial canthoplasty.

BLEPHAROPHIMOSIS

Blepharophimosis is a congenital malformation involving the orbital region which is usually associated with ptosis of the upper eyelids and epicanthal folds. The tissues of the medial canthal region encroach upon the ocular globe, covering the caruncle and a portion of the sclera (epiblepharon). The bridge of the nose appears flattened and widened. The eyes thus appear to be far apart, whereas in reality in most cases only the intercanthal distance is increased (telecanthus), and epicanthal folds are present; only in severe cases of blepharophimosis is there a minor degree of orbital hypertelorism. The diminution of the transverse dimension of the palpebral fissure is accompanied by a diminution in the vertical dimension of the palpebral fissure caused by the eyelid ptosis. There is almost always an absence of the supratarsal fold in the upper eyelid; the eyebrows are arched, as is usually seen in severe ptosis.

Because of the lateral (temporal) displacement of the medial canthi, the lacrimal puncta are also laterally displaced. Shortage of skin is frequent, particularly in the lower lid. Epicanthal folds may be present, but there is nearly always an excess of skin and also of subcutaneous tissue between the skin and the underlying skeletal structures of the nose.

As in many other congenital syndromes, the malformation is rarely an isolated developmental anomaly. Auricular deformities and anomalies of the forehead are frequent. The patient has a characteristic posture, maintaining his neck extended backward in order to be able to see below his ptotic eyelids. The patient may appear mentally retarded, although in many cases his intellectual development may be higher than the average.

Genetic Aspects. According to Callahan (1974), Dimitry (1921) studied five generations of patients with blepharophimosis and coined the term from two Greek words—*blepharon* (eyelids) and *phimosis* (stricture). Dimitry's studies suggested that the malformation occurs more frequently in males, although it is not sex-linked. Owens, Hadley, and Kloepfer (1960) confirmed Dimitry's observation that the hereditary pattern is usually transmitted as an autosomal dominant with 100 per cent penetrance. Chromosome studies have been negative.

In the American and British literature, the treatment of patients with blepharophimosis has been reported by Berke (1953), Hughes (1955), Johnson (1956, 1964), Lewis, Arons, Lynch, and Blocker (1967), Fox (1963), and Mustardé (1963).

Classification and Treatment. Callahan (1974) has recognized the characteristic features and the required treatment of three types of blepharophimosis (Fig. 28–83).

BLEPHAROPHIMOSIS TYPE I. Type I blepharophimosis is characterized by large epicanthal folds extending upward from the lower lid with epicanthus inversus, a downward slant of the medial canthi. The eyelids are shortened in their horizontal dimension, and the upper eyelids are ptotic.

Three essential operative procedures for the correction of this deformity are advocated:

1. Elimination of the epicanthal folds by the quadrilateral flap technique of Mustardé (see Fig. 28–78) or by the double-opposing Z-plasty technique (see Fig. 28–81).

2. Resection of bone through the upper portion of the lacrimal groove. The medial canthal tendons and the adjacent periorbita are tucked into the bony window by means of transosseous wiring.

3. Correction of the ptosis. In the absence of adequate levator action, the ptosis is corrected by frontalis slings using whatever method the surgeon prefers (see p. 931).

BLEPHAROPHIMOSIS TYPE II. Type II blepharophimosis is characterized by the absence of epicanthal folds and telecanthus without

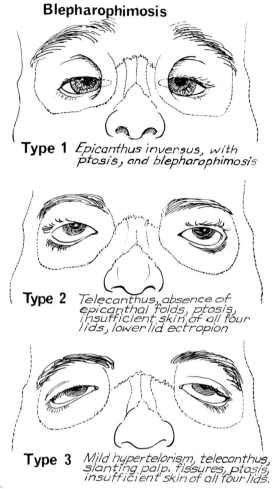

Blepharophimosis

Type 1 *Epicanthus inversus, with ptosis, and blepharophimosis*

Type 2 *Telecanthus, absence of epicanthal folds, ptosis, insufficient skin of all four lids, lower lid ectropion*

Type 3 *Mild hypertelorism, telecanthus, slanting palp. fissures, ptosis, insufficient skin of all four lids.*

FIGURE 28–83. Types of blepharophimosis. (After Callahan, 1974.)

skeletal deformities and without an increased distance between the medial orbital walls. Patients show ptosis of the upper lids, no levator function, and shortness of skin. Two procedures are necessary for the correction of this type of deformity:

1. Skin grafts must be added to each of the four lids.

2. Callahan (1974) advocated fixation of the medial canthal tissues into the bony openings of the medial orbital wall and fixation by transnasal wiring. In our own clinic, we prefer to displace the medial orbital walls nasally (medially) after osteotomy in addition to the fixation. Exenteration of the ethmoid cells may be required to facilitate the displacement. The medial canthi are reattached by transosseous wiring, which also maintains the medial displacement of the medial orbital walls.

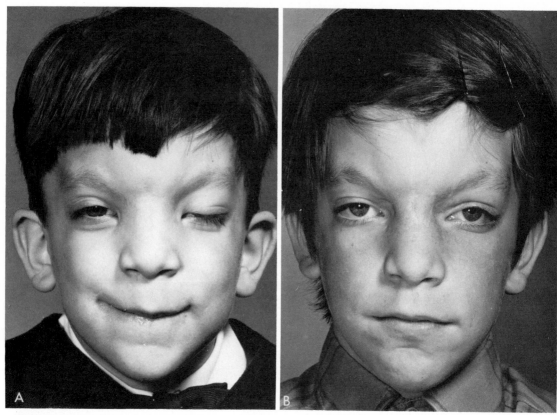

FIGURE 28-84. Corrective surgery for blepharophimosis. *A,* A patient aged 5 years with typical characteristics of blepharophimosis. *B,* Appearance of the patient six years later following bilateral opposing Z-plasties, medial displacement of the medial orbital walls after osteotomy, and resection of a central segment of bone. Sufficient levator muscle activity was present to correct the ptosis by levator resection. Patient has slight degree of orbital hypertelorism. (From Converse, J. M., Ransohoff, J., Mathews, E. S., Smith, B., and Molenaar, A.: Ocular hypertelorism and pseudohypertelorism. Plast. Reconstr. Surg., *45:*2. Copyright 1970, The Williams & Wilkins Company, Baltimore.)

3. The ptosis is corrected with frontalis slings.

BLEPHAROPHIMOSIS TYPE III. This type is characterized by the lack of epicanthal folds, telecanthus, antimongoloid slanting of the palpebral fissures, and a minor degree (type I) of orbital hypertelorism which is confirmed by radiologic studies (see Chapter 56). In addition to the grafting of the eyelids and the correction of the ptosis, the entire orbital contents must be moved medially in order to correct the orbital hypertelorism. This type of blepharophimosis is preferably treated according to the technique employed in the correction of orbital hypertelorism (see Chapter 56). Figure 28–84 shows a patient in whom bilateral double-opposing Z-plasties and medial displacement of the medial orbital walls after resection of a central segment from the midline of the nose corrected the deformity. In this case there was sufficient levator activity to permit levator resection to correct the ptosis.

Surgical Correction of the Oriental Eyelid

BURGOS T. SAYOC, M.D.

Surgery of the Oriental eyelid may encompass many types of surgical procedures, depending on the objectives and motivation of the patient and the operating surgeon. The facial features of Occidentals and Orientals are different in many respects. The Oriental eye has an epicanthus of variable degree, a narrow palpebral fissure, and a slight to an accentuated fullness of the upper eyelid (Fig. 28–85). If the intention is to westernize the Oriental eyelid, the surgical procedures, in addition to correction of the superior palpebral (supratarsal) fold, might include removal of the epicanthus and the supraorbital fat pad, construction of a much longer fold, and excision of the skin in the upper lid to give an impression of slightly more deep-seated eyeballs. The epicanthus, if exaggerated, can be removed by inserting a piece of cartilage or a Silastic implant to raise the bridge of the nose. Surgery of the Oriental eyelid then becomes a long and rather complicated process. To westernize Oriental features, a rhinoplasty must be done as well. Yet even when all these procedures are performed the characteristic Oriental features remain. This section will be confined to a detailed discussion of the construction of the supratarsal fold. It is mainly for this surgical procedure that Oriental patients consult the plastic surgeon.

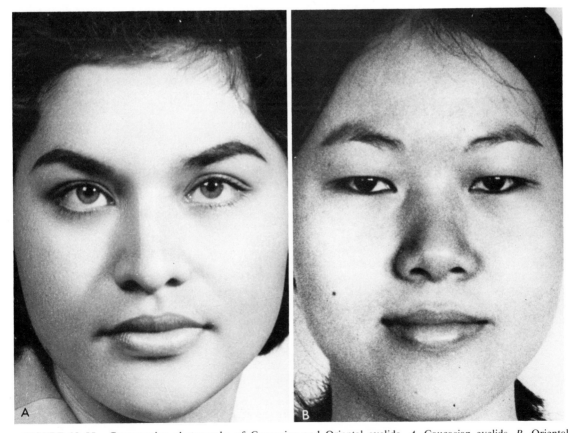

FIGURE 28–85. Comparative photographs of Caucasian and Oriental eyelids. *A*, Caucasian eyelids. *B*, Oriental eyelids. Note epicanthus, narrower palpebral fissure, full upper eyelid, and absence of the superior palpebral (supratarsal) fold.

947

The eyes undeniably play a large part in the expression of human emotion. The evolution of the human eye and its adnexa has given rise to diverse prototypes characteristic of each race. The Greek eye, which is horizontally set, neither too deep nor too shallow in the eye socket, with well-formed eyelids, long lashes slightly tilted upward, and wide palpebral fissures, has been taken as representative of the Occidental eye. The slit or almond-shaped eye of the Oriental appears somewhat obliquely set, with acute corners. The palpebral opening is much narrower, and the upper eyelid covers almost half the iris at 12 o'clock. The slanted Oriental eye gives a charming, intriguing, exotic effect which many Western women have desired. By and large, the Oriental eyelid is devoid of the supratarsal fold. Because of this anatomical variation, a Filipino director of the Manila School of Fine Arts has expressed the opinion that the Oriental eyes are not as expressive as the nonslit eyes of the Occidentals.

GENERAL CONSIDERATIONS

The main fold of the skin of the upper eyelid is of considerable topographic interest. A horizontally curved palpebral or orbital-palpebral infold, superior and inferior, divides the lid into tarsal and orbital areas. The tarsal portion overlies the tarsal plate and globe, while the orbital portion is related to the space between the tarsal margin and the bony margin.

Whitnall (1932) stated, "The superior palpebral fold is deep; it lies 2 or 3 mm above the highest point of cutaneous insertion of the levator palpebrae superioris, the contraction of which causes it to become deeply recessed, as the orbicularis oculi is thinnest along this line. The skin of the orbital region of the lid above this sags forward in the middle age when it has lost its elasticity, to form a fold which covers the tarsal region even as low down as the eyelashes. It is most marked on the lateral side and may even form a kind of lateral epicanthus in an old subject."

Sappey (1874–1875) stated that the superior and inferior palpebral folds exactly superimpose the lines of reflection of the conjunctiva onto the globe (fornices). According to Charpy (1878), they indicate the limit between the smooth and the folded parts of the membrane. These authors, however, do not explain the absence of the superior palpebral (supratarsal) folds in Oriental slit eyes. According to our clinical observations, even when the eyes are closed, the supratarsal fold can be identified by a somewhat horizontal cutaneous line, which is produced and indicated by the highest cutaneous insertion of the terminal fibers of the levator muscle.

ANATOMICAL CONSIDERATIONS

The levator palpebrae superioris muscle is the special elevator muscle of the upper lid which lies in the orbit; only its terminal part enters the lid. It arises at the apex of the orbit. Its cutaneous insertion is into the skin of the tarsal part of the lid by means of the vertically radiating fibers of the delicate connective tissues; this is the primary and essential attachment of the horizontally disposed fasciculi of the orbicularis oculi muscle, which sweep over the bare superficial face of the tarsal plate in their downward course.

In the downward course, the lower fibers pass into the lower third of the face of the tarsal plate and mingle with the bulbs of the cilia. Müller's muscle enters the upper margin of the tarsal plate.

Note the different measurements of the tarsal plate of the upper eyelid (Table 28–2).

The osseous connections are effected by the medial and lateral horns to the corresponding orbital margins at their midpoints and to the commissures of the lids.

Action of the Levator Palpebrae Superioris. By the contraction of the muscle belly of the levator of the upper eyelids, the transversely disposed aponeurosis is swung backward over the globe like the visor of a helmet, pulling

TABLE 28–2. *Average Dimensions of the Tarsal Plate*

CAUCASIAN EYELID	ORIENTAL EYELID
Length: 30–32 mm Width: nasal, 5 mm middle, 10–12 mm temporal, 4–4.5 mm	Length: 28–30 mm Width: nasal, 4 mm middle, 8–10 mm temporal, 3–3.5 mm

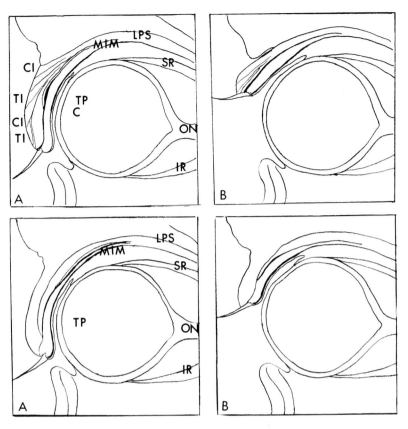

FIGURE 28–86. Sayoc's concept of anatomical variations between the Caucasian and Oriental eyelid. *Upper,* sagittal section of Caucasian eyelid, showing insertion of septum orbitale to levator aponeurosis above the upper edge of the tarsal plate. *Lower,* sagittal section of Oriental foldless eyelid. *A,* Closed position. *B,* Open position. (LPS, levator palpebrae superioris; ON, optic nerve; IR, inferior rectus muscle; CI, cutaneous insertion of the aponeurosis of LPS; TP, tarsal plate; SR, superior rectus muscle, TI, tarsal insertion of the aponeurosis of the LPS; MIM, Müller's involuntary muscle.)

with it the skin of the lid into which its terminal fibers are inserted, thus deepening and forming the superior palpebral fold. At the same time, the tarsal plate is raised both by the terminal fibers attached to the lower part of its anterior aspect and by the conjoint action of the involuntary palpebral muscle (Müller's) inserted into its margin, and the loose conjunctiva of the superior fornix is pulled up by the facial attachment of the levator muscle sheath. In the Oriental slit eye, the cutaneous insertion of the terminal fibers of the levator palpebrae superioris is absent (Fig. 28–86). The variations are listed in Table 28–3. There are no appreciable differences between male and female eyelids, and anatomical studies have included individuals whose ages range from 15 to 55 years.

There are no gross anatomical differences between the lower eyelids of Caucasians and Orientals.

The Oriental craving to acquire an Occidental appearance leads the patient to request esthetic surgery to establish supratarsal folds, with subsequent removal of the epicanthal folds when necessary, thus giving an illusion of larger eyes with exposed caruncles.

There is usually a psychosocial motivation behind the desire of the Oriental to acquire an Occidental appearance.

CONSTRUCTION OF THE SUPRATARSAL FOLD

Preliminary Examination. In constructing a supratarsal fold, one must consider the external appearances of the following structures of the upper eyelids: the skin, the orbicularis oculi muscle, the levator palpebrae superioris, and the tarsal plates. The following observations must be made:

1. Congenital or acquired ptosis, with or without levator action, either unilateral or bilateral, may be mistaken for the characteristic Oriental eyelid.

2. The texture of the skin of the lids should be evaluated. The presence of sagging skin in patients over 30 years of age may necessitate modification of the technique, depending on the degree of sagging and the presence of baggy eyelids.

3. Chronic infection of the eyelids—con-

TABLE 28–3. *Anatomical Differences*

CAUCASIAN EYELID	ORIENTAL EYELID
Well developed	Less developed
Supratarsal fold present	No fold present
With deep-seated look	With full upper lid look
Wider and longer palpebral fissure	Narrower and shorter palpebral fissure
Corneal overlap about 3 mm with iris well exposed	Corneal overlap 5 mm or more with iris at 12 o'clock border or partly hidden
Canthal angles obtuse	Canthal angles somewhat acute
Epicanthus rare	Epicanthus very common
Caruncle well exposed	Caruncle partly or wholly hidden
Eyelashes longer and roots well exposed, tilted slightly	Eyelashes shorter and roots usually covered by sagging skin, not tilted
Languorous appearance	No languorous appearance; mysterious look
Past middle age, sagging starts over the preseptal portion of the orbicularis muscle just above the fold line	Sagging starts at the edge or just above the ciliary line
Insertion of levator to skin present	Insertion of levator to skin absent
Lid fold is formed when levator contracts	No lid fold formed, instead skin rolls in upward
Septum orbitale interrupted by the insertion of the aponeurosis of levator to the skin	Septum orbitale not interrupted as it inserts on the aponeurosis of the levator muscle
Presence of full upper eyelid rare	Presence of full upper eyelid common
Septum orbitale inserts usually high, about 10–12 mm above superior border of tarsus	Insertion on aponeurosis usually low, just above superior border of tarsus (5–7 mm)
When lids are closed, palpebral fissure appears horizontal, although temporal portion is 1 mm higher than nasal portion.	When lids are closed, edge appears slightly slanting in temporal portion, because it is higher by 2–3 mm, giving what is called Oriental slant

junctivitis, infection of the lacrimal glands or passages, and blepharitis marginalis—should be corrected before surgery is undertaken.

4. Blepharospasm, if present, should be taken into consideration before surgery is done.

5. Any abnormality of either eyelid should be studied carefully, for it will influence the symmetry of the lids.

Preparation. Before surgery is begun, the height and shape of the future lid fold is estimated. This depends on the esthetic sense of the surgeon. For an oval face with large eyes, a larger fold is desirable; for the round face with small eyes, a smaller fold is more pleasing. The patient sits comfortably on a chair with the head rested and the eyes closed, as in sleep. With the use of a curved malleable wire or tissue forceps and slight pressure on the planned line of incision, a temporary lid fold is formed as the patient is asked to open the eyes, looking straight ahead in the primary gaze position. The crease is then marked from its nasal to its temporal end. Measurements are made and the line of incision drawn. Similar measurements and lines are made on the contralateral eyelid.

Anesthesia. Local anesthesia is used. A few drops of 0.5 to 1 per cent tetracaine (Pontocaine) are instilled into the conjunctival sac. Anesthetic solution is infiltrated along the line of incision (2 per cent procaine hydrochloride or lidocaine, 1 drop of epinephrine 1:1000 to

every 5 ml). Two ml of the solution is sufficient to prevent pain for approximately one hour.

Procedure. With an eyebrow pencil, the height and shape of the intended fold is drawn

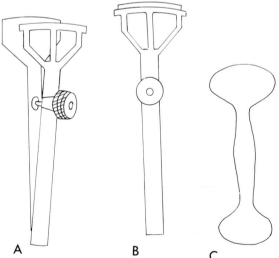

FIGURE 28–87. The Sayoc eyelid fixation forceps (*A*, opened; *B*, closed). The lower plate is smoothly curved to fit the lid above the eyeball below. The upper arm has three teeth beneath its upper edge. The forceps was designed specifically for the construction of the supratarsal fold in Oriental eyelids and in sagging eyelids. The eyeball protector (*C*) is inserted into the upper conjunctival sac and placed over the eyeball after the skin incision is made, and it stays in place until after the dermis is sutured to the tarsal plate. The larger plate is for use in adults, the smaller in children.

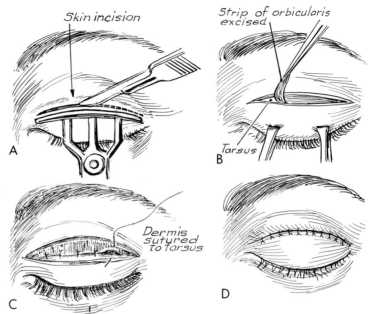

FIGURE 28–88. *A,* Line showing the height and shape of the fold to be constructed. Sayoc's lid fixation forceps in place, indicating just above it the incision made through the skin, subcutaneous tissue, and orbicularis down to the anterior surface of the tarsal plate. *B,* The narrow strip of orbicularis muscle (1 to 2 mm) excised from the nasal to the temporal ends of the incision. *C,* Suturing of the dermal layer of the lower skin flap to the anterior surface of the exposed tarsus. *D,* Closed incision. The eyelid with a supratarsal fold.

on both eyelids. The upper eyelid is grasped with a Sayoc fixation lid forceps (Figs. 28–87 and 28–88) devised for the operation. The incision is made in a single stroke from the nasal to the temporal end of the line, through the skin, subcutaneous tissues, and orbicularis muscle, down to the tarsus (Fig. 28–88, *A*).

A narrow (2 to 3 mm) strip of orbicularis muscle extending from the nasal to the temporal end is excised on the edge of the lower flap to make the orbicularis muscle thinner horizontally at this point to simulate the anatomy of the Occidental lid in this particular area (Fig. 28–88, *B*).

The dermal layer of the lower skin flap is anchored to the anterior surface of the exposed tarsus with 7-0 braided silk or 6-0 chromic catgut using an atraumatic needle (Fig. 28–88, *C*). Care is taken that the needle does not go through the whole thickness of the tarsus. Three to five such buried sutures are inserted.

The incision is closed with 6-0 braided silk, continuous or interrupted, or intracutaneously (Fig. 28–88, *D*). Narrow strip dressings are applied to the incision in such a way that they do not interfere with the opening and closing of the eyes. This allows the patient to be ambulatory. The supratarsal fold is thus formed (Fig. 28–89).

The patient with only one foldless eyelid may insist that the operation be confined to that side only. However, after operating on several such cases, the author found that an unsatisfactory asymmetry resulted and since then has abandoned the practice of operating

only on one side. The usual procedure is to obtain the outline and size of the natural fold of the one side and to apply it to the foldless eyelid. The operations on the two eyelids are done simultaneously. Boo-Chai (1964), using a conjunctival approach, has reported good results with operations done for unilateral foldless eyelids. Nevertheless, the patient has to wait for some months for bilateral symmetry.

Postoperative Care. The patient is usually kept overnight just to ensure that if anything untoward happens within 24 hours, it an be treated at once. Only under special circumstances do patients stay in the clinic only a few hours.

The patient is immediately given analgesics for pain. The wound is cleansed and the dressing changed 6 to 12 hours after surgery to avoid serum or blood clotting between the lids of the wound on the suture line.

The wound is cleansed daily with hydrogen peroxide, Merthiolate, and an antibiotic ointment without any strip dressing at all after 12 to 24 hours. The sutures are removed on the fourth or fifth day after operation.

Complications

ECCHYMOSIS. When local anesthesia is given, the needle may puncture a vessel in the orbicularis muscle, causing bleeding and hematoma formation immediately in spite of the epinephrine in the anesthetic solution. To minimize this situation, care is exercised so that the point of the needle is placed just beneath the

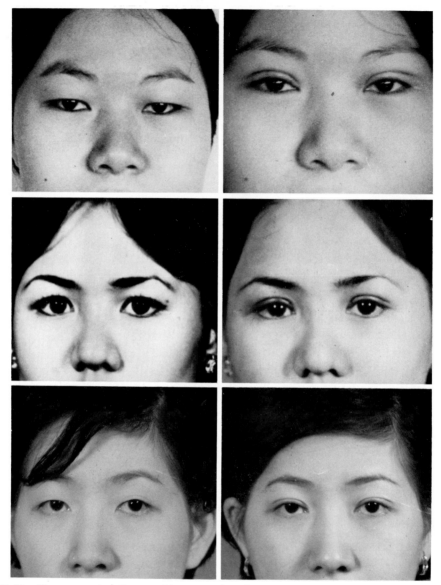

FIGURE 28–89. Three examples of successful construction of supratarsal folds in three patients: preoperative (left) and postoperative (right) views.

skin. If a hematoma forms during the operation, the hematoma in the muscle is excised and the bleeding point cauterized. If it occurs 24 to 48 hours after surgery, the wound is reopened, the blood clot removed, and the wound edges reapproximated as previously mentioned. If untreated, the hematoma will produce a noticeable discoloration in the upper and lower eyelids, the typical "black eye."

SUBCONJUNCTIVAL HEMORRHAGE. Sometimes when the septum orbitale is inadvertently incised, subconjunctival hemorrhage occurs within 24 to 48 hours or even before the surgery is completed. An eyedrop preparation with prednisolone is given, and ophthalmic ointment is massaged into the conjunctival sac while the eyes are closed. To minimize such a complication, care should be exercised that the septum orbitale is not incised or damaged.

GAPING WOUND. When the sutures are removed on the fourth or fifth day, a thin, dry film of serum or blood clot may be found incarcerated between the edges of the wound; the wound may gape and heal by second intention. To prevent this, blood clots are searched for on the first dressing change, which is done 6 to 12 hours after surgery, and thereafter during daily dressings.

DISCOLORATION. Despite the utmost care, mild to severe discoloration may occur, more so when there has been slight hemorrhage or hematoma. A treatment is instituted similar to that for ecchymosis.

SHALLOW LID FOLD OR TEMPORARY LID FOLDS. The presence of a hematoma and edema immediately after surgery may dislodge some or all of the sutures inserted intradermally in the lower flap or from their anchorage to the tarsal plate, so that when the wound heals no adhesion is formed between the tarsus and the skin. Thus, the folds may not be formed at all, or they may not be sufficiently deep and may soon disappear. A secondary operation is undertaken after one month, and during the operation it is made certain that the intradermal and the tarsus sutures are sufficiently strong not to give way.

When the incision line for the lid fold construction is made higher than 10 mm from the lid margin on Filipinos, or on any Oriental for that matter, there is the danger that the lower skin flap may be anchored or sutured to the septum orbitale as it joins the aponeurosis of the levator. Hence, only a shallow lid fold is formed. With the passage of time, the supraorbital fat may push the septum orbitale forward and downward. This may eventually dislodge or remove the adhesions that have formed between the skin, orbicularis muscle, and septum orbitale. The fold thus formed may become shallower (less pronounced) and in time may disappear completely.

SCARS. Some surgeons may take more than a single stroke to make the incision. Use of the lid fixation forceps helps to avoid this, because it fixes the skin and makes it easier to cut in one long stroke drawn from the nasal to the temporal end. If the incision is done in the reverse direction, a serrated wound may result and may eventually produce an irregular or thick scar. Removal of the sutures earlier than three days may produce a gaping wound which

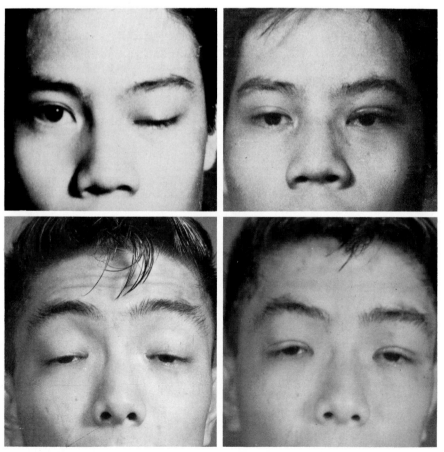

FIGURE 28–90. Two examples of simultaneous construction of the supratarsal fold combined with a ptosis operation. *Above,* Unilateral ptosis. *Below,* Bilateral ptosis.

will subsequently heal with an unacceptable scar. Removal of the sutures later than five to seven days may leave stitch marks or epithelized tunnels.

POSTOPERATIVE ASYMMETRIC LID FOLDS. The patient looks for symmetry with a critical attitude. A slight difference in the size and shape of the lid folds will provoke a complaint immediately after surgery and constantly thereafter. If after one month when the major part of the edema has subsided the patient still complains of asymmetry, reoperation is indicated and justified. The patient should be asked which side's appearance is preferred (Sayoc, 1969).

Other Indications for Construction of the Supratarsal Fold. Although plastic surgical construction of the supratarsal fold was originally conceived for the foldless eyelids of Orientals, experience has taught that it has other uses as well.

CONGENITAL PTOSIS. It is well known that in congenital ptosis with or without levator action the involved lid does not have a superior palpebral fold. In the management of ptosis, esthetic improvement is just as important as the restoration of function; hence, simultaneous construction of the superior palpebral fold is necessary to give cosmetically acceptable results, whether the ptosis is unilateral or bilateral (Fig. 28–90) (Sayoc, 1956).

FULL UPPER EYELID (Sayoc, 1967). In the full upper eyelid, with or without a fold, the insertion of the septum orbitale occurs farther down on the aponeurosis of the levator or on the superior border of the tarsus, so that the supraorbital fat falls down as low as the insertion. This gives a baggy or full upper eyelid, which is also common among Orientals. Surgical management includes removal of the supraorbital fat, relocation of the insertion of the septum orbitale to a higher level, and simultaneous construction of the superior palpebral fold (Fig. 28–91) (see also Chapter 37, p. 1895).

BLEPHARODERMACHALASIS (Sayoc, 1962). In persons past middle age, the excess skin associated with aging is excised, regardless of the absence or presence of the lid fold. The lid fold is then formed because the intradermal anchorage of the lower flap to the tarsus will keep the skin of the lower flap taut and, at the same time, prevent the preseptal skin from falling down to the ciliary border. This minimizes premature sagging after surgery. Better results are obtained if, in the excision of the excess skin, 2 mm of skin below the original fold are included in the lower incision. In anchoring the

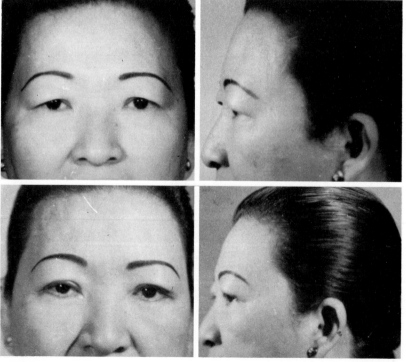

FIGURE 28–91. Front and lateral views of a patient with full upper eyelids. A slight improvement was achieved by constructing lid folds. In persons past middle age, the excess skin is excised and a superior palpebral fold is constructed as previously described.

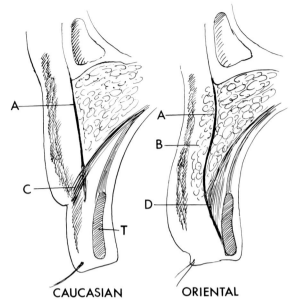

CAUCASIAN   ORIENTAL

FIGURE 28–92. Anatomical variations in the Caucasian and Oriental eyelids. *A,* The septum orbitale. *B,* The submuscular fat. *C,* The expansion of the levator palpebrae superioris muscle extending through the septum orbitale and orbicularis oculi muscle to attach to the skin of the supratarsal fold in the Caucasian lid. *D,* In the Oriental lid, the levator expansion terminates at the septum orbitale. (After Fernandez.)

lower flap intradermally to the tarsus, the flap is pulled back to the original height of the fold, giving a better result than simple excision of the excess skin (see also Chapter 37, p. 1895).

ASYMMETRIC LID FOLDS (Sayoc, 1969). When found in either Oriental or Occidental eyes, asymmetric lid folds indicate different levels of cutaneous insertion of the levator in the right and left eyelids. In this case, the patient is asked which fold is preferred. That measurement is then used for operating on both eyelids. In the asymmetric lid folds which

arise as a complication of plastic construction of the supratarsal fold, the same surgical approach is followed.

THE FERNANDEZ TECHNIQUE

Fernandez (1960) (Fig. 28–92) described one of two procedures, a simple or a radical one according to the desires of the patient and the appearance of the eyelids. In the simple procedure he forms only the supratarsal fold. He makes an incision 5 to 7 mm from the ciliary border and removes an ellipse of skin 7 to 8 mm in height. Under the inferior skin margin, the orbicularis muscle fibers and the septum orbitale are split, exposing the supraorbital fat and beneath this the levator palpebrae superioris expansion. The levator expansion is then sutured to the dermis of the skin below the incision with three 5–0 white nylon sutures. The skin is closed with a continuous or interrupted 6–0 nylon suture (Fig. 28–93).

The more radical procedure is performed when the patient desires a more Occidental look, has fatty eyelids, and is willing to accept a longer period of convalescence. The skin lines are outlined 7 to 8 mm from the ciliary border; a Z-plasty for the epicanthal fold is also outlined. An elliptical piece of skin is removed medially as far as the angle of the eye and laterally as far as the eyebrow. A bridge of tissue 7 or 8 mm in extent is left at the lateral canthus to allow for lymphatic drainage. The septum orbitale is incised and the supraorbital fat and levator palpebrae superioris muscle identified and separated. The supraorbital fat is removed, and the inferior thickened edge of the levator is dissected free and sutured to the

FIGURE 28–93. Operation for the formation of a supratarsal fold. Skin is incised. A strip of orbicularis muscle and septum orbitale is excised and excess orbital fat is removed. The levator muscle is sutured to the skin at the lower border of the skin incision. Note two-layer closure. (After Fernandez.)

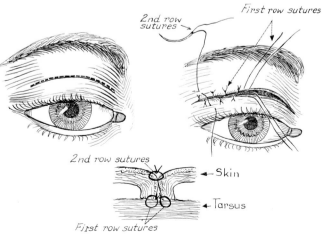

subcutaneous tissues and the deepest fibers of the dermis at the edge of the lower incision. A Z-plasty is completed, with the lower flap based medially and the upper laterally. The skin is closed with a continuous 6–0 nylon suture.

Deformities of the Eyebrow

MARK K. H. WANG, M.D., W. BRANDON MACOMBER, M.D., AND RAY A. ELLIOTT, JR., M.D.

Distortion of the Eyebrow. A common injury to the passenger who has been projected through the windshield in an automobile crash is a rather typical pattern of avulsion of soft tissue of the skull, especially just above, through, or below the eyebrows. Initially, the wounds should be carefully cleansed and bleeding controlled, as residual hematoma results in an ugly, discolored, thickened scar with distortion of the eyebrows.

Vertical displacements that result can usually be corrected by a Z-plasty procedure (Fig. 28–94), while horizontal displacement can be corrected by scar revision and realignment of the parts. These procedures should be performed 6 to 12 months following the accident, after the scar tissue has softened.

Defects of the Eyebrows. These important features can be lost through a variety of causes, such as avulsion injury, thermal or radiation burns, operations for neoplasm, or diseases such as syphilis, leprosy, and alopecia areata.

Tanzer (1962) reviewed the techniques of eyebrow reconstruction. In 1849 Jobert used a flap along the temporal hairline for reconstruction. Monks (1898) and Esser (1917) advocated an artery island flap to transplant temporal skin and hair into the supraorbital region.

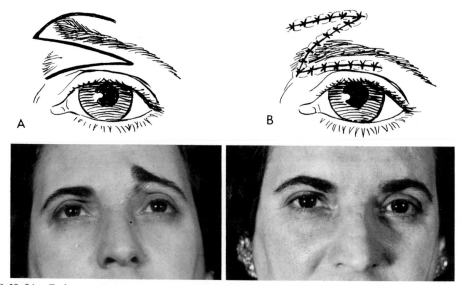

FIGURE 28–94. Z-plasty technique to correct distortion of left eyebrow. *A,* Outline of Z-plasty. *B,* The flaps are transposed, restoring the contour of the eyebrow. The photographs illustrate the restoration of eyebrow contour by Z-plasty.

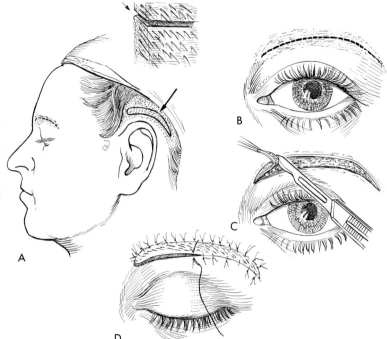

FIGURE 28-95. Reconstruction of an eyebrow by a scalp graft. *A,* Removal of a strip of scalp from the temporal area. *B,* An incision is made in the supraorbital area to receive the scalp transplant. *C,* A strip of skin is removed, providing a bed for the graft. *D,* The scalp graft sutured in position.

Morax (1919) formed a flap by splitting the unaffected brow. In 1920 Wheeler emphasized the use of scalp grafts.

GRAFTING FOR EYEBROW RECONSTRUCTION

The success of an eyebrow graft (Fig. 28–95) depends heavily on the state of the recipient bed. A scarred, fibrotic brow is inimical to successful grafting. The scarred tissue must first be removed and the area recovered by an advancement or rotation flap or by a thick split- or full-thickness skin graft. A hair-bearing graft is cut in a vertical direction from behind the ear and transplanted. The vertical incision provides the proper slant of the hairs, which in the eyebrow are directed upward and laterally. An ink mark at one end prior to transfer helps orient the graft, which is cut to a pattern made from the contralateral eyebrow and is up to 4 or 5 mm in width; after the pattern is removed, it is reversed in order to provide the shape of the contralateral eyebrow. If the eyebrows are missing on both sides, a curved line along the superciliary ridge is used as a guide. If additional width is needed, it is preferable to do a second similar procedure. Before transfer, the graft is partly defatted without disturbing the hair bulbs and then sutured in place with 6–0 sutures. Because the scalp graft is only partly

defatted, it depends for its survival upon revascularization from the edges of the host bed. The survival of the scalp grafts in eyebrow reconstruction is quite unpredictable; large grafts may be successful against all expectations.

Scalp grafts are usually successful when their width does not exceed 5 to 10 mm. The hairs usually require periodic trimming, as they grow excessively long.

Brent (1975) advocated a technique which he termed "medial accentuation" and "strip coupling." He places several narrow grafts in separate incisions and then joins them at a second stage (Fig. 28–96).

For better vascularization between graft and recipient site, the area of contact can be increased by a slight variation in technique. The recipient area is opened by two separate cuts through the same skin incision, making an inverted "V" with the apex at the skin. Thus, with spreading, a "W" is formed in cross section. The graft, stabilized by two skin hooks, is incised in its long axis through the subcutaneous and dermal layers without damage to the hair follicles, leaving the epidermis intact to form a "W" (Fig. 28–97). The graft is placed in the recipient site, sutured with 6–0 silk, and splinted with a moderate pressure dressing, which is changed on the fifth to seventh day.

Delayed Grafting. Karfik and Smahel (1969) have reported that a delay of four or

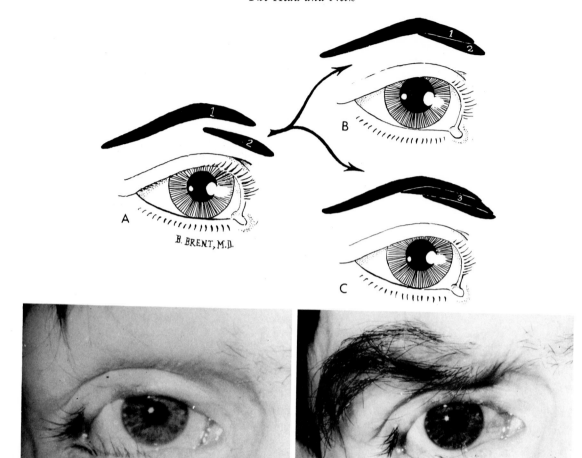

B. BRENT, M.D.

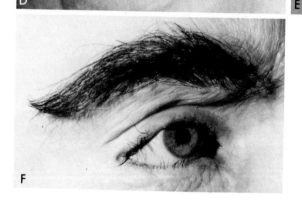

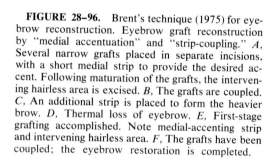

FIGURE 28–96. Brent's technique (1975) for eyebrow reconstruction. Eyebrow graft reconstruction by "medial accentuation" and "strip-coupling." *A*, Several narrow grafts placed in separate incisions, with a short medial strip to provide the desired accent. Following maturation of the grafts, the intervening hairless area is excised. *B*, The grafts are coupled. *C*, An additional strip is placed to form the heavier brow. *D*, Thermal loss of eyebrow. *E*, First-stage grafting accomplished. Note medial-accenting strip and intervening hairless area. *F*, The grafts have been coupled; the eyebrow restoration is completed.

five days between the incision and preparation of the recipient site and the transplantation of the hair-bearing scalp graft has increased the results of the "take" of the graft.

Combined Composite Scalp and Full-Thickness Skin Graft. Longacre, de Stefano, and Holmstrand (1962) advocated, in patients in whom additional skin grafting was indicated, a full eyebrow reconstruction by planning a combined composite (scalp) and full-thickness (postauricular skin) graft, removed in continuity from behind the ear as a single graft. The numerous vascular connections between the large full-thickness skin graft and the recipient bed appear to enhance the vascularity of the scalp graft and thereby ensure the successful take of the transplant.

FLAP FROM THE OPPOSITE EYEBROW

If a graft has been tried without success, if the recipient site is unsuitable, or if the medial aspect of the contralateral eyebrow is missing, a flap from the contralateral eyebrow may be indicated. The unaffected brow is split longitudinally and rotated on a glabellar pedicle to the opposite side (Fig. 28–98). The flap, because of its narrowness, is susceptible to necrosis; the result may be two brows, neither of which retains a normal shape. The best indication for this method is loss of the medial aspect of the brow.

SCALP FLAPS

Use of a flap of scalp tissue from the temporal area is the most reliable method of resurfacing the eyebrow. It is successful when the flap is transferred immediately; when the distance between donor and recipient areas is greater than

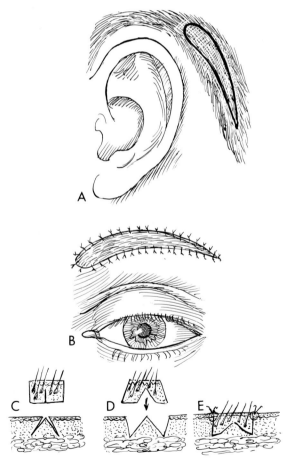

FIGURE 28–97. A technique to increase the area of contact between the scalp graft and host bed. *A*, Design of the scalp graft. *B*, The graft sutured in position. *C*, Prior to insertion, the graft is partly split on its undersurface; two divergent incisions are made in the host bed. *D*, The graft and host bed ready for insertion of the graft. *E*, The graft in position.

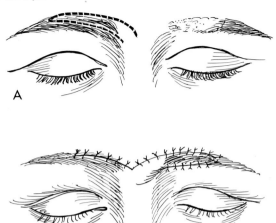

FIGURE 28–98. Flap from the contralateral eyebrow transposed to provide the missing medial portion of the defective eyebrow.

usual, the transfer should be delayed by the outline delaying technique (see Chapter 6, p. 197), because the pedicle is long and narrow (Fig. 28–99). After transfer, the remainder of the pedicle of the flap is returned to its original site. It is often necessary to trim the hairs, since they tend to grow to excessive lengths. This technique appears to be the most reliable in terms of attaining an adequate eyebrow, particularly if the recipient site is scarred.

In the Monks-Esser island flap (Figs. 28–100 and 28–101), the desired brow configuration is mapped on the shaved temporal area, allowing sufficient length for transfer. The island of scalp is centered over the frontal branch of the superficial temporal artery. The vascular pedicle may be dissected out, but it is simpler and safer to include the vascular pedicle in a pedicle of subcutaneous tissue and fascia approximately 1 cm in width (Fig. 28–102). After the recipient area is prepared, the pedicle is introduced into the defect through a subcutaneous tunnel. The donor area is closed and the graft sutured in position. Postoperatively, the transplanted scalp tissue may be edematous and cyanotic, and it requires careful and regular observation. The patient's head is elevated and the flap "milked" with applicator sticks. The hair may also be temporarily lost, as in most hair-bearing grafts.

Microvascular free scalp flaps (see Chapter 14) can also be employed.

THE SCALPING FLAP FOR EYEBROW RECONSTRUCTION

When the scalp has been destroyed over the portion that would serve as a donor area for a

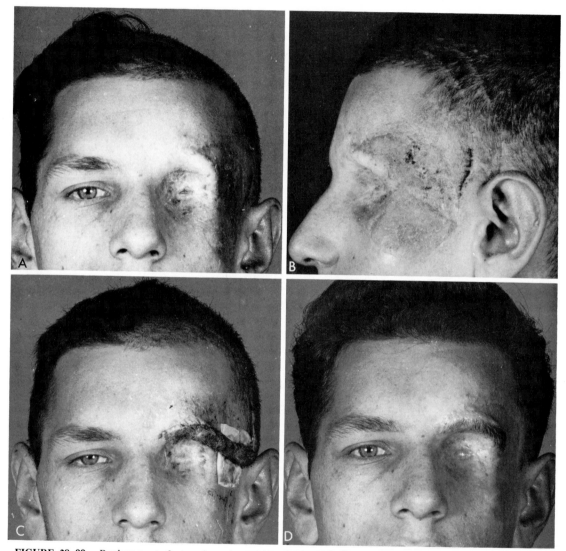

FIGURE 28–99.   Replacement of an eyebrow by a delayed temporal scalp flap. *A*, The left orbit was exenterated and skin grafted; the eyebrow was destroyed by radiation. *B*, A long temporal scalp flap was delayed. *C*, Scalp flap after transfer. *D*, Result obtained. The donor area was closed by direct approximation of the wound edges. (From Kazanjian and Converse.)

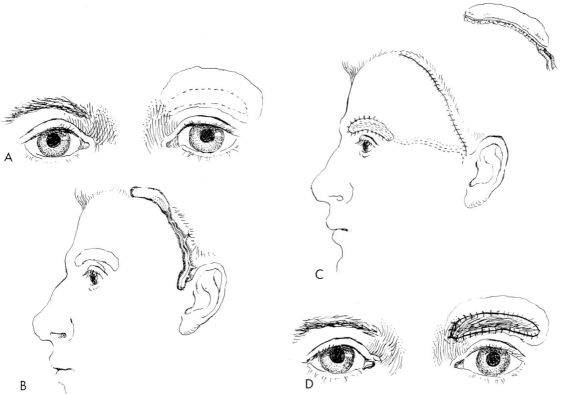

FIGURE 28–100. Artery island flap for eyebrow reconstruction. *A*, Skin grafting the left supraorbital area following burns. The eyebrow was destroyed. *B*, Outline of the flap and the dissected superficial temporal vessels. *C*, The scalp on a vascular pedicle. *D*, The scalp flap in position, restoring the left eyebrow.

flap and when the eyebrow cannot be reconstructed by scalp grafts because of an inhospitable recipient site, a scalping flap (see Chapter 29, p. 1234), usually employed in nasal reconstruction, is a useful procedure. A portion of the scalping flap used to reconstruct the nose has also been detached, after the pedicle of the flap has been severed and before it is returned to the scalp and forehead donor area, and used to reconstruct an eyebrow.

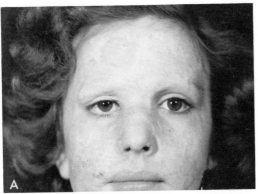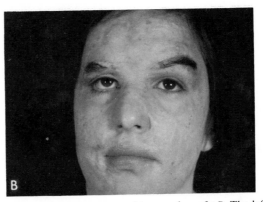

FIGURE 28–101. Reconstruction of both eyebrows. *A*, The right eyebrow was restored by a scalp graft. *B*, The left eyebrow was restored by an artery island flap.

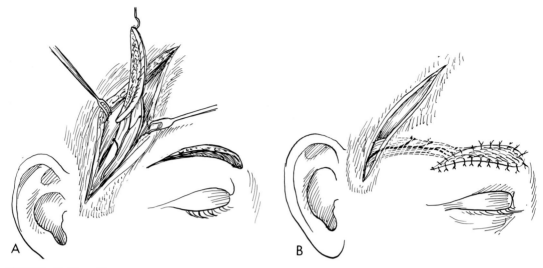

FIGURE 28–102. The artery island scalp flap with a subcutaneous pedicle. *A*, The superficial temporal vessels are included in a pedicle of subcutaneous tissue. *B*, The scalp flap is in position, having been introduced into the recipient bed via the subcutaneous route.

The Orbit

ANOPHTHALMOS AND MICROPHTHALMOS

BYRON SMITH, M.D.,
AND AUGUSTUS J. VALAURI, D.D.S.

Anophthalmos (anophthalmia) is defined as a condition in which no ocular globe, however small, can be found in the orbit. It is difficult to distinguish between a true anophthalmos and an extreme degree of microphthalmos, in which there is a small ocular globe. The answer lies in microscopic examination of serial sections of the orbital contents, a procedure which is impractical in the living.

A variety of developmental mishaps may lead to the suppression of an eye. In primary anophthalmos, the single originating fault is a failure of the optic pit to deepen and form an optic outgrowth from the forebrain. In secondary anophthalmos, there is complete suppression or abnormal development of the entire forebrain; absence of the eye is merely the consequence of the lack of development of the entire region and is one of a host of concomitant abnormalities. A third type of anophthalmos may also be recognized, in which an optic vesicle forms but subsequently degen-

erates and disappears. This type is linked with extreme degrees of microphthalmos and is designated as consecutive or degenerative anophthalmos.

In *primary anophthalmos,* the cause probably is germinal, since in a typical case no other defect is present. Moreover, there are clinical and experimental records of an occasional familial and hereditary character in which the *ectodermal* elements alone are missing. The orbit, eyelids, lacrimal apparatus, conjunctival sac, extrinsic ocular muscles, and their nerves are all self-determining and can develop without any stimulus from the optic vesicle. The lens, not being self-determining but arising from the surface ectoderm only, in response to a stimulus received from the optic vesicle, is absent. The cornea and sclera, on the other hand, form normally as condensations around an optic cup, but even in its absence there usually appears to be some attempt at a mesodermal condensation. The relationships of parts and the balance of growth between them are obviously interfered with by the absence of an optic cup, around which the subsidiary mesodermal structures should group themselves. As a result, the orbit is present but usually slightly smaller than normal. The upper and lower eyelids are present, but the palpebral aperture is small. The lids are often ad-

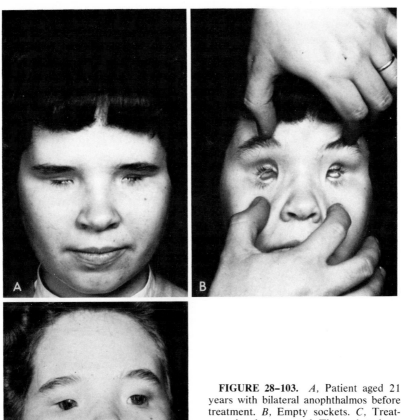

FIGURE 28–103. *A*, Patient aged 21 years with bilateral anophthalmos before treatment. *B*, Empty sockets. *C*, Treatment has been started. The sockets have been enlarged and prosthetic eyes inserted.

herent at their margins but can be separated without cutting; eyelashes, meibomian glands, and lacrimal puncta are usually present, though the puncta may be absent; there is a small conjunctival sac; the lids appear concave and are usually closed (Fig. 28–103); the lacrimal gland is present, and tears issue from the conjunctival sac when the child cries. The brain in primary anophthalmos shows no abnormality other than atrophy of the central optic paths from disuse.

The clinical appearance of true anophthalmos in man corresponds very closely with the findings of experimental embryologists (Fig. 28–104).

Secondary anophthalmos due to complete suppression or gross abnormality of the front end of the medullary tube is better known to experimental teratologists than to clinicians, since the monstrosities produced are not usually viable.

Degenerative or consecutive anophthalmos is a term used to include the cases in which an optic outgrowth appears to have formed and subsequently to have degenerated. Embryos are occasionally found in which a great disparity of size is noted between the two optic cups, one being normal and the other stunted and not in contact with the surface ectoderm. Such an eye might be expected either to attain an extreme degree of microphthalmos or to become swamped by the growth of surrounding parts and to disappear almost completely.

If the fate of the ectodermal optic outgrowth is followed a stage further (after invagination), there is a group of abnormalities arising in man between the 7-mm and 14-mm stages. This growth period includes the time between in-

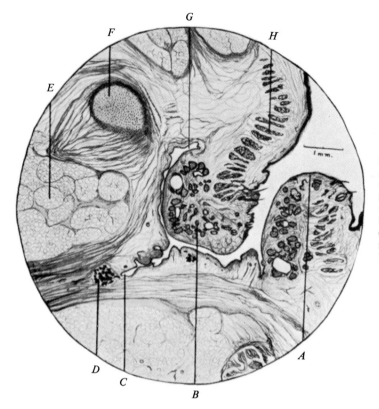

FIGURE 28–104. Section through the lids and orbital contents in a case of anophthalmos. *A*, lower lid; *B*, upper lid; *C*, lower conjunctival fornix; *D*, accessory lacrimal gland; *E*, orbital fat; *F*, nodule of cartilage; *G*, upper conjunctival fornix; *H*, fibers of orbicularis oculi muscle. (From Mann, I.: Developmental Abnormalities of the Eye. Philadelphia, J. B. Lippincott Company, 1957.)

vagination of the optic vesicle and complete closure of the embryonic cleft. These abnormalities lead to gross defects of the entire ocular globe, known clinically as microphthalmos with orbital cysts, and typical coloboma of retina, choroid, and iris.

Microphthalmos has been described as a uniocular congenital deformity in which lack of development of one eye is in striking contrast to the development of the other. In some cases it may be said that the eye is not present at all, though a firm cystic tumor occupying the normal site of the globe in the orbit has sometimes been mistaken for an eye. Fuchs (1924) described such a cyst as being attached to the lower lid, where it is seen glimmering with a bluish luster. When opened, the cyst contains a rudimentary retina, floating in a serous fluid. In cases of less severe deformity, coloboma or congenital fissure of the iris and of the optic nerve is usually present. Some observers claim that associated deformities are less frequent in patients with microphthalmos than in patients with anophthalmos. In microphthalmos, a cyst of the lower eyelid which contains a rudimentary eye is nearly always found. In almost all patients, other congenital stigmas are seen, of which a miniature orbit is the commonest. Other defects in the order in which they may occur are cleft lip, cleft palate, nasal cleft,

supernumerary auricle, and supernumerary digits.

Etiology. In 1903 von Hippel laid the foundation for the modern view that the defect is due to an inherent abnormality of growth in the optic cup itself. He pointed out the hereditary nature of the condition but still considered that persistence of mesoderm played a large part in failure of closure. He was the earliest observer to realize that, since coloboma is hereditary in rabbits, specimens at various stages of embryonic development can be obtained for examination. By this means, he entirely disproved the inflammatory theory and laid the foundation for the work of Koyanagi (1921) and von Szily (1913), whose embryologic researches are the most accurate and illuminating in the entire field of teratology. Their conclusions are:

1. The fault is primarily ectodermal, the persistence of mesoderm being secondary and not present in every case.

2. The affected strain shows transmission of the typical coloboma of choroid, retina, and iris, coloboma of optic nerve, and orbital cysts interchangeably, but never of cyclopia and anophthalmos.

3. The condition is mendelian recessive.

Incidence. True congenital anophthalmos is rare, but microphthalmos occurs frequently in

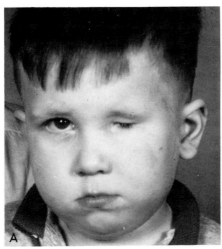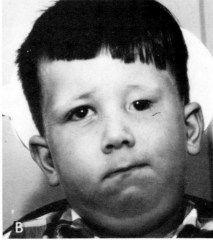

FIGURE 28–105. *A*, Child aged 9 years with congenital microphthalmos of the left eye, showing a collapse of the upper lid and a concave lower lid. *B*, Patient during treatment with prosthetic expanders.

degrees varying from a nubbin to a complete miniature ocular globe. The deformity is usually unilateral, occasionally bilateral (Figs. 28–105 and 28–106). Collins between 1887 and 1897 could find only 30 cases of bilateral and 12 of unilateral anophthalmos in the literature. In 1900 von Hippel raised the recorded number of bilateral cases to 64 and of unilateral to 23, a somewhat similar proportion. In 15 of the latter, the other eye showed congenital anomalies. Sex incidence was not significant, and heredity was a rare factor. Our own experience has been in accord with these findings.

Treatment. Microphthalmos and anophthalmos are deformities that are distressing to the parents and affect the psychologic develop-ment of the afflicted child. Correction of the deformity is a difficult problem.

MICROPHTHALMOS. In the favorable case, with a miniature eye in the socket, treatment consists of placing a small, plastic, concave-convex conformer in the conjunctival socket within the first four weeks of life. The conformer must be changed to one of a larger size approximately every two weeks. The sequence is continued with increasing intervals until past puberty. A peg can be attached to the anterior surface of the prosthesis as an aid in its manipulation. Pressure can also be transmitted to the conformer through this attachment.

Depending on the degree of microphthalmos, expansion of the cul-de-sac with graduated prostheses may be of prime importance. In the average case of microphthalmos,

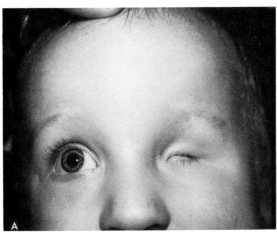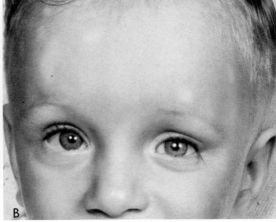

FIGURE 28–106. *A*, Child aged 2½ years with congenital anophthalmos of the left eye, concave, closed lids, and a small palpebral fissure. *B*, Patient with ocular prosthesis after five months of treatment, showing the growth of the lids and an almost normal palpebral fissure.

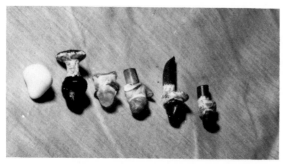

FIGURE 28–107. Graduated expanders employed during treatment of the patient shown in Figure 28–105. Note the size and the form of the cul-de-sac during pressure expansion.

a sufficient cul-de-sac is present to accommodate an adequate prosthesis without utilizing an expansion technique. The orbit and the palpebral fissure are usually near normal size.

A shell prosthesis is fashioned. Before prosthetic fittings are begun, the position of the cornea should be established to prevent irritation from the posterior surface of the shell. It is important to stain the cornea after fitting to be certain that it is not abraded by the prosthesis. Usually two or three fittings are necessary before a satisfactory prosthesis is achieved. The size and motility of the microphthalmic eye will determine the motility of the prosthesis. Muscle surgery is required in some cases. In unilateral microphthalmos, the motility can only be expected to approach that of the uninvolved eye. There is usually an associated ptosis. The procedure used to correct the ptosis is determined by the type of ptosis involved, as discussed earlier in the chapter.

ANOPHTHALMOS. In congenital anophthalmos the problem is much more involved. A contracted bony orbit is usually associated with the anophthalmos, with a small palpebral opening, scant eyelashes, and ptosis. The first corrective measure should be the enlargement of the socket. Surgery should be avoided as long as possible. Forcing dental molding compound into the contracted socket produces a progressive enlargement, and the dental compound provides a pattern from which an acrylic prosthesis can be made. The prosthesis is placed in the socket and initially held in place with a moderately compressive dressing. A stem on the prosthesis protruding through the palpebral opening facilitates secure fitting. The orbital expansion with the compound implant is repeated at suitable intervals over a period of months until a socket of adequate size is obtained (Figs. 28–107, 28–108, and 28–109).

In some patients an impasse is reached. The conjunctival socket will not accept a larger conformer than can be passed through the narrow palpebral fissure, and a lateral canthoplasty must be done to elongate the palpebral fissure. If a simple canthoplasty is not sufficient, a more expansive lateral canthoplasty extending lateral to the bony margin of the orbit is done. The raw area is lined with a split-thickness buccal mucous membrane graft. The expansion of the palpebral fissure will permit the fitting of a more suitable prosthesis.

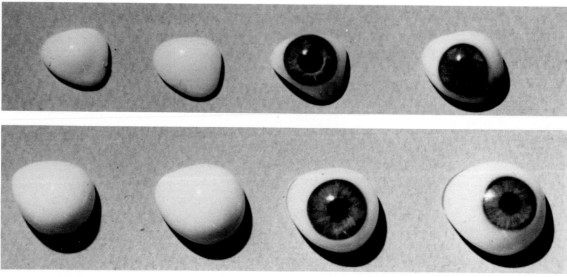

FIGURE 28–108. Prostheses used for expansion treatment of patient shown in Figure 28–106. Note the progressive change of size from 9 mm wide and 6 mm vertically to 16 mm wide and 11 mm vertically in a period of five months.

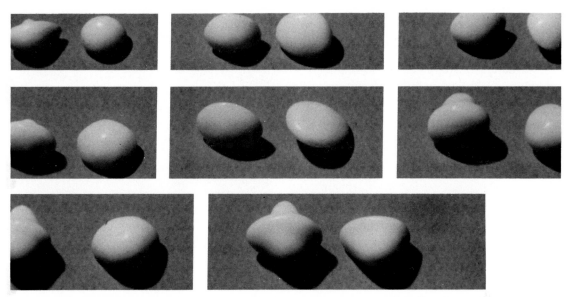

FIGURE 28–109. Prostheses used for expansion treatment of a patient with bilateral anophthalmos.

When mechanical expansion is not possible, more radical surgery may be required. Smith and Cole suggested cutting through the periosteum along the orbital margins and burring away as much bone as possible to enlarge the bony socket. The raw areas are covered with buccal mucous membrane grafts to enlarge the cavity in order that an artificial eye more comparable in size to the opposite eye may be fitted. Hartman (1962) stated that Strampelli enlarges the entire conjunctival sac by cutting through the conjunctiva along the tarsal edge of both upper and lower eyelids. He carefully undermines and cuts free the conjunctiva around the entire 360 degrees, working toward the center and allowing it to bunch up as a central stump. Both eyelids are completely everted and held in this extended position until the large, thin, labial mucous membrane graft which was applied over the raw area has healed. An orbital socket large enough to contain a satisfactory artificial prosthesis, with some possibility of motion, is obtained. Craniofacial surgical techniques may also be employed to expand the orbit (see Chapter 56).

During treatment a number of complications may arise; the most frequent and troublesome is lack of retention of the conformer. In order to overcome this obstacle, various devices have been tried, the simplest being that of taping the eyelids in order to maintain the prosthesis within the socket. In the early stages, under general anesthesia, positive pressure can be exerted by means of a dental compound stick, softened, yet with enough body to force the soft tissues to expand inside the cul-de-sac.

This phase of the expansion is rapid. The dental compound is often self-retentive; it may be maintained by means of a tight bandage with pressure applied to a peg left on the stick and extending outward through the palpebral opening. Complications arising from the bandage or tape have given some concern, especially during warm weather. The skin under the tape or bandage may show a contact dermatitis and delay further treatment.

When the socket has attained a relatively satisfactory size and the tissue tone is good, impressions are taken with a rubber base material or a plastic base using a hand syringe and a shell conformer as a carrier tray. The shell conformer is fitted inside the lids; through an opening in its stem, a hypodermic syringe needle is inserted, and impression material is injected into the socket in a manner similar to the way an impression is taken for a contact lens. From this impression a wax pattern is made and fitted in the orbital socket; proper adjustments are made to the shape and contour by adding or shaping wax. The pattern is then invested and "cured" into scleral material with a peg or handle attached to the anterior surface; the "cured" sclera is highly polished and fitted into the socket. This operation is repeated a number of times until the desired size and maximum expansion are attained.

In the various stages retention of the prosthesis may become a problem. Many solutions have been offered: head caps of different sorts with bars and universal joints (Roger Anderson type appliances); fixation of the prosthesis to the teeth by means of dental splints and orthodontic tubes (Figs. 28–110 and 28–111); eyeglasses with extensions from the frame to support the eye prosthesis. However ingenious these appliances may be, without the parents' cooperation treatment would be fruitless. It is of utmost importance, therefore, to talk to the parents and ensure their cooperation before treatment is begun.

The complication of entropion occurs frequently and may be caused by too large a conformer. The eyelashes begin to point toward the palpebral fissure rather than away from it. When the entropion is allowed to progress, the cilia become plastered to the anterior face of the prosthesis with dried secretion, causing discomfort and an unpleasant appearance. This complication is an indication either to proceed with caution in enlarging the size of the conformer or of the need to enlarge the conjunctival fornices. Eyelash curlers are of assistance.

Lateral orbitotomy facilitates the accommodation of a definitive prosthesis, and a suspension operation may be required to correct the ptosis.

Observation of the results obtained in several of our patients with the pressure technique for the correction of anophthalmos indicates that growth of the cul-de-sac and orbital region of the face has been stimulated. It is reasonable to assume that early treatment with positive pressure followed by intermittent passive pressure from the prosthesis should stimulate normal development of the orbit and its surrounding structures.

Surgical expansion of the anophthalmic orbit. The degree of expansion of the small orbit in the anophthalmic patient is limited. While the conjunctival sac can be expanded, expansion is limited and arrested by the resistance of the bone. The surgical expansion of the anophthalmic orbit has been achieved through an intracranial approach (see Chapter 56).

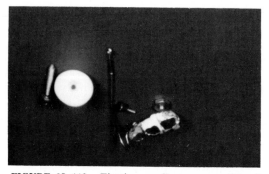

FIGURE 28–110. Fixation appliance supporting the eye prosthesis by means of a dental splint and orthodontic tube.

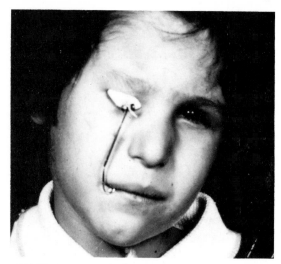

FIGURE 28–111. Patient wearing appliance shown in Figure 28–110.

SOCKET RECONSTRUCTION

Successful reconstruction of the anophthalmic socket for the maintenance of an artificial eye depends upon a cavity of sufficient size and shape to maintain the prosthetic device. This necessitates the presence of eyelids and fornices of sufficient depth to keep the prosthesis within the socket. A socket may be lined with skin or mucous membrane; the best socket has a mucous membrane lining. A skin socket is dry and has some tendency to accumulate desquamated epidermis, producing a foul odor.

Surgical Management. The surgical technique in socket reconstruction is contingent upon whether total or partial socket reconstruction is required. The simplest type of socket revision is the type in which there is sufficient socket lining but the lining is in the wrong position. The surgical revision of such a socket is done by undermining the socket lining and thinning it and dissecting the fornices into the proper shape, repositioning the mucous membrane or conjunctiva by placing a conformer within the socket and maintaining its position until healing has taken place. The assurance of the proper positioning of the conformer during the healing process necessitates careful fixation. The technique is relatively simple (Fig. 28–112). After the socket has been dissected and designed in proper configuration, an incision is made through the lower lid overlying the inferior orbital rim (Fig. 28–112, *A, B*). In the middle third of the inferior orbital rim, a drill hole is placed through the rim from the outside to the inside (Fig. 28–

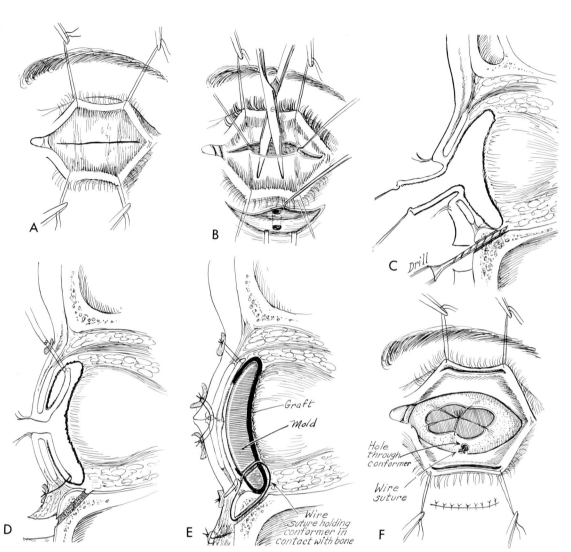

FIGURE 28–112. *A,* Contracted socket showing obliteration of the fornices. The horizontal line across the center represents the line of incision across the dome of the socket. Traction sutures are placed in the lid to exert traction on the mucous membrane lining the socket during dissection. *B,* The wound edges are retracted with dissecting hooks, and the membrane is undermined from the incision toward the lid margin. The socket is then dissected downward toward the orbital rim and upward and outward in all directions to prepare a cavity to receive the conformer. A horizontal incision is made over the orbital margin approximately 10 mm below the lid edge, after the margin has been cleared of periosteum. The drill hole is placed in the position shown by the dotted lines. *C,* A cross section of the orbit and lids, showing the dissection of the new socket cavity and the retracted conjunctiva between the lid margins. The drill hole is shown in its position across the angle of the orbital margin near its midpoint. *D,* The dissected conjunctiva is then retracted and sutured as shown by interrupted sutures tied over rubber plates on the outer surface of the lid margin. A cross section of the drill hole and its relationship to the lower socket margin are shown. *E,* The conformer is in place surrounded by a graft of skin or mucous membrane. The drill hole in the bone is connected to a drill hole through the lower portion of the conformer by a wire suture; the knot of the suture is tied and tucked into the hole within the conformer in order to avoid irritation of the soft tissues. The suture across the inner palpebral fissure maintains the central lid adhesion until healing has taken place. The lid adhesion is left for approximately two months. *F,* The conformer is shown in place with the wire suture maintaining the lower margin of the conformer in approximation to the lower orbital rim. The skin wound is closed with interrupted 6–0 silk sutures. The incisions for the lid adhesion are shown along the lid margin. At the termination of two months, the lid adhesion is severed, the wire is removed, and the conformer is replaced by an artificial eye.

112, *B, C*). A stainless steel wire is then passed through this hole and into the socket, and the other end of the wire is passed over the inferior orbital rim into the socket. The prepared conformer is perforated, and the wire is then passed from behind forward through the hole in the conformer and twisted with the other end of the wire (Fig. 28–112, *D, E*). This pulls the conformer down toward the orbital rim and maintains it in an upright position. The wire knot is tied within the socket and tucked into the hole in the conformer. The best type of conformer is made of gutta-percha and is prepared at the time of surgery. The graft may be sutured to itself after it has been wrapped around the conformer raw surface outward (Fig. 28–112, *F*).

If the upper half of the socket is normal and the lower half deficient, the dissection consists of making an incision along the lower lid margin, thinning out the lower lid, and extending the dissection down to the inferior orbital rim bone. The partially covered conformer is then placed in the socket and wired. Because of the fact that some lids tend to contract in a vertical fashion during the healing process, it is advisable to perform a tarsorrhaphy over the central third of the lid during the healing process. This adhesion is maintained for eight weeks or longer. After the socket has healed and softened, the adhesion is opened, the wire cut, and the conformer removed. The socket should not be left without some type of a prosthetic device during the postoperative phases.

When the lining is missing in the upper fornix, the surgery required to reconstruct the fornix is somewhat more difficult. The dissection in the upper lid is extended upward (Fig. 28–112, *C* to *F*), and attempts are made to preserve the levator if at all possible. After the dissection has been completed, a conformer is fashioned with a drill hole for fixation to the lower orbital rim. The upper part of the conformer is covered with a graft and inserted and wired into proper position.

Complete restoration of the socket combines the two previously described techniques, and the conformer is completely covered with a graft rather than being partially covered. If the Castroviejo mucotome (see Fig. 28–61) is used to obtain the graft from the oral cavity, a 0.3-mm thickness graft is used. Ordinarily the membrane must be 0.3-mm thick or more, or else it does not handle with ease. A moderate pressure dressing is applied. The dressing is changed in 48 hours.

Mustardé (1975) has advocated transplanta-

tion of septal cartilage in the lower lid to prevent the fold that forms under the artificial eye in the lower lid.

EXOPHTHALMOS

JOHN MARQUIS CONVERSE, M.D.,
AND SERGE KRUPP, M.D.

Exophthalmos may be defined as an excessive proptosis of the ocular globe and orbital contents from the orbital cavity.

Exophthalmos occurs in the following conditions:

1. Increase of the orbital contents, such as occurs in thyrotoxic ophthalmopathy (Fig. 28–113), intraorbital tumors, or arteriovenous aneurysm.

2. Decrease in the size of the orbital cavity:

A. Reduction of the volume of the orbit by intraorbital tumors, fractured fragments, osteomas, mucocele of the frontal sinus, and fibrous dysplasia.

B. Decrease in the size of the orbit in patients with craniofacial dysostosis; the orbit fails to develop and is incapable of lodging the orbital contents, which are expelled (see Chapters 53 and 56).

The plastic surgeon may be called upon to correct thyrotoxic exophthalmos of varying degrees. It has been stated (Naffziger, 1948, 1954; Ogura and Walsh, 1962; Low, 1967) that surgery should not be performed for cosmetic reasons only. An increasing demand for improvement in appearance and the development of operations of diminished risk have led to the more frequent performance of corrective decompression operations.

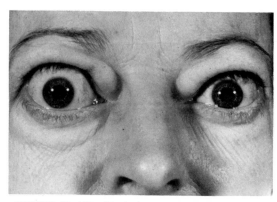

FIGURE 28–113. Typical appearance of patient with thyrotoxic exophthalmos. (Courtesy of Dr. Thomas C. Naugle, Jr.)

According to Mayo (1914), in the late 18th century Morgagni and Parry had already mentioned a connection between hyperthyroidism and exophthalmos. But the credit belongs to Graves (1840) and von Basedow (1840) for having recognized the clinical entity of thyrotoxic exophthalmos. Robert Graves in 1840 wrote of his findings in three patients: "The eyes assumed a singular appearance, for the eyeballs were apparently enlarged, so that when she slept or tried to close her eyes, the lids were incapable of closing. When the eyes were open, the white sclerotic could be seen for a breadth of several lines, around the cornea." In 1840, von Basedow recorded his findings in four patients. In the United States, the clinical entity is usually designated as Graves' disease.

Later it was realized that the exophthalmos persists and may even occur or progress after hyperthyroidism has been controlled by thyroidectomy (Dollinger, 1911; Kuhnt, 1912; Böhm, 1929; Andersson, 1932; Guyton, 1946; Wood, 1936; Craig and Dodge, 1952a, b; Heydenreich and coworkers, 1966; Kuehn and coworkers, 1966; Long and Ellis, 1966; Long, 1967). Additional endocrine factors from the pituitary gland were studied, such as TSH (thyroid stimulating hormone) (Albert, 1945; Canadell, 1959; Dobyns and Steelman, 1953; Pochin, 1944; Sedan and Harter, 1966; Smelser, 1943; Sonnenberg and Money, 1960; Valenti and Cordella, 1967a, b); EPS (exophthalmos producing substance) and LATS (long-acting thyroid stimulator) (McKenzie, 1961; Adams, 1961); and other steroids (Alterman, 1954; Slansky and coworkers, 1967). A combination of hormones (Smelser and coworkers, 1958; Soler Sala and coworkers, 1968) was found to participate in malignant exophthalmos. It has also been suggested that Graves' disease may be one of the autoimmune disorders, with possible links to rheumatoid arthritis and systemic lupus erythematosus (Eversman and coworkers, 1966; Werner, 1967).

Orbital Pathology in Graves' Disease

The orbital pathology in Graves' disease and the tissue alterations which result in exophthalmos have been reviewed by Wybar (1957), Smelser (1961), and Riley (1972). It has been reported that mast cells, mucopolysaccharides, and water content are increased in orbital tissues. An inflammatory infiltration, consisting predominantly of lymphocytes and plasma cells, is found in all orbital tissues. An etiologic role has been ascribed to mast cells in the production of mucopolysaccharides and the resultant exophthalmos. The extraocular muscles are usually involved, and the extraocular muscle imbalance is another complicating factor.

At present Graves' disease is universally considered a multisystem disease of unknown etiology (Chopra and Solomon, 1970), characterized by (1) hyperthyroidism associated with diffuse hyperplasia of the thyroid gland, (2) infiltrate ophthalmopathy, and (3) infiltrate dermopathy (pretibial myxedema) (Odell and coworkers, 1970).

The role of the nervous system has been invoked. Hyperthyroidism and exophthalmos appear to be aggravated by psychologic stress. Emotional disturbances may have a deleterious effect on the immunologic surveillance system, either directly or indirectly by the corticotropin releasing hormone–ACTH–adrenal cortex system or by the release of thyrotopin releasing hormone (TRH).

Two factors are of paramount interest: the orbital pathology and the endocrine and immunologic factors responsible for the exophthalmos (Naffziger, 1933; Walsh and Ogura, 1957; Ogura and Walsh, 1962; Eversman and coworkers, 1966; Werner, 1967).

Thyrotoxic Exophthalmos

The exophthalmos in Graves' disease is usually bilateral (see Fig. 28–113), but in some patients it may be unilateral (see Fig. 28–119) (Andersson, 1932; Rintoul, 1968). It is more common in the female than in the male, the ratio being about 6:1, but in the male it usually leads to more complications (von Graefe, 1867).

According to Means (1941), the severe form of thyrotoxic exophthalmos is observed in about 4.5 per cent of the cases of hyperthyroidism. Craig and Dodge (1952b) and Poppen (1950) reported that only 1 per cent of the cases develop malignant exophthalmos. If the increasing proptosis in malignant thyrotoxic exophthalmos is not arrested, a progressive fullness of the eyelids occurs, followed by lacrimation and epiphora. With increasing proptosis, the lids are unable to cover the globe, resulting in dryness and ulceration of the cornea. The scleral conjunctiva appears watery, and later there is the development of chemosis of the conjunctiva of the lower eyelid. Diplopia and lack of parallelism of the ocular globe due to muscular imbalance are followed by increasing limitation of movements of the globe, and ultimately only downward movements are retained. With increasing proptosis, edema extends to both upper and lower lids, and varying degrees of retinal hemorrhage, papillitis, and rapid loss of vision may ensue. There is always the danger of either perforation of the globe or panophthalmitis and death caused by infection (Würdemann and Becker, 1906; Merrill and Oaks, 1933; Naffziger, 1933).

Classification of Exophthalmos in Graves' Disease. The American Thyroid Association has adopted a system of classification of exophthalmos. Class I is termed mild; Class 2 represents the earlier involvement of soft tissue; Class 3 indicates proptosis; Class 4 has extraocular muscle involvement; in Class 5 the cornea is involved; and in Class 6 the optic nerve is threatened.

Early Methods of Treatment. In severe cases of malignant thyrotoxic exophthalmos, the death of the patient was expected; consequently, enucleation of the affected eye (or eyes) was performed as a life-saving procedure during the nineteenth century and extending into the 1930's (Merrill and Oaks, 1933). Lorenz in 1857 had performed an enucleation in an attempt to decompress the orbit.

Palliative operations on the eyelids, such as tarsorrhaphy (Eagleton, 1912; Kuhnt, 1912; Juler, 1915) and canthotomy (von Graefe, 1867; Kuhnt, 1912) or surgical division of the cervical sympathetic nerves, proved to be of little value in the severe cases (Dollinger, 1911; Hirsch and Urbanek, 1930; Naffziger, 1933). The latter procedure was advocated by the French school (Jaboulay and Poncet, 1897; Jaboulay, 1898; Jonneseo, 1897; Reclus and Faure, 1897) to induce Horner's syndrome and was performed in the United States by Mayo (1914), in Germany by Balacescu (1902), and in Great Britain by Juler (1915).

The Development of Decompression Operations. The various techniques which have been employed for the decompression of the orbit in Graves' disease are summarized in Figure 28–114.

In 1888 Krönlein advocated a temporal approach to enter the orbital cavity for removing a dermoid cyst. On October 20, 1911, Dol-

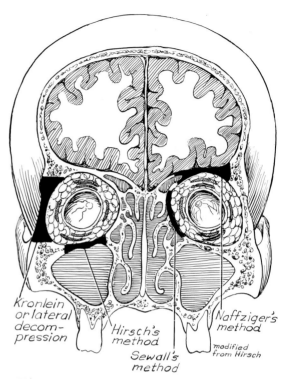

FIGURE 28–114. Composite drawing illustrating various techniques for decompression of thyrotoxic exophthalmos.

linger from Budapest performed the first recorded orbital decompression in a case of severe thyrotoxic exophthalmos using a Krönlein-type approach by removing a triangular portion of the lateral wall. The temporal decompression of the orbital contents saved the patient's vision and life. Kuhnt in 1912 recommended recourse to this procedure only in the severe cases of exophthalmos in Graves' disease. Eagleton (1912) also advocated decompression in severe malignant thyrotoxic exophthalmos by a Krönlein procedure. Tinker (1912) suggested removal of the floor, in addition to temporal decompression, to obtain further enlargement of the orbit but did not perform such an operation. The temporal decompression was later performed by Ask (1932), Thomas and Woods (1936), Spaeth (1939), McCravey and Mather (1940), Guthrie (1941), and Adler (1944), each of whom operated upon no more than three patients.

Moore in 1920 was the second surgeon to attempt orbital decompression in Graves' disease. He made an incision along the entire lower fornix, incising the septum orbitale and removing the orbital fat for additional decompression. The procedure gave only slight relief.

The temporal access to the orbital cavity for enlargement in severe cases of exophthalmos

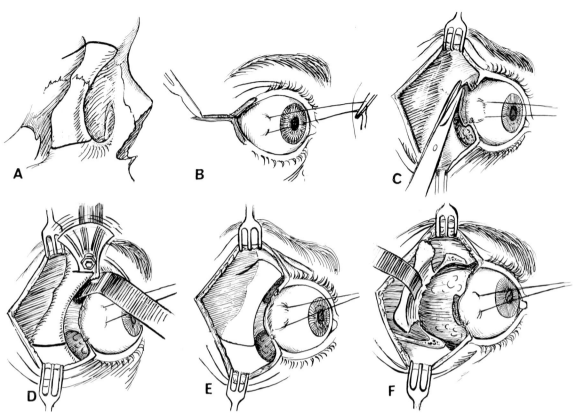

FIGURE 28–115. Lateral decompression: the Krönlein-Berke operation. *A*, The lines of osteotomy. *B*, T incision for exposure. *C*, The lateral tendon and lateral canthal raphé are raised from the bone, and the check ligament of the lateral rectus muscle is severed. *D* to *F*, The section of the lateral wall, the out-fracture, and removal.

in Graves' disease was popularized by Swift (1935), who approached the lateral orbital wall through a T-type incision. The technique was later standardized by Berke (1954) (Fig. 28–115) as an approach for the resection of intraorbital tumors. Guyton reported satisfactory results with this method in 1946.

In 1942 Welti and Offret reported another modification of the temporal decompression of the orbital cavity in Graves' disease. A curved incision exposed not only the lateral wall of the orbit but also part of the floor of the orbit, which could be resected, as well as the floor of the frontal sinus and even part of the orbital roof, without entering the cranial cavity. Schimek (1972) has also advocated additional resection of the floor of the orbit to obtain a satisfactory decompression.

Hirsch and Urbanek in 1930 described a new technique for decompression of the orbital cavity. By a Caldwell-Luc type of approach, they removed the orbital floor, preserving the infraorbital nerve (see Fig. 28–114). This operation proved to be a success. Meesmann

in 1940 also resected the infraorbital nerve to achieve additional decompression.

In 1936 Sewall enlarged the orbit by removing the ethmoid cells through a curved incision over the frontal process of the maxilla to obtain access to the lamina papyracea (see Fig. 28–114). This method was also successful and was used by Kistner (1939), Schall and Regan (1945), and Boyden (1956). The technique did not receive full recognition, however, until Walsh and Ogura in 1957 and Ogura and Walsh in 1962 in their series of operations proved the value of the procedure. They resected the orbital floor as well as the ethmoids and the lamina papyracea.

Naffziger in 1931 chose to solve the problem of orbital decompression in severe thyrotoxic exophthalmos by an intracranial approach to the orbital roof, which was resected (see Fig. 28–114). Later this type of operation was modified in 1944 by Poppen, who approached the orbital roof in a similar fashion. Poppen enlarged the resection of the orbital roof into the ethmoids and the frontal sinus. The Poppen modification was adopted by Craig and Dodge (1952a), who extended the decompression to include the sphenoid ridge (see Fig. 28–120).

The disadvantage of the Naffziger operation and the Poppen modification is the resulting contact of the brain with the orbital contents, which receive the pulsations of the brain.

Naffziger deserves credit for having shown the medical world that the eye, even in the severest type of Graves' exophthalmos, can be saved if the diagnosis is correct and the patient is operated upon before the late, even life-threatening, complications such as ulcerative keratitis and panophthalmia have destroyed the ocular globe. The Naffziger operation in its original description was used successfully by Semmes (1932), Bothman (1934), Rosenbaum (1937), Cairns (1938), Kistner (1939), Niall (1939), McCravey and Mather (1940), Daily and coworkers (1942), Simpson (1942), Moffat (1943), Savin (1943), and Bardram (1944).

Indications for Surgical Decompression of the Orbit. Surgical decompression in the severe type of exophthalmos in Graves' disease is performed if other forms of treatment have failed to control the exophthalmos. These include radioactive isotopes (^{131}I); thyroidectomy (Andersson, 1932; Mueller and associates, 1967; Naffziger, 1954; Sedan and Harter, 1966); radiation treatment of the pituitary gland (Heydenreich and coworkers, 1966; Kuehn and coworkers, 1966; Ljungren and Walander, 1959; Sedan and Harter, 1966); and hormonal or other forms of treatment (Ljungren and Walander, 1959; Slansky and coworkers, 1967; Werner, 1967).

Although Graves' disease may be controlled by these various forms of therapy, the proptosis of the orbital contents may persist.

The objectives of surgical decompression of the orbit are: (1) to restore or preserve the threatened vision, the function of the extraocular muscles, and the ability to occlude the eyelids; (2) to relieve the increased orbital tension by allowing the periocular tissues to herniate into an enlarged orbital space; (3) to attain a satisfactory cosmetic result; (4) to avoid surgical trauma to an already injured eye; (5) to prevent immediate or late postoperative complications (Naffziger, 1948, 1954; Welti and Offret, 1942; Craig and Dodge, 1952; Walsh and Ogura, 1957; Kroll and Casten, 1966; Long, 1967; Low, 1967).

With growing experience over the years it has become obvious that the indications for decompression of the orbital cavity in severe exophthalmos in Graves' disease are divided into primary and secondary considerations. The primary indications are related to preservation of eye function; the secondary indications are related to the effects of the disease process (Naffziger, 1948, 1954; Berke, 1954; Ogura and Walsh, 1962; Chilaris and Taptas, 1965; Kroll and Casten, 1966; Ogura, 1968).

The primary indications for the operation are increasing exposure of the cornea with impending ulcerative keratitis, and increasing loss of visual acuity by papillitis and hemorrhages into the fundus (Naffziger, 1948; Ogura and Walsh, 1962; Ogura, 1968).

Secondary considerations for operative decompression are relief of increasing exophthalmos, increasing loss of function of the extraocular muscles, and chemosis of the conjunctiva and orbital edema (Naffziger, 1948, 1954; Ogura and Walsh, 1962; Ogura, 1968).

Choice of Surgical Procedure for Orbital Decompression. The treatment of exophthalmos in Graves' disease is essentially palliative: (1) enlargement of the orbital space to permit expansion of the orbital contents, and (2) removal of orbital fat and excess skin, as is done in cosmetic blepharoplasty.

The Naffziger-Poppen-Craig intracranial approach is indicated in malignant exophthalmos, a condition less commonly seen than formerly; the greater risk involved in the intracranial approach is responsible for its decreased popularity. The Krönlein-Berke approach and its modifications provide adequate access for decompression of the orbital contents. The procedure also provides access to the orbital floor and the frontal sinus and allows inspection of the optic foramen.

The transantral decompression leaves no visible scar, does not alter the nasal physiology, and provides ample space for herniation of the orbital contents into the ethmoids and the maxillary sinus. In the hands of experienced surgeons, it is recognized as a simple procedure without serious complications. Its disadvantages, however, are a lack of control of hemorrhage and the indirect inspection of the orbital contents it allows; it is a technique best performed by otolaryngologists accustomed to working in deep cavities with head mirror illumination.

MEDIAL DECOMPRESSION THROUGH AN EXTERNAL INCISION: THE SEWALL OPERATION. The external approach through an incision extending through the skin and subcutaneous tissues over the frontal process of the maxilla and curving upward below the eyebrow and supraorbital rim leaves an inconspicuous scar. The ethmoid cells can be removed under direct vision; control of hemorrhage is assured, and the approach allows a direct inspection of the orbital cavity and the cribriform plate.

Major complications in the subcranial types of operations are unusual. In nearly all cases, transient diplopia occurs. Should this condition become persistent, corrective extraocular muscle surgery is required. Extraocular muscle imbalance is more frequent in the advanced cases, in which intrinsic degenerative changes have occurred in the musculature (Naffziger, 1948, 1954; Walsh and Ogura, 1957; Low, 1967).

LATERAL DECOMPRESSION: THE KRÖNLEIN-BERKE OPERATION. Under general anesthesia with the cornea protected by occlusive sutures through the lids or by a scleral lens, a horizontal incision is made through the skin for a distance of 3 cm or more in length from the lateral canthus to the temporalis fascia (Fig. 28–115, *A, B*). The tissues are widely undermined. The muscle can now be retracted, and the entire temporal aspect of the lateral wall of the orbit is exposed. The soft tissues are widely retracted, exposing the rim of the orbit in its supraorbital, lateral, and inferior aspects. An incision through the periosteum is now made immediately medial to the edge of the orbital rim. The periorbita is elevated, the lateral tendon and lateral canthal raphé are raised and freed from the bone, and the check ligament of the lateral rectus muscle is severed (Fig. 28–115, *C*). The orbital contents are thus separated from the lateral orbital wall and retracted; the lateral orbital wall thus retracted is sectioned with the Stryker oscillating saw and fractured outward through the thinner bone at the base (Fig. 28–115, *D* to *F*).

As mentioned earlier in the text, additional decompression can be obtained by removing the floor of the frontal sinus and also by resecting the floor of the orbit, as advocated by Schimek (1972). The extent of exophthalmos is measured by the Hertl exophthalmometer.

MEDIAL DECOMPRESSION THROUGH A MAXILLARY SINUS APPROACH: THE WALSH-OGURA OPERATION (1957). The operation is done through a Caldwell-Luc approach. A large opening is made through the anterior wall of the maxillary sinus. The operation is usually performed under general anesthesia with an intratracheal tube. The location of the ethmoidal sinus is indicated by the point at which the superior-posterior and medial walls of the maxillary sinus come together. A line is drawn anteriorly along the junction of the superior medial wall to the point where the superior medial and anterior walls join. At the midpoint along this line an opening is made into the ethmoid labyrinth, and ethmoidal cells are opened until the point of junction of the superomedial and posterior walls is reached. At this point a transverse bony ridge is seen, under which are located the second division of the fifth nerve and the terminal branch of the internal max-

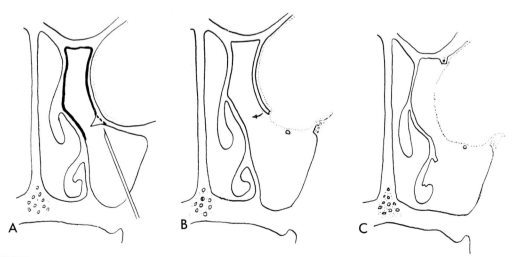

FIGURE 28–116. Medial decompression through a maxillary sinus approach: the Walsh-Ogura operation. *A,* The maxillary sinus is entered through a Caldwell-Luc approach. The ethmoid sinus is entered, and the ethmoid cells are exenterated. A bony ridge obstructs further exposure of the remaining ethmoid cells and must be resected (see text). *B,* The floor of the orbit is removed, the arrow indicates the in-fracture of the lamina papyracea. *C,* Extent of the decompression. In this drawing the lamina papyracea has been resected rather than in-fractured. (Courtesy of Dr. Joseph H. Ogura.)

illary artery (Fig. 28–116, *A*). The bony ridge obstructs further exposure of the remaining ethmoid cells. The ridge is removed with a chisel, thus permitting complete exposure of the whole ethmoid labyrinth. The lamina papyracea is used as a landmark, and all of the posterior ethmoidal cells are removed as far as the anterior face of the sphenoid. It is essential to remain medial to the lamina papyracea in performing the exenteration, because of the close relationship of the optic foramen with the posterior portion of the lamina papyracea. The other precaution is to avoid perforating the roof of the ethmoid, thus entering the anterior cranial fossa; another precaution is to remain medial to the cribriform plate in order to avoid cerebrospinal rhinorrhea. The floor of the orbit is then removed after raising the periorbita and also the lining of the maxillary sinus (Fig. 28–116, *B*); both of these structures are preserved, as well as the infraorbital nerve. The fragile lamina papyracea is fractured medially (Fig. 28–116, *B*) or resected (Fig. 28–116, *C*) except for its posterior portion, which is in close proximity to the optic nerve.

Several posterior-anterior incisions are made through the periorbita, care being taken to avoid injury to the medial and inferior rectus muscles and the inferior oblique muscle; the orbital fat will be seen to herniate into the maxillary and ethmoid sinuses. A window into the maxillary sinus is made under the inferior turbinate, and the mucoperiosteal incision line over the maxillary sinus is closed (Figs. 28–117 and 28–118).

THE EXTERNAL APPROACH TO THE ETHMOID SINUS AND ORBITAL FLOOR. A curved incision extending from the medial portion of the eyebrow and immediately below it downward across the frontal process of the maxilla is the type of incision employed for an operation rarely performed today, the external ethmoidectomy. After incision of the periosteum and subperiosteal elevation extending backward to the anterior lacrimal crest, the lacrimal sac is elevated from the lacrimal groove. Periorbital elevation is continued backward over the lamina papyracea upward from under the roof of the orbit and over the orbital floor; adequate exposure is obtained. The ethmoid sinus is entered through the anterior portion of the lamina papyracea, which is resected along with the cells of the ethmoid labyrinth, except for the posterior portion of the lamina papyracea to avoid injury to the optic nerve, as previously mentioned. Resection is then extended downward and laterally to include the floor of the orbit. In cases in which the exophthalmos is moderate, a depression fracture of the floor of the orbit can be achieved and will provide sufficient decompression; in more severe cases the floor of the orbit is resected in its entirety.

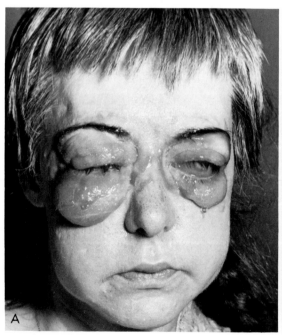 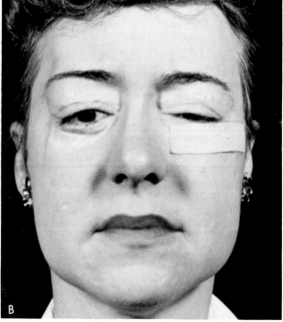

FIGURE 28–117. *A,* Extreme chemosis and exophthalmos. *B,* Appearance after decompression of the orbit. The adhesive is placed to support the lower eyelid during the period of healing. (Courtesy of Dr. Joseph H. Ogura.)

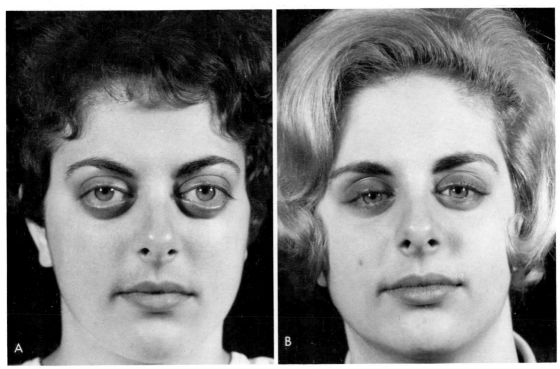

FIGURE 28–118. *A,* Moderate exophthalmos. *B,* Result obtained by medial orbital decompression. (Courtesy of Dr. Joseph H. Ogura.)

If the exposure of the orbital floor is found to be inadequate, a second subciliary incision is made and the orbital floor is further exposed. The periorbita is incised as described in the Walsh-Ogura operation to allow extrusion of the orbital fat. This approach facilitates the operation for surgeons who are not accustomed to working in cavities, as are the otolaryngologists (Fig. 28–119).

COMPLICATIONS. Possible complications during the operation include penetration into the anterior cranial fossa through the roof of the ethmoid sinus or the cribriform plate, with consequent dural tears and cerebrospinal rhinorrhea; optic nerve injury; and medial or inferior rectus muscle or inferior oblique muscle injury. However, complications are infrequent in the subcranial operations. Accidental avulsion of the infraorbital nerve results in loss of sensibility in its area of distribution.

Postoperative edema may be quite severe.

PRESENT-DAY TECHNIQUES. As stated earlier in the chapter, Naffziger (1948, 1954), Ogura and Walsh (1962), and Low (1967) stated that orbital decompression should not be undertaken for cosmetic reasons alone. An increased demand for improvement in appearance and the development of subcranial opera-

tive procedures have promoted the more frequent performance of decompression operations by this approach.

The Naffziger operation, employed also by Poppen (1944) and modified by Craig and Dodge (1952a) (Fig. 28–120), involves the intracranial-extradural removal of the roof of the orbit, the sphenoid ridge, and the lateral orbital wall. The Naffziger intracranial approach is less employed than formerly. Malignant exophthalmos is a rarity in the present era; patients are usually not allowed to progress to such a severe degree of exophthalmos.

The Krönlein-type approach, modified by Berke for his approach to intraorbital tumors, the transantral Walsh-Ogura procedure, and decompression through an external incision by ethmoidectomy and resection of the orbital floor are the most popular contemporary techniques for orbital decompression in Graves' exophthalmopathy.

Castañares (1971) attempted to relieve exopthalmos by diminishing the amount of orbital fat; the results shown are questionable. The authors have also employed this technique to improve the appearance of patients who have had thyrotoxic exophthalmos and who have been treated by radioactive iodine without im-

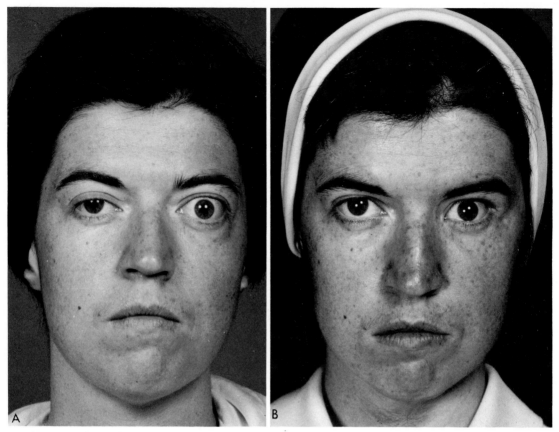

FIGURE 28–119. Unilateral thyrotoxic exophthalmos relieved by medial decompression and removal of the orbital floor through an external excision. *A,* Preoperative. *B,* Postoperative. (Patient of Drs. John M. Converse and Byron Smith.)

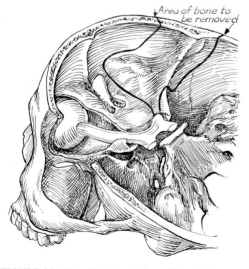

FIGURE 28–120. Decompression of the orbit by removal of the orbital roof: the Naffziger operation modified by Craig and Dodge. As outlined in the drawing, the operation involves the intracranial-extradural removal of the roof of the orbit, the sphenoid ridge, and the lateral orbital wall.

provement in the exophthalmos (Fig. 28–121). Extreme prudence must be exerted in performing cosmetic blepharoplasty in patients with exophthalmos. One of the complications is upper lid retraction (or levator spasm).

UPPER LID RETRACTION IN GRAVES' DISEASE

The exophthalmos and other signs of infiltrative ophthalmopathy seen in Graves' disease do not always disappear with routine nonsurgical therapy. Although congestion and edema of the lids, conjunctiva, and orbit are partly responsive to systemic or repository steroid therapy, extraocular imbalance, restriction of upward gaze, and the puffy swelling of the lids, as well as varying degrees of exophthalmos, remain unchanging features in Graves' disease.

The exact mechanism responsible for eyelid retraction is not fully understood; spasm or

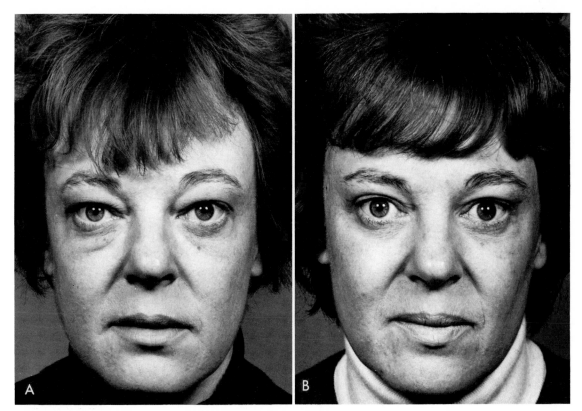

FIGURE 28–121. Improvement following resection of excess skin and orbital fat in a patient whose thyrotoxic exophthalmos had not been entirely relieved by treatment with radioactive iodine.

overactivity of the musculature of the eyelid has been presumed to cause the deformity, consisting in an altered position of the eyelid. The disorder is almost always bilateral, rarely unilateral, frequently symmetric, and occasionally asymmetric.

Upper eyelid retraction may be caused by overactivity or spasm of Müller's muscle and/or the levator palpebrae superioris muscle. Aside from the undesirable appearance, corneal and conjunctival exposure mandate surgical correction.

Surgical Correction. Lid retraction is not an indication for orbital decompression, although decompression may make the lid retraction less obvious. Retraction of the upper eyelid has been treated by weakening of the levator, as advocated by Moran (1956) and Berke (1965).

The surgical approach to two muscles, Müller's muscle and the levator palpebrae superioris muscle, was undertaken by Henderson (1965, 1967).

Müller's muscle is made up of smooth muscle fibers innervated by the sympathetic nervous system; the levator muscle is a striated type of muscle, innervated by the third cranial nerve.

Putterman and Urist (1972) have described a technique for distinguishing between the eyelid retraction due to overaction of Müller's muscle alone and that secondary to the combined overaction of both Müller's muscle and the levator muscles. This is determined first by completely excising Müller's muscle and observing the height of the lid. If the lid is insufficiently lowered, further lowering is obtained by partial tenotomy of the levator aponeurosis.

In order to obtain a block anesthesia of the upper eyelid, Putterman and Urist employ the sensory nerve block described by Hildreth and Silver (1967). A 25-gauge needle is inserted 4 cm into the orbit, the needle penetrating immediately below the midsuperior orbital rim and hugging the roof of the orbit. Xylocaine, 2 per cent, is injected in a dose of 0.5 ml. Anesthesia of the upper eyelid is obtained while preserving the motility of the lid.

The patient is then placed in a sitting position, and the levels of the upper eyelids are compared with each other in the primary position of gaze and on looking up and down. The upper lid is everted over a Desmarre retractor, thus exposing the superior tarsal border. The important structures above the tarsus are the conjunctiva, Müller's muscle, and the levator aponeurosis. Müller's muscle attaches to the superior tarsal border, whereas the levator aponeurosis extends over the anterior surface of the tarsus and inserts into the inferior border of the tarsus as well as into the skin.

The lid being everted, an incision is made 2 mm above the superior tarsal border at its lateral aspect. Scissors are inserted between the plane of the conjunctiva and layer by layer along the central part of the lid. This procedure gradually lengthens the tendon and allows the lid to come down slowly. The patient is again checked in a sitting position several times during the levator stripping procedure to evaluate the position of the lid. If the lid level continues to be high, additional levator fibers are stripped. If the lid level is higher temporally than nasally, additional stripping can be done on the temporal half of the levator aponeurosis.

Defects of the Lacrimal System

JOHN MARQUIS CONVERSE, M.D., AND BYRON SMITH, M.D.

ANATOMICAL CONSIDERATIONS

The lacrimal apparatus (Fig. 28–122) is a bipartite system consisting of a secretory and an excretory division.

The Lacrimal Secretory System. The lacrimal secretory system is made up of two distinct glands: basic secretors and reflex secretors (Viers, 1955; Jones, 1974b).

1. BASIC SECRETORS. Mucin-secreting goblet cells of the conjunctiva, which contribute most of the lubrication of the lids, also form the inner or fixed polysaccharide layer of the precorneal film. Accessory lacrimal glands (Krause, Wolfring), about 50 in number, are located in the subconjunctival tissue of the upper lid. These form the intermediate layer of the precorneal film. Oil secretors are made up almost entirely of tarsal (meibomian) glands. These basic secretors are the only secretors functioning during sleep.

2. REFLEX SECRETORS. The second group of secretors is made up of reflex secretors. The main lacrimal gland lodged in the lacrimal fossa in the lateral portion of the lacrimal roof has two to six excretory ducts. The accessory palpebral gland has 15 to 40 loosely knit lobules, each of which has a small excretory duct that empties into one of the main gland's ducts and into the conjunctival sac just above the superolateral portion of the tarsus.

The Lacrimal Excretory System. Movement of tears is produced by the opening, closing, and medial movement of the lids each time a person blinks. The tears collect along the border of each lid, and excessive fluid moves

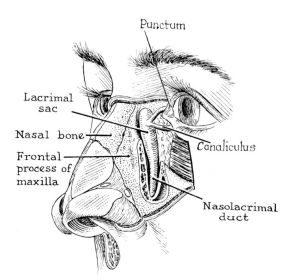

FIGURE 28–122. The lacrimal apparatus.

toward the upper and lower puncta and the lacrimal lake medially. During blinking, the pressure of the lid against the globe is increased. The muscles of the lid also furnish the motor power for the lacrimal pump. The canaliculi are about 10 mm long and consist of a vertical part 2 mm long and a horizontal component 8 mm long. The vertical part of each canaliculus begins with the punctum and lies in the apex of the lacrimal papilla. It is about 3 mm in diameter and is surrounded by a ring of connective elastic tissue. The lumen widens to form the ampulla, which is 2 to 3 mm in its greatest diameter. The horizontal part with the ampulla is 8 mm long and 0.5 mm in diameter. In 90 per cent of patients, both canaliculi join to form a single common duct that opens into the lacrimal sac just posterior and superior to the center of the lateral wall of the sac. The canaliculi are lined with stratified squamous epithelium.

The Lacrimal Sac and the Nasolacrimal Duct. The lacrimal sac lodged in the lacrimal groove and the nasolacrimal duct are anatomically a single structure, with a wide fundus that extends 3 to 5 mm above the level of the medial canthus and a narrowing below, called the isthmus, at the point where it enters the osseous nasolacrimal duct (Fig. 28–122). The combined length of the lacrimal sac and nasolacrimal duct is about 30 mm. The general direction is slightly outward and backward as the nasolacrimal duct descends into the nasal cavity.

Epiphora. Epiphora, the accumulation of tears which are not evacuated from the lacrimal lake and spill over the lower eyelid onto the cheek, is a troublesome complication for the patient. The causes are varied. Paralysis of the orbicularis oculi muscle in facial paralysis prevents the contact of the puncta with the ocular globe and results in paralysis of the lacrimal pump system (see Chapter 36). Obstruction of any portion of the lacrimal excretory system also results in epiphora. It is of interest, however, that epiphora may be absent even in cases in which the lacrimal sac has been destroyed; if infection ensues, epiphora appears and is troublesome.

EXCRETORY DISORDERS AND DEVELOPMENTAL DEFECTS

The excretory portion or lacrimal passages are formed from a thickening of ectoderm in the naso-optic fissure. This cord buries itself in the mesenchyme, separating from the surface ectoderm as the lateral nasal and maxillary processes fuse. The cord thickens as it develops and divides to form the duct and canaliculi extending through the mesenchyme from the medial canthus to the nasal fossa. Normally the passages canalize just before birth.

The puncta may be absent or may appear only as a surface dimple separated slightly from the canaliculus. In adults it may be difficult to distinguish between congenital absence of the puncta and acquired stenosis. Membranous closure of the puncta may be treated by establishing an opening using the dissecting microscope. It is often clinically impossible to determine whether the canaliculi are absent or have failed to reach the surface. If an opening cannot be found, retrograde probing becomes necessary. A skin incision is made down to the lacrimal sac, and a probe is passed through the common canaliculus. If a duct is located, the probe is passed toward the punctum, and an incision is made over the probe. A small polyethylene tube is inserted and left in place for approximately eight weeks. If both puncta are located, one can use a single piece of silicone tubing which bridges between the two puncta so that the ends lie in the lacrimal sac (Fig. 28–123). The tubing is not uncomfortable and is easily removed when desired. If no canaliculi are found, a conjunctivodacryocystostomy, or direct connection of the lacrimal sac to the conjunctival sac, is required.

A membrane at the lower end of the nasolacrimal duct is the commonest developmental defect; this may be explained by the fact that

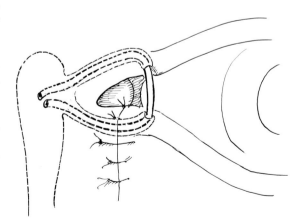

FIGURE 28–123. Another technique of maintaining the patency of the canaliculus after repair consists in placing a silicone tube in a circular fashion into the upper and lower canaliculi.

this portion is the last to canalize. Relief is usually achieved by passing a small probe down the passage and perforating the membrane. If this fails, it may be concluded that a more extensive defect is present.

Abnormalities of the lacrimal system in craniofacial malformations have been studied by Whitaker and others (1974).

Diagnostic Tests. The plastic surgeon dealing with malunited naso-orbital fractures or penetrating lacerations which have obstructed or injured the excretory lacrimal system at some point along its course should evaluate its patency. For this purpose there are two simple tests.

THE DYE TEST. A drop of methylene blue is injected into the lower canaliculus, or a drop of 2 per cent fluorescein solution is placed in the conjunctival sac. A cotton-tipped applicator is placed in the inferior meatus, under the inferior turbinate, where the cotton retrieves the dye if the nasolacrimal system is patent, the dye exiting through the valve of Hasner in the inferior meatus. If no dye is detected on the cotton, the test is considered negative; the epiphora is then considered to be caused by lacrimal duct obstruction.

THE DYE DISAPPEARANCE TEST. The rate at which the dye disappears from the conjunctival sac will also indicate that the ducts are opened or closed. This test is not, however, as reliable as the dye test described above.

The valve of Hasner, the opening of the nasolacrimal duct into the nasal cavity, is situated anteriorly to the highest point of the cavity of the inferior turbinate. In some cases, the inferior meatus is narrow, and a cotton-tipped applicator may penetrate with difficulty into the meatus. A copper wire applicator with a small amount of cotton is moistened with a 5 per cent cocaine solution and is carefully introduced under the inferior turbinate. A solution of 0.5 per cent to 2 per cent fluorescein solution is placed in the conjunctival sac. If the cotton is stained with dye, the staining should occur within 3 minutes, showing that the nasolacrimal excretory system is patent.

There are a number of other tests (the Schirmer #1 and #2 tests) employed by ophthalmologists to differentiate pseudoepiphora or paralysis of the reflex secretors from other types of excretory deficiencies.

CANALICULUS TEST. This test is employed to evaluate canalicular patency. Saline solution in a 2-ml syringe with a lacrimal canula is injected into a canaliculus; if it returns through the opposing canaliculus, it is evidence that the ducts are open as far as the common canaliculus and that they communicate with each other.

REPAIR OF THE LACRIMAL APPARATUS

The plastic surgeon is frequently involved in treating disturbances of the lacrimal system caused by trauma. In all acute trauma involving the naso-orbital area, injury to the lacrimal system must be considered a possibility. Verification of the integrity of the lacrimal system should be a routine diagnostic procedure.

Injuries to the lacrimal system occur most frequently in naso-orbital fractures caused by glass fragment laceration in automobile accidents, by sports injuries, by razor or knife lacerations, and by fragments impelled by high explosives. Early recognition and adequate repair of these injuries will do much to prevent disability from epiphora and late infection.

Immediate diagnosis and treatment may be rendered impossible when hemorrhage, ecchymosis, and local tissue swelling are severe. In such cases, the diagnosis and treatment may be deferred for a few days, the patient being maintained under antibiotic therapy, until the swelling has partially subsided. In some cases, early treatment may not be possible. Fortunately, with present-day reconstruction techniques, later treatment of lacrimal defects is usually successful.

Injury to the secretory portion of the lacrimal system is rare because the lacrimal gland is protected by the bony orbital rim. If the gland is destroyed, the accessory lacrimal glands usually supply adequate moisture.

Nasolacrimal duct interruption should be suspected in any fracture of the middle third of the face. If the nasolacrimal duct becomes blocked a chronic dacryocystitis will ensue.

Cicatricial Stenosis of the Punctum. Stenosis of the punctum may result from lacerations of the lid. Isolated closure or stenosis of the punctum may be alleviated by a vertical stab in the papilla lacrimalis but may require retrograde probing for accurate location and surgery. Jones (1962) advocated the "1 snip" operation, in which a vertical 2-mm cut is made in the conjunctival wall of the canaliculus. He feels this technique is superior to the "3 snip" operation (Stallard, 1940), as it preserves the capillary attraction value of the vertical canaliculus and the pumping action of the ampulla.

Transection of the Canaliculus. Transection of the lid margin between the punctum and the medial canthus is not infrequent in lacerations and in accidents in which the lower eyelid may be avulsed. The continuity of the lid margin, canaliculus and lower portion of the medial canthal tendon is disrupted. The orbicularis muscle tends to enlarge the area of laceration and produce ectropion. Cicatricial coloboma is frequent when the wound has not been treated primarily.

The punctum can usually be located, and a punctum dilator will facilitate the placing of a probe through the punctum to locate the lateral lumen of the canaliculus.

Patients with traumatic canalicular section or obstruction have been treated by end-to-end anastomosis over a silicone tube with 7–0 sutures under visual magnification by means of loupes or the operating microscope. Identification of the lumen by direct examination may be aided by the injection of a colored fluid into the sac or into the punctum of the unaffected canaliculus. Sufficient data are not available to determine the success rate of end-to-end anastomosis.

The Worst (1962) pigtail probe is a sharply curved instrument which is inserted into the punctum of the unaffected canaliculus, into the common canaliculus, and back through the severed canaliculus, where it emerges into the area of the laceration. Beard (1967) confirmed excellent results with the use of this probe. In expert hands this instrument is useful; however, considerable damage may be the consequence of inexpert use of the instrument.

If the tendon is difficult to locate, an additional incision is made over the frontal process of the maxilla, and the proximal portion of the tendon is exposed and dissected as shown in Figure 28–124.

Many patients with an inferior canalicular obstruction appear to be able to compensate by means of drainage through the upper canaliculus. Some patients do not have a major complaint of epiphora. In most cases in which canalicular obstruction is a major problem, conjunctivodacryocystorhinostomy is the only solution (see p. 987).

Dacryocystitis. As mentioned earlier, a multiplicity of factors may cause interference with lacrimal function: eversion of the puncta from the ocular globe due to entropion or ectropion; cicatricial stricture of a canaliculus; injury of the sac either by direct penetration of a foreign body or by a comminuted fragment of bone; obstruction of the nasolacrimal duct.

The sac becomes dilated when the nasolacrimal duct is obstructed, and part of its contents flows back through the lacrimal puncta into the palpebral fissure. Fluid injected into the lower canaliculus should normally pass through the lacrimal system and appear when the patient blows his nose. If, on pressure over the sac, the fluid flows back and is clear and thin, there may be obstruction without infection. If the sac is very dilated, it is a sign that the lacrimal flow has been chronically interrupted, a condition designated as a mucocele.

The enlarged sac or mucocele forms a visi-

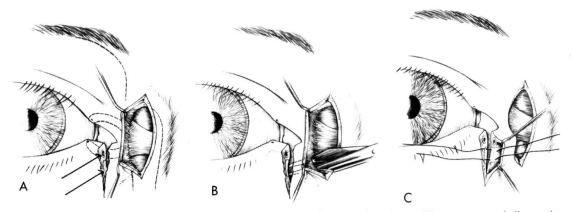

FIGURE 28–124. Treatment of a sectioned canaliculus and medial canthal tendon. *A,* The upper arrow indicates the sectioned canaliculus; the lower arrow indicates the sectioned portion of the medial canthal tendon. An incision has been made medially to expose the uninjured portion of the tendon. *B,* The dissection extended laterally facilitates exposure of the severed tendon. *C,* The severed tendon is sutured. The canaliculus is sutured after a polyethylene catheter has been inserted through the punctum into the lateral and medial portions of the severed canaliculus. (After Smith and Cherubini, 1970.)

ble and palpable mass in the medial canthal region. A viscous fluid characteristic of the presence of a mucocele may be expressed by pressure over the swollen sac.

Distention of the lacrimal sac may cause kinking of the common canaliculus; when this occurs, the fluid becomes trapped in the lacrimal sac, and the resulting distention causes pain. Because it is not possible to aspirate the sac contents through the kinked common canaliculus, direct aspiration through the skin with a needle may relieve the acute distention and also release the mechanically angulated and secondarily obstructed canaliculus. Instruments can usually be introduced through the canaliculus after such aspiration.

Attacks of acute dacryocystitis associated with redness, swelling, and pain may occur with associated edema of the entire orbital region and closure of the eyelids over the globe. Hot applications and antibiotics are indicated; incision and drainage are essential when the purulent collection has become fluctuant. A suppurating lacrimal sac is a source of constant danger, because even a slight abrasion of the cornea may become infected and ulcerated.

TREATMENT OF DACRYOCYSTITIS. When dilatation of the lacrimal punctum is required, a topical anesthetic solution is injected into the canaliculus, and a thin probe is introduced. The probe is directed vertically, rotated 90 degrees, and then advanced medially while the canaliculus is stretched (Fig. 28–125). The probing must be done carefully in the manner described to prevent the probe from striking a fold of mucosa and perforating the canaliculus. The probe is pressed forward until it reaches the sac. Penetration into the sac is evidenced by contact of the tip of the probe with the bony wall of the orbit; the handle is elevated vertically and inclined slightly forward, directly into the duct. After the lacrimal sac has been reached, it is advisable to withdraw the probe and inject saline or an anesthetic solution through the canaliculus; if the fluid passes into the nose, further probing should be discontinued, for free passage of the solution indicates elimination of the obstacle in the nasolacrimal duct.

The treatment of chronic dacryocystitis is surgical, replacing the former method of periodic probing to relieve obstruction. However, extirpation of the sac may be necessary when it is irretrievably damaged by multiple lacerations and scarring or by prolonged suppuration and necrosis.

Dacryocystorhinostomy and Dacryocystectomy. Dacryocystorhinostomy is a frequent operation in patients with nasolacrimal apparatus obstruction. The indications for dacryocystorhinostomy according to Jones (1974b) are: (1) as an initial procedure in lacerations of the common canaliculus; (2) in acute and chronic dacryocystitis; (3) in complete obstruction of either the lacrimal sac or the nasolacrimal duct; (4) in paralysis of the lacrimal pump, such as occurs in facial paralysis; (5) in nasoorbital fractures in which the continuity of the nasolacrimal duct may be interrupted at some point.

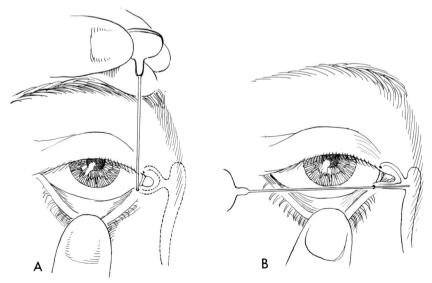

FIGURE 28–125. Probing the canaliculus. Successive positions assumed by the probe, first vertically (left), then horizontally (right).

Dacryocystectomy is generally condemned by those who prefer dacryocystorhinostomy. Dacryocystectomy is still required, however, in patients in whom the sac has been badly damaged by fracture and in patients in whom dacryocystorhinostomy has failed.

TECHNIQUE OF DACRYOCYSTECTOMY. A few drops of methylene blue solution are injected through the lower punctum and canaliculus into the lacrimal sac with a lacrimal canula and syringe to identify the sac. The cutaneous incision should be at least 7 mm from the medial canthus, the incision beginning at the level of the medial canthal tendon and extending downward about 25 mm. The incision is extended down to the periosteum, and a periosteal elevator is used to raise the periosteum backward to the lacrimal crest, which is exposed. The insertions of the inferior and superior preseptal muscles on the anterior lacrimal crest are detached. Jones (1974b) advises removing the upper 5 mm of the anterior lacrimal crest in order to simplify the removal of the upper part of the nasolacrimal duct. The sac is extracted subperiosteally from the wall of the lacrimal groove in the upper part of the nasolacrimal duct. The lateral wall of the sac is then exposed, starting below by the exposure of the nasolacrimal duct. The common canalicus is identified by means of a No. 1 Bowman probe. The duct is then severed immediately lateral to its entrance into the sac. After the sac is completely freed, the nasolacrimal duct is severed with small curved scissors as far down in the canal as possible, and the remaining mucosa is thoroughly curetted. The methylene blue is of great assistance in locating the sac in naso-orbital fractures in which the sac may have been damaged and surrounded by scar tissue. The edges of the cutaneous incision are approximated with fine caliber suture material.

TECHNIQUE OF DACRYOCYSTORHINOSTOMY WITH A TOTALLY EPITHELIUM-LINED PASSAGE INTO THE NASAL CAVITY. A technique which is applicable in patients in whom local fractures and fibrosis have not occurred to complicate the operative procedure is the following: the medial wall of the lacrimal sac and the adjacent nasal mucous membrane may be vertically split and both the anterior and posterior flaps sutured to the margins of the nasal mucosal opening in the nose (see Fig. 28–160).

Toti (1904) introduced dacryocystorhinostomy, allowing the tears to enter the nose by perforating the lacrimal groove. Mosher (1915, 1923) improved upon this procedure by a technique in which the anterior margin of the opening in the sac was approximated with catgut sutures to the anterior margin of the bony opening. Further modifications of this operation by Dupuy-Dutemps and Bourguet (1921), having a much higher percentage of success, consisted in careful approximation of the nasal mucous membrane to the edges of the lacrimal sac.

This technique (see Fig. 28–160), when feasible, is the best because it ensures an epithelial-lined passage between the lacrimal sac and the nasal cavity. The operation may be performed under general anesthesia or preferably under local anesthesia with intravenous infusion of drugs that produce subliminal anesthesia.

A skin incision is made 11 mm medial to the medial canthus. The incision begins slightly below the level of the medial canthal tendon and extends downward and slightly outward over a distance of approximately 25 mm. The incision extends through the skin only; the wound edges are retracted, and the strands of superficial fascia are spread apart with scissors. The angular vein may be located as it crosses the medial canthal tendon and may be retracted, thus avoiding cutting the vein and the subsequent profuse hemorrhage (Jones, 1974b). A subperiosteal dissection is then started beneath the point where the medial canthal tendon attaches to the bone. The periosteal incision is made after retraction of the soft tissues to expose the area. The periosteum is incised about 5 mm medial to and below the margin of the anterior lacrimal crest. The periosteum is elevated posteriorly over the lacrimal groove as far back as the posterior lacrimal crest and downward as far as possible into the nasolacrimal canal.

The nasal cavity is now inspected with the aid of a nasal speculum and headlight illumination. If the middle turbinate is hypertrophied, its anterior tip should be resected; if a septal deviation is present, it should be remedied.

A solution of procaine-adrenaline is then injected beneath the mucoperiosteum lining the frontal process of the maxilla. An incision is made near the base of the frontal process, and subperiosteal elevation is extended upward and backward to the area of the lacrimal groove. A tent-shaped piece of gauze soaked in adrenalin solution is then placed into this tunnel and left in position until the operation reaches the point at which the nasal mucosa must be incised.

With adequate retraction, the bone forming the anterior lacrimal crest and the wall of the lacrimal groove is removed, exposing the gauze which protects the nasal mucosa. The opening into the nasal cavity may be made with an osteotome, a trephine, or a burr activated by an electric motor or an air driven turbine. The most important area to remove is that portion of bone situated in front of the posterior lacrimal crest. The bone is removed under the medial canthal tendon, which is not severed. This technique is possible in the nontraumatized patient; after a naso-orbital fracture, detachment of the tendon is a necessary procedure. Bone is then removed from the nasolacrimal canal for a distance of at least 5 mm below the opening of the common canaliculus into the lacrimal sac. A Bowman probe is inserted through one canaliculus, and the medial wall of the lacrimal sac is tented medially. An opening is made into the lacrimal sac with a pointed knife blade immediately lateral to the tip of the probe. Scissors are then inserted, and the incision is extended to the top of the fundus and to the botton of the nasolacrimal duct.

A parallel incision is made through the nasal mucoperiosteum. The posterior flaps are then sutured with fine plain catgut sutures on a small atraumatic needle. The anterior flaps are now approximated. The wound edges are sutured. It may be necessary to make T or H incisions in the mucosal flaps to facilitate the suturing, but when the medial wall of the nasolacrimal canal has been removed, the suturing is facilitated and such incisions are not required. A cross-cut may be necessary occasionally at the upper end of the anterior nasomucosal flap to provide more mobility.

DACRYOCYSTORHINOSTOMY FOLLOWING NASO-ORBITAL FRACTURES. The technique of dacryocystorhinostomy described in the previous section of the text presupposes favorable conditions for achieving epithelial continuity from the lacrimal sac into the nose and the preparation of anterior and posterior flaps. When the medial orbital wall is disrupted or disorganized as a result of a malunited fracture, the bony landmarks are lost, and the lacrimal sac may be injured; the ideal operation cannot be achieved. In many cases only a posterior flap can be joined with a flap from the nasal mucous membrane; in other cases only an anterior flap can be sutured to the nasal mucous membrane. Whenever possible, however, both anterior and posterior flaps should be sutured.

COMPLICATIONS OF DACRYOCYSTORHINOSTOMY. Although Toti (1904) revolutionized the treatment of obstructive epiphora by approaching the lacrimal sac from an external excision and establishing a communication between the lacrimal sac and the nasal cavity for the drainage of the lacrimal secretions, no sutures were employed to establish the continuity of the structures. In 1921 Dupuy-Dutemps and Bourguet advocated edge-to-edge suture of the sac to the mucous membrane of the nose through the communicating bony opening in order to avoid cicatricial occlusion. Failures in dacryocystorhinostomy are more frequent following severe malunited fractures with anatomical disorganization of the area than in cases in which the nasolacrimal duct is obstructed without fracture of the naso-orbital area. Failures are the result of faulty technique: inability to establish a completely closed tract between the lacrimal sac and the nasal mucous membrane; inadequate intranasal surgery resulting in the lacrimal sac evacuating itself into an ethmoid cell instead of the open nasal cavity; a fenestration into the nose either too small or inappropriately placed. As emphasized by the description of the operation advocated by Jones (see above), it is essential that the lacrimal sac be opened from the nasolacrimal duct through the fundus and that the bony ostium be sufficiently large to allow the sac to be completely incorporated within the ostium.

In cases in which dacryocystorhinostomy has failed, Welham and Henderson (1947) recommended visualization of the lacrimal apparatus by dacryocystography prior to surgery. If sufficient lacrimal sac is present, the area is explored and every effort is made to obtain lacrimal sac–nasal mucous membrane continuity.

Canaliculodacryocystorhinostomy. This technique is done when a stricture is present at the junction of the common canaliculus and the lacrimal sac.

A dacryocystorhinostomy is first done. After the posterior flaps of the lacrimal sac and the nasal mucosa have been sutured, a Bowman probe (No. 1) is passed through either canaliculus through the obstruction, and the end of the probe is then seen to tent the common canaliculus into view in the lacrimal sac. The common canaliculus can then be excised, leaving a round hole about 3 mm in diameter. A polyethylene or silicone tube is threaded through both canaliculi, leaving a loop of tubing at the puncta, and the ends of the tubing are drawn into the nose and out through the nostril where they are taped to the cheek. The tubing is removed after a period of three months. A Jones tube is an excellent alternative (see following section).

The technique of Werb (1971) and Quickert and Dryden (1970) consists of placing a probe into either canaliculus through the site of obstruction.

Conjunctivodacryocystorhinostomy. This procedure (Jones, 1962) is indicated when both canaliculi are obliterated. It may also be used in patients with facial paralysis and paralysis of the lacrimal pump resulting from paralysis of the orbicularis oculi muscle.

A dacryocystorhinostomy is performed as described earlier in the text, suturing together the posterior lacrimal sac and nasal mucosal flaps. Jones emphasizes that it is important not to detach the medial canthal tendon. The medial half or all of the caruncle, if it is a large one, is resected. Care is taken to remove as little conjunctiva as possible. If the caruncle is small and flat, no removal is necessary. A hypodermic needle (22-gauge), 30 mm long and slightly curved, is inserted 2.5 mm posterior to the cutaneous margin of the medial canthus. The concavity of the needle faces anteriorly, and the needle is pushed in a direction that will cause its point to penetrate into the nose at a spot situated immediately anterior to the sutured posterior flaps, midway between the fundus and the isthmus, penetrating into the nasal cavity immediately anterior to the body of the middle turbinate. If necessary, the anterior portion of the middle turbinate should be resected.

A sharp pointed knife (such as a cataract knife) is used to penetrate the conjunctival sac into the lacrimal sac; the knife incises the passageway above and below just enough to allow the insertion of a Pyrex tube. The tube should be about 8 mm in length with a 4-mm collar outside and a beveled nasal end. It is threaded over a No. 2 Bowman probe, which is then passed through the new opening in the nose (Fig. 28–126). If the tube presses against the nasal septum, a shorter tube should be used. A 6–0 silk suture is tied around the collar of the tube, and a needle anchors the tube to the skin of the canthus, where it is tied to prevent dislodgement. After a period of from one to three weeks, the Pyrex tube may be replaced by one with a smaller collar or shorter length. As Jones (1974b) has stated, the Pyrex tube has the following three advantages: (1) it is not hydrophilic; (2) it does not plug up easily; and

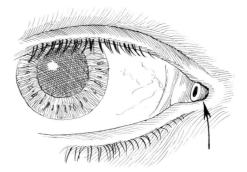

FIGURE 28–126. Pyrex tube for the maintenance of a conjunctivodacryocystorhinostomy (Jones, 1962). The technique is employed when the canaliculi and lacrimal sac are destroyed; it establishes a direct communication between the conjunctival sac and nasal cavity.

(3) it does not irritate the tissues. The intranasal negative pressure at the nasal end during inspiration is an important factor in assisting the lacrimal flow through the tube.

Postoperative care. Postoperative care is the most important part of the procedure. The length of the tube should be carefully determined. Intranasal examination will show how far the tube extends. It should not extend more than 3 mm. The tube should be removed, and another tube should be selected which will protrude intranasally 1 or 2 mm. During the following one to six weeks, the 4-mm collar tube may be exchanged for one with a 3.5-mm collar. The patient must be told not to blow his nose. Should he be obliged to blow his nose or to sneeze, he should be taught to close his eyelids tightly and hold his finger over the end of the tube. If the tube becomes obstructed, a fine wire should be run through it. This can be done by the surgeon or by a member of the family who is taught to perform this procedure. Saline irrigation may be necessary to reopen the tube in case it is obstructed; if there is a mild suppurative condition, the saline irrigation and the alleviation of any intranasal or sinus condition are required to prevent secretions from plugging the nasal end of the tube.

Should the tube become extruded, the patient should be seen within 24 hours. The conjunctivorhinostomy opening is dilated with a probe, and the tube is reinserted. Anesthesia can be administered by placing a few drops of proparacaine drops into the conjunctival sac and inserting applicators of 5 per cent cocaine solution intranasally. Conjunctivitis may occur and is usually due to the formation of granulation tissue around the tube in the early stages.

The tube should be removed and cleansed, and the patient should be seen frequently until the condition has been relieved. While the tube is being cleaned, a dilator should be inserted to prevent the constriction of the passageway.

The Pyrex tube technique requires an intact medial (or nasal) margin of the lower eyelid. Reconstruction of a defective eyelid should precede any attempt at placing a Pyrex tube.

The Pyrex tube technique has been used by Jones in 500 patients. He reports no failures (Jones, 1974b). After a period of about six months, the tube may begin to loosen and may extrude itself. The patient should be taught to remove it and reinsert it immediately. As in all constructed passageways, stenosis is always a danger if the tube is left out too long. After a variable period of time, however, the patient each day can increase the intervals before he reinserts the tube, until he only wears it at night or eventually discards the tube entirely.

The patient shown in Figure 28–127, *A* was the victim of an automobile accident and suffered a naso-orbital fracture with comminution of the right medial orbital wall, penetrating laceration by a piece of the windshield through the

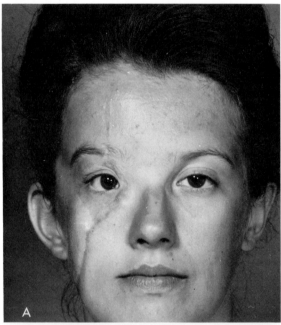
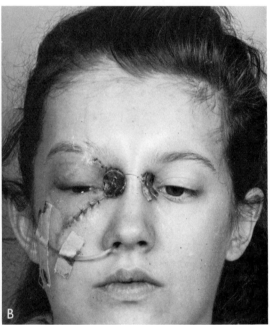

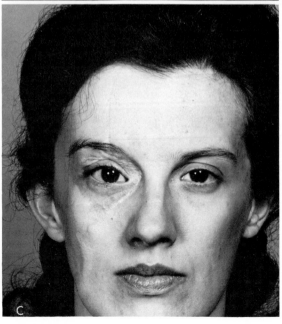

FIGURE 28–127. *A,* The patient, a 17 year old adolescent female, was a victim of an automobile accident when she was projected through the windshield after striking the dashboard. She suffered a naso-orbital fracture involving the medial wall of the right orbit, severe lacerations of the forehead and cheek, and a penetrating laceration through the medial canthus. Obstruction of the right lacrimal system resulted in a mucocele which can be seen as a swelling immediately below the medial canthus. Note also the telecanthus on the right side. *B,* After reduction of the naso-orbital fracture and reestablishment of the position of the medial orbital wall, the mucocele was resected. A conjunctivorhinostomy was then performed, placing silicone tubing as illustrated in Figure 28–128. The patient is shown with the tubing taped to the cheek. The cheek laceration has been repaired, and the canthal plates maintained by transosseous wiring (see Fig. 28–158) are in position. *C,* Reestablished medial canthal region after medial canthoplasty five years after surgery. A Jones Pyrex tube had been placed and maintained in position for a period of two years. The patient no longer needs the Jones tube, as the conjunctivorhinostomy remains patent. (From Converse, J. M., and Smith, B.: Naso-orbital fractures and traumatic deformities of the medial canthus. Plast. Reconstr. Surg., *38*:147, 1966.)

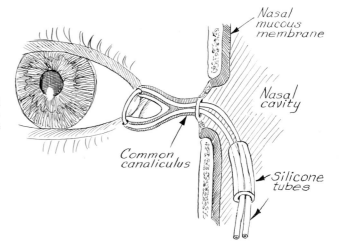

FIGURE 28–128. Silicone catheter placed through the upper and lower puncta into the canaliculi and maintaining the continuity between the common canaliculus and the nasal opening.

right medial canthus and cheek, section of the medial canthal tendon, and disruption of the lacrimal apparatus. The lacrimal sac can be seen as a swelling which has migrated below the level of the medial canthus. After reconstruction of the right medial orbital wall, the lacrimal sac, which was isolated from the nasolacrimal duct and canaliculi, was resected. The medial canthal tendon was reattached to the medial orbital wall by transosseous wiring (Fig. 28–127, *B*; see also Fig. 28–158). In order to establish an epithelized conduit from the conjunctival sac to the nasal cavity, a silicone catheter was threaded through both lacrimal puncta into the common canaliculus and into the nose, the ends of the catheter being brought out through the right nostril and taped to the cheek (Figs. 28–127, *B* and 28–128).

This procedure was not successful, and three months later a conjunctivorhinostomy was performed and a Pyrex tube inserted. The appearance of the patient is shown one year later (Fig. 28–127, *C*).

This case emphasizes an important point in the treatment of anatomical disruption of the medial canthus involving the lacrimal system, the medial canthal tendon, the medial wall, and (often) the floor of the orbit and nasal skeleton: a one-stage operative procedure gives the best results. This case is also an example of the contrast between the management of conjunctivorhinostomy in a severely disrupted medial canthal region and that of conjunctivodacryorhinostomy in less damaged or virginal tissues. (See also Malunited Fractures of the Medial Orbital Wall, page 1005.)

Malunited Fractures
of the Orbit

JOHN MARQUIS CONVERSE, M.D.,
BYRON SMITH, M.D.,
AND DONALD WOOD-SMITH, F.R.C.S.E.

High-speed automobile collisions are the most common cause of severe comminuted fractures involving the upper portion of the midface, including the orbits and structures between the orbits. Because this area of the face contains important functional structures, patients who

have not received expert early treatment may be left with a gross deformity. Inadequate primary treatment of an orbital fracture, greatly delayed treatment, severe comminution, and loss of bone all can contribute to a residual orbital deformity and disorganization of orbital structures. Lesions of the lacrimal apparatus interfering with lacrimal function, extraocular muscle imbalance, and diplopia are frequent sequelae of malunited orbital fractures. Malunited orbital fractures are frequently associated with malunited naso-orbital and maxillary fractures.

MALUNITED FRACTURES OF THE ORBITAL ROOF

Deformities of the roof of the orbit usually involve the prominent supraorbital ridge, frontal bone, and frontal sinus. Traumatic defects are seen particularly in the thin portion of the orbital plate of the frontal bone situated in the medial aspect of the orbital roof. Enophthalmos and the transmission of the pulsations of the brain to the ocular globe are signs of such a defect when it is of moderate size. Exophthalmos may result from massive herniation of the brain into the orbit in large defects.

Large orbital roof defects are repaired through an intracranial approach similar to that employed for the treatment of orbital hypertelorism. The technique of combined craniofacial exposure was described by Tessier and his associates (1967) and Converse and his associates (1970) and was reviewed by Converse, Wood-Smith, McCarthy, and Coccaro (1974). An area of frontal bone sufficient to provide exposure is resected. The frontal lobe is raised, the area of elevation remaining lateral to the cribriform plate. A plane of cleavage is usually found quite readily between the dura and periorbita. A thin iliac bone graft taken from the medial aspect of the ilium, or a split rib graft in the child, is placed over the bony defect of the orbit. The pressure of the brain maintains the bone graft without the need for interosseous wire fixation. The frontal bone segment is replaced into the frontal defect.

In two patients a small defect was repaired by the authors through an orbital approach. An incision was made immediately below the supraorbital rim. The periorbita was raised until the defect was reached, and the periorbita was separated from the dura over the extent of the defect. The dura was also separated over the intracranial surface of the bone along the edge of the defect by means of an angulated elevator. A thin bone graft was placed into the defect, bridging over the defect and resting on the anterior cranial fossa.

The pulley of the superior oblique muscle is often damaged owing to its proximity with the surface of the roof and contact with the bony fragment. Transitory diplopia usually results from this specific injury.

The sixth cranial nerve may also be traumatized in orbital injuries, resulting in paralysis of the lateral rectus muscle and limitation of ocular abduction. A period of six months should elapse to allow for recovery before corrective muscle surgery is undertaken. Prism vergence tests should be made, and if spontaneous recovery has not occurred, surgical treatment must be considered. In lateral rectus paralysis, strips of the superior and inferior rectus muscles may be transplanted to the tendon of the lateral rectus; this procedure is usually combined with recession of the insertion of the medial rectus. In some instances, recession of the medial and lateral rectus muscles can also be achieved without disturbing the vertical muscles.

Fortunately, the compensatory power of the binocular fusion mechanism tends to overcome diplopia. However, in some instances, injury to the oculorotary muscles is sufficiently severe to render ineffective the compensatory power of the binocular fusion mechanism.

MALUNITED FRACTURES OF THE ORBITAL FLOOR

Deformities and functional impairment are late complications which can be reduced by early diagnosis and treatment; however, often the diagnosis is obscured by more severe cranial and facial injuries which demand priority treatment.

Occasionally, despite early treatment of the orbital fracture, progressive ocular muscle imbalance and enophthalmos ensue.

The authors have treated many complicated malunited blowout fractures, often accompanied by malunited fractures of other facial bones, as well as injuries of the soft tissues. The treatment of malunited orbital fractures has been reviewed (Converse, 1974; Converse and coworkers, 1967, 1975).

These patients show a variety of deformities and functional disturbances: impairment of oculorotary action with resultant diplopia, enophthalmos (Fig. 28–129), depression of the zygomatic prominence, ptosis of the upper eyelid, downward displacement of the orbital contents, medial canthal deformities, shortening of the horizontal dimensions of the palpe-

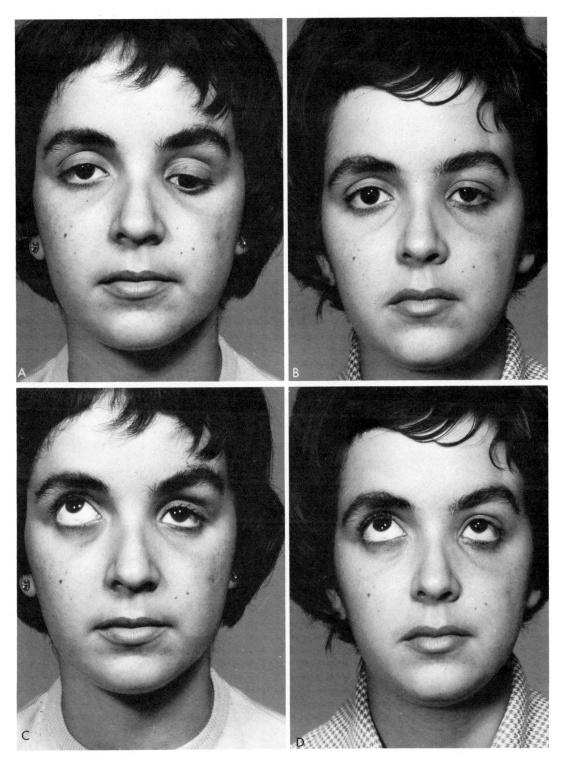

FIGURE 28–129. *A*, Patient four months after blowout fracture of the left orbit. Note the deepened supratarsal fold and the downward rotation of the left ocular globe. *B*, Two months after operation. Note the improved position of the left ocular globe and the restored supratarsal fold. *C*, The patient's left eye shows limited oculorotary movement in the upward gaze. *D*, Improved oculorotary movement of the left eye in the upward gaze after surgery. (From Converse, J. M., Cole, J. C., and Smith, B.: Late treatment of blowout fracture of the floor of the orbit. A case report. Plast. Reconstr. Surg., *28*:183, 1961.)

bral fissure, shortening of the vertical dimension of the lower eyelid, saddle deformity of the nose, widening of the nasal bony bridge, and, occasionally, deformities of the supraorbital arch.

Functional disturbances may include diminution of vision and blindness or loss of the eye. Blindness or loss of the eye is remarkably infrequent, in view of the severity of some of the injuries sustained. Epiphora resulting from interruption of the continuity of the lacrimal apparatus and cystic dilatation of the lacrimal sac (mucocele) requires treatment. Lacerations through the eyelids may result in severe structural disorganization and may sever the canaliculi, the medial canthal tendon, or the levator palpebrae superioris. These associated injuries have been discussed in Chapter 25 and in the earlier part of this chapter.

True ptosis of the upper eyelid is to be differentiated from pseudoptosis resulting from the downward displacement of the eyeball and enophthalmos. True ptosis results from loss of function of the levator palpebrae superioris muscle. This may occur following transection of the muscle or the aponeurosis, intramuscular hematoma resulting in subsequent fibrosis, or an injury to the third cranial nerve.

The most frequent sequelae of inadequately treated blowout fractures of the orbital floor are diplopia and enophthalmos.

Diplopia. Permanent diplopia is usually produced by interference with the oculorotary mechanism by entrapment of orbital structures in blowout fractures. The patient has diplopia because he is unable to rotate the affected eye in various directions. The degree of diplopia is dependent upon the degree of oculorotary disturbance. Thus, in the patient shown in Figure 28–129, inability to rotate the ocular globe resulted in diplopia except when the patient compensated by tilting her head backward and looking toward the left. Relief of this type of diplopia is obtained by releasing the orbital contents from the area of entrapment and repairing the orbital floor defect.

Many fractures of the orbital floor occur without blowout fracture. In most zygomatic fractures and fractures involving the rim of the orbit without blowout fracture, diplopia is transitory and is attributed to hematoma causing muscular imbalance by elevating the ocular globe or to injury of the extraocular musculature temporarily affecting the oculorotary mechanism. In patients with malunited fracture of the zygoma with separation of the frontozygomatic suture line and downward displacement of the orbital floor, after a period of transitory diplopia there is often an accommodation of the extraocular musculature. In addition, a remarkable degree of binocular fusion compensates for the ptosis of the ocular globe, permitting single vision. Most of these patients complain of diplopia when fatigued in the same manner that a person with a weakened musculature of the lower extremity will limp with fatigue. They incur a temporary loss of the capacity for binocular fusion which ensures single vision.

Malunited depressed fractures of the orbital floor are frequently accompanied by restriction of the superior rectus and superior oblique muscles. This is not usually the result of direct involvement of the muscle but is indicative of the relative inelasticity of the inferior rectus. In early cases we have found the inferior rectus and inferior oblique muscles incarcerated in the fracture site. In late cases, these muscles and surrounding tissues become so incorporated in scar tissue that the eye cannot be rotated upward (see Fig. 28–129). The eye cannot be rotated upward when the forced duction test with forceps applied to the tendon of the inferior rectus attempts upward rotation. This test affords a means of differentiating contracture or fibrosis of the inferior rectus from weakness or paralysis of the superior rectus.

Trauma and fracture affect the extraocular muscles by causing edema, ecchymosis, hematoma, displacement, and entrapment. The intimate anatomical relationship of the inferior rectus and inferior oblique muscles to the common fracture site is one of the reasons for their vulnerability. The inferior oblique muscle arises from the orbital floor near the temporal margin in the lacrimal groove. It passes posteriorly, superficial to the belly of the inferior rectus muscle, and inserts into the sclera behind the equator deep to the belly of the lateral rectus. The sheath of the inferior rectus muscle is loosely attached to that of the inferior oblique. While the muscles themselves may not be entrapped, the fascial expansions may be tethered to the fracture site.

TESTS FOR DIPLOPIA. Inasmuch as diplopia is a subjective condition, the tests for its analysis depend upon the cooperation of the patient. Subjective results from tests for diplopia must therefore be correlated with objective findings for proper diagnosis and treatment.

The occlusion test. Alternating a small cover in front of the eyes permits the patient to advise the examiner about what happens to the double image. Persistence of the double image when one eye is occluded means that diplopia

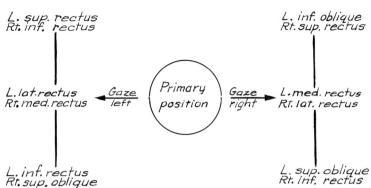

FIGURE 28–130. Schematic representation of the action of the yoke of the eye muscles in various positions of gaze.

is monocular rather than binocular; disappearance of one image indicates binocular diplopia. The image seems to move when the occluding apparatus is rapidly alternated from one eye to the other. The apparent motion of the image is opposite to the direction of movement of the eyeball. This test enables the examiner to observe the motion of the eye and to draw conclusions as to whether the deviation is horizontal or vertical or a combination. The amount of ocular deviation in the various fields of gaze may be estimated by testing with prisms (Fig. 28–130). Interpretation of the findings leads to a presumptive diagnosis as to the specific muscles involved. The occlusion test is reliable because it offers both a subjective and an objective analysis.

The red glass test. Simple red filter placed in front of the one eye helps the patient to describe the displacement of images. Although a diplopia field may be plotted by means of this test, it is not as accurate as the cover or occlusion test. The red glass may be modified so that its image is perceived as a line rather than a point. This modification is known as the Maddox rod test and has the advantage of separating the horizontal from the vertical displacement by observation of the line in the vertical and horizontal meridians, respectively.

Other tests. Numerous mechanisms such as Polaroid filters, complicated machines, perimeters, and other orthoptic devices aid in the refinement of diplopia analysis. These complicated tests are unnecessary in the average case of diplopia resulting from orbital fracture.

MONOCULAR DIPLOPIA. Monocular diplopia is a one-eyed phenomenon and consequently represents a visual rather than an oculorotary disturbance. If functional, the condition is managed as any other psychosomatic disorder. Organic monocular diplopia is caused by any alteration or obstruction along the visual axis which is conducive to duplication or

multiplicity of monocular retinal images. Abrasions of the cornea, opacities in the cornea, lens, or transparent media, aberrations in the iris diaphragm, displacement of the lens, disturbance of the retina and choroid, and other similar conditions may contribute to monocular diplopia. Organic monocular diplopia is purely an ophthalmologic problem.

BINOCULAR DIPLOPIA. Temporary diplopia, as stated in Chapter 25, is a frequent phenomenon after any fracture involving the orbit. In many cases, however, extraocular muscle injury requires secondary surgery for restoration of function for esthetic reasons.

Binocular double vision is caused by images upon noncorresponding retinal points in both eyes. These images, transmitted to consciousness under normal circumstances, are the fused images from corresponding points of the retina. Essentially, the sharply focused fused images received by the cerebral cortex from the macular areas are those registered in the area of consciousness. Images received from noncorresponding points on the peripheral retina are poorly perceived in consciousness and are used as a means of orientation rather than attentive fixation.

A normal person can observe the diplopia arising as a result of peripheral images being focused upon noncorresponding retinal points. Most of us are not plagued with this type of diplopia (physiologic diplopia) because we have learned to suppress the peripheral images. Ordinarily, we see but a single image; if one tries, however, physiologic diplopia may occur. This simple experiment is conducted by holding a pencil in a central position about 2 feet in front of the eyes and focusing across the room. The pencil is seen double. Likewise, focusing on the pencil and observing objects across the room produces a double image of the distant objects.

Occasionally, the patient discovers physiologic diplopia and suffers from its symptoms until explanations and reassurances lead the patient back to normal peripheral visual suppression.

Suppression is a psychologic mechanism by which the individual learns to ignore ocular images. Suppression may be central, peripheral, or both. Suppression is one means by which a person may learn to overcome double vision caused by extraocular muscle imbalance.

Binocular diplopia due to deviation of the visual axes, secondary to extraocular muscle imbalance, is the diplopia usually encountered following orbital fracture. Ocular deviation and diplopia resulting from organic muscle changes are caused by conditions which include edema, hemorrhage, laceration, fibrosis and disturbances in the nerve supply, and displacement of the eyeball. Deviation may also follow diminution of visual acuity because the normal mechanism is not sufficiently stimulated to bring about binocular vision. Ocular deviation may also occur in the presence of good vision in each eye as a result of a defect in the fusion mechanism.

Individuals with normal vision and a normal fusion mechanism become conscious of double vision when the visual axes are carried beyond the range of normal fusion. Even slight restriction of extraocular muscular activity in orbital fractures may result in diplopia. Individuals with defective vision or poor fusion tolerate extreme limitations of ocular motility without diplopia. Because the range of vertical fusion is much less than that of horizontal fusion, the binocular mechanism is less tolerant of vertical imbalance.

Horizontal deviations frequently develop secondary to the vertical deviation; this is partially the result of direct involvement of the horizontally acting muscles. Secondary actions of the vertically acting muscles are also influential in the superimposed horizontal deviation.

Enophthalmos. Enophthalmos in excess of 5 mm is disfiguring. The deformity seen in the malunited blowout fracture is characteristic (see Fig. 28–129, *A*). The ocular globe appears depressed and recessed; the horizontal length of the palpebral fissure is diminished; and the superior tarsal fold is deepened and the upper lid droops. The latter finding has been mistakenly interpreted as ptosis caused by severance of the levator palpebrae superioris aponeurosis or by a nerve injury. As reviewed previously in Chapter 25, enophthalmos can be attributed to one of a number of factors:

1. Escape of orbital fat into the maxillary sinus after rupture of the periorbita, as occurs in severe blowout fractures.

2. Enlargement of the size of the orbital cavity. The increased volume of the orbital cavity is the result of gross downward displacement of the orbital floor; the orbital fat thus distributed in a large orbital cavity no longer maintains adequate protrusion of the globe, and enophthalmos ensues.

3. Entrapment of the inferior rectus muscle in the blowout fracture area. Enophthalmos may occur immediately after blowout fracture; the ocular globe is pushed backward with the soft tissues of the orbit, and the tethered structures maintain the backward (enophthalmic) position of the globe. This complication seems to occur more frequently in the "pure" type of fracture of the orbital floor.*

4. Atrophy of orbital fat resulting from injury, hematoma, low grade infection, and fibrosis. Although these factors are difficult to evaluate, they must also be considered among the causes of enophthalmos.

Transient enophthalmos or retraction of the globe may occur as a result of normal extraocular muscle pull against a shortened or fibrotic opposing extraocular muscle. This is a characteristic sign in the globe retraction commonly observed in Duane's syndrome. It is also observed in any condition in which one or more of the extraocular muscles has sustained fibrosis or shortening. As the opposing muscle or muscles contract, the globe is pulled backward into the orbit, because the offending muscle fails to relax as countertraction is applied by the stimulated opponent muscle. This may be demonstrated by either or both of the vertical or horizontal rotators of the eyeball.

MEASUREMENT OF ENOPHTHALMOS. Determination of the degree of enophthalmos is based upon the relative position of a line projected from the lateral orbital margin to the profile of the zenith of the cornea. When there is bone loss and displacement, fixed points on the affected and unaffected sides cannot be used in diagnosis. In such cases, the degree of ocular protrusion or recession is determined by differences in the number of millimeters required to focus an instrument on each cornea.

ROENTGENOGRAPHIC STUDIES. Roentgenographic examination offers additional orbital

---

*The "pure" blowout fracture occurs without fracture of the orbital rim, whereas the orbital rim, as well as the floor, is fractured in the "impure" type of fracture (see Chapter 25).

information and employs five projections: the Caldwell, the Waters, the lateral, the optic canals, and the base views. Tomograms are essential to define the anatomical changes in the bony orbit (see Chapters 24 and 25) and to provide information concerning associated fractures of the other orbital walls.

SURGICAL TREATMENT OF MALUNITED FRACTURES OF THE ORBITAL FLOOR

Restoration of Orbital Architecture and Release of Entrapped Structures. The objective treatment is the release of the entrapped orbital tissues and the restoration of the architecture of the orbit. Once this has been achieved, additional surgery may be required to correct deformities or malfunction of the ocular adnexa.

The fracture site is approached through a lower eyelid incision in most of our patients with blowout fracture of the orbital floor. The various approaches to the orbital floor have been reviewed in Chapter 25.

In the late treatment of malunited fractures, the authors prefer an eyelid incision which provides better exposure of the orbit and periorbital structures and avoids loss of orbital fat, a precious tissue in patients with enophthalmos.

Surgical exploration through fibrosed tissues is laborious. Subperiosteal elevation from the orbital rim backward to the area of fracture is followed by elevation over the nonfractured medial and lateral aspects of the orbital floor. Painstaking elevation of the periorbita from the fracture area is then done. The orbital contents which have prolapsed into the maxillary sinus are extracted from the opening. When this is done gently with the aid of visual magnification (binocular loupes), it is occasionally possible, by preserving the mucous membrane of the sinus, to avoid a wide area of communication with the maxillary sinus. Preservation of the infraorbital nerve is necessary to avoid permanent anesthesia of the upper lip and cheek.

Correction of Diplopia. After separation of the entrapped orbital contents from the infraorbital nerve, it is essential to verify that they have been freed and that oculorotary movement has been restored. The forced duction test should be done to verify that free oculorotary movements are fully restored. The periorbita should be raised from the orbital walls as extensively as possible. Because an associated fracture of the medial wall

is frequent, an adhesion in this area may be responsible for persistent impairment of oculorotary movements after freeing the floor.

The exposure of the floor must often be extended into the posterior reaches of the orbital cavity. The most frequent cause of failure is fear of freeing posteriorly entrapped tissues.

Restoration of free oculorotary movements to the ocular globe is the first and most important step toward rehabilitation of the patient with a malunited orbital floor blowout fracture. The next step is to restore the continuity of the orbital floor and relieve the enophthalmos, if possible.

Correction of Enophthalmos. The cause of enophthalmos must be determined. Is it caused by prolapse of the orbital contents through a large fracture in the floor, or is it a result of a fracture of the lateral or medial walls or the roof of the orbit?

The architecture of the orbit must be restored by means of bone grafts, inorganic implants, or osteotomies.

The continuity of the orbital floor must be reestablished and the size of the orbital cavity must be reduced when it is enlarged. Jackson (1968), in a study of 33 patients in whom no graft or implant had been used to repair the orbital floor, observed that enophthalmos developed in 20 patients. When the volume of the orbital cavity is diminished by bone grafting or inorganic implants, the orbital fat will then suffice for an adequate degree of protrusion of the eyeball; the eyeball will be raised, the deepened supratarsal fold reduced, and the enophthalmos partially or completely corrected (Figs. 28–129, 28–131, and 28–132).

If enophthalmos is present, the periorbita should be raised from the orbital floor and walls as extensively as possible, sparing the apex of the orbit. An additional incision immediately below the supraorbital rim is usually required in order to raise the periorbita from the roof of the orbit. This procedure not only assists in liberating the orbital contents from their retracted positions but also establishes a plane beteen the periorbita and the orbital walls for the placement of implant material.

INORGANIC AND AUTOGENOUS TRANSPLANTS. Inorganic implants (Teflon, Silastic, Supramid) have all been employed successfully in the orbit. The implant is cut to size and placed over the orbital floor; in order to avoid slippage, a tongue is cut along the anterior margin of the implant and slipped under the forward edge (see Chapter 25, Fig. 25–33). Silastic implants are variously shaped to fit in

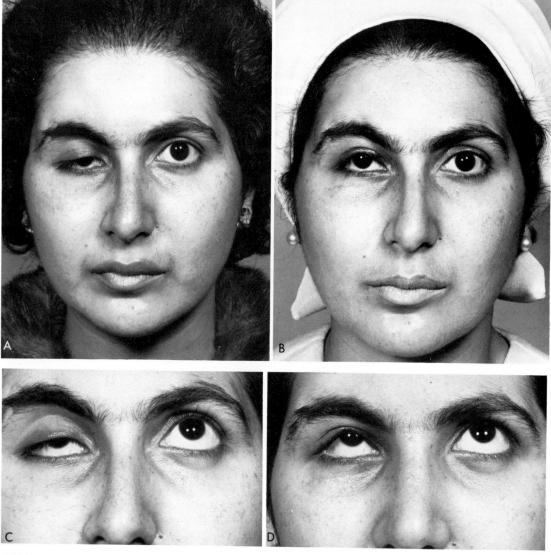

FIGURE 28–131. Late correction of enophthalmos. *A,* Patient with blowout fracture of the right orbit of many months' duration. The patient shows the typical enophthalmos with pseudoptosis of the upper eyelid. *B,* Correction after release of the entrapment of the orbital contents in the area of the blowout and bone grafting of the floor of the orbit. The size of the orbital cavity was reduced by a bone graft, and this resulted in an appreciable correction of the enophthalmos. *C,* Limitation in the upward rotation of the right ocular globe. *D,* Improvement obtained after the release of the structures entrapped in the orbital floor. (From Converse, J. M.: *In* Georgiade, N. G. (Ed.): Plastic and Maxillofacial Trauma Symposium. Vol. 1. St. Louis, Mo., C. V. Mosby Company, 1969.)

the orbit in order to reduce the size of the orbital cavity and to cause the ocular globe to protrude. Silastic implants have been employed by Spira, Gerow, and Hardy (1974) to correct moderate enophthalmos. Fascia lata has been employed, but partial absorption of the transplant requires overcorrection (Converse and coworkers, 1961).

When there is a wide area of communication between the orbit and the maxillary sinus, bone grafting may be preferable, the autogenous bone graft being less prone to infection than an inert implant. If additional implant material is required, it may be added in a later operative procedure.

Autogenous costal cartilage was employed extensively in orbital reconstruction by La-Grange (1918) in the wounded of World War I

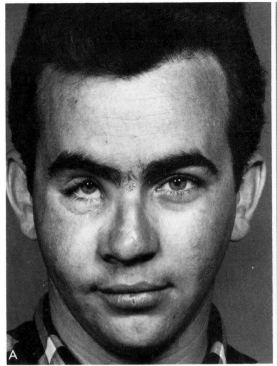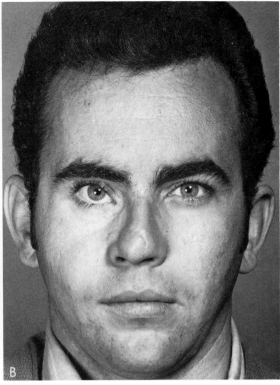

FIGURE 28–132. Late correction of enophthalmos. *A*, The patient had suffered a blowout fracture of the right orbit with esotropia and limitation of motion of the ocular globe. *B*, Result obtained after the release of the entrapped structures, placing Silastic implants over the orbital floor, and medial canthoplasty. The improvement of the enophthalmos was moderate.

and is a satisfactory transplant. Although cartilage is not as resistant to infection as bone, it is particularly indicated in extensive prolapse of the orbital floor. Dingman and Grabb (1974) employed irradiated cartilage allografts as implant material.

Bone grafts may not be successful because of inadequate contact between the graft and host bone in old malunited fractures. In severe malunited fractures with large bony defects, bone grafts provide the safest and best means of reconstruction.

Evaluation of the amount of implant material to be placed into the orbital cavity can be made by observing the gross changes which occur in the repaired orbit; the ocular globe protrudes and fills the supratarsal fold. Comparison with the unaffected eye provides a guide to the amount of implant material required to achieve the correction.

FORWARD TRACTION TEST. Late correction of enophthalmos is difficult to achieve. Some information concerning the prognosis of the surgical correction of enophthalmos may be obtained by the forward traction test (Fig. 28–133). This test is done by applying two forceps to the eyeball, one to the lateral rectus and the other to the medial rectus muscle. Forward traction is then exerted. If the ocular globe cannot be advanced readily, the prognosis for surgical improvement of the enophthalmos is poor; the musculature and other soft tissue structures, which have become fibrosed and shortened, oppose surgical correction.

CORRECTION OF ENOPHTHALMOS IN THE NONSEEING EYE. In the patient with a nonseeing eye or prosthetic eye, the posterior reaches of the orbit may be approached by raising the periorbita along the lateral wall of the orbit, as the danger of causing blindness, ever present in the seeing eye, is nonexistent (Fig. 28–134). Silastic implants may be placed in the posterior aspect of the orbital cone medially and laterally after raising the periorbita from the orbital wall. A technique utilized by Smith, Obear, and Leone (1967) consists of placing Pyrex glass beads in the apex of the orbit. These are introduced, after elevation of

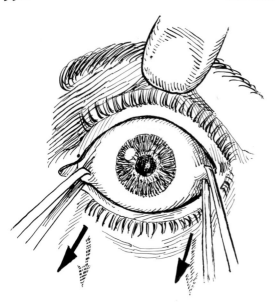

FIGURE 28–133. The forward traction test. Two forceps grasp the medial and lateral recti muscles and exert a forward traction on the eyeball. Freedom of forward displacement of the orbital contents is a favorable prognostic sign for the correction of enophthalmos by orbital implants; resistance to forward traction is a poor prognostic sign. (From Converse, J. M., Smith, B., Obear, M., and Wood-Smith, D.: Orbital blow-out fracture: A ten-year survey. Plast. Reconstr. Surg., *39*:20, 1967.)

the periorbita, with the aid of a suction tip which carries the bead until the suction is interrupted, at which time it is deposited into the orbital apex over the lateral orbital wall (Fig. 28–135), or by means of a tube and a ramrod (Fig. 28–136). Pyrex beads are added until an adequate projection of the eyeball is obtained.

In the correction of enophthalmos in the anopthalmic orbit, Iverson, Vistnes, and Siegel (1973) advocated the subperiosteal injection of RTV (room temperature vulcanizing) Silastic along the superior, lateral, and inferior walls of the orbit. In their evaluation studies, the technique gave a result superior to that obtained following the insertion of Pyrex beads.

RESULTS. In the majority of our patients, complete correction of the enophthalmos was not achieved. Most patients, however, were improved by placing implants over the orbital floor, the lateral orbital wall, and (prudently) over the lamina papyracea behind the lacrimal sac (see Figs. 28–129, 28–131, and 28–132). It is essential to recall that the optic foramen is situated near the medial orbital wall; implants placed posteriorly along this wall risk injuring the nerve. The lateral orbital wall, because it is

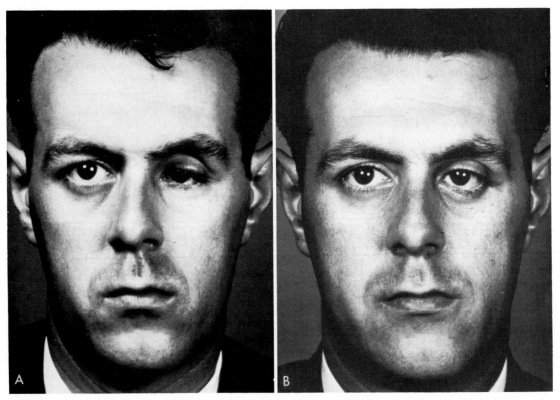

FIGURE 28–134. Treatment of enophthalmos in a patient with a nonseeing eye. *A,* The patient has suffered a blow-out fracture of the left orbit with esotropia, limitation of motion of the ocular globe, and enophthalmos. *B,* Correction of the enophthalmos by the technique shown in Figure 28–135. Subsequent extraocular muscle surgery corrected the esotropia.

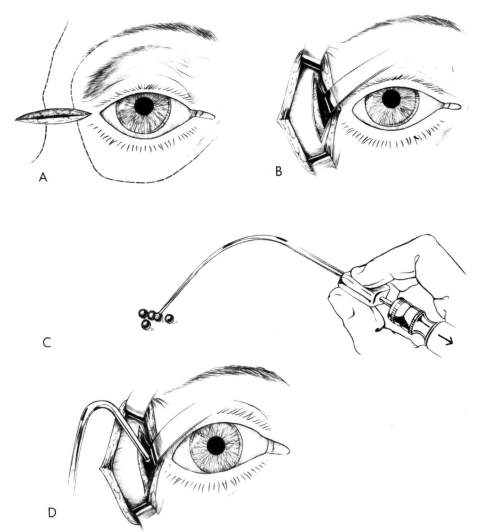

FIGURE 28–135. Pyrex bead method for correction of enophthalmos in a nonseeing eye. (After Smith, Obear and Leone, 1967.) *A*, Horizontal incision made at the lateral canthus. *B*, Subperiosteal exposure of the lateral wall of the orbit back to the apex. *C*, Pyrex beads are picked up by means of a suction tip. *D*, A Pyrex bead is being introduced into the apex of the orbit on the end of the suction tip. When it has reached its destination, the suction is released and the bead is deposited.

situated in an anterolateral-posteromedial plane, is the most favorable site for implants; it is also removed from the optic foramen. In patients with residual enophthalmos, contour restoration of a malunited depressed zygoma should be done with prudence; an increased projection of the zygoma will cause the enophthalmic eye to appear relatively more enophthalmic.

The problem of correction of established severe enophthalmos is a difficult one. In a malunited fracture with entrapment of the orbital contents, restoring the free oculorotary movements is obviously the first step. In persistent enophthalmos following release of the entrapped tissues, the degree of correction will depend upon the response of the orbital contents to the transplants or implants placed to

reduce the volume of the orbit: the lateral wall build-up will project the ocular globe forward; raising the level of the orbital floor will elevate the ocular globe and also assist in the forward projection. The thickness of the implants must be evaluated carefully. The only means of estimating the amount of increased projection is clinical experience.

In a series of 50 patients (Converse and coworkers, 1967) who had been referred following unsuccessful primary or late treatment, longitudinal studies were obtained. The mean time interval between the accident and primary repair was 3½ weeks. The patients were first seen at a mean time interval of one month after trauma; the range extended to 20 years after fracture. Of the 14 patients who had previous surgery for fracture of the floor of the orbit, ten

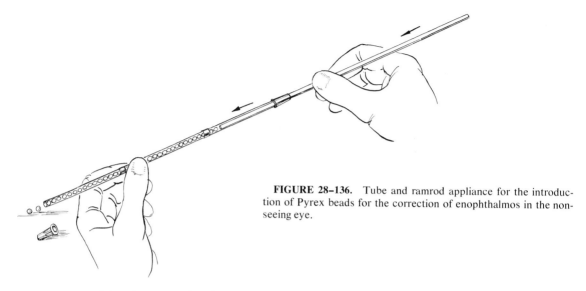

FIGURE 28–136. Tube and ramrod appliance for the introduction of Pyrex beads for the correction of enophthalmos in the non-seeing eye.

underwent additional surgery for the treatment of blowout fractures; four patients required additional surgery for one or more of the complications resulting from blowout fractures.

The most common finding was double vision; the second was enophthalmos. Similar observations were made by Hakelius and Pontén (1973), who observed an incidence of permanent diplopia in 24 per cent of the patients in whom treatment was delayed.

Five patients had visual impairment, and 15 had ptosis on the involved side. None of the patients complained subjectively of the infraorbital anesthesia; this clinical finding was elicited only by direct questioning and objective examination. Patients who had associated facial bone fractures had more obvious facial asymmetry, lacrimal obstruction, ptosis of the globe, ptosis of the lid, and canthal displacement.

Radiographic examination was positive for fracture of the orbital floor in all of the patients before surgical treatment and proved to be most informative.

Late primary surgical repair of the fracture was performed in 35 patients. Only three patients were not operated upon for secondary exploration of the orbital floor fracture but were treated for other concomitant complications of the blowout fracture. All of these fractures were repaired through a transcutaneous lower eyelid approach. The surgical release of incarcerated muscle and fascial expansions from the healed bony fragments impacted around them was necessary in all of the eight patients previously repaired only through a maxillary sinus approach (Caldwell-Luc).

Three of the patients operated upon primarily required secondary operations to correct progressive enophthalmos and diplopia; one patient was operated upon two months after the primary repair, one after six months, and the third two years after primary repair. The first patient required secondary operation because of posterior migration of a Teflon implant and reexposure of the blowout fracture area. This defect was repaired with an iliac bone graft after removal of the Teflon implant. The second patient had been repaired primarily with a silicone plate; a persistent 5-mm enophthalmos required correction with an iliac bone graft at six months. This patient still has a residual 3-mm enophthalmos, but the associated recession of the zygomatic prominence renders it less obvious.

Postoperative examinations were done one month, three months, six months, and one year after surgery. When the preoperative findings were compared to the findings after one year, eight patients were cured of all their symptoms, 38 improved, and two were unchanged; in two patients the appearance was not improved. Additional surgery was required in 22 cases; the total number of surgical procedures was 34.

Correction of Other Deformities and Functional Impairment

EXTRAOCULAR MUSCLE IMBALANCE. Most frequent of these sequelae is muscle imbalance. Secondary muscle imbalance occurs in the ptotic ocular globe only when the eye is enophthalmic. Muscle surgery is planned once the muscle pattern has been established as a permanent deviation. The time of the first muscle surgery in late repairs may be anywhere from the first month to three months after the treatment of the orbital floor fracture.

Second and third muscle operative procedures are often necessary. The aim of these procedures is to obtain fusion in the primary and eyes-down positions, which are the most functional positions for speaking, eating, and reading. To achieve this result, it may be necessary to sacrifice fusion in eyes-up position, a very unphysiologic one at best.

It is not infrequent that extraocular muscle surgery is indicated in the unaffected eye in order to obtain binocular fusion.

INTRAOCULAR PRESSURE. Intraocular pressure is a complication which should not occur if an excessively large transplant or implant is avoided. If the patient complains of pain, the retinal vessels should be examined. Pressure should be relieved, if indicated, to avoid possible blindness.

MEDIAL AND LATERAL CANTHAL DEFORMITIES. These are sequelae of orbital fractures more frequently found in association with multiple midfacial bone fractures and naso-orbital fractures. Zygomatic fractures and dislocations dislodge the lateral raphé and lateral canthal tendon, and an antimongoloid slant of the lid may result. Complete detachment of the lateral tendon and raphé produces a rounded lateral canthus and decreased intercanthal distance.

As discussed early in the chapter, the medial canthal tendon inserts on the lacrimal crest anteriorly, and the deep head of the pretarsal muscle (the tensor tarsi) inserts on the posterior lacrimal crest. Naso-orbital fractures involving the frontal process of the maxilla, lacrimal bones, or nasal bones disrupt the stability of the medial support of the lid. The medial canthus is pulled laterally and, occasionally, downward (see Fig. 28–148). When untreated, naso-orbital fractures may result in traumatic telecanthus, an increased distance between the medial canthi. The treatment of canthal deformities is described in a later section of this chapter.

VERTICAL SHORTENING OF THE LOWER EYELID. Exposure of the sclera below the limbus of the globe in the primary position (the "scleral show" or "white eye" syndrome) may result from scar contracture (vertical shortening of the lower eyelid), from downward and backward displacement of the fractured inferior orbital rim, or from suturing the periorbita to the septum orbitale after placement of the implant. Release of the scar tissue and replacement of the orbital rim into the corrected position restore the lid to normal position. If the fractured rim is malunited, release of the septum orbitale attachment from the orbital rim and restoration of the orbital rim by a bone graft are procedures which can elevate the lid margin. If primary operative procedures fail, a tarsoconjunctival graft from the same or opposite upper eyelid may increase the vertical dimension of the lower lid and raise the lid margin up to 4-mm.

INFRAORBITAL NERVE ANESTHESIA. Infraorbital nerve anesthesia may be very disconcerting to some patients. The area of sensory loss usually extends from the lower lid

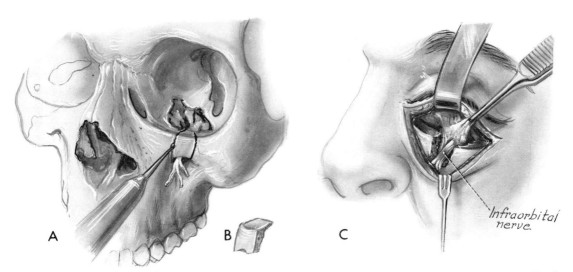

FIGURE 28–137. Decompression and identification of the infraorbital nerve. *A,* When difficulty is encountered in dissecting the infraorbital nerve in the orbital fracture area, the nerve is exposed at the infraorbital foramen, and a section of bone is outlined for removal to uncover the infraorbital canal. *B,* A block of bone is removed and set aside for later replacement. *C,* The infraorbital nerve is traced back to the blowout fracture area and dissected from the orbital contents. The block of bone illustrated in *B* is then replaced. (From Converse, J. M., Smith, B., Obear, M. F., and Wood-Smith, D.: Orbital blow-out fracture: A ten-year study. Plast. Reconstr. Surg., *39:*20, 1967.)

over the cheek and lateral ala to the upper lip. Release of the infraorbital nerve from the pressure of bone fragments within the canal may be indicated (Fig. 28–137). Sensation may recur spontaneously as late as one year after fracture.

TREATMENT OF EXTENSIVE LOSS OF THE ORBITAL FLOOR. Extensive loss of the orbital floor may result from destructive injuries such as gunshot wounds or from comminution of the floor of the orbit followed by sequestration of bone fragments after infection and suppuration.

When the floor of the orbit is removed in a surgical procedure, such as the resection of the maxilla for carcinoma, the periorbita and the orbital fascia, including the suspensory ligament of Lockwood, are undisturbed. Progressive sagging of the orbital contents results in the ocular globe being situated at a lower level than the contralateral unaffected eye. As the extraocular musculature is not appreciably disturbed, diplopia does not usually follow. These patients usually complain of transient diplopia only when fatigued.

As a result of direct injury to the periorbita, orbital fascia, and inferior oblique and inferior rectus muscles, scar tissue contraction may not only interfere with ocular rotary movements of the eye but also, by progressive contraction, result in a fixed downward displacement and rotation of the ocular globe and a vertical shortening of the lower lid (Fig. 28–138).

The bony defect may involve a major portion of the orbital floor in its maxillary and zygomatic portions and also a major portion of the body of the zygoma. Extensive reconstruction may be required when there is major bone loss (Fig. 28–139). The surgical approach is through preexisting scars or through a lower eyelid incision. Dissection of the orbital contents is often done with difficulty in such cases. The peripheral limits of the orbital contents are exposed and freed. Usually a shelf or orbital floor is found medially and laterally. Elevation of the orbital contents is extended posteriorly

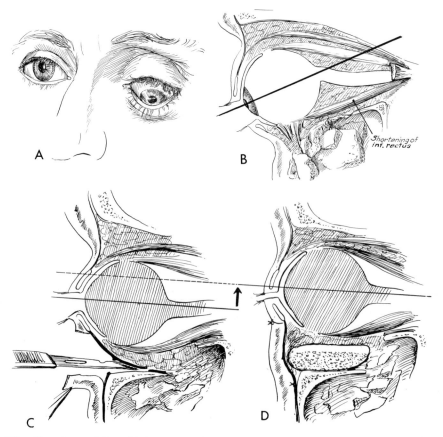

FIGURE 28–138. The release of the orbital structures in a malunited blowout fracture. *A,* The ocular globe is maintained in downward rotation by the entrapped structures. Note the deepened supratarsal fold and the deep fold in the lower lid, which is also shortened by the downward and backward traction of the entrapped structures upon the septum orbitale. *B,* Sagittal section illustrating the entrapment in a massive fracture. *C, D,* Exploration and correction following insertion of an iliac bone graft.

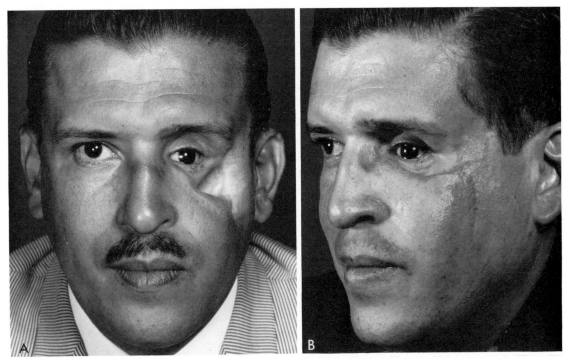

FIGURE 28–139. Loss of a major portion of the floor of the orbit and zygoma as a result of a gunshot wound. *A,* Patient with a large defect in the zygomatic area involving a major portion of the floor of the orbit and loss of the ocular globe. The patient is wearing a prosthetic eye. *B,* After reconstruction of the orbital floor by means of a bone graft, filling of the bony defect of the zygoma with bone chips, and repair of the soft tissues by advancing cheek tissue and employing a temporal flap to restore the lateral portion of the lower eyelid.

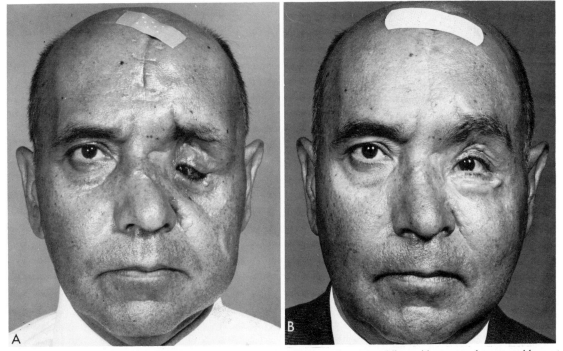

FIGURE 28–140. Extensive disorganization of the orbital floor. *A,* An automobile accident caused a severe blowout fracture of the floor of the orbit, severance of the medial canthal tendon and lacrimal sac, and esotropia. The patient also had a craniotomy for evacuation of a subdural hematoma. *B,* After medial canthoplasty and dacryocystorhinostomy, the ocular globe was released from its entrapment in the orbital floor, and a bone graft was placed to restore the orbital floor. Suture of the levator aponeurosis with levator resection was also done to correct the traumatic ptosis. After this operation, the patient had additional surgery elsewhere, and an inorganic implant was placed over the orbital floor. Note that the orbital implant is being extruded.

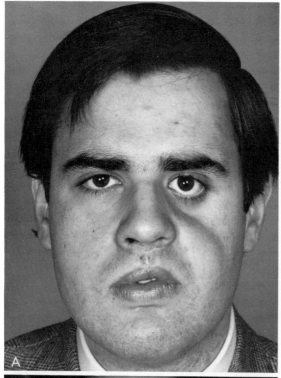
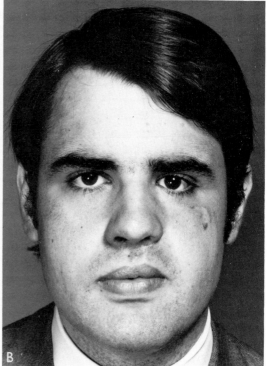
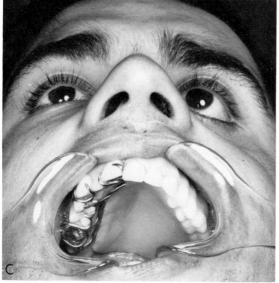

FIGURE 28–141. Loss of the entire floor of the orbit. *A,* After resection of the maxilla and floor of the orbit at another institution for fibrous dysplasia of the left maxilla. Note the drooping of the left eyelid and depression of the infraorbital region. *B,* Result obtained after reconstruction of the floor of the orbit and upper portion of the maxilla by bone grafting according to the technique illustrated in Chapter 30 (Fig. 30–255). *C,* The obturator is employed to close the gap in the palate, restore the dentition, and maintain the contour of the lower portion of the cheek.

until a posterior shelf is encountered. The freed orbital contents are then raised, and a bone graft consisting of the inner table of the ilium with attached cancellous bone is placed across the floor. Reconstruction of the orbital floor, orbital rim, and infraorbital portion of the maxilla and the zygoma by bone grafts can be achieved. In large defects, inorganic implants

tend to be unstable and extrude (Fig. 28–140); bone grafts may be preferable.

A patient who has lost the entire left half of his maxilla was successfully reconstructed by the technique illustrated in Figure 28–141. A prosthodontic obturator provided the continuity of the missing left half of the hard palate and the contour of the cheek and acted as a

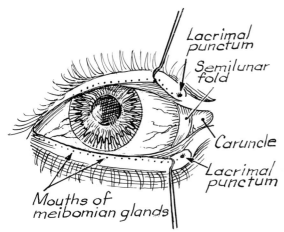

FIGURE 28–142. Superficial structures of the medial canthus.

denture, while the bone grafts successfully restored the orbital floor, upper maxilla, and a portion of the zygoma.

MALUNITED FRACTURES OF THE MEDIAL ORBITAL WALL

Medial orbital wall fractures occur in orbital floor fractures and are a hidden cause of enophthalmos (see Chapter 25). In their more severe form, they are usually associated with naso-orbital fractures.

Because of the presence of the lacrimal system in the medial canthal area (Fig. 28–142), the treatment of malunited fractures involving the medial wall may be quite complex. In addition, the proximity of the anterior cranial fossa may also complicate the treatment.

Naso-orbital fractures may also impair the physiology of the accessory sinuses, as the nasofrontal duct, the ostia of the ethmoidal cells, and the ethmoidal cells themselves may be disrupted (Fig. 28–143).

The most vulnerable structures, however, are the anatomical complex formed by the lacrimal sac lodged in the lacrimal groove and the nasolacrimal duct and the tendinous structures which surround the sac (Figs. 28–144 and 28–145).

A malunited fracture of the medial orbital wall in the portion formed by the lamina papyracea may have occurred in conjunction with a blowout fracture of the orbital floor and a naso-orbital fracture and remained undetected. Such a fracture should be considered if late enophthalmos develops after what had appeared to be satisfactory treatment of an orbital floor fracture.

Malunited fracture of the medial orbital wall may result from backward displacement of comminuted fragments of the nasal bones and frontal processes of the maxilla. These fragments may enter the orbital cavity, injuring the lacrimal sac (see Fig. 28–145, *B*) or they may be forced into the ethmoidal labrynth, outfracturing the medial orbital wall and reducing the horizontal dimension of the orbit.

The Deformity of a Malunited Naso-orbital Fracture. In untreated or maltreated naso-orbital fractures, the patient has a characteristic appearance; the bony bridge of the nose is depressed and widened, and the eyes appear far apart (Fig. 28–146). In severe midfacial fractures associated with naso-orbital and bilateral orbital fractures, the degree of deformity is such that the patient is unrecognizable (Fig. 28–147). Traumatic telecanthus is caused by an increase in the distance between the me-

FIGURE 28–143. The structures involved in a naso-orbital fracture seen from the medial aspect of the lateral nasal wall. Above, the frontal sinus and the nasofrontal duct. An anterior ethmoidal cell, the agger nasi cell, and the other anterior ethmoidal cells as well as their ostia are indicated.

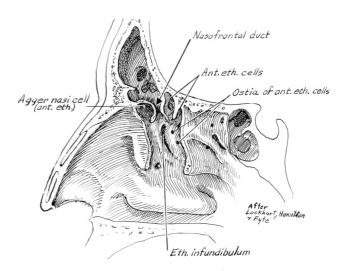

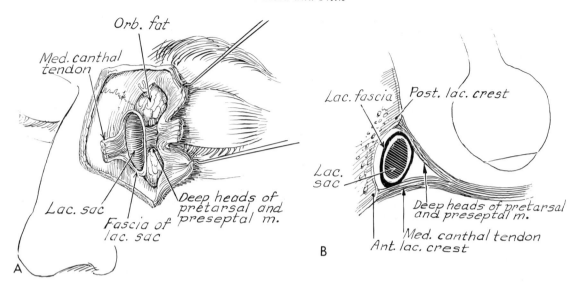

FIGURE 28–144. The left medial canthal region. The medial canthal tendon and the deep heads of the pretarsal and preseptal muscles embrace the lacrimal sac.

dial canthi (intercanthal distance), resulting from fracture displacement of the bones forming the skeletal framework of the nose and medial orbital walls. The medial canthi are deformed; cutaneous scars and epicanthal folds may be present; and the function of the lacrimal apparatus is disturbed. The deformity may be unilateral or bilateral. The pseudohyperteloric appearance of the orbits is increased by the flattening of the bony dorsum of the nose.

Roentgenographic studies and tomography at the plane extending through the lacrimal groove are of assistance in diagnosis.

THE BONY DEFORMITY. The crushing type of injury resulting from a striking force over the bridge of the nose, when the impact is a violent one, fractures, disorganizes, and displaces the skeletal structures of the nose. The displacement is backward into the interorbital space and the orbits. The types of fractures have

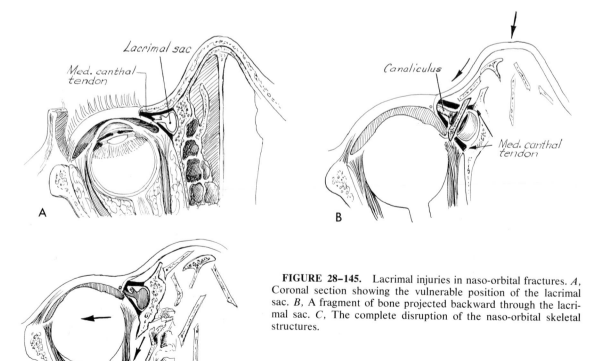

FIGURE 28–145. Lacrimal injuries in naso-orbital fractures. *A,* Coronal section showing the vulnerable position of the lacrimal sac. *B,* A fragment of bone projected backward through the lacrimal sac. *C,* The complete disruption of the naso-orbital skeletal structures.

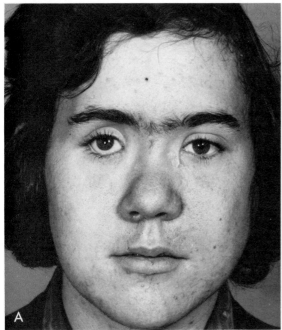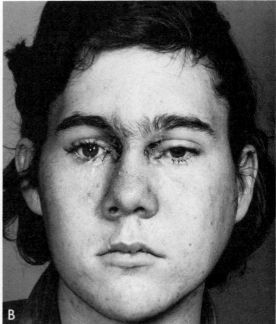

FIGURE 28–146. The deformity of naso-orbital fracture. *A*, Typical deformity. The nose is flattened, and the eyes appear far apart because of the telecanthus. The caruncles are covered. The epicanthal fold is the result of the penetration of a piece of glass which occurred in the head-on automobile crash. Note also the loss of the horizontal dimension of the right palpebral fissure. The right eye had been enucleated at the time of the primary treatment. *B*, The patient underwent treatment at the time when this text was being prepared. The patient is shown ten days after operation. Double-opposing Z-plasties corrected the epicanthal fold in the left medial canthus. The overlapping malunited fragments of the left medial orbital wall were removed. The right medial orbital wall was defective and was restored by means of a bone graft. Both lacrimal sacs were found to be badly damaged. Bilateral conjunctivodacryocystorhinostomies were performed, and a Jones Pyrex tube was inserted bilaterally. The bone graft restoring the right medial orbital wall was maintained in fixation by the technique shown in Figure 28–155. The right medial canthal tendon was reinserted to the bone graft, and the left medial canthal tendon was reinserted to the medial orbital wall by means of transosseous wiring. An iliac bone graft was used to restore the dorsum of the nose and was maintained by transosseous wiring (the cantilever technique). The canthal buttons were maintained by transosseous wiring (see Fig. 28–162).

been discussed in Chapter 25. In view of the complexity of malunited fractures and their repair, it is useful to remind the reader of the surgical pathology of these fractures.

Traumatic telecanthus is produced by three varieties of backward displacement of the bony structures and injury to the medial canthal tendon, the lacrimal sac, and the posterior heads of the pretarsal (tensor tarsi) and preseptal muscles (see Fig. 28–145).

In a first type of fracture, the nasal bones and frontal process of the maxilla are splayed outward. The bones fill the medial portion of the orbital cavity, being pushed backward along the lateral surface of the medial orbital wall, severing the medial canthal tendon, and traversing the lacrimal sac or severing the canaliculi (see Fig. 28–145). Considerable increase in the thickness of the medial orbital wall may result from overlapping bone fragments. Loss of bone in the area may also result from injudicious debridement and removal of bone fragments or the expulsion of bone fragments into the nasal cavity at the time of frac-

ture. Injury to the medial rectus muscle has been noted in this type of fracture (Fig. 28–145, *C*).

In a second type of fracture, the bones enter the interorbital space, comminuting the ethmoid cells and out-fracturing the medial wall of the orbit. The medial canthal deformity is the result of lateral displacement of the medial canthal tendon with a loose fragment of comminuted bone upon which the tendon is still attached; the unopposed contraction of the orbicularis muscle pulls the structures laterally (Fig. 28–148).

THE MEDIAL CANTHAL DEFORMITY. The medial canthus has lost its angular shape, and the caruncle is often no longer visible (see Fig. 28–148), being covered by an epicanthal fold of skin and subcutaneous tissue. This results in a shortening of the horizontal dimension of the palpebral fissure, a laxity of the eyelids, and a tendency to eversion of the lower eyelid margin. The punctum is no longer in contact with the ocular globe, and epiphora results.

Downward displacement of the fractured

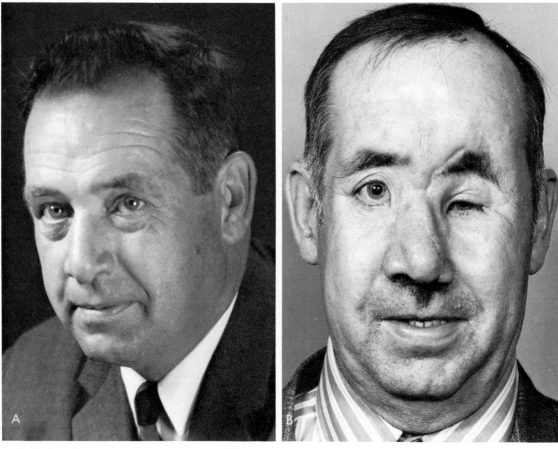

FIGURE 28–147. *A*, Portrait of patient prior to automobile crash. *B*, Photograph when the patient was first seen with malunited naso-orbital and bilateral orbital fractures. Note the total disorganization of the upper and midfacial skeletal framework, the severity of the deformities, and the tragic change in the patient's appearance.

fragment upon which the medial canthal tendon is inserted results in a canthus inversus deformity.

Comparison of the traumatic telecanthus, when the naso-orbital fracture is unilateral, with the unaffected side demonstrates the lateral displacement of the medial canthus (Figs. 28–149 and 28–150). In bilateral fractures, the telecanthus is obvious. Clinical examination usually shows the extent of the bony displacement and deformity. Roentgenographic examination and, in particular, tomography of the interobital space are of assistance in demonstrating the nature of the bony deformity.

EPICANTHAL FOLDS AND CUTANEOUS SCARS. Epicanthal folds usually result from lacerations through the medial canthal region, the excess skin resulting from backward displacement of the nasal bony bridge; the skin of the nose flows over into the naso-orbital valley. An epicanthal fold may also form at the time of surgery when the medial canthus is replaced into its corrected position; the excess skin forms the fold.

DISTURBANCE OF THE LACRIMAL APPARATUS. Malfunction of the lacrimal apparatus may be present even in the absence of severance or interruption of any portion of the lacrimal system. As was previously mentioned, relaxation of the medial canthal tissue and the inability of the orbicularis oculi muscle to maintain normal muscle tone between the medial canthal tendon and the lateral canthal tendon causes a relaxation of the lower eyelid, eversion of the lacrimal punctum, and inadequate evacuation of the tears from the lacrimal lake. Interference with the function of the orbicularis oculi muscle also hampers the evacuation of tears from the lacrimal sac into the nasolacrimal duct, the evacuation being largely dependent on the contraction of the orbicularis oculi fibers over the lacrimal sac (the lacrimal pump).

Interruption of the continuity of any portion

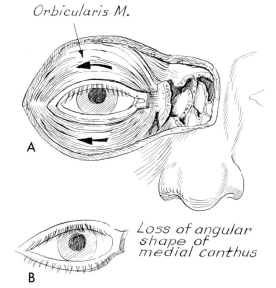

Orbicularis M.

Loss of angular shape of medial canthus

B

FIGURE 28–148. *A,* Traction exerted by the orbicularis oculi muscle upon the medial canthus when the medial canthal tendon is severed or detached. *B,* This results in a characteristic deformity of the medial canthus and a diminution of the horizontal dimension of the palpebral fissure. (From Converse, J. M., and Smith, B.: Naso-orbital fractures and traumatic deformities of the medial canthal region. Plast. Reconstr. Surg., *38*:147, 1966. Copyright © 1966. The Williams & Wilkins Company, Baltimore.)

of the lacrimal system may occur at the level of the canaliculi, the common canaliculus, the lacrimal sac, or the nasolacrimal duct. The canaliculi are usually severed by some sharp object, such as a piece of glass lacerating the medial portion of the lids and the lacrimal sac. The naso-lacrimal duct may be obstructed or lacerated along its course through the lateral wall of the nose or at its point of exit below the inferior turbinate.

As previously stated, the lacrimal sac becomes distended when the nasolacrimal duct is obstructed and fills with mucoid fluid. This is readily expressed when pressure is exerted over the medial canthal region. Such a mucocele of the lacrimal sac is manifested by a swelling at the medial canthus, which adds to the distortion of the area resulting from the fractures and the detachment or severance of the medial canthal tendon. The lacrimal sac may be dilated and displaced (Fig. 28–151).

EXTRAOCULAR MUSCLE INJURY. The insertion of the inferior oblique may be disrupted, as the medial portion of the floor of the orbit is frequently involved in the fracture. The inferior rectus or its check ligament is also vulnerable.

PTOSIS OF THE UPPER LID. A number of patients with malunited naso-orbital fractures also have ptosis of the upper lid from injury, hematoma, or a severance of the levator palpebrae superioris muscle or its aponeurosis (Converse and Smith, 1966) (Fig. 28–152).

CONCOMITANT ORBITAL FRACTURE. In pa-

FIGURE 28–149. Traumatic telecanthus. *A,* Deformity resulting from fracture of the left nasal bone and frontal process of the maxilla. Bone fragments fill the medial portion of the orbital cavity. *B,* The left medial canthus is displaced laterally. (From Converse, J. M.: Two plastic operations for the repair of orbit following severe trauma and extensive comminuted fracture. Arch. Ophthalmol., *31*:323, 1944.)

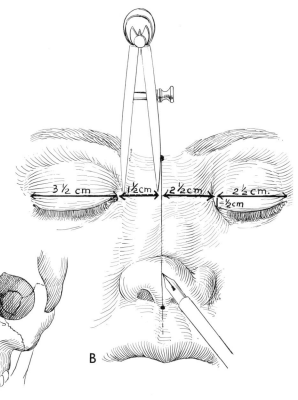

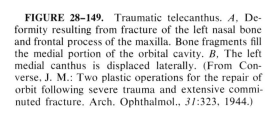

A

B

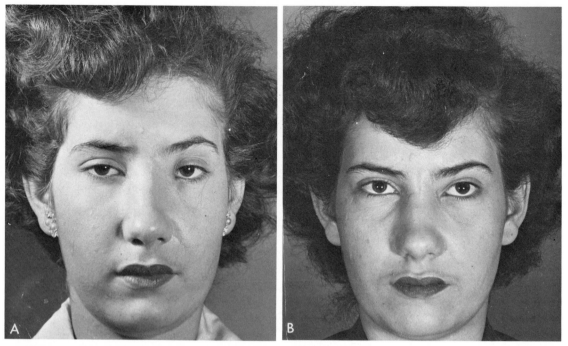

FIGURE 28–150. Deformity of the left medial canthal area after comminuted fracture of the left nasal bones and frontal process of the maxilla. *A,* Typical deformity of the left medial canthus, which is displaced forward, laterally, and downward. *B,* Result obtained after canthoplasty and dacryocystorhinostomy. (From Converse, J. M., and Smith, B.: Canthoplasty and dacryocystorhinostomy in malunited fractures of the medial wall of the orbit. Am. J. Ophthalmol., *35*:1103, 1952.)

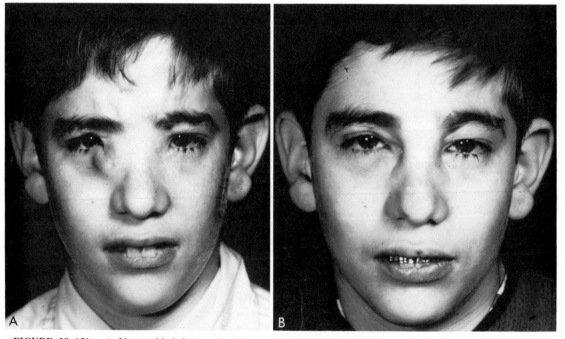

FIGURE 28–151. *A,* Naso-orbital fracture having caused obstruction of the nasolacrimal ducts. The patient has dilated lacrimal sacs in addition to the telecanthus. *B,* Result obtained following bilateral dacryocystorhinostomy and restoration of the bony contour of the nasal bones and medial orbital walls.

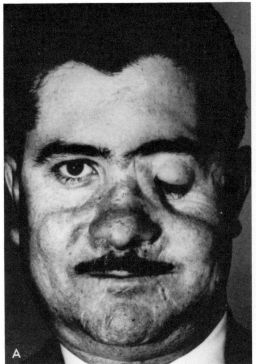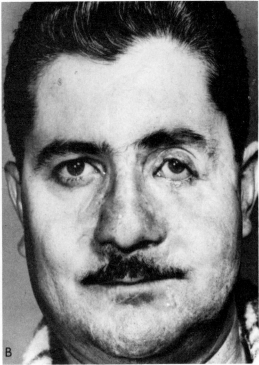

FIGURE 28–152. *A,* A 30 year old motorcycle policeman sustained typical naso-orbital fractures with comminuted fragments of the nasal bones and frontal process of the maxilla, which were pushed into the medial portion of the orbit and interorbital space. He also sustained a fracture of the floor of the left orbit and severance of the levator palpebrae superioris muscle aponeurosis. *B,* After reconstruction of the medial wall of the left orbit, contour-restoring bone grafting of the nose, bone grafting of the floor of the left orbit, and first stage repair of the levator muscle. Further surgery is required to restore the left upper eyelid. (From Converse, J. M., and Smith, B.: Naso-orbital fractures. Trans. Am. Acad. Ophthmol. Otolarygnol., *67:*662, 1963.)

tients who have suffered severe trauma or an orbital fracture, a blowout fracture is often a frequent associated fracture (Figs. 28–152 and 28–153). When orbital fractures occur bilaterally concomitantly with naso-orbital fractures and are not treated aggressively in the early stage, the resulting deformity may be extremely difficult to correct.

Treatment. Treatment of malunited naso-orbital fracture should not be undertaken until the progressive softening of the tissues and a restoration of blood and lymphatic vessel continuity have occurred. A concomitant malunited blowout fracture should be treated during the same operating session in order to release the inferior rectus and inferior oblique muscle entrapment and to reestablish the continuity of the orbital floor.

Lacrimal probes introduced through the lower or upper punctum and canaliculus are employed to test the continuity of the canaliculi. When the nasolacrimal duct is obstructed,

the lacrimal sac is usually dilated and forms a mucocele. Contrast media may also be injected through the punctum, and roentgenograms show the outline of the lacrimal apparatus.

Surgical correction involves four different types of surgical procedures that are best performed in the same operating session, whenever possible. Staged procedures have the inconvenience that each is made more difficult by the scar tissue resulting from the previous operation; however, staged procedures may be necessary in severe injuries.

1. CORRECTION OF THE CUTANEOUS EPICANTHAL FOLD. The double-opposing Z-plasty technique (Converse, 1964), modified as shown in Figure 28–81, is most effective in correcting the epicanthal fold associated with naso-orbital fractures. Mustardé's (1959) rectangular flap technique for the correction of the congenital type of epicanthal fold may also be employed.

2. RESTORATION OF THE BONY CONTOUR OF THE AREA. This requires osteotomy, re-

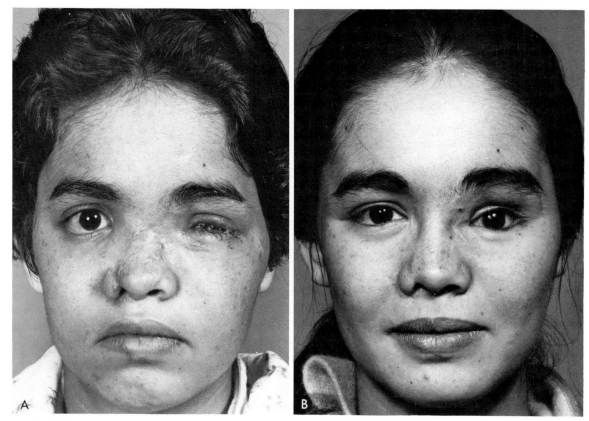

FIGURE 28–153. *A,* Twenty one year old Filipino patient. Naso-orbital fracture one month after the accident with loss of the left ocular globe, medial canthal deformity from posteriorly displaced comminuted bone fragments, and left lacrimal duct obstruction. *B,* Result obtained after dacryocystorhinostomy and reattachment of the medial canthal tendon, nasal contour restoration by bone grafting, provision of an ocular prosthesis, and intraorbital silicone implants to correct the enophthalmos. (From Converse, J. M., and Smith, B.: Proceedings of the 8th International Congress of Otorhinolaryngology, Tokyo, October, 1965.)

placement of displaced bone, and reduction of the thickness of the medial orbital wall resulting from overlapping fractured fragments. Occasionally the medial orbital wall may require reconstruction by a bone graft if it has been severely comminuted or destroyed. Restoration of contour of the bony bridge of the nose by bone grafting is usually required. Realignment of the bony portion of the nasal pyramid after osteotomy may be necessary.

3. REESTABLISHMENT OF CONTINUITY OF THE LACRIMAL SYSTEM. The reestablishment of function of the nasolacrimal apparatus is an integral and essential aspect of the treatment of malunited naso-orbital fractures when the lacrimal system is damaged.

4. MEDIAL CANTHOPLASTY AND CANTHOPEXY. This is achieved by reattachment of the medial canthal tendon by means of wire fixation of the tissues of the medial canthus to the bone of the medial orbital wall after removal of all scar tissue and realignment of displaced bone fragments.

Canthopexy, Dacryocystorhinostomy, Bone Grafting: A One-Stage Procedure

An incision made through the skin and periosteum over the frontal process of the maxilla provides a suitable approach to the area (Fig. 28–154). If a Z-plasty procedure is required to correct an epicanthal fold, the Z-plasty incisions can also be employed as the route of approach. The periosteum is raised backward over the anterior lacrimal crest, the lacrimal groove, and the lamina papyracea of the ethmoid bone. Identification of the lacrimal apparatus may be extremely tedious when the area is filled with scar tissue left in the wake of penetrating lacerated wounds. Staining the lacrimal sac by the injection of a solution of methylene blue through the lower or upper punctum and canaliculus and placing a lacrimal probe through the same route may aid in the identification of the structures during the surgical exploration of the area.

The protruding and overlapping bone fragments are exposed. When severe comminution has resulted in destruction of a section of the medial orbital wall or when the bone has been reduced to mere pulp, an iliac bone graft is maintained in position by transosseous transnasal wires (Fig. 28–155). Malunited segments of bone, including the medial portion of the orbital floor, should be freed by means of an osteotome and wired into their original anatomical position (Fig. 28–156). Replacement of the medial canthus into its corrected position is achieved by the reattachment of the remnants of the medial canthal tendon to the medial orbital wall. The stump of the tendon can usually be found and traction exerted upon it to mobilize the canthus in a medial direction. In locating the stump of the medial canthal tendon amid the mass of scar tissue, the tip of a curved hemostat is placed into the conjunctival sac at the medial canthus (Fig. 28–157) to indicate the position of the stump and/or the tissues of the medial canthus to be reattached to the bone.

Often in long-standing deformities, heavy scar tissue lies between the medial canthus and the medial orbital wall. Resection of this tissue is essential if the canthus is to be reapproximated to the orbital wall and the depth of the naso-orbital valley regained. Traction is exerted to approximate the tissues to the bone, and the tip of the curved hemostat placed into the conjunctival sac in the medial canthal area assists in this approximation. Difficulty may be experienced in mobilizing the canthus toward

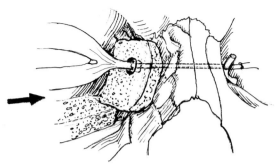

FIGURE 28–155. Schematic representation of the use of a bone graft to reconstruct the medial wall of the orbit, thus furnishing an area of purchase for the medial canthal tendon. The bone graft and the medial canthal tendon are maintained in fixation by transosseous wiring. A batten of stout wire provides fixation on the contralateral side. The wire can be inset into the bone to avoid excessive protrusion under the skin.

the medial orbital wall. The scar tissue is the result of fractures of the orbital rim, penetrating lacerations, or previous unsuccessful attempts at surgical correction and must be resected.

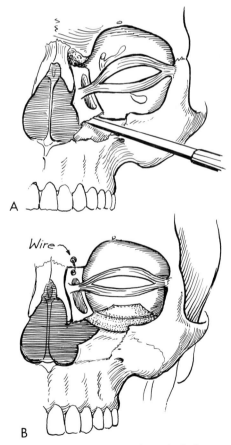

FIGURE 28–156. Osteotomy for malunited naso-orbital fracture. *A,* An osteotome frees the malunited fragment. *B,* Wire fixation maintains the fragment. A bone graft is placed to reconstruct the floor of the orbit following a concomitant malunited orbital fracture.

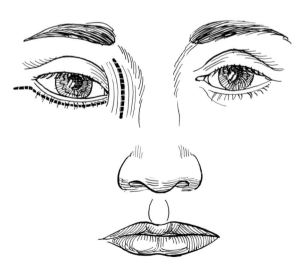

FIGURE 28–154. Outline of incision over the frontal process of the maxilla for the approach to the medial canthal area and the medial wall of the orbit. The subciliary incision for the approach to the orbital floor is also indicated.

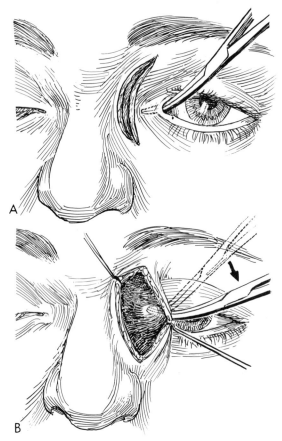

FIGURE 28–157. A curved hemostat is placed in the conjunctival sac at the medial canthus to assist in locating the medial canthal tendon.

If difficulty is experienced in moving the canthus inward, the septum orbitale should be detached as widely as possible. In severe deformities the periorbita should be raised from the periphery of the orbital cavity, with the exception of the apex, as described earlier in the text under treatment of enophthalmos. This procedure is effective in releasing the canthus, thus permitting its replacement into the corrected position.

Before reattaching the medial canthal tendon to the medial orbital wall, a dacryocystorhinostomy, if required, should be performed (see Fig. 28–160). Dacryocystorhinostomy (see p. 985) restores the continuity of the lacrimal system by short-circuiting the tears into the nasal cavity. This operation, as well as other operations on the lacrimal system, is best done concomitantly with procedures to restore the medial canthal region; the dacryocystorhinostomy is not done until the wires for the canthopexy are in position (see Fig. 28–158).

When the lacrimal sac is destroyed, badly damaged, or grossly displaced, the sac should be resected. The common canaliculus, point of juncture of the superior and inferior canaliculi, may be introduced into the nasal cavity through an opening made in the lateral wall of the nose in an attempt to reestablish lacrimal continuity. Techniques for the restoration of the continuity of the lacrimal system were discussed earlier in the chapter (see p. 985).

Transosseous Wiring for Medial Canthopexy. Contact lenses are placed to protect the cornea during the procedure. If the bony landmarks (anterior and posterior lacrimal crests) have been preserved, which is usually not the case in malunited naso-orbital fractures, a drill hole is made through the anterior lacrimal crest on each side (Fig. 28–158, *A*). The hole must be wide enough to permit the passage of the transosseous wires. The drill point is then placed obliquely backward through the left hole, drilling through the perpendicular plate of the ethmoid at a point posterior to the lacrimal crests. This procedure is often necessary because the perpendicular plate may be thickened by overlapping malunited fragments in severe naso-orbital fractures. The more posterior position of the opening through the perpendicular plate will assist in maintaining the position of the medial canthi. Having thus established a passageway through the interorbital space, two doubled wires folded upon themselves are passed through with a large 3/8 curved needle or an instrument, such as Mustardé's awl. The needle should be passed in such a way that it curves backward to penetrate through the hole in the perpendicular plate. The two doubled wires are cut; thus four separate wires are available (Fig. 28–158, *A*). Two of the wires will be twisted around each other after one of them has been threaded through the stump of the medial canthal tendon by means of a curved cutting needle (Fig. 28–158, *B, C*); the cut ends of the wires are bent flat against the bone. On the contralateral side, a similar procedure is executed, tightening the wires and snugging the medial canthal tendon into the bony openings. The other two wires are threaded into the eye of a curved needle and brought out through the skin immediately above and below the medial canthus on each side; they serve to anchor an acrylic button which maintains the skin of the area against the bone and prevents hematoma formation (Fig. 28–158, *D, E*).

An additional wire may be passed through the transosseous passage between the holes in the medial orbital walls to aid in the fixation of

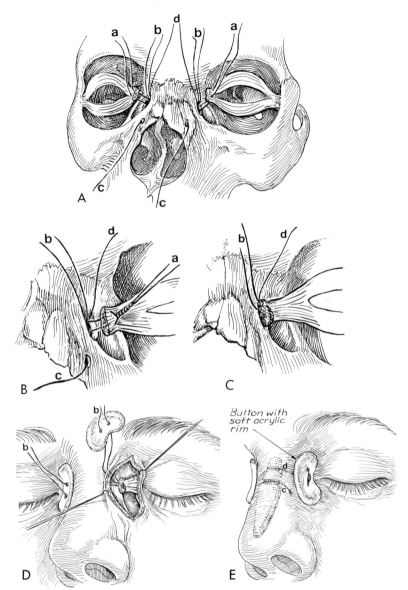

FIGURE 28–158. Respective positions of the transosseous wires. The four wires placed high on the anterior lacrimal crest are used as follows: two wires (*a*) for fixation of the medial canthal tendons (high to correct the canthus inversus deformity), and two others (*b*) for the canthal buttons. The other wires (*c* and *d*) will be looped around an iliac bone graft. The drawing represents a medial orbital wall with well-preserved anatomical landmarks. In malunited naso-orbital fractures, the landmarks are not present, as the bones are telescoped and overlapped. Even the lamina papyracea is thickened. The point of reattachment in these cases should be high and posterior in order to reestablish the naso-orbital valley.

a bone graft; a second transosseous wire is placed through the nasal bones (Fig. 28–158, *A, E*). Thus two additional wires, one above the other, ensure firm fixation of a bone graft and prevent its lateral tilt or displacement. The bone graft serves to reestablish the projection of the dorsum and to assist in improving the patient's appearance.

In severely comminuted naso-orbital fractures, anatomical landmarks, such as the anterior and posterior lacrimal crests and lacrimal groove, have been effaced. The overlapping bone fragments have thickened the orbital wall, including the thin lamina papyracea. In such cases the point of reinsertion of the medial canthus should be more posterior to produce upward, inward, and posterior traction

in order to restore the naso-orbital valley and attempt to reproduce the traction exerted by the head of the pretarsal muscle (Horner's tensor tarsi muscle).

When the reattachment of the medial canthal tendon to the anterior lacrimal crest is possible, the function of the orbicularis muscle as the lacrimal pump is preserved; the anterior lacrimal crest provides a solid point of attachment.

In the first canthoplasties (Converse, 1944; Converse and Smith, 1952), prior to using through-and-through transosseous wiring, stainless steel wire looped through two holes drilled through the medial orbital wall was employed (see Fig. 28–82, *C*). A small, curved needle was used to loop the wire through the

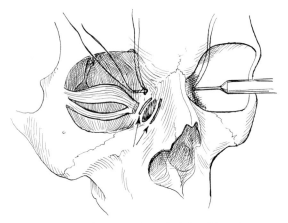

FIGURE 28-159. In unilateral deformities the reattachment of the medial canthal tendon should be placed upwards and backwards if the medial orbital wall is comminuted, thickened and has lost the anatomical landmarks shown in the drawing.

upper hole and out through the lower hole. The technique of through-and-through wiring has become a routine technique in both unilateral and bilateral deformities (Converse and Smith, 1962, 1963, 1964; Converse, 1974).

The operation is completed by the approximation of the skin incision. The canthus is maintained snugly approximated to the bone by means of specially fabricated, perforated, transparent acrylic buttons (see Fig. 28-158, *E*). The acrylic buttons are now made with a rim of soft acrylic a few millimeters wide, to prevent the edges of the buttons from cutting into the adjacent skin (see Fig. 28-166). After the ends of the wires are placed, the twisting of the wires on each side controls the amount of pressure exerted by the plates. The pull-out wires are usually left in position for a period of approximately 14 days before being cut and removed.

In unilateral deformities, the reattachment of the medial canthal tendon should be placed upward and backward (Fig. 28-159) if the medial orbital wall is comminuted and thickened and has lost the anatomical landmarks shown in the drawing.

Dacryocystorhinostomy Combined with Medial Canthoplasty and Canthopexy. All of the procedures described earlier in the text are completed with the exception of the final tightening of the wires for the canthopexy. After the subperiosteal exposure of the medial orbital wall (Fig. 28-160, *A*), a circular section of bone about 10 mm in diameter is removed from an area slightly below and anterior to the

lacrimal groove by an osteotome or, preferably, by means of a motor- or turbine-driven trephine (Fig. 28-160, *B*); the opening is made without cutting through the nasal mucous membrane. The trephine opening is enlarged to a diameter of 15 to 20 mm (Fig. 28-160, *C*), and a dacryocystorhinostomy procedure is then done. A vertical I-shaped incision is made through the wall of the lacrimal sac (Fig. 28-160, *C*), and a similar incision is made through the nasal mucous membrane. The posterior flaps of nasal mucous membrane and lacrimal sac wall are sutured first with fine caliber chromic catgut (Fig. 28-160, *D*). In malunited naso-orbital fractures, completion of the suturing of the anterior flaps of nasal mucous membrane and lacrimal sac is postponed until the transnasal wires are twisted and the medial canthal tendon is reattached to the orbital wall (Fig. 28-160, *E, F*).

Conjunctivodacryorhinostomy and Conjunctivorhinostomy: the Jones Tube. If sufficient lacrimal sac tissue is preserved, a conjunctivo-dacryorhinostomy may be performed (see p. 987). When the lacrimal sac is destroyed or must be resected, canaliculorhinostomy is feasible if the common canaliculus is intact, as described earlier in the text. Often, however, in malunited naso-orbital fractures, the lacrimal structures cannot be utilized. In such cases, conjunctivorhinostomy as described earlier in the chapter is indicated.

Contour Restoration of the Nasal Dorsum. In malunited naso-orbital fractures, it is usually necessary to increase the projection of the nasal dorsum of the nose by an iliac bone graft in the same stage, because the scars resulting from the canthoplasties will render a subsequent bone grafting procedure more difficult. The fixation of the graft is maintained by a transosseous and circumferential wire (see Fig. 28-158, *E*). As stated previously, the wire is passed through a tunnel drilled through the nasal bones, looped over the bone graft, and twisted into one of the perforations. The periosteum over the bony bridge is raised, and all deep scar tissue should be resected until bare bone is exposed before placing the bone graft (Fig. 28-161).

In instances when scars overlying the bony bridge of the nose require resection and repair, it is relatively easy to restore the contour of the depressed bony dorsum by a bone graft under direct vision. Should the soft tissue be inadequate, a forehead flap can provide extra tissue.

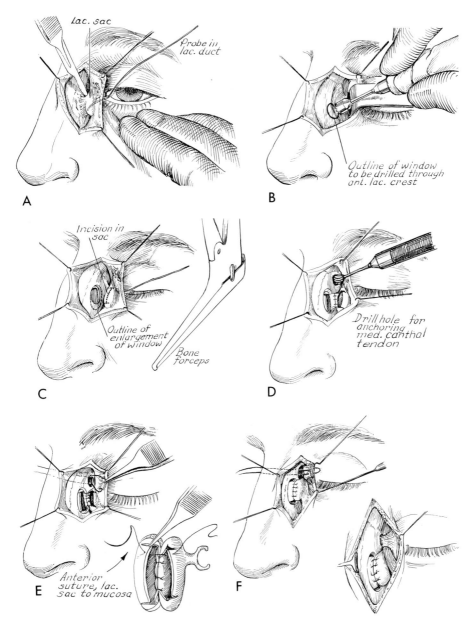

FIGURE 28–160.   A technique of dacryocystorhinostomy combined with medial canthoplasty and canthopexy. *A*, Exposure of the medial orbital wall. The lacrimal probe placed into the lower lacrimal punctum (or an injection of methylene blue into the sac) helps to identify the lacrimal sac. The sac is dissected from the scar tissue resulting from the fracture. The sac is being raised from the lacrimal groove. *B*, A circular section of bone approximately 10 mm in diameter is removed from an area situated slightly below and anterior to the lacrimal groove without perforating the nasal mucoperiosteum. *C*, The bony opening is enlarged to a diameter of 15 to 20 mm, the diameter of the sac which is usually dilated by the accumulation of secretion as a result of the obstruction of the nasolacrimal duct (mucocele). A vertical I-shaped incision is made through the sac and through the nasal mucoperiosteum. *D*, The posterior nasal flap is sutured to the posterior flap of the lacrimal sac. A drill hole is prepared for the attachment of the medial canthal tendon. *E*, The suture of the anterior flaps is begun. The transosseous wires have been passed through the medial canthal tendon. *F*, Suture is completed. The wires are twisted, and traction is exerted from the contralateral medial wall to maintain the fixation of the medial canthal tendon and canthus.

Medial Canthoplasty for Canthus Inversus after Naso-orbital Fracture. The lacrimal sac has not been damaged in the patient shown in Figure 28–161, but the medial canthal tendon has been displaced downward as a result of malunited fracture; a canthus inversus, the downward tilt of the medial canthus, has resulted. When the displaced bone can be replaced by osteotomy, as shown in Figure 28–156, the canthus may return to its anatomical

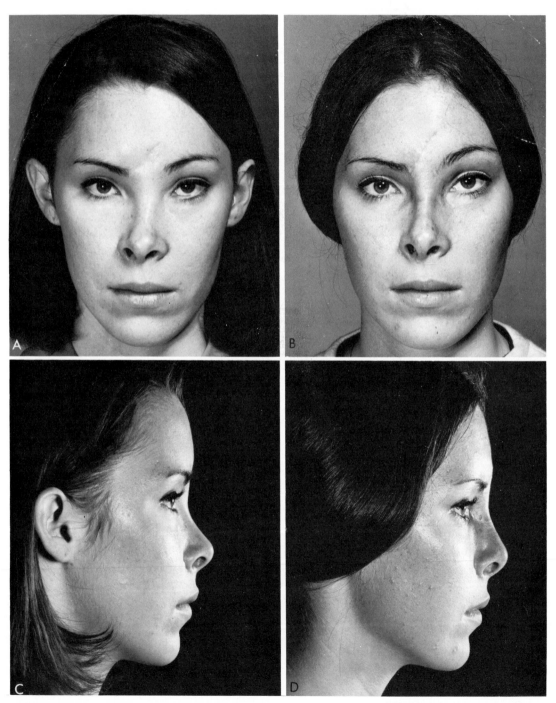

FIGURE 28–161. Contour restoration of the nose by bone grafting in conjunction with medial canthoplasties. *A,* Naso-orbital fracture, associated with a depressed fracture of the glabellar portion of the frontal bone, incurred in an automobile accident. *B,* A dacryocystorhinostomy was required on the left side, and bone grafting to the glabellar and nasal areas was done in the same operative procedure. *C,* Preoperative. *D,* Postoperative.

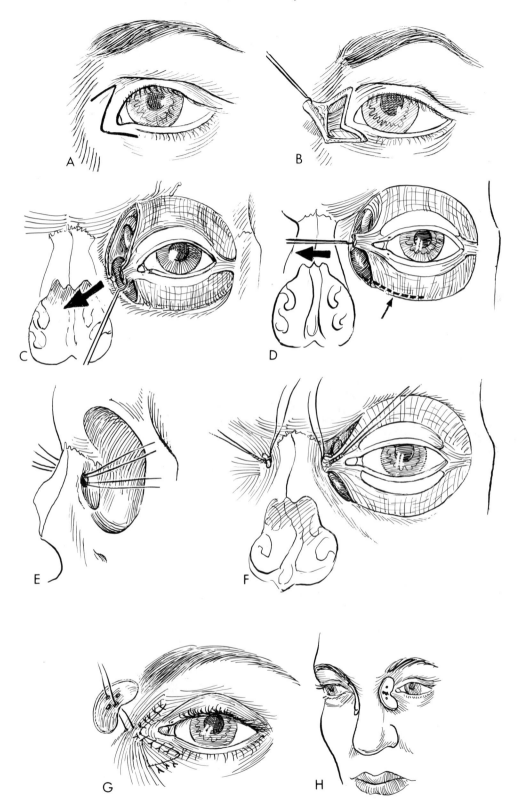

FIGURE 28–162. Correction of canthus inversus. *A*, Z-plasty incision. *B*, Elevation of flaps. *C*, Note the inferiorly displaced insertion of the medial canthal tendon. *D*, Repositioning of the medial canthal tendon. Dotted line indicates release of the septum orbitale. *E, F*, Transnasal wiring to secure the tendon in the new position. *G*, Approximation of wound edges. *H*, Appearance with canthal buttons in position.

position. The depression of the bony dorsum of the nose gives the appearance of a minor degree of telecanthus. There is also a slight deviation of the nose and depressed fracture in the glabellar region. A corrective rhinoplasty and lateral osteotomies, straightening the septum, a cantilever iliac bone graft over the dorsum of the nose, an onlay bone graft over the depressed glabella, and medial canthoplasties (Fig. 28–162) were performed in a single operative stage.

The Coronal Flap for Exposure in Malunited Naso-orbital Fractures. Use of the coronal scalp flap (see Chapter 56), although it is a somewhat indirect approach, gives adequate exposure of the naso-orbital area, the roof of the orbit, and the medial and lateral walls. This approach facilitates the peripheral raising of the periorbita, an important precaution in order to achieve successful canthopexy and approximate each canthus to the medial orbital walls. The lateral nasal incision is required if a dacryocystorhinostomy is indicated.

COMPLICATED CASES OF MALUNITED ORBITAL AND NASO-ORBITAL FRACTURES

Some cases are complicated not only by the presence of concomitant orbital and naso-orbital fractures but also by loss of the ocular globe, loss of soft and hard tissue of the nose, depressed fracture or loss of the frontal bone, fracture-dislocation of the entire orbit, or traumatic orbital hypertelorism.

One of the most complicated cases was that of the patient shown in Figure 28–163. The patient was injured in an automobile accident; after striking the dashboard, she was projected through the windshield, suffering multiple lacerations, loss of the right eye, and a blowout fracture of the right orbital floor. She also sustained a laceration through the levator aponeurosis, with resulting ptosis of the left upper lid, as well as loss of the nasal bones and an appreciable amount of nasal soft tissue, with consequent foreshortening of the nose. The medial orbital walls had been splayed outward

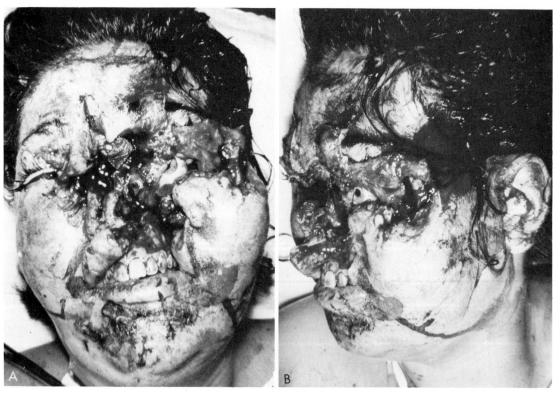

FIGURE 28–163. *A, B,* Severe facial injuries incurred by an 18 year old girl who was projected against the dashboard of the automobile and through the windshield in a head-on crash. The nasal bones were pulverized and projected into the interorbital space; the right eye required enucleation; the levator palpebrae superioris aponeurosis of the left upper eyelid was severed; the maxilla suffered multiple fractures; and the right lacrimal system was obstructed. (Figs. 28–163, *A,* 28–164, 28–167, and 28–168 from Converse, J. M.: Surgical elongation of the traumatically foreshortened nose: The perinasal osteotomy. Plast. Reconstr. Surg., *47:*539. Copyright 1971, The Williams & Wilkins Company, Baltimore.)

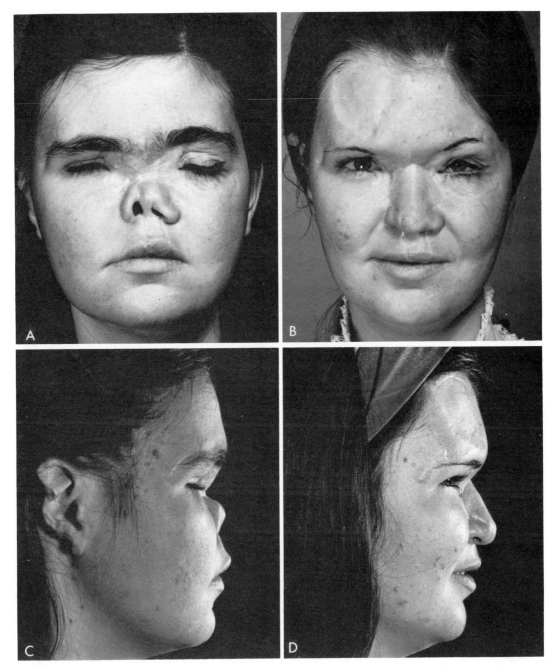

FIGURE 28–164. *A,* After primary surgery done in the local hospital. Note the severe foreshortening of the nose, the traumatic telecanthus, the loss of the right eye, and the ptosis of the left upper eyelid. *B,* Early result following the procedures shown in Figures 28–165, 28–167, and 28–168. A dacryocystorhinostomy was done on the right side, and a shortening of the levator aponeurosis remedied the ptosis of the left upper eyelid. *C,* Preoperative profile view. *D,* Postoperative profile appearance.

as a result of the severe trauma, causing traumatic telecanthus.

After treatment in the local hospital, the patient was referred to us with the residual deformity shown in Figure 28–164, *A, C*. The traumatic telecanthus was severe; the right oc-

ular globe had been enucleated; the left upper lid was ptotic; and the nose was grossly foreshortened.

In a first stage, a skin flap was raised through a trapdoor flap, exposing the interorbital space over the depressed nasal dorsum

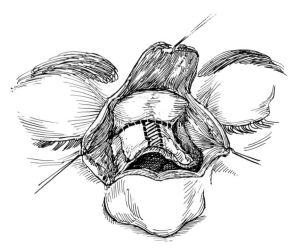

FIGURE 28–165. Stage 1. In a first procedure, the traumatic telecanthus was corrected by raising a skin flap to expose the interorbital area. Both medial orbital walls were exposed. A transverse osteotomy, the resection of bone from the midline, and the medial mobilization of the medial orbital walls reduced the traumatic telecanthus. A dacryocystorhinostomy was performed on the right side, and the medial canthal tendons were reattached after freeing the periorbita. The nose was then divided by a transverse incision, and the tip of the nose was swung down into its anatomical position.

(Fig. 28–165). The medial orbital walls were exposed. After a transverse osteotomy at the naso-frontal junction and resection of a central segment of bone, an osteotomy of the medial orbital walls was done, and they were moved medially. The floor of the right orbit was repaired by an iliac bone graft.

The telecanthus and increased distance between the medial orbital walls were manifest. Subperiosteal elevation along the medial orbital walls showed multiple fractures and loss of the anatomical landmarks (anterior lacrimal crest, lacrimal groove, posterior lacrimal crest).

Projecting fragments of bone along the medial orbital walls were removed; a section of bone was removed from the small amount of bone remaining between the medial orbital walls (Fig. 28–165), and a submucous resection of what remained of the greatly thickened septum was done. An osteotomy of the medial walls was performed, freeing them so that they could be moved medially to correct the telecanthus. Drill holes were made through each medial wall, and four transosseous wires were passed from side to side for the triple purpose of (1) maintaining the medial displacement of the medial orbital walls, (2) reattaching the medial canthal tendons, and (3) placing the canthal buttons. A dacryocystorhinostomy was performed on the right side.

The first stage in the reconstruction was completed by the passage of the wires through the skin of the medial canthus on each side, the suture of the skin incision, and the tightening of the transosseous wires over the acrylic canthal buttons (Fig. 28–166).

The lower portion of the nose was swung downward, drawbridge fashion, so that the tip of the nose assumed a position slightly overcorrecting the above foreshortening (Fig. 28–167). Mucous membrane was sutured to the skin along the edges of the defect. The downward position of the lower portion of the nose was maintained by dental compound softened in warm water, molded into the defect, and hardened with cold saline solution. A second mold was made and was sent to the laboratory to be duplicated in acrylic and serve as the definitive mold, which was worn by the patient for a period of three months (Fig. 28–167, *C*).

The principle of dividing the nose and tilting the tip downward to lengthen a nose shortened by the loss of tissue was employed by Szymanowski (1870), Nélaton and Ombrédanne (1904), and Gillies (1920).

During the next three months, an artificial eye was fitted on the right side, and a levator shortening operation corrected the ptosis of the upper lid on the left side.

The telecanthus correction having brought

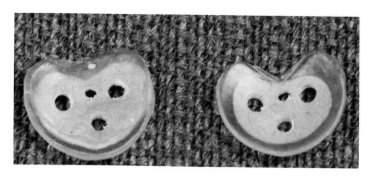

FIGURE 28–166. New type of canthal buttons. The rim of the button is made of soft acrylic, which lessens the risk of excessive pressure of the rim against the soft tissues. (Fabricated by Augustus J. Valauri, D.D.S.)

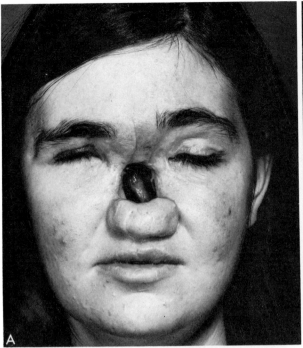

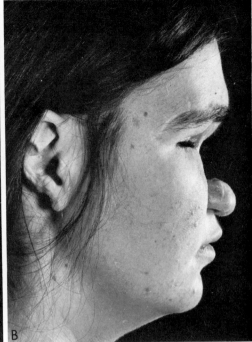

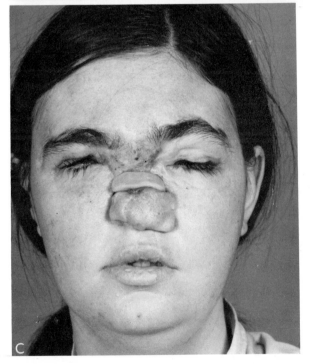

FIGURE 28–167. *A, B,* The patient shown in Figures 28–163 and 28–164 following the procedures illustrated in Figure 28–165. An acrylic mold was placed in the nasal opening to prevent the upward retraction of the tip and was maintained for a period of three months prior to further reconstructive surgery. *C,* Note the acrylic mold placed in the defect to prevent the recurrence of the nasal foreshortening.

about an improvement, the second stage of the nasal reconstruction was started by raising a trapdoor flap from the tip of the nose, hinged on the edge of the defect (Fig. 28–168). The tip cartilages being thus exposed, the nasal tip was remodeled under direct vision; cartilage was excised and sutured with plain catgut sutures. The trapdoor flap was then reflected to serve as lining for the defect, and was sutured to a similar trapdoor flap from the upper portion of the nose and to smaller flaps on each side of the defect. A scalping forehead flap (see Chapter 29, p. 1234) furnished the covering flap.

In a third stage of the reconstruction, a costal cartilage graft was removed, shaped, and introduced between the flaps to provide shape

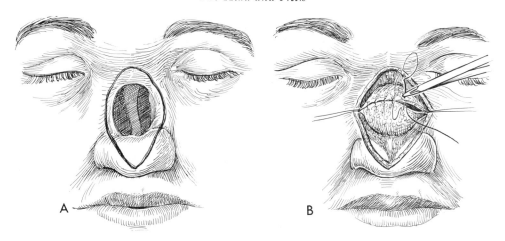

FIGURE 28–168. *A,* An ellipse of skin was outlined and used to provide an adequate lining four months after the procedure shown in Figure 28–165. *B,* The flaps are hinged on the edge of the defect and sutured. The nasal tip was remodeled under direct vision, and a scalping forehead flap provided the cutaneous cover.

and support for the nasal dorsum. The patient's final appearance one year later is shown in Figure 28–169, *B.*

In the patient shown in Figure 28–170, *A,*

the reconstruction of the frontal bone was achieved by means of a contoured and shaped iliac bone graft which restored the glabellar-frontal area and also the supraorbital arches

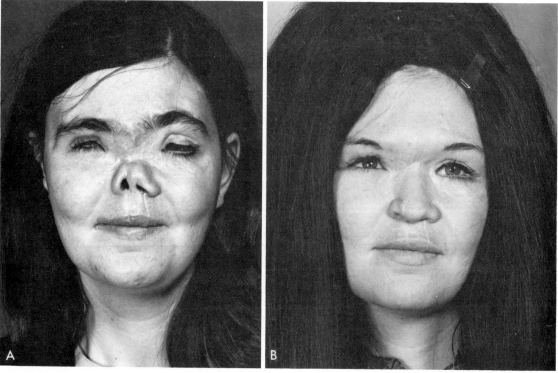

FIGURE 28–169. Comparative views of the patient before (*A*) and after (*B*) the reconstructive procedures. A costal cartilage graft furnished the skeletal framework of the nose.

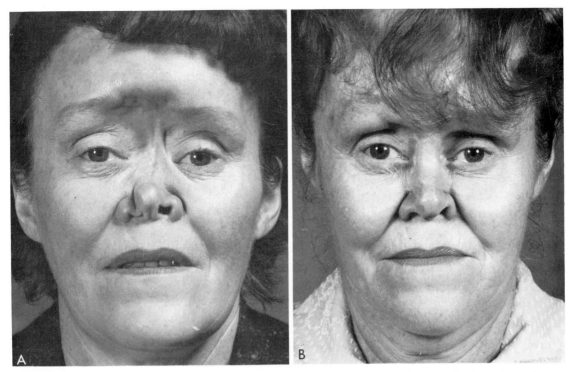

FIGURE 28–170. *A*, Extensive naso-orbital and frontal bone fractures resulted in the deformity shown in this 35 year old patient. *B*, After reconstruction of the defect of the frontal bone and the supraorbital arches by means of an iliac bone graft and restoration of the contour of the nose by two consecutive, superimposed scalping flaps completed by a small Silastic implant.

(Fig. 28–170, *B*). (For the technique of frontal bone reconstruction by means of iliac bone grafts, see Chapter 27.)

The most difficult problem was the naso-orbital deformity. The medial orbital walls were intact and the lacrimal system patent on both sides; the medial orbital walls, however, had been badly comminuted and splayed apart. An osteotomy of each medial wall was performed. After resection of the obstructing remnants of nasal septum, the medial walls were displaced medially and maintained by means of transos-

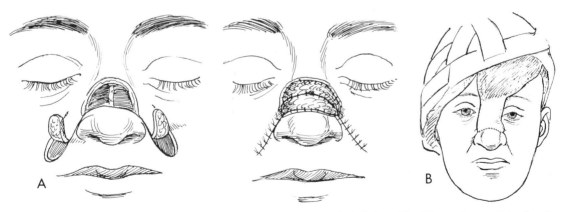

FIGURE 28–171. *A*, In an older patient, nasolabial flaps which can be imbricated furnish an adequate lining for elongation purposes. This technique was employed in the patient shown in Figure 28–170. *B*, The scalping flap in position, providing the cutaneous covering. Because of extensive soft tissue loss, two successive scalping flaps were superimposed; a second scalping flap was placed over the tissue provided by the first scalping flap after dermabrasion.

seous wiring, which also reattached the medial canthal tendons. The telecanthus was thus corrected.

The nose was scarred extra- and intranasally, and tissue loss was responsible for the foreshortening of the nose.

In the older patient, nasolabial flaps may be utilized for the restoration of the defective nasal lining (Fig. 28–171, *A*). The nose was divided, and the nasolabial flaps provided adequate lining (Fig. 28–171, *A*). In the same stage, a scalping forehead flap furnished the surface skin (Fig. 28–171, *B*). A first flap did not provide sufficient tissue bulk; after it has been in place for a period of three months, it was dermabraded, and a second scalping flap taken from the contralateral side of the forehead was placed over the abraded initial flap. A small Silastic implant was placed for final contour restoration.

MALUNITED FRACTURES OF THE ZYGOMA AND THE LATERAL WALL OF THE ORBIT

The zygomatic or zygomaticomaxillary area, located in the lateral portion of the midface skeleton, is formed by a skeletal framework consisting of the zygoma (malar bone) and the zygomatic process of the maxilla; these bones are covered by the origins of the masseter, the zygomatic head of the quadratus labii superioris and zygomaticus muscles, the lateral portion of the orbicularis oculi muscle, the subcutaneous tissues, and skin.

The prominence of the upper part of the cheek is formed by the zygoma (the cheek bone or malar bone); the most prominent point of the zygoma is sometimes referred to as the "tubercle" of the zygoma. Loss of the prominence due to malunited fracture of the zygoma results in a noticeable deformity.

Deformity and functional disturbances resulting from malunited fracture vary according to the type of fracture, whether a fracture-dislocation or a comminuted fracture and, in particular, whether there is a downward displacement with loss of continuity of the lateral orbital wall and lateral portion of the orbital floor.

Other functional disturbances also occur in fractures of the body of the zygoma and of the zygomatic arch, for the displaced bone may press against the coronoid process of the mandible, thus interfering with mandibular function. This complication is particularly frequent following depressed fractures of the zygomatic arch.

Depressed Malunited Fractures of the Zygoma with Loss of Continuity of the Lateral Orbital Wall. In malunited fractures of the zygomatic bone with downward displacement, the zygoma is detached from the frontal bone, and there is a gap in the continuity of the lateral wall of the orbit. The lateral canthus and the attachment of the lateral canthal tendon and raphé are displaced downward (Fig. 28–172). Inasmuch as the lateral position of the floor of the orbit is formed by the zygoma, in fractures of considerable severity the comminution may extend to the entire orbital floor with prolapse into the maxillary sinus and enlargement of the size of the orbital cavity. The insertion of Lockwood's suspensory ligament of the globe on the lateral wall of the orbit is also displaced downward with the bone, thus accentuating the prolapse of the orbital contents. An antimongoloid slant of the palpebral fissure and lateral canthus and vertical shortening of the lower lid and ectropion are charac-

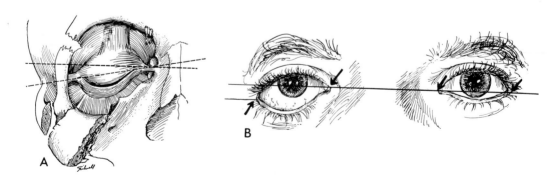

FIGURE 28–172. Deformity resulting from malunited fracture of the zygoma with frontozygomatic separation. *A*, Malunited compound fracture of the zygoma, frontozygomatic separation, and downward displacement of the lateral canthus. *B*, The downward displacement of the lateral canthus and vertical shortening of the lower lid.

teristic deformities (Fig. 28–173), in addition to the flatness of the zygomatic prominence resulting from the malunited fractured zygoma. In malunited downward fracture-dislocation of the zygoma and separation of the frontozygomatic junction, the orbital cavity is enlarged, and enophthalmos may result.

TREATMENT

Osteotomy and reduction. This method of treatment is indicated when the zygoma is depressed and separated from the frontal bone, leaving a gap in the lateral orbital wall.

Blind transcutaneous osteotomy of the malunited zygoma is dangerous, because the force required to sever the bony connections of the zygoma to the surrounding bones may cause radiating fractures and hemorrhage in the vicinity of the optic nerve. Blindness is an occasional complication of the fractured zygoma.

The safe technique is by direct exposure of the area through selective incisions (Fig. 28–174). The osteotomy can then be done under direct vision (see also Chapter 24, Figs. 24–155 and 24–156).

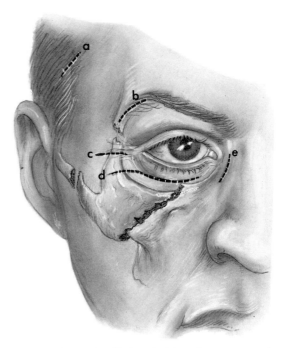

FIGURE 28–174. Various incisions for exposure of a malunited zygomatic fracture. A coronal scalp flap may also be indicated in extensive defects.

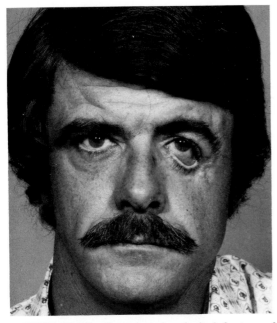

FIGURE 28–173. Comminuted malunited fracture of the left zygoma. Typical deformity: antimongoloid slant, vertical shortening, and ectropion of the lower lid. The ocular globe is supported by a large silicone implant. There was a wide gap in the lateral wall (15 mm). The patient had been operated upon when this text was being sent for publication. The silicone implant had begun to collapse into the maxillary sinus and was removed; an osteotomy was done, and the infraorbital rim was raised. A large iliac bone graft restored the floor, and another restored the lateral wall which had been partially destroyed. Because of exposure of bone after correction of the ectropion (some eyelid tissue had been destroyed), a temporal flap was employed (see Fig. 28–54).

Through a lower eyelid incision, subperiosteal exposure of the rim and floor of the orbit is obtained (Fig. 28–174). An incision in the lateral portion of the eyebrow gives subperiosteal exposure of the frontozygomatic junction. A transverse osteotomy of the floor of the orbit, extending across the floor and upward through the lateral wall, is complemented by an anteroposterior osteotomy of the orbital rim through a short skin incision, exposing the zygomaticomaxillary junction. The zygoma can then be replaced through the temporal approach, if necessary (Fig. 28–175, *A*). Fixation is established by interosseous wiring at the frontozygomatic and the maxillozygomatic junction (Fig. 28–175, *B*). Bone grafts supplement the missing bone, if necessary, and fill any bony gaps.

If the zygoma and lateral orbital wall have been comminuted, considerable bone loss and/or malposition of bone will require osteotomies and bone grafts. In such cases additional exposure is required. A scalp flap is raised through a coronal incision, and the frontalis and temporalis muscles are raised subperiosteally in order to obtain exposure of the lateral orbital wall. Wire fixation of the sectioned fragments and bone grafts will ensure the stability of the reconstruction, which may, in certain cases, involve a major portion of the lateral orbital wall. Usually in these cases, the floor of the orbit is also comminuted and requires bone graft reconstruction.

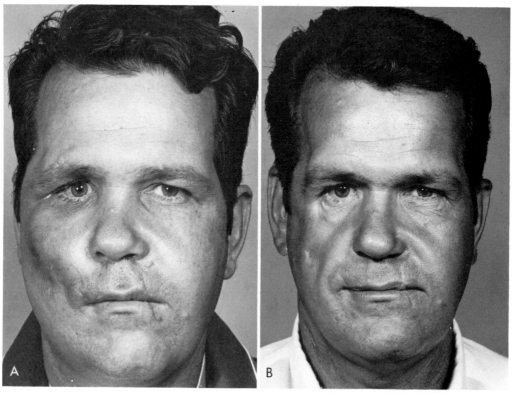

FIGURE 28–175.   *A*, Comminuted malunited fracture of the zygoma with frontozygomatic separation. Note the lateral canthal deformity on the right side. *B*, After osteotomy and wire fixation of the fragments. Patient also had a blowout fracture through the lateral orbital wall. The area of the blowout was bone-grafted. A coronal scalp flap provided adequate exposure.

Although the coronal incision through the scalp is more anterior than the coronal suture, the name persists. It is preferable to the bifrontal flap, in which the incision is made close to the hairline; a receding hairline will eventually uncover the residual scar. The scalp flap raised subperiosteally exposes the frontal bone, the nasal bones, the walls of the orbit (with the exception of the floor), and the zygoma.

Malunited Blowout Fracture of the Lateral Orbital Wall.   Mention must be made of a rare type of fracture, the blowout fracture of the lateral wall of the orbit. Tomographic investigations of patients with enophthalmos and malunited fractures of the zygoma and lateral orbital rim have suggested that a blowout may have taken place through the thin portion of the lateral wall, posterior to the thick orbital rim formed by the orbital process of the zygoma. The lateral wall becomes thin more posteriorly, and this is the site of such a fracture (see Chapter 25, Fig. 25–6). Usually, the lateral wall is fractured into multiple small pieces, and an "impure" type of blowout fracture occurs.

Clinical findings during craniofacial operations performed for severe midfacial fractures also include an extrusion of orbital contents through this area. The findings suggest that the orbital process of the zygoma, when fractured, causes comminution of the thinner sphenoid bone, thus facilitating the extrusion of orbital fat into the temporal fossa when the periorbita has been torn. Intraocular injuries or loss of the ocular globe are frequent in such severe injuries.

The approach to the lateral orbital wall through a coronal scalp incision, by raising the periosteum and temporalis muscle, is the preferable technique of exposure. This approach, combined with the lower eyelid incision approach, provides excellent exposure for reduction osteotomy and bone grafting. Fixation of the sectioned bone fragments and bone grafts is provided by interosseous stainless steel wire.

In the patient shown in Figure 28–175, open reduction and wire fixation were required to reposition the malunited zygoma. The tomogram having shown a blowout fracture of the lateral wall and extruded orbital contents, exposure of the area of fracture was followed by repair by means of an iliac bone graft.

Depressed Malunited Fractures of the Zygoma without loss of Continuity of the Lateral Orbital Wall. There are two types of depression deformities of the zygoma. In type I, the maxillary process of the zygoma and the zygomatic process of the maxilla are depressed into the maxillary sinus, and the fractured bone is dislocated laterally; the resulting deformity is seen as a depression in the infraorbital region of the cheek (Fig. 28–176). In type 2, the zygoma is depressed, causing loss of the cheek bone prominence and a generalized appearance of flatness (Fig. 28–177). Because of the relaxation of the musculature caused by the downward displacement of the bony origins of these structures, additional effects, such as accentuation of the nasolabial fold, drooping of the upper lip, and deviation of the lip to the unaffected side, also occur.

TREATMENT

Contour restoration. In malunited fracture with no loss of continuity in the lateral orbital wall (in some cases the separation between the frontal bone and zygoma has been corrected in a prior operation), the patient shows recession of the infraorbital margin, slight ectropion, and flatness of the malar prominence.

When little or no functional disturbance has occurred, loss of the cheek prominence requires correction, and contour restoration is achieved by bone grafting over the malunited zygoma. Bone grafts were employed for the restoration of zygomatic contour by Murphy as early as 1915. Often a bone graft is required to restore the level of the depressed orbital floor. A thin bone graft from the medial aspect of the iliac bone is placed over the orbital floor after the periorbita has been raised and is shaped so that it will protrude anteriorly to the depressed orbital rim and thus correct this deformity, as well as improve the ectropion caused by backward traction on the septum orbitale.

Iliac bone grafts are preferred to other transplants or implants for contour restoration after fracture in the treatment of traumatic depression of the zygoma. Bone grafts are placed subperiosteally over the depressed zygoma by an extraoral or an intraoral approach after being suitably shaped and fitted over the host bone. Inorganic implant material (Silastic) has been employed in minor defects but is not favored for major defects.

The extraoral approach. In considering restoration of zygomatic contour by bone grafts, if the depressed area extends laterally to the tuberosity of the zygoma, an external incision is made horizontally in one of the crease lines lateral to the lateral canthus. An excellent external incision for approach is through the

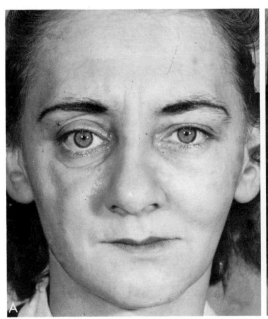 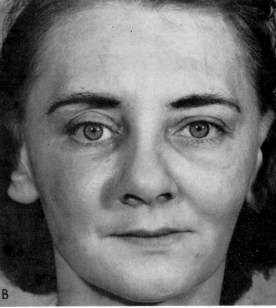

FIGURE 28–176. Malunited fracture of the zygoma: contour restoration by bone grafting through the intraoral approach. *A,* Type of deformity obtained when the fracture results in a rotation of the zygoma with a backward displacement of the maxillary process of the zygoma and a lateral displacement of the frontal process of the zygoma. The displacement produces a depression in the infraorbital region. *B,* Result obtained by contour-restoring bone grafting through the intraoral approach. (From Converse, J. M.: Restoration of facial contour by bone grafts introduced through the oral cavity. Plast. Reconstr. Surg., 6:295, 1950.)

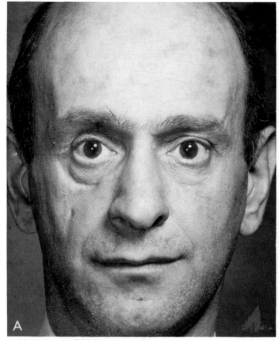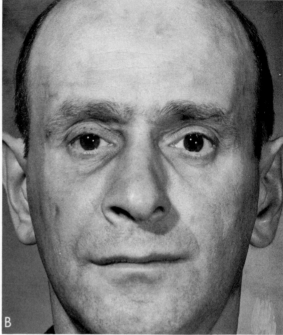

FIGURE 28–177. Malunited fracture of the zygoma: contour restoration by bone grafting through the intraoral approach. *A,* Depression over the right zygomaticomaxillary area resulting from a malunited fracture after fist blows. *B,* Restoration of contour obtained by iliac bone grafts placed over the right maxilla and zygoma after elevation of the periosteum. (From Converse, J. M.: Restoration of facial contour by bone grafts introduced through the oral cavity. Plast. Reconstr. Surg., 6:295, 1950.)

lower eyelid, which provides wide exposure and an inconspicuous postoperative scar (see Fig. 28–174).

The periosteum over the depressed zygoma is incised and raised, and a suitably shaped iliac graft of cortical and cancellous bone is inserted to restore the cheekbone contour.

When a major defect is present following destructive trauma, a partial coronal scalp flap is raised on the affected side; if sufficient exposure is not obtained, a full coronal flap is raised. The temporal fascia is incised as in the Gillies (temporal) approach for reduction of a fractured zygoma; the periosteal elevator is passed down to the zygomatic arch between the two layers, superficial and deep, of the temporalis fascia. The periosteum over the zygomatic arch and zygoma is incised and elevated, exposing the area. This route provides good exposure for the introduction of contour-restoring bone grafts (split rib or iliac bone). The placement of the grafts may be checked through a lower eyelid incision.

The intraoral approach (Converse, 1950). The intraoral approach is another choice for exposure of the malunited zygoma for osteotomy and replacement and also for the introduction of contour-restoring bone grafts. The approach is particularly indicated in type 2 malunited frac-

tures of the zygoma. The procedure permits a direct view of the maxilla and zygoma from the pyriform aperture medially to the infraorbital margin superiorly. The incision in the oral mucosa of the lip is placed lateral to the frenulum on the affected side above the vestibular cul-de-sac (Fig. 28–178, *A*). The periosteum is incised and elevated after the mucosa is dissected from the orbicularis oris muscle, thus exposing the defect (Fig. 28–178, *B*). Wide exposure of the maxilla is obtained; the zygoma may be approached by extending the periosteal elevation laterally. The infraorbital nerve and vessels are avoided by carefully raising the periosteum around the neurovascular bundle and preserving its attachment to the elevated soft tissues. The bony defect may then be inspected under adequate lighting.

Most defects are repaired by one main bone graft consisting mostly of cancellous bone, which is placed over the defect. Additional fragments of cancellous bone are packed beneath and around this onlay of bone in the intervening crevices to further improve the bony contour. The vestibular incision is sutured with 4–0 plain catgut sutures, and an external pressure dressing is applied to immobilize the grafts and prevent hematoma formation. The eyelids should be sutured to avoid corneal

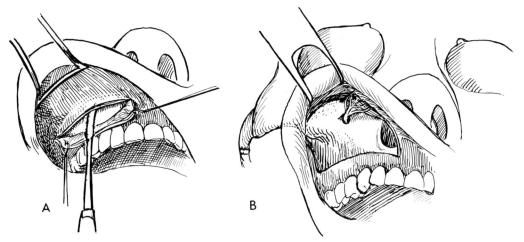

FIGURE 28–178. The intraoral approach to the maxilla and zygoma. *A,* The incision through the mucosa has been made on the labial aspect of the oral vestibule. A flap of mucous membrane has been raised from the orbicularis muscle. *B,* The periosteum has been incised and elevated. The subperiosteal exposure has been extended to the infraorbital nerve which is spared. The subperiosteal exposure is also extended to the edge of the pyriform aperture and laterally over the zygoma.

abrasion under the pressure dressing. Further dressings are unnecessary after fixation of the graft, which usually occurs as early as one week postoperatively.

Smaller defects of the maxilla above the alveolar process, in the region of the anterior wall of the maxillary sinus or the pyriform aperture, can also be readily repaired by this technique. Although the lower rim of the orbit may be approached through the oral route, it is best exposed by an incision in the lower eyelid.

Although the onlay bone autografts will occasionally show some degree of absorption, they are the preferred material for contour restoration. A second onlay bone graft, placed over the first, if necessary, will usually provide definitive contour restoration.

MALUNITED FRACTURE-DISLOCATION OF THE ORBIT

In unusual cases, the entire orbit is displaced by fracture. Such fracture-dislocations are seen following comminuted midfacial fractures combined with fracture of the frontal bone. The orbit is downwardly displaced and occasionally rotated upon itself. The patient shown in Figure 28–179, *A* had been treated for multiple facial fractures resulting from a shot-put injury. The sequela was a downward dislocation of the right orbit. In such cases, a craniofacial approach similar to that employed for the treatment of orbital hypertelorism pro-

vides the only means of obtaining a satisfactory correction (Fig. 28–179, *B*).

The Rectangular Orbital Osteotomy. As illustrated in Figure 28–180, a segment of the frontal bone, large enough to afford exposure of the roof of the orbit by subperiosteal elevation of the frontal lobe, is removed. The frontal lobe is raised and retracted, exposing the roof of the orbit and preserving the cribriform plate. An osteotomy of the roof of the orbit, lateral wall, zygoma, maxilla, and medial orbital wall is performed, sparing the apex of the orbit and the optic nerve. An upward displacement of the functional orbit is then accomplished after the resection of the required segment of frontal bone to permit elevation of the orbit, as outlined in Figure 28–180, *A.* This frontal bone segment is then placed into the secondary defect located inferiorly in the zygoma and maxilla (Fig. 28–180, *B*).

TRAUMATIC ORBITAL HYPERTELORISM

Traumatic orbital hypertelorism is rare. The aftermath of untreated naso-orbital fractures is usually telecanthus, an increased distance between the medial canthi and medial orbital walls.

The patient shown in Figure 28–181 is believed to represent the only case of traumatic orbital hypertelorism described in the medical literature. In this patient, orbital hypertelorism

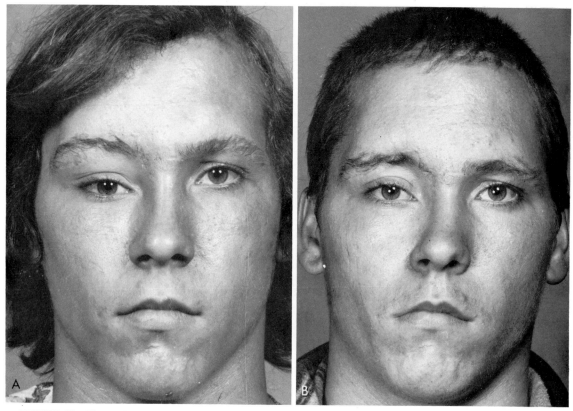

FIGURE 28–179. *A*, Fracture-dislocation of the right orbit with downward displacement. *B*, Result obtained from operation illustrated in Figure 28–180.

occurred as a result of an automobile accident at the age of one year. At this age, the patient's nasofrontal area was splayed apart at the metopic suture of the frontal bone and the orbits were displaced laterally. The patient received neurosurgical care, and a bone graft was placed in the median defect. The patient

was seen at the age of 14 years with orbital hypertelorism.

The technique for the correction of traumatic orbital hypertelorism is similar to that employed in congenital orbital hypertelorism (Tessier and coworkers, 1967, 1973; Converse and coworkers, 1970). The technique em-

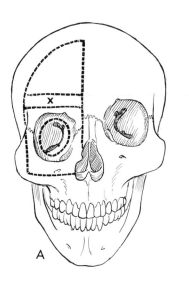

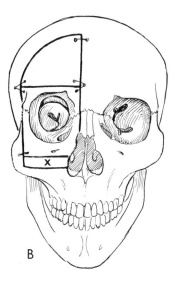

FIGURE 28–180. Rectangular orbital osteotomy to correct downward displacement of the orbit. *A*, Outline of the osteotomy lines and of the area of the frontal bone resected. *B*, The orbit is displaced upward; the resected segment of frontal bone is placed in the resulting maxillozygomatic defect. (Drawing courtesy of Dr. Paul Tessier.)

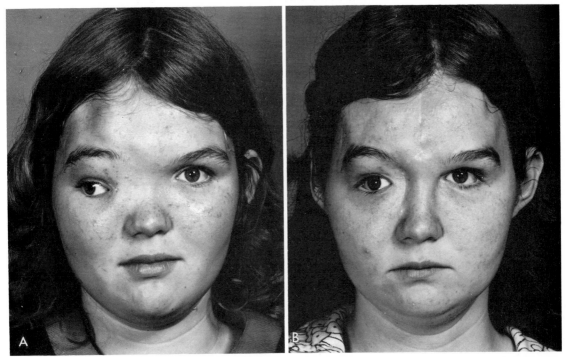

FIGURE 28–181. *A*, Patient with traumatic orbital hypertelorism. In this unusual case, the orbits were splayed apart in an automobile accident at the age of 1 year. Note the wide interorbital space and the exotropia of the right ocular globe. *B*, Postoperative result prior to extraocular surgery to correct the residual exotropia of the right ocular globe and a medial canthoplasty. Future surgery is planned.

ployed is a modification of Tessier's technique with preservation of the cribriform plate and of the continuity of the olfactory nerves (Converse and associates, 1970). The preoperative planning, which includes cephalometric tracings, and the operative technique are described in Chapter 56.

The operation is considerably more laborious than in the congenital type. The scarred tissues, including adherent dura, and, in the case of the patient shown, destruction of a portion of the dura and frontal lobe, demand more caution during the operation than when operating within the virginal tissues of the patient with congenital orbital hypertelorism. When a large dural or frontal lobe defect is found initially, it may be advisable to repair the dura by a dermis or fascia graft and postpone the osteotomy. A two-stage correction may thus be required in traumatic orbital hypertelorism, similar to the two-stage procedure originally described by Tessier and his associates in 1967.

The postoperative care should include antiepileptic therapy, as patients undergoing craniofacial operations for the correction of posttraumatic deformities frequently have epileptic seizures during the postoperative period.

An improvement in the patient's appearance was obtained following this procedure (Fig. 28–181, *B*). The patient was noted to have enophthalmos resulting from the original injury which could not be corrected. At the time the postoperative photograph was taken, further surgery was being planned, including canthoplasties and extraocular muscle surgery. (Additional details concerning the craniofacial approach may be found in Chapter 56.)

REFERENCES

Ackerman, L. V., and de Regato, J. A.: Cancer—Diagnosis, Treatment and Prognosis. St. Louis, Mo., C. V. Mosby Company, 1947, p. 139.

Adams, D. D.: Bioassay of long-acting thyroid stimulator (L.A.T.S.). The dose response relationship. J. Clin. Endocrinol. Metab., *21*:737, 1961.

Adler, F. H.: The role of exophthalmos: The diagnosis and treatment of Graves' disease. West Virginia Med. J., *40*:316, 1944.

Albert, A.: The experimental production of exophthalmos in Fundulus by means of anterior pituitary extracts. Endocrinology, *37*:389, 1945.

Alterman, K.: Exophthalmos: Its reaction to adrenocortical function. I. Experimental exophthalmos. II. Clinical exophthalmos. Acta Endocr. (Suppl), *20*:59, 1954.

Andersson, E.: Ein Fall von schwerem Exophthalmus auf

Grund von Morbus Basedowi bei einem 69 -jährigen Manne operiert nach Dollinger. Acta Ophthalmol., *10*:396, 1932.

Ask, F.: Cited in Andersson (1932).

Bakamjian, V. Y., and Souther, S. G.: Use of temporal muscle flap for reconstruction after orbito-maxillary resection for cancer. Plast. Reconstr. Surg., *56*:171, 1975.

Balacescu, J.: Die totale und bilateral resection des sympathicalis cervicalis beim Morbut Basedowii. Arch. Klin. Chir., *67*:501, 1902.

Bardram, M. T.: Progressive exophthalmos. Acta Ophthalmol., *22*:1, 1944.

Bartisch, G.: Ophthalmodoulia, Das Ist Augendienst. Dresden, 1583, Pf. 11, p. 217.

Basedow, C. von: Exophthalmos durch Hypertrophie des Zellgewebes in der Augenhöhle. Wochenschr. Ges. Heilk., *6*:197, 220, 1840.

Beard, C.: Repair of traumatic defects of the lacrimal system (acute). *In* Proceedings of the Second International Symposium on Plastic and Reconstructive Surgery of the Eye and Adnexa. St. Louis, C. V. Mosby Company, 1967, p. 171.

Beard, C.: Ptosis. St. Louis, Mo., C. V. Mosby Company, 1969.

Beard, C., and Fox, S.: Spontaneous lid repair. Am. J. Ophthalmol., *58*:947, 1964.

Beare, R.: Basal cell carcinoma. Proc. R. Soc. Med., *66*:691, 1973.

Berke, R. N.: An operation for ptosis utilizing the superior rectus muscle. Trans. Am. Acad. Ophthalmol., *53*:499, 1949.

Berke, R. N.: A simplified Blaskovics operation for blepharoptosis. Arch Ophthalmol., *45*:460, 1952.

Berke, R. N.: A modified Krönlein operation. Trans. Am. Acad. Ophthalmol., *51*:193, 1953.

Berke, R. N.: A modified Krönlein operation. Arch. Ophthalmol., *51*:609, 1954.

Berke, R. N.: Complications in ptosis surgery. *In* Fasanella, R. M. (Ed.): Management of Complications in Eye Surgery. Philadelphia, W. B. Saunders Company, 1957, p. 71.

Berke, R. N.: Results of resection of the levator muscle through a skin incision in congenital ptosis. A.M.A. Arch. Ophthalmol., *61*:177, 1959.

Berke, R. N.: Types of operation indicated for congenital and acquired ptosis. *In* Troutman, R. C., Converse, J. M., and Smith, B. (Eds.): Plastic and Reconstructive Surgery of the Eye and Adnexa. Washington, D.C., Butterworth, 1962.

Berke, R. N.: Complications in ptosis surgery. *In* Fasanella, R. M. (Ed.): Complications in Eye Surgery. 2nd Ed. Philadelphia, W. B. Saunders Company, 1965.

Birge, H. L.: Cancer of the eyelids, basal cell and mixed basal squamous cell epithelioma. Arch. Pathol., *19*:700, 1938.

Blair, V. P., Brown, J. B., and Hamm, W. G.: Correction of ptosis and of epicanthus. Arch. Ophthalmol., *7*:831, 1932.

de Blaskovics, L.: Uber totalplastik des untern Lides. Bildung einer hinteren Lidplatte durch. Transplantation eines Tarsus-und. Bindehautstriefeus aus dem Oberlide. Z. Augenheilk., *40*:222, 1918.

de Blaskovics, L.: New operation for ptosis with shortening of the levator and tarsus. Arch. Ophthalmol., *52*:563, 1923.

Bock, E.: Die Propfung von Haut und Schleimhaut auf ocultistischen Gebiete. Vienna, W. Braumuller, 1884.

Böhm, F.: Der Exophthalmus, seine Diagnose und Be-handlung in der Chirurgie. Munch. Med. Wochenschr., *76*:51, 1929.

Boniuk, M., and Zimmerman, L. E.: Eyelid tumors with reference to lesions confused with squamous cell carcinoma. II. Inverted follicular keratoses. Arch. Ophthalmol., *69*:698, 1963.

Boniuk, M., and Zimmerman, L. E.: Eyelid tumors with reference to lesions confused with squamous cell carcinoma. III. Keratoacanthoma. Arch. Ophthalmol., *77*:29, 1967.

Boo-Chai, K.: Plastic construction of the superior palpebral fold. Plast. Reconstr. Surg., *31*:74, 1964.

Bothman, L.: Endocrines in ophthalmology with reports of cases of exophthalmos and cataracts following thyroidectomy. Illinois Med. J., *65*:226, 1934.

Bowman, W.: Cited by Bader: Report of a chief operation performed at the Royal London Ophthalmic Hospital for the quarter ending 25th of September 1857, II Eyelid. 51 Operations. Royal London Ophthal. Hosp. Rep., *1*:34, 1859.

Boyden, G. L.: An otolaryngologic approach to malignant exophthalmos. Trans. Am. Laryngol. Rhinol. Otol. Soc., *66*:227, 1956.

Brent, B.: Personal communication, 1974.

Brent, B.: Reconstruction of ear, eyebrow, and sideburn in the burned patient. Plast. Reconstr. Surg., *55*:312, 1975.

Burian, F.: Operations in blepharoptosis: Fascial and synthetic slings and dermomuscular suspension. *In* Troutman, R. C., Converse, J. M., and Smith, B. (Eds.): Plastic and Reconstructive Surgery of the Eye and Adnexa. Washington, D.C., Butterworth, 1962.

Cairns, H.: *In* Brain, W. R.: Exophthalmic ophthalmoplegia. Quart. J. Med., *7*:293, 1938.

Callahan, A.: Personal communication, 1956.

Callahan, A.: Ptosis associated with congenital defects; blepharophimosis, epicanthus and other syndromes. *In* Symposium on Surgery of the Orbit and Adnexa. Transactions New Orleans Academy of Ophthalmology. St. Louis, Mo., C. V. Mosby Company, 1974.

Campbell, H. H.: Reconstruction of the maxilla. Plast. Reconstr. Surg., *3*:66, 1948.

Campbell, H. H.: Surgery of lesions of the upper face. Am. J. Surg., *87*:676, 1954.

Canadell, J. M.: Exophtalmie et Thyrostimuline. Extrait de la 5ème Réunion des Endocrinologistes de Langue Française, 1959, p. 178.

Castanares, S.: Blepharoplasty in exophthalmos. Plast. Reconstr. Surg., *47*:215, 1971.

Charpy, W.: Elements of Anatomy. 8th Ed. New York, W. Wood and Company, 1878.

Chilaris, G., and Taptas, J.: Surgical treatment of malignant exophthalmos. Arch. Soc. Ophthal. Grèce du Nord., *14*:169, 1965.

Chopra, I. J., and Solomon, D. H.: Graves' disease with delayed hyperthyroidism; onset after several years of euthyroid ophthalmopathy, dermopathy and high serum LATS. Ann. Intern. Med., *73*:985, 1970.

Cirincione, G.: Sulla blefaro plastica. Clin. Ocul., Palermo, *2*:449, 1901.

Cole, J. G.: Lateral Canthoplasty. Manual, Am. Acad. Ophthalmol. Otolaryngol., 1961, p. 104.

Cole, J. G.: Eyelid surgery. *In* Troutman, R. C., Converse, J. M., and Smith, B. (Eds.): Plastic and Reconstructive Surgery of the Eye and Adnexa. Washington, D.C., Butterworth, 1962.

Collins, E. T.: On anophthalmos. Ophthal. Hosp. Rep., *11*:429, 1887.

Collins, E. T.: Microphthalmos with cystic protrusion for the globe. Ophthal. Hosp. Rep., *17*:254, 1897.

Converse, J. M.: Two plastic operations for the repair of orbit following severe trauma and extensive comminuted fracture. Arch. Ophthalmol., *31*:323, 1944.

Converse, J. M.: Restoration of facial contour by bone grafts introduced through the oral cavity. Plast. Reconstr. Surg., *6*:205, 1950.

Converse, J. M.: Introduction to plastic surgery. *In* Converse, J. M. (Ed.): Reconstructive Plastic Surgery. Philadelphia, W. B. Saunders Company, 1964, p. 16, Fig. 1–17.

Converse, J. M.: Surgical elongation of the traumatically foreshortened nose. The perinasal osteotomy. Plast. Reconstr. Surg., *47*:539, 1971.

Converse, J. M.: Deformities of the eyelids and orbital and zygomatic region. *In* Kazanjian, V. H., and Converse, J. M. (Eds.): Surgical Treatment of Facial Injuries. The Williams & Wilkins Company, Baltimore, 1974.

Converse, J. M., and Smith, B.: Canthoplasty and dacryocystorhinostomy in malunited fractures of the medial wall of the orbit. Am. J. Ophthalmol., *35*:1103, 1952.

Converse, J. M., and Smith, B.: An operation for congenital traumatic hypertelorism. *In* Troutman, R. C., Converse, J. M., and Smith, B. (Eds.): Plastic and Reconstructive Surgery of the Eye and Adnexa. Washington, D.C., Butterworth, 1962, p. 104.

Converse, J. M., and Smith, B.: Naso-orbital fractures (symposium: midfacial fractures). Trans. Am. Acad. Ophthalmol. Otolaryngol., *67*:622, 1963.

Converse, J. M., and Smith, B.: Deformities of the eyelids and orbital region. *In* Converse, J. M. (Ed.): Reconstructive Plastic Surgery. Philadelphia, W. B. Saunders Company, 1964, pp. 645–661.

Converse, J. M., and Smith, B.: Naso-orbital fractures and traumatic deformities of the medial canthus. Plast. Reconstr. Surg., *38*:147, 1966.

Converse, J. M., Cole, G., and Smith, B.: Late treatment of blowout fracture of the floor of the orbit. A case report. Plast. Reconstr. Surg., *28*:183, 1961.

Converse, J. M., Smith, B., Obear, M. F., and Wood-Smith, B.: Orbital blowout fracture: A ten-year survey. Plast. Reconstr. Surg., *39*:20, 1967.

Converse, J. M., Ransohoff, J., Mathews, E. S., Smith, B., and Molenaar, A.: Ocular hypertelorism and pseudohypertelorism. Plast. Reconstr. Surg., *45*:1, 1970.

Converse, J. M., Wood-Smith, D., McCarthy, J. G., and Coccaro, P. J.: Craniofacial Surgery. Clinics in Plastic Surgery, *1*:499, 1974.

Converse, J. M., Smith, B., and Wood-Smith, D.: Deformities of the midface resulting from malunited orbital and naso-orbital fractures. Clinics in Plastic Surgery, *2*:107, 1975.

Craig, W. M., and Dodge, H. W., Jr.: Surgical treatment of progressive exophthalmos. Trans. Am. Surg. Assoc., *70*:70, 1952a.

Craig, W., and Dodge, H. W., Jr.: The surgical treatment of malignant exophthalmos. Surg. Clin. North Am., *32*:991, 1952b.

Cutler, W. L., and Beard, C.: A method for partial and total upper lid reconstruction. Am. J. Ophthalmol., *39*:1, 1955.

Daily, R. K., Daily, L., Walker, J. D., and Peterson, H. J.: Exophthalmic ophthalmoplegia. South. Med. J., *35*:344, 1942.

Davis, J. S.: Plastic Surgery: Its Principle and Practice. Philadelphia, P. Blakiston's Son & Company, 1919.

Dayton, G. O., and Hanafee, W. N.: Oribital venogram in surgery of the orbit. Am. J. Ophthalmol., *67*:512, 1969.

Del Regato, J. A.: Roentgen therapy of carcinoma of the skin of the eyelids. Radiology, *52*:564, 1949.

Dimitry, T. J.: Hereditary ptosis. Am. J. Ophthalmol., *45*:4656, 1921.

Dingman, R. O., and Grabb, W. C.: Personal communication, 1974.

Dobyns, B. M., and Steelman, S. L.: The thyroid stimulating hormone of the anterior pituitary as distinct from the exophthalmos producing substance. Endocrinology, *52*:705, 1953.

Dollinger, J.: Die Druckentlastung der Augemhöhl durch Entfernung der äusseren Orbitalwand bei hochgrädigem Exophthalmus (Morbus Basedowii) und konsekutive Hosnhauterkrankung. Dtsch. Med. Wochenschr., *37*:1888, 1911.

Driver, J. R., and Cole, H. N.: Epithelioma of the eyelids and canthus: Report of a series of 324 cases. Am. J. Roentgenol., *41*:616, 1939.

Dupuy-Dutemps, L.: Autoplastie palpébro-palpébrale intégrale. Réflection d'une paupière détruite dans toute son épaisseur par greffe cutanée et tarso-conjonctivale prise à l'autre paupière. Ann. Ocul., *164*:915, 1921.

Dupuy-Dutemps, L., and Bourguet, J.: Plastic operation for chronic dacryocystitis. Bull. Acad. Nat. Med., *86*:293, 1921.

Eagleton: Cited in Tinker (1912).

Elschnig, A.: Ueber Ptosisoperationen (Ptosisoperation mit Freier Fascientransplantation). Med. Klin., Berlin, *9*:1536, 1913.

Esser, J. F. S.: Island flaps. N.Y. Med. J., *106*:264, 1917.

Esser, J. F. S.: Ueber eine gestielte ueber-pfanzung eines senkcrechtangelegten keils aus dem oberen Augenlid in das gleichseitige unterlid oder umge-kehrt. Klin. Monatsbl. Augerheilk., *63*:379, 1919.

Esser, J. F. S.: Esser Inlay. Leiden, Holland, E. J. Brill, 1940.

Eversbusch, O.: Zur operation der congenitalen Blepharoptosis. Klin. Monatsbl. Augenheilk., *21*:100, 1883.

Eversman, J. J., Skillern, P. G., and Senhauser, D. A.: Hashimoto's thyroiditis and Graves' disease with exophthalmos with hyperthyroidism. Cleveland Clin. Quart., *33*:179, 1966.

Fasanella, R. M.: Personal communication, 1973.

Fasanella, R. M., and Servat, J.: Levator resection for minimal ptosis: Another simplified operation. Arch. Ophthalmol., *65*:493, 1961.

Fernandez, L. R.: Double eyelid operation in the Oriental in Hawaii. Plast. Reconstr. Surg., *25*:257, 1960.

Fox, S. A.: Primary congenital entropion. Arch. Ophthalmol., *56*:839, 1956.

Fox, S.: Blepharophimosis. Am. J. Ophthalmol., *55*:469, 1963.

Fricke, J. C. G.: Die Bildung neuer Augenlider (Blepharoplastik) nach Zerstoerungen und dadurch hervorgebrachten Auswaertswendungen derselben. Hamburg, Perthes und Besser, 1829.

Friedenwald, J. S., and Guyton, J. S.: Simple ptosis operation: Utilization of the frontalis by means of a single rhomboid shaped suture. Am. J. Ophthalmol., *31*:411, 1948.

Fuchs, E.: Textbook of Ophthalmology. Philadelphia, J. B. Lippincott Company, 1924.

Gillies, H. D.: Plastic Surgery of the Face. London, Frowde, Hodder and Stoughton, 1920.

Ginsberg, J.: Present status of meibomian gland carcinoma. Arch Ophthalmol., *73*:271, 1965.

Gradenigo, P.: Scritti oftalmologici del conte Pietro Gradenigo. Padua Stabilimento della Societa Cooperativa Tipografica, 1904, pp. 115, 157, 158.

Graefe, A. von: Ophthalmologische Miheilungen. Berl. Klin. Wochenschr., *4*:319, 1867.

Graefe, C. F. von: De Rhinoplastice. Berlin, Reimer, 1818, p. 13.

Graves, R.: Clinical lectures. Med. Classics, *5*:22, 1840.

Guthrie, D.: Surgical treatment of goiter. N.Y. State Med. J., *41*:2315, 1941.

Guyton, J. S.: Decompression of orbit. Surgery, *19*:790, 1946.

Hakelius, L., and Pontén, B.: Results of immediate and delayed surgical treatment of facial fractures with diplopia. J. Maxillofac. Surg., *1*:150, 1973.

Hardin, C. A., and Robinson, D. W.: The surgical treatment of extensive skin cancer of the lower eyelid. J. Kansas Med. Soc., *52*:260, 1951.

Hartman, D. C.: Anophthalmos and microphthalmos. *In* Troutman, R. C., Converse, J. M., and Smith, B. (Eds.): Plastic and Reconstructive Surgery of the Eye and Adnexa. Washington, D.C., Butterworth, 1962.

Helsham, R. W., and Buchanan, G.: Keratoacanthoma of oral cavity. Oral Surg., *13*:844, 1950.

Henderson, J. W.: Relief of eyelid retraction; a surgical procedure. Arch. Ophthalmol., *74*:205, 1965.

Henderson, J. W.: Corrective surgery for endocrine lid retraction. *In* Proceedings of the Second International Symposium on Plastic and Reconstructive Surgery of the Eye and Adnexa. St. Louis, Mo., C. V. Mosby Company, 1967, p. 490.

Hess, H.: Eine Operationsmethode gegen Ptosis. Arch. Augenheilk., 1893.

Heydenreich, A., Morczek, A., and Kurrals, U.: Behandlung des malignen Exophthalmus. Dtsch. Gesundheitsw. Wesen., *21*:1236, 1966.

Hildreth, H. R., and Silver, B.: Sensory block of the upper eyelid. Arch. Ophthalmol., *77*:230, 1967.

Hippel, E. von: Anatomische Untersuchungen über angeborene Korektopie. Arch. Ophthalmol., *51*:132, 1900.

Hippel, E. von: Embryologischen Untersuchungen über die Entstehungweise der typischen augeborenen Spaltbildung (Colobome) des Augapfels. Arch. Ophthalmol., *55*:507, 1903.

Hirsch, O., and Urbanek, K.: Behandlung eines exzessiven exophthalmus (Basedow) durch Entfernung von Orbitalfett von der Kieferhohle aus. Monatsschr. Ohrenheilk., *64*:212, 1930.

Hollander, L., and Krugh, F. J.: Cancer of the eyelid. Am. J. Ophthalmol., *27*:244, 1944.

Holmström, H., Bartholdson, L., and Johanson, B.: Surgical treatment of eyelid cancer with special reference to tarsoconjunctival flaps. A follow-up on 193 patients. Scand. J. Plast. Surg., *9*:107, 1975.

Huffstadt, A. J. C., and Heybroek, G.: Total reconstruction of the lower eyelid. Arch. Clin. Neerl., *18*:33, 1966.

Hughes, W. L.: New method for rebuilding lower lid. Arch. Opthalmol., *17*:1008, 1937.

Hughes, W. L.: Reconstructive Surgery of the Eyelids. St. Louis, Mo., C. V. Mosby Company, 1943, 2nd Ed., 1954.

Hughes, W. L.: Surgical treatment of congenital palpebral phimosis. The V-Y operation. Arch. Ophthalmol., *54*:586, 1955.

Hunt, H. B.: Cancer of the eyelid, treated by radiation with consideration of irradiation cataract. Am. J. Roentgenol., *57*:160, 1947.

Hutchinson, J.: Senile freckles–melanotic staining–epithelial cancer. Arch. Surg. (Lond.), *5*:257, 1894.

Iliff, C. E.: A simplified ptosis operation. Am. J. Ophthalmol., *37*:529, 1954.

Isaksson, I., and Johanson, B.: Structure, function and methods in relation to congenital ptosis. *In* Troutman, R. C., Converse, J. M., and Smith, B. (Eds.): Plastic and Reconstructive Surgery of the Eye and Adnexa. Washington, D.C., Butterworth, 1962.

Ischreyt, G.: Verfahren fuer der plastichen Ersatz des Unterlides. Munch. Med. Wochenschr., *59*:479, 1912.

Iverson, R. E., Vistnes, L. M., and Siegel, R. J.: Correction of enophthalmos in the anophthalmic orbit. Plast. Reconstr. Surg., *51*:545, 1973.

Jaboulay, A.: Le traitement du goitre exophthalmique par la section du sympathique cervical. Presse Med., *61*:81, 1898.

Jaboulay, A., and Poncet, M. A.: Le traitement chirurgical du goitre exophthalmique par la section ou la résection du sympathique cervical. Bull. Acad. Méd., *38*:121, 1897.

Jackson, A.: Results of treatment of orbital fractures. Proc. R. Soc. Med., *61*:497, 1968.

Jobert, A. J.: Traité chirurgie plastique. J. B. Ballière, 1849, Vol. 1, p. 503.

Johnson, C. C.: Operations for epicanthus and blepharophimosis. Evaluation and method for shortening medial canthal ligament. Am. J. Ophthalmol., *41*:71, 1956.

Johnson, C. C.: Surgical repair of the syndrome of epicanthus inversus, blepharophimosis, and ptosis. Arch. Ophthalmol., *71*:510, 1964.

Jones, H. W.: One stage composite lower lid repair. Plast. Reconstr. Surg., *37*:346, 1966.

Jones, L. T.: The cure of epiphora due to canalicular disorders, trauma, and surgical failures on the lacrimal passages. Trans. Am. Acad. Ophthalmol., *66*:506, 1962.

Jones, L. T.: Orbital anatomy. *In* Proceedings of the Second International Symposium on Plastic and Reconstructive Surgery. St. Louis, Mo., C. V. Mosby Company, 1967, p. 20.

Jones, L. T.: Levator resection. *In* Callahan, A.: Ptosis associated with congenital defects: Blepharophimosis, epicanthus and other syndromes. Chapter 21 in Symposium on Surgery of the Orbit and Adnexa. Transactions of the New Orleans Academy of Ophthalmology. St. Louis, Mo., C. V. Mosby Company, 1974a.

Jones, L. T.: Lacrimal surgery. *In* Symposium on Surgery of the Orbit and Adnexa. Transactions of the New Orleans Academy of Ophthalmology. St. Louis, Mo., C. V. Mosby Company, 1974b.

Jonneseo, T.: La résection totale et bilatéral du sympathique cervical (traitement du goitre exophthalmique). Ann. Ocul. (Paris), *117*:161, 1897.

Juler, F. A.: Acute purulent keratitis in exophthalmic goiter, treated by repeated tarsorrhaphy, resection of cervical sympathetics and x-rays. Retention of vision in one eye. Trans. Ophthalmol. Soc. U.K., *33*:58, 1915.

Karfik, V., and Smahel, J.: New method of transplantation of skin with hair. Rozhl. Chir., *48*:233, 1969.

Kazanjian, V. H.: Deformities of the eyelids, orbital and zygomatic regions. *In* Kazanjian, V. H., and Converse, J. M. (Eds.): The Surgical Treatment of Facial Injuries. The Williams & Wilkins Company, Baltimore, 1949, p. 548.

Kistner, F. B.: Decompression of exophthalmos. Report of three cases. J.A.M.A., *112*:37, 1939.

Köllner, P.: Verfahren für den plastischen. Ersatz des Unterlids. Munch. Med. Wochenschr., *58*:2166, 1911.

König, E.: Die Körpereignee frei Fascienverpflanzung. Vienna, Urban & Schwarzenberg, 1928.

Koyanagi, Y.: Embryologische Untersuchungen über die Genese der Augen—Kolobome und des Mikrophthalmus mit Orbitacyste. Graefes Arch. Ophthalmol., *104*:1, 1921.

Kroll, A. J., and Casten, V. G.: Dysthyroid exophthalmos. Palliation by lateral orbital decompression. Arch. Ophthalmol., *76*:205, 1966.

Krönlein, R.: Zur pathologie und Behandlung der Dermoidcysten der orbita. Beitr. Klin. Chir., *4*:149, 1888.

Kuehn, P. G., Newell, R. C., and Reed, J. F.: Exophthalmos in a woman with lingual, subhyoid and lateral-lobe thyroid glands. New Engl. J. Med., *274*:652, 1966.

Kuhnt, H.: Zur Behandlung der Hornhautulzeration bei hochgradigem Basedow—Exophthalmos. Z. Augenheilk., *27*:1912.

Kwitko, M. D., Boniuk, M., and Zimmerman, L. E.: Eyelid tumors with reference to lesion confused with squamous cell carcinoma. I. Incidence and error in diagnosis. Arch. Ophthalmol., 69:693, 1963.

Lacassagne, A.: Répartition des différentes variétés histologiques d'epithéliomas de la peau suivant les régions anatomiques, le sexe et l'âge. Ann. Dermatol. Syph., 4:497, 613, 722, 1933.

LaGrange, F.: De l'anaplerose orbitaire. Bull. Acad. Med. Paris, 80:641, 1918.

Landolt, M.: Un nouveau cas de blépharoplastie suivant notre procédé. Arch. Ophtalmol., 1:111, 1881.

Lawson, G.: On the transposition of portions of skin for the closure of large granulating surface. Trans. Clin. Soc. London, 4:49, 1871.

LeFort, L. C.: Blépharoplastie par un lambeau complétement détaché du bras et reporté à la face. Bull. Mem. Soc. Chir., 1:39, 1872.

Lewis, S. R., Arons, M. S., Lynch, J. B., and Blocker, T. G.: The congenital eyelid syndrome. Plast. Reconstr. Surg., 39:271, 1967.

Lexer, E.: Ptosisoperation, Herstellung der Oberlidfalte und Herstellung des Unterlides durch Faszienzügel. Klin. Mbl. Augenheilk., 70:464, 1923.

Ljungren, H., and Walander, A.: Transantral dekompression vid malign exophthalmus. Nord. Med., 61:436, 1959.

Long, J. C.: Lateral decompression of the orbit for thyroid exophthalmos. In Proceedings of the Second International Symposium on Plastic and Reconstructive Surgery of the Eye and Adnexa. St. Louis, Mo., C. V. Mosby Company, 1967, p. 463.

Long, J. C., and Ellis, G. D.: Temporal decompression of the orbit for thyroid exophthalmos. Am. J. Ophthalmol., 62:1089, 1966.

Longacre, J. J., de Stefano, G. A., and Holmstrand, K.: Reconstruction of the eyebrow: graft versus flap. Introducing the concept of the combined composite scalp and postauricular skin graft. Plast. Reconstr. Surg., 30:638, 1962.

Lorenz (1857): Cited by Merrill, H. G., and Oaks, L. W.: Extreme bilateral exophthalmos. Report of 2 cases with autopsy findings in one. Am. J. Ophthalmol., 16:231, 1933.

Low, J. G.: Transcranial decompression for relief of exophthalmos. In Proceedings of the Second International Symposium on Plastic and Reconstructive Surgery of the Eye and Adnexa. St. Louis, Mo., C. V. Mosby Company, 1967, p. 478.

McCravey, A., and Mather, J. R., Jr.: Treatment of exophthalmos by decompression of the orbit: Report of two cases. Arch. Neurol. Psychiatr., 43:187, 1940.

McGregor, I. A.: Eyelid reconstruction following subtotal resection of upper or lower lid. Br. J. Plast. Surg., 26:346, 1973.

McKenzie, J. M.: An evaluation of the thyroid activator of hyperthyroidism. In Pett-Rivers, R. (Ed.): Transactions of the Fourth International Goiter Conference. Vol. 11. New York, Pergamon Press, 1961, p. 210.

Macomber, W. B., Wang, M. K. H., and Gottlieb, E.: Epithelial tumors of the eyelids. Surg. Gynecol. Obstet., 98:331, 1954.

Macomber, W. B., Wang, M. K. H., and Sullivan, J. G.: Cutaneous epithelioma. Plast. Reconstr. Surg., 24:545, 1959.

Mayo, C. H.: The surgical treatment of exophthalmos. J.A.M.A., 63:1147, 1914.

Means, J. H.: The eye problems in Graves' disease. Illinois Med. J., 80:135, 1941.

Meesmann, A.: Operative Behandlung des malignen Exophthalmus. Zentralbl. Ges. Ophthal., 45:166, 1940.

Merrill, H. G., and Oaks, L. W.: Extreme bilateral exophthalmos. Report of two cases with autopsy with findings in one. Am. J. Ophthalmol., 16:231, 1933.

Millard, D. R.: Oriental peregrinations. Plast. Reconstr. Surg., 16:337, 1955.

Moffat, P. M.: Thyrotoxicosis in relation to ophthalmology. Trans. Ophthalmol. Soc. U.K., 63:19, 1943.

Monks, G. H.: The restoration of a lower lid by a new method. Boston Med. Surg. J., 139:385, 1898.

Moore, R. F.: Exophthalmos and limitation of the eye movements of Graves' disease. Lancet, 199:701, 1920.

Moran, R. E.: The correction of exophthalmos and levator spasm. Plast. Reconstr. Surg., 18:411, 1956.

Morax, V.: Plastic operations on the orbital regions including restoration of the eyebrows, eyelids, and oral cavity. The Bowman Lecture. Trans. Ophthalmol. Soc. U.K., 39:5, 1919.

Morax, V.: Cancer de l'appareil visuel. Paris, G. Doin, 1926, pp. 1-136.

Mosher, H. P.: An operation for draining the lachrymal sac and nasal duct into the unciform fossa. Laryngoscope, 25:739, 1915.

Mosher, H. P.: The combined intranasal and external operation on the lacrimal sac. Ann. Otol. Rhinol. Laryngol., 32:1, 1923.

Mueller, W., Schemmel, K., Uthgenannt, H., and Weissbecker, L.: Die Behandlung des malignen exophthalmos durch totale Thyroidektomie. Dtsch. Med. Wochenschr., 92:2103, 1967.

Murphy, J. B.: Old compound fracture of the right malar bone resulting in loss of the external wall of the orbit. Outward dislocation of the eyeball. Unsuccessful paraffin injection. Successful bone transplantation. Clin. John B. Murphy, 4:Feb., 1915.

Mustardé, J. C.: The treatment of ptosis and epicanthal folds. Br. J. Plast. Surg., 12:252, 1959.

Mustardé, J. C.: Epicanthus and telecanthus. Br. J. Plast. Surg., 16:346, 1963.

Mustardé, J. C.: Repair and Reconstruction in the Orbital Region. A Practical Guide. Baltimore, The Williams & Wilkins Company, 1966.

Mustardé, J. C.: Personal communication, 1974.

Mustardé, J. C.: Personal communication, 1975.

Naffziger, H. C.: Progressive exophthalmos following thyroidectomy: Its pathology and treatment. Ann. Surg., 94:582, 1931.

Naffziger, H. C.: Pathologic changes in the orbit in progressive exophthalmos with special reference to alterations in the extraocular muscles and the optic discs. Arch. Ophthalmol., 9:1, 1933.

Naffziger, H. C.: Exophthalmos, some surgical principles of surgical management from the neurosurgical aspect. Am. J. Surg., 75:25, 1948.

Naffziger, H. C.: Progressive exophthalmos. Ann. R. Coll. Surg. Engl., 17:25, 1954.

Naquin, H. A.: Orbital reconstruction utilizing temporalis muscle. Am. J. Ophthalmol., 41:519, 1956.

Nélaton, C., and Ombrédanne, L.: La Rhinoplastie. Paris, G. Steinheil, 1904.

Niall, F.: Persistent and progressive exophthalmos: The relationship to Graves' disease. Trans. Ophthalmol. Soc. Aust., 1:55, 1939.

Odell, W. D., Fisher, D. A., Korenman, S. G., et al.: Symposium on hyperthyroidism. Calif. Med., 113:35, 1970.

Ogura, J. H.: Transantral orbital decompression for progressive exophthalmos. A follow-up of 54 cases. Med. Clin. North Am., 52:399, 1968.

Ogura, J. H., and Walsh, T. E.: The transantral orbital decompression operation for progressive exophthalmos. Laryngoscope, 72:1078, 1962.

Owens, N., Hadley, R. C., and Kloepfer, H. W.: Hereditary blepharophimosis, ptosis, and epicanthus inversus. J. Int. Coll. Surg., *33*:558, 1960.

Pack, G. T., and Ariel, I. M.: Treatment of Cancer and Allied Diseases. 2nd Ed. Vol. 3, Tumors of the Head and Neck. New York, Hoeber-Harper, 1959, p. 466.

Paufique, L., and Tessier, P.: Reconstruction totale de la paupière supérieure. *In* Troutman, R. C., Converse, J. M., and Smith, B. (Eds.): Plastic and Reconstructive Surgery of the Eye and Adnexa. Washington, D.C., Butterworth, 1962.

Payr, E.: Plastischen erfolgreicher Ersatz aller 4 Augenlider (von 3 durch Fernplastik aus den Arm). Arch. Klin. Chir., *152*:532, 1928.

Pochin, E. E.: Exophthalmos in guinea pigs injected with pituitary extracts. Clin. Sci., *3*:75, 1944.

Poncept, A., and Dor, L.: De la Botromycose humaine. Rev. Chir., *17*:996, 1897.

Poppen, J. L.: Exophthalmos. Diagnosis and surgical treatment of intractable cases. Am. J. Surg., *64*:64, 1944.

Poppen, J. L.: The surgical treatment of progressive exophthalmos. J. Clin. Endocr., *10*:1231, 1950.

Putterman, A.: Treatment of epiphora with absent lacrimal puncta. Arch. Ophthalmol., *89*:125, 1973.

Putterman, A. M., and Urist, M.: Surgical treatment of upper eyelid retraction. Arch. Ophthalmol., *87*:401, 1972.

Quickert, M. H., and Dryden, R. M.: Probes for intubation in lacrimal drainage. Trans. Am. Acad. Ophthalmol. Otolaryngol., *74*:431, 1970.

Reclus, F., and Faure, J. P.: Réséction bilaterale du grand sympathique cervical dans le goitre exophthalmique. Ann. Ocul. (Paris), *118*:38, 1897.

Reeh, M. J.: Treatment of Lid and Epibulbar Tumors. Charles C Thomas, Springfield, Ill., 1963, pp. 75–88.

Reeh, M. J.: Discussion of paper by Smith, B., and Obear, M. F.: The bridge flap technique for reconstruction of upper lid defects. Trans. Am. Acad. Ophthalmol. Otolaryngol., *71*:897, 1967.

Reese, A. B.: Tumors of the Eye. New York, Hoeber-Harper, 1953.

Reverdin, J. L.: Greffe epidermique. Expérience faite dans le service de M. le docteur Guyon à l'hôpital Nécker. Gas. L'op., *43*:15 Disc. 35. 1870 (Reported on Dec. 15, 1869).

Riley, F. C.: Orbital pathology in Graves' disease. Mayo Clin. Proc., *47*:973, 1972.

Rintoul, A. J.: Unilateral proptosis. Proc. R. Soc. Med., *61*:545, 1968.

Risdon, F.: Plastic operations about the orbit. Bull. Acad. Med. Toronto, *18*:139, 1945.

Rosenbaum, J. A.: A case of malignant exophthalmos. Can. Med. Assoc. J., *36*:12, 1937.

Rycroft, B.: Tearing–Management with transantral vidianectomy. *In* Troutman, R. C., Converse, J. M., and Smith, B. (Eds.): Plastic and Reconstructive Surgery of the Eye and Adnexa. Washington, D.C., Butterworth, 1962.

Sappey, P. C.: Anatomie, Physiologie, Pathologie ref. Varffpeaux Lymphatiques considerés chez l'homme et les vertebrés ref. Paris, Delahaye, 1874–1885.

Savin, G. H.: Thyrotoxicosis in relation to ophthalmology. Trans. Ophthalmol. Soc. U.K., *63*:9, 1943.

Sayoc, B. T.: Simultaneous construction of the superior palpebral fold in ptosis operation. Am. J. Ophthalmol., *41*:1040, 1956.

Sayoc, B. T.: Blepharodermachalasis. Am. J. Ophthalmol., *53*:879, 1962.

Sayoc, B. T.: Full upper eyelid. Am. J. Ophthalmol., *6*:155, 1967.

Sayoc, B. T.: Asymmetrical lid folds. Phil. J. Ophthalmol., *1*:122, 1969.

Schall, L. A., and Regan, D. J.: Malignant exophthalmos. Ann. Otol. Rhinol. Laryngol., *54*:37, 1945.

Schimek, R. A.: Surgical management of ocular complications of Graves' disease. Arch. Ophthalmol., *87*:655, 1972.

Sedan, R., and Harter, M.: Irradiation interstitelle hypophysaire dans l'exophtalmologie oedemateuse maligne. Neurochirurgie, *12*:226, 1966.

Semmes, R. E.: In discussion of paper of Dinsmore, Naffziger, and Jones. J.A.M.A., *99*:645, 1932.

Sewall, E. C.: Operative control of progressive exophthalmos. Arch. Otolaryngol., *24*:621, 1936.

Simington, J.: Personal communication to Fasanella, 1972.

Simpson, W. L.: In discussion of paper of Daily, Daily, Walker, and Peterson. South. Med. J., *35*:352, 1942.

Slansky, H. H., Kolbeit, G., and Gartner, S.: Exophthalmos induced by steroids. Arch. Ophthalmol., *77*:579, 1967.

Smelser, G. K.: Water and fat content of orbital tissues in guinea pigs with experimental exophthalmos produced by extracts of anterior pituitary gland. Am. J. Physiol., *140*:308, 1943.

Smelser, G. K.: Experimental studies on exophthalmos. Am. J. Ophthalmol., *54*:929, 1961.

Smelser, G. K., Ozanics, V., and Zugibe, F. T.: The production of exophthalmos in the absence of adrenal and ovarian hormones. Am. Rec., *131*:701, 1958.

Smith, B.: Eyelid surgery. Surg. Clin. North Am., *38*:367, 1959.

Smith, B.: Personal communication, 1974.

Smith, B.: Personal communication, 1975.

Smith, B., and Cherubini, T. D.: Oculoplastic Surgery. St. Louis, Mo., C. V. Mosby Company, 1970, pp. 20–27.

Smith, B., and Obear, M. F.: Bridge flap technique for reconstruction of large upper lid defects. Trans. Am. Acad. Ophthalmol. Otolaryngol., *71*:897, 1967.

Smith, B., Obear, M., and Leone, C. R.: The correction of enophthalmos associated with anophthalmos by glass bead implantation. Am. J. Ophthalmol., *64*:1088, 1967.

Soler Sala, J. M., Noguer, L. A., and Lillo, J.: Consideraciones Sobre el Exoftalmos Endocrino. Arch. Soc. Oftal. Hisp.-Am., *28*:171, 1968.

Sonnenberg, M., and Money, W. L.: Chemical derivatives of thyroid stimulating hormone preparations. *In* Modern Concepts of Thyroid Physiology. Ann. N.Y. Acad. Sci., *86*:625, 1960.

Spaeth, E. B.: The Principles and Practice of Ophthalmic Surgery. Philadelphia, Lea & Febiger, 1939, pp. 65, 66. 2nd Ed., 1948.

Spira, M., Gerow, F. J., and Hardy, S. B.: Correction of post-traumatic enophthalmos. Acta Chir. Plast., *16*:107, 1974.

Stallard, H. B.: Operations for epiphora. Lancet, *2*:743, 1940.

Stellwag von Carion, K.: Rückblicke auf die augenärztlichen Pfropfungsversuche und ein neuer Fall von Schleimhautübertragung. Allg. Wien. Med. Ztg., *34*: 341, 1889.

Stetson, C. G., and Schulz, M. D.: Carcinoma of the eyelid. Analysis of 301 cases and review of the literature. N. Engl. J. Med., *241*:725, 1949.

Swift, G. W.: Malignant exophthalmos and operative approach. West. J. Surg., *43*:119, 1935.

Szily, A. von: Weitere Beitrage zu den embryologischen

Grundlagen der Missbildungen des Auges. Erklaung der angerborenen umschrieben Loch- oder Gruben-bildungen an der Papille. Berl. Ophthalmol. Ges. Heidelberg, *39*:344, 1913.

Szymanowski, J. von: Handbuch der operativen Chirurgie. F. Vieweg. u. Sohn, Braunschweig, 1870.

Tanzer, R. C.: Reconstruction of eyebrow and eyelashes. *In* Troutman, R. C., Converse, J. M., and Smith, B. (Eds.): Plastic and Reconstructive Surgery of the Eye and Adnexa. Washington, D.C., Butterworth, 1962, p. 154.

Teale, T. P.: On relief of symblepharon by transplantation of the conjunctiva. Ophthal. Hosp. Rev., *3*:253, 1860.

Tenzel, R. R.: Personal communication to Fasanella, 1970.

Tessier, P., Guiot, G., Rougerie, J., Delbet, J. P., and Pastoriza, J.: Ostéotomies cranio-naso-orbital-faciales. Hypertélorisme. Ann. Chir. Plast., *12*:103, 1967.

Tessier, P., Guiot, G., and Derome, P.: Orbital hypertelorism. II. Definitive treatment of orbital hypertelorism by craniofacial or by extracranial osteotomies. Scand. J. Plast. Reconstr. Surg., 7:39, 1973.

Thomas, H. M., Jr., and Woods, A. C.: Progressive exophthalmos following thyroidectomy. Bull. Johns Hopkins Hosp., *59*:99, 1936.

Thomson, H. G.: Reconstruction of the orbit after radical exenteration. Plast. Reconstr. Surg., *45*:119, 1970.

Tillett, C. G., and Tillett, G. M.: Silicone sling in the correction of ptosis. Am. J. Ophthalmol., *62*:521, 1966.

Tinker, M. B.: The surgical treatment of exophthalmos. Sec. on Ophthalmol., J.A.M.A., *58*:353, 1912.

Toti, A.: Nuovo metodo conservatore di cura radicale delle suppurazioni croniche del sacco lacrimal (dacriocistorhinostomia). Clin. Med., *10*:385, 1904.

Traub, E. F.: Diagnosis and treatment of carcinoma of the eyelid. J.A.M.A., *154*:9, 1954.

Valenti, G., and Cordella, M.: Sugli affetti di un beta—bloccante adrenergico sullo esoftalmo spetimentale da triiodotironin. Ann. Ottal., *93*:1037, 1967a.

Valenti, G., and Cordella, M.: Esoftalmo sperimentale de triiodotironina, da STHC e da proprietiouracile dopo timectomia. Ann. Ottal., *93*:1025, 1967b.

Viers, E. R.: The Lacrimal System. New York, Grune & Stratton, 1955.

Wadsworth, J. A. C.: Exenteration. *In* Symposium on Surgery of the Orbit and Adnexa. Transactions of the New Orleans Academy of Ophthalmology. St. Louis, Mo., C. V. Mosby Company, 1974.

Wallace, H. J.: The conservative treatment of haemangiomatous nevi. Br. J. Plast. Surg., *6*:78, 1953.

Walsh, T. E., and Ogura, J. H.: Transantral orbital decompression for malignant exophthalmos. Laryngoscope, *65*:544, 1957.

Wang, M. K. H., Macomber, W. B., and Elliott, R. A., Jr.: Tumors of the eyelids and orbit. *In* Converse, J. M. (Ed.): Reconstructive Plastic Surgery. W. B. Saunders Company, Philadelphia, 1964, pp. 662–693.

Webster, J. P.: Temporalis muscle transplants for defects following orbital exenteration. *In* Trans. Internatl. Soc. Plast. Surg. Baltimore, The Williams & Wilkins Company, 1957.

Welham, R. A. N., and Henderson, P.: Failed dacryocystorhinostomy. Trans. Am. Acad. Ophthalmol. Otolaryngol., *78*:OP 824, 1974.

Welti, H., and Offret, G.: A propos des exophthalmies malignes basedowiennes. Ann. Endocr. (Paris), *3*:186, 1942.

Werb, A.: Personal communication to L. T. Jones, 1971.

Werner, S. C.: Management of the active severe eye changes of Graves' disease. Trans. Am. Acad. Ophthalmol. Otolaryngol., *71*:631, 1967.

Wheeler, J. M.: Restoration of the margin and neighboring portion of the eyelid by a free graft from the lower part of the eyebrow and the skin directly below it: Report of an illustrative case. J.A.M.A., *75*:1055, 1920.

Wheeler, J. M.: Plastic operations about the eye. Proc. Internatl. Congr. Ophthalmol., 1922, p. 443.

Wheeler, J. M.: Halving wounds in facial plastic surgery. Proc. 2nd Congr. Pan-Pacific Surg. Assoc., 1936, p. 229.

Wheeler, J. M.: Collected Papers of John Martin Wheeler, M.D. New York, 1939.

Whitaker, L. A., Katowitz, J. A., and Randall, P.: The nasolacrimal apparatus in congenital facial anomalies. J. Maxillofac. Surg., *2*:59, 1974.

Whitnall, E.: The structure and muscle of the eyelids. *In* Anatomy of the Human Orbit. London, W. H. Milford, 1932, pp. 129–162.

Wolfe, J. R.: A new method of performing plastic operation. Med. Times Gaz., *1*:608, 1876.

Wood, A. C.: The ocular changes of primary diffuse toxic goitre. Rev. Med., *25*:113, 1936.

Worst, J. G. F.: Method of reconstructing torn lacrimal canaliculus. Am. J. Ophthalmol., *53*:520, 1962.

Würdemann, H. V., and Becker, W.: A typical exophthalmic goiter from endothelioma of the pituitary and thyroid bodies. Death from general sepsis. Autopsy. Ophthalmology, *2*:411, 1906.

Wybar, K. C.: The nature of endocrine exophthalmos. Ophthalmology, *49*:119, 1957.

Wynn-Williams, D.: Surgical treatment of malignant diseases of the peri-orbital area. Br. J. Plast. Surg., *20*:315, 1967.

Youens, W. T., Westphal, C., Barfield, F. T., Jr., and Youens, H. T., Jr.: Full thickness lower lid transplant. Arch. Ophthalmol., *77*:226, 1967.

Zimmerman, L. E.: Tumors of the eye and adnexa from the Armed Forces Institute of Pathology. Int. Ophthalmol. Clin., *2*:239, 1962.

CHAPTER 29

CORRECTIVE AND RECONSTRUCTIVE SURGERY OF THE NOSE

JOHN MARQUIS CONVERSE, M.D.,
DONALD WOOD-SMITH, F.R.C.S.E.,
BROMLEY S. FREEMAN, M.D.,
W. BRANDON MACOMBER, M.D.,
AND MARK K. H. WANG, M.D.

Corrective Rhinoplasty

JOHN MARQUIS CONVERSE, M.D.

The nose, the most prominent and characteristic feature of the human face, is readily injured, is often congenitally malformed, and is subject to benign and malignant tumors. One of the most frequently performed operations in plastic surgery is that of modifying the shape of the nose by a corrective operation for the improvement of form and function.

Deformities of the nose involve the skeletal framework of the nose, which may be malformed; the covering soft tissues of the nose, which may be scarred or defective; the lining of the nasal vestibules and nasal fossae; and the nasal septum, which may be deviated. Other pathology of the nose and sinuses may coexist with hypertrophy of the turbinates.

Following severe accidents or resection of the nose for malignant disease, the full thickness of the nasal tissues requires reconstruction.

HISTORICAL CONSIDERATIONS

Corrective surgery of the external nose is required for both functional and esthetic reasons.

Little faith in the success of purely corrective procedures was expressed by Nélaton and Ombrédanne in their textbook *La Rhinoplastie* published in 1904: "The surgeon could not pretend to correct a slight malformation. If a nose be slightly deviated or humped, or show a slight saddle deformity—these are unfortunate defects... but we do not believe that the correction of such defects can be achieved by surgery." Nasal corrective operations were being developed by other surgeons, however, during this period. A review of the literature of the last decade of the 19th century and the early part of the 20th century indicates that nasal corrective procedures were initiated mostly through externally placed incisions.

In the United States, corrective nasal surgery was pioneered by a small number of surgeons, among whom Roe, Goodale, and Mosher are outstanding. Roe appears to have been the first to employ an intranasal approach as early as 1887. Extracts from some of Roe's papers reveal his understanding of both the functional and psychologic aspects of corrective rhinoplasty (Converse, 1970).

If the deformity of the nose is found to be associated with a local disturbance inside the nose, obstructing the passages, we should invariably remove or correct this local condition, whether it be deviation or thickening of the septum, enlargement of the turbinates, a polyp or other growths, or even adenoids and large tonsils. To preserve perfect nasal respiration is of the utmost necessity, not only to the health and comfort of the patient, but to the satisfactory correction of the nasal deformity.

While symmetrical relations to the different portions of the nose to one another are of the greatest importance, the symmetrical relation as to the size and shape of the nose to the general contour of the face must also be carefully considered, in order to approach the ideal from an artistic point of view.

We are able to relieve patients of a condition which would remain a lifelong mark of disfigurement, constantly observed, forming a never ceasing source of embarrassment and mental distress to themselves, amounting, in many cases, to a positive torture, as well as often causing them to be objects of greater or less aversion to others.

These quotations from Roe's writings could have been written in a present-day paper. Because of his technical skill and his esthetic sense, Roe achieved international fame. Roe was the first surgeon to use an intranasal approach, but it was Joseph who popularized corrective nasal surgery through internally placed incisions. His influence was predominant during the first third of this century. His teachings were collected in a textbook published in 1931. The Joseph technique was introduced in the United States by Aufricht and Safian. The literature concerned with corrective nasal plastic surgery is abundant. A comprehensive bibliography was compiled by McDowell, Valone, and Brown (1952).

Prior to the undertaking of corrective rhino-

plastic procedures, an understanding of the anatomy and physiology of the nose is a prime requisite.

ANATOMY OF THE NOSE

The nose is in the shape of a pyramid. The nasal pyramid is an osteocartilaginous structure, covered with soft tissues which include skin, subcutaneous tissue, muscle, and epithelium. The surface anatomy of the nose is shown in Figure 29–1; the osteocartilaginous framework of the nose is illustrated in Figure 29–2.

The nasal pyramid has two openings at its base, the external nares (see Fig. 29–16). These inlets for the nasal airway admit air into the nasal vestibules, delimited posteriorly by the internal nares, frequently referred to as the nasal valves (Mink, 1920). It is these valvelike structures that control the air flow into the nasal fossae proper, paired cavities separated in the midline by the nasal septum (see Fig. 29–17). The convergence and divergence of the nasal valves open and close the internal nares, thus controlling the air flow into the nasopharyngotracheal airway. The nasal fossae drain the accessory sinuses and the lacrimal apparatus. A small portion of the nasal mucous membrane near the cribriform plate is specifically olfactory in function. Irregularities of the shape of the nose, both external and internal, may disturb nasal physiology.

The Covering Soft Tissues of the Nose. At the tip, the skin of the nose is tightly bound to the alar cartilages; in contrast, the skin and musculature are loosely attached and mobile over the lateral cartilages and nasal bones. The skin is rich in sebaceous glands over the lower portion of the nose. The arteries and veins of the nose are situated in the soft tissues; the plane of dissection in nasal operations should therefore be close to the osteocartilaginous framework to avoid injury to the vessels and unnecessary bleeding.

Essential External Landmarks of the Nose. The dorsum of the nose, also termed the bridge, is formed in part by the bony nose and in part by the cartilaginous nose. It is essential that a uniform terminology be employed to designate the various portions of the nose. The nasofrontal angle is the area where the nose joins the forehead, the root of the nose

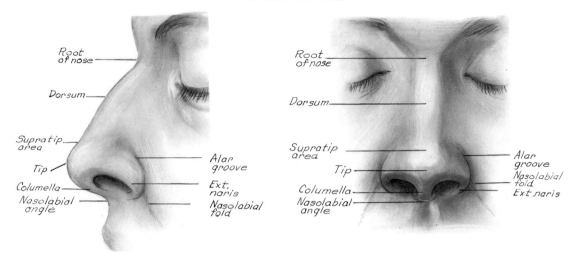

FIGURE 29–1.   External anatomy of the nose.

(the radix nasi). Nasion is an anthropometric point, a bony landmark (see Fig. 29–1).

Above (cephalad to) the tip of the nose is the supratip area. This area usually overlies the septal angle of the septal (or quadrangular) cartilage of the septum. The "septal angle" is a convenient term for the angle formed by the caudal and dorsal borders of the septal cartilage (Converse, 1955).

The tip of the nose is formed by the junction of the two alae of the nose. Confusion has resulted from the use of the term "lobule," which has been variously applied to the tip of the nose as well as to the resilient or flexible cartilaginous portion of the nasal pyramid. The noun "lobule" originates from the ancient Greek *lobos,* which became in late Latin *lobus,* a term which designated a hanging structure such as the lobe of the ear. A lobule is therefore a small lobe. The nose consists of fixed and mobile structures. The fixed structures are the bony pyramid and the cephalic portion of the lateral (upper lateral) cartilages, and the mobile structures are the caudal cartilaginous structures: the alar (lower lateral) cartilages forming the tip of the nose, the caudal portion of the septum, and the columella (see Fig. 29–7). If one wishes to use the term "lobule," it can be accepted as a descriptive term for the lower mobile part of the nose (Natvig, 1975).

The base of the nasal pyramid is formed by the nostrils and the columella. The nostrils can also be designated as the external nares in contradistinction to the internal nares. The external naris is prolonged medialward by a ridge which forms the anterior limit of the floor of the nose and rejoins the columella.

The nostrils are the point of entry of the air into the nose. The columella joins the tip of the nose to the upper lip and separates the two external nares. The base of the columella forms the nasolabial angle. Subnasale is a skeletal anthropometric point and is not the columella-labial angle, also referred to as the nasolabial angle, which is formed by soft tissue and the underlying skeletal structures.

Other essential landmarks of the external nose include the alar groove, which is at the junction of the ala with the cheek and which in its midportion meets the nasolabial fold. The alar groove extends over the cephalic border of the alar cartilage, where it forms a shallow furrow.

The Bony Structures of the Nose.   The anatomy of the nose varies from individual to individual within the same ethnic group and according to the individual's ethnic background. Variations include those found in the bony skeletal framework (the nasal bones may be absent) and those found in the structures forming the cartilaginous framework.

The bony portion of the nose is formed by the paired nasal bones; these are joined in the midline and are supported posteriorly by the nasal spine of the frontal bone and laterally by the frontal process of the maxilla. The osseous lateral walls of the nose are formed by the nasal bones and frontal processes of the maxilla.

The nasal bones are quadrangular, thick and narrow above, and thin and wide below (Figs.

29–2 and 29–3); their anterior surface is concave from above downward in the upper portion, convex from side to side. The thicker and stronger cephalic portion of the nasal bones is further reinforced by the nasal spine of the frontal bone, which lends additional support to this part of the bony bridge. The caudal borders of the nasal bones show a concave curve, the lateral portion of each bone extending downward along the edge of the pyriform aperture (Fig. 29–3, *B*). The frontal process of the maxilla is a plate of bone, thick below and thinner above, which projects upward and medially from the body of the maxilla, forming the edge of the pyriform aperture (Fig. 29–3, *C*), the lower boundary of the lateral nasal wall. The posterior border of the frontal process of the maxilla, with the neighboring lacrimal bone, forms the lacrimal groove (Fig. 29–3, *C*).

The frontal process of the maxilla forms the anterior lacrimal crest. The medial canthal tendon inserts upon this crest; some of its fibers insert on the anterior slope of the crest, and some reach the suture line between the nasal bone and the frontal process.

The Cartilaginous Structures of the Nose

THE LATERAL (UPPER LATERAL) CARTILAGES. During embryologic development, the nasal cartilages are formed from a portion of the chondrocranium, the cartilaginous nasal capsule, a paired structure. This explains embryologic abnormalities such as duplication of the septum or duplication of the entire nose.

The lateral cartilages are paired structures, roughly triangular in shape (thus their appellation "triangular cartilages"), attached to the nasal bones and frontal processes of the maxilla above and to the septal cartilage in the midline (Fig. 29–4). The mode of attachment of the lateral cartilages to these structures and to the septum is described later in the text. As the lower third of the lateral cartilage is reached, they diverge from the septum and thus become mobile and constitute the nasal valves of the nose.

The lower portion of each lateral cartilage is thicker and turns on itself, forming a cuff (Fig. 29–4, *A, B*). This characteristic was described by Testut and Jacob (1929) and other anatomists, who also described small sesamoid cartilages which are present between the lateral cartilage and the alar cartilage that overlaps the lateral cartilage. The small sesamoid cartilages appear to act as roller bearings, facilitating the movement of the alar cartilage over the lateral cartilage.

The lateral margin of the lateral cartilage is joined to the edge of the pyriform aperture except in its lower portion, where the area of the junction varies (Fig. 29–4, *C*).

The cartilages of the nose are subjected to movements by the nasal musculature (Fig. 29–5) and play an important role in nasal physiology. The closure of the nasal valves is effected by the compression of the cephalic portion of the lateral crura of the alar cartilages which overlap the lateral cartilages. Van Dishoek (1937) studied the action of these muscles. The preservation of the mobility of the caudal

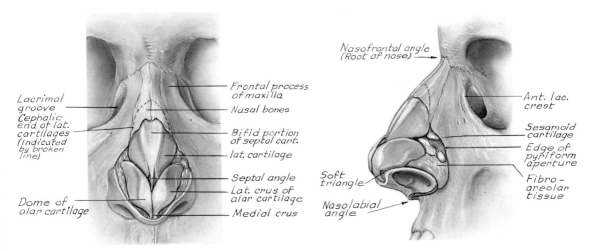

FIGURE 29–2. Structural framework of the nose. See also Figure 29–4.

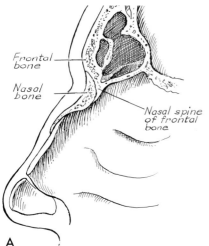

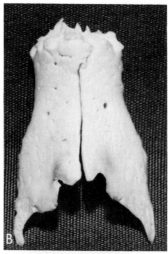

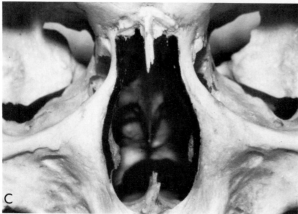

FIGURE 29–3. The bony framework of the nose. *A*, Sagittal section illustrating the thicker cephalic portion of the nasal bones reinforced by the nasal spine of the frontal bone. *B*, The nasal bones. *C*, The pyriform aperture.

portion of the nose is essential for the function of these muscles. Their function is inhibited in facial paralysis; the cartilages of the nose are immobile due to paralysis of the musculature, and an inadequate nasal airway is noted on the paralyzed side (Fig. 29–6).

The alar cartilages are connected to the lateral cartilages by loose connective tissue which facilitates their cephalic displacement over the lateral cartilages.

The cartilaginous external nose is situated caudad and anterior to the pyriform aperture. The pyriform aperture, the base of the nasal pyramid, is a pear-shaped opening to the nasal fossae. It is bounded above by the lower borders of the nasal bones and laterally by the frontal processes of the maxilla, the thin, sharp margins of which extend downward, where they curve medially to join each other at the anterior nasal spine.

THE NASAL SEPTUM AND THE SEPTAL CARTILAGE. The nasal septum is a median struc-

ture which divides the nasal cavity into two lateral chambers. The septal framework is composed of bony and cartilaginous constitutents: the four bony components of the osseous septum (the perpendicular plate of the ethmoid, the vomer, the nasal crest of the maxilla, the nasal crest of the palatine bone) and the septal cartilage. The septal cartilage has a posterior extension into the ethmoid plate (Fig. 29–7).

The septal cartilage is a quadrangular lamina which forms the major portion of the framework of the caudal portion of the septum; it protrudes in front of the pyriform aperture. The septal angle is located immediately cephalad to the alar cartilages in an area referred to as the supratip area. The lower portion of the septal cartilage is firmly bound to the vomer and the premaxillary wings, the perichondrium of the cartilage being continuous with the periosteum of the vomer. The caudal part of the septal cartilage becomes

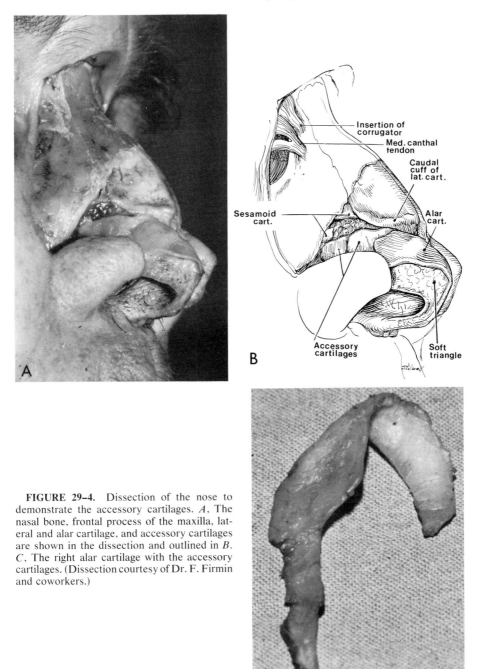

FIGURE 29–4. Dissection of the nose to demonstrate the accessory cartilages. *A*, The nasal bone, frontal process of the maxilla, lateral and alar cartilage, and accessory cartilages are shown in the dissection and outlined in *B*. *C*, The right alar cartilage with the accessory cartilages. (Dissection courtesy of Dr. F. Firmin and coworkers.)

more mobile and flexible. The perichondrium of the septal cartilage extends outward to join the periosteum of the wider groove in the premaxillary wings and the flat surface of the nasal spine, thus simulating a joint capsule within which lateral movements of the septal cartilage are possible. The plasticity of this portion of the septum, known as the mobile septum, increases the flexibility of the septal cartilage. The caudal margin of the septal cartilage is separated from the columella by the juxtaposition of two mucocutaneous flaps which form the membranous septum. The layers of the membranous septum extend forward, di-

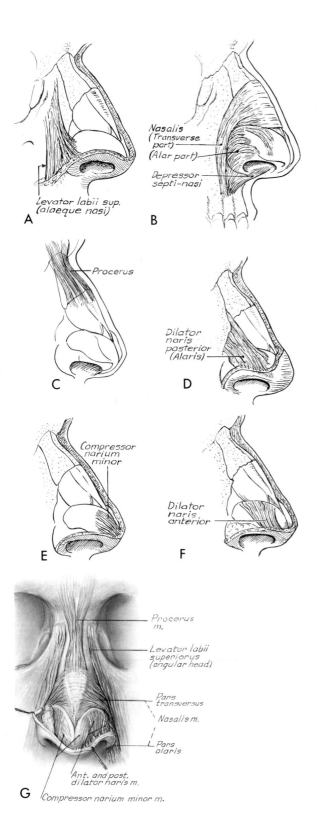

FIGURE 29–5.   The muscles of the nose.

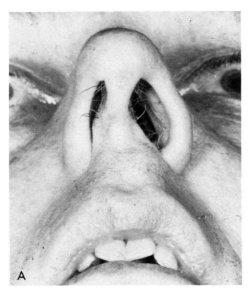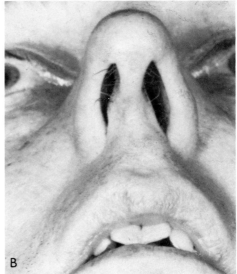

FIGURE 29–6. Loss of function of the ala in facial paralysis *A*, The nose during inspiration. On the unaffected left side, the naris opens; on the paralyzed right side, the ala is immobile. *B*, The paralyzed right ala remains collapsed during expiration.

verging to join with the cutaneous covering of the medial crura, which constitute the skeletal support of the columella.

The mobility of the lower portion of the septal cartilage and of the membranous septum permits side to side movement and, together with the resilient lateral and alar cartilages, accounts for the shock-absorbing role of these

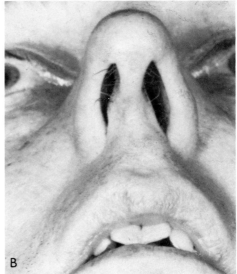

FIGURE 29–7. The line X indicates the line of demarcation between the fixed and the resilient portion of the nasal septum.

structures in preventing nasal fractures as well as more severe craniofacial injuries.

The cephalic portion of the dorsal border of the septal cartilage, intimately connected with the cephalic portion of the lateral cartilages, extends under the nasal bones, where it is received in a shallow bony groove. The posterior border is connected to the perpendicular plate of the ethmoid; the posterior extension of the septal cartilage separates a portion of the ethmoid plate from the vomer (see Fig. 29–7).

THE CENTRAL PILLAR OF THE NOSE. The cephalic portion of the septal cartilage is usually thicker, constituting at its junction with the ethmoid plate a strong, fixed, central pillar supporting the nasal bones. The preservation of the central pillar is of considerable importance in rhinoplasty when all of the structures of the nose have been mobilized and only the central pillar remains to support the dorsum.

RELATIONSHIP OF THE LATERAL CARTILAGES TO THE BONY PYRAMID. The relationship of the lateral cartilages to the nasal bones is established during the embryologic development of these structures. The nasal bones develop from the membrane on the surface of the cartilaginous nasal capsule, thus accounting for the extension of the lateral cartilage under the nasal bones (Straatsma and Straatsma, 1951; Converse, 1955). The overlapping of the nasal bones over the cephalic portion of the lateral cartilages may extend over an area of 8 to 10 mm (see Fig. 29–2; Fig. 29–8). The fusion of the perichondrium and the periosteum through dense connective tissue results in an intimate relationship between cartilage and bone. The overlapping area is oval in shape. The maximum length of the oval is at the junction of the nasal bones; as the frontal process is reached, the overlap is only a few millimeters. The extent of this anatomical neighborliness may be observed when the nose is dissected. The upper portion of each lateral cartilage is exposed when the overlying nasal bone is removed. This intimate relationship is of clinical significance in fractures and in nasal plastic operations, for it explains why the lateral cartilage is displaced medially with the bony lateral wall following lateral osteotomy.

RELATIONSHIP OF THE LATERAL CARTILAGES TO THE SEPTUM. The septal cartilage extends upward beneath the nasal bones for a distance equal to that of the lateral cartilages. As mentioned above, the septal cartilage is thicker near its junction with the perpendicular plate of the ethmoid, a portion of the septum often designated as the "tubercle" of the septum. The increased thickness of the septum extends to the dorsal border of the cartilage in this area.

The dorsal border of the cartilaginous nasal septum undergoes alteration in width and con-

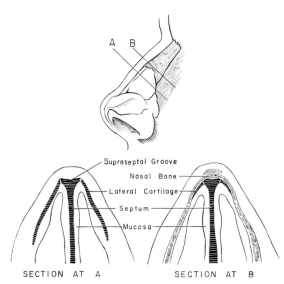

Supraseptal Groove
Nasal Bone
Lateral Cartilage
Septum
Mucosa

SECTION AT A   SECTION AT B

FIGURE 29–8. Serial sections of the external nose through a frontal plane. The upper drawing illustrates the levels A and B at which cross sections have been made. The sectional view *A* demonstrates the relationship of the lateral and septal cartilages. The sectional view *B* shows the relationship to the lateral and septal cartilages with the nasal bones (see the dotted line in Fig. 29–2).

figuration toward the nasal bones, bifurcating into a Y, forming a supraseptal groove between the limbs of the Y (see Figs. 29–2 and 29–8). The groove is readily seen and palpated in some individuals, but it is usually not distinguishable on the surface, being masked by the perichondrium, connective tissue, aponeurosis of the nasalis muscle, and subcutaneous tissue. The supraseptal groove is wide near the junction with the nasal bones and fades away toward the septal angle.

The nasal hump, often a prominent portion of the dorsum, is formed by the nasal bones, the widened portion of the septal cartilage, and the lateral cartilages. The dorsal hump is fusiform, narrow above, wide near the junction of the lateral cartilages and nasal bones, and narrow above the septal angle.

The lateral and septal cartilages are intimately connected near the nasal bones. In the series of sections obtained from cadaver dissections (Converse, 1955), there was a gross appearance of cartilaginous continuity. Histologic examination, however, showed a separation between the ends, bound together by dense connective tissue; continuity of the perichondrium was seen in every specimen. In the specimens studied by Straatsma and Straatsma (1951) and by Natvig, Sether, Gingrass, and Gardner (1971), continuity of the septal and lateral cartilages was seen on histologic examination. However, Natvig (1975) has reexamined a series of specimens and confirmed the findings of Converse (1955).

The septal and lateral cartilages are separated by a narrow cleft which becomes wider towards the septal angle. Fibroareolar tissue in this area permits inward and outward movement of the lateral cartilages. The mobile caudal portion of the lateral cartilages activated by the nasal musculature regulates the flow of air that penetrates into the nasal fossae and constitutes the internal nares (the nasal valves).

In the course of a corrective rhinoplasty, the integrity of the nasal valve must be preserved.

THE ALAR (LOWER LATERAL) CARTILAGES. The alar cartilages are paired structures which form the cartilaginous framework of the tip of the nose (see Fig. 29–2). Each cartilage consists of two portions, a medial crus and a lateral crus, which are joined at the most prominent point of the tip of the nose, the dome of the alar cartilage. The medial crura curve downward to form the skeletal framework of the columella. As they extend downward, they diverge at their lower ends (the feet of the me-

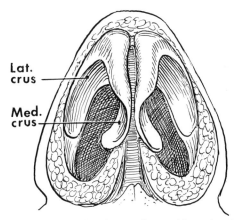

FIGURE 29–9. The alar cartilages. Note the downward curve of the caudal portions and the flare of the medial crura.

dial crura), the maximal divergence being reached at the widened base of the columella. Each medial crus is intimately joined to the skin of the columella.

The size, shape, and orientation of the alar cartilages, particularly the lateral crura, vary. The medial crura assume various curves and shapes (Natvig, 1975).

In dissected specimens, when viewed from their caudal aspect (the "worm's eye view"), the lateral crura and the domes show a distinct downward curve of their caudal portions (Fig. 29–9). The caudal margin is lower than the dome and the more cephalic portion of the lateral crus.

The lateral portion of the lateral crus, which occupies little more than the medial half of the ala, is joined to the edge of the pyriform aperture by accessory and sesamoid cartilages.

THE ACCESSORY CARTILAGES OF THE NOSE. The term "sesamoid" may be applied to the minuscule cartilages between the lateral and alar cartilages and also the small cartilages in the superolateral portion of the ala. The term "accessory" cartilages is suggested to designate the larger cartilages which join the lateral crus to the edge of the pyriform aperture through the continuity of the perichondrium of these structures. Described by Testut and Jacob (1929) and in many anatomical texts, their presence has been confirmed by dissections done by Firmin and collaborators (1974) and in our own dissections.

Although variable in size and shape, the accessory cartilages establish a bridge between the alar cartilage and the edge of the pyriform aperture (Fig. 29–10). The accessory cartilages are joined to each other and to the lateral crus by the continuity of the perichondrium (Fig. 29–11). Thus the alar cartilage and its accessory cartilages form a cartilaginous three-quarter ring at the base of the nasal pyramid (Fig. 29–12).

The Nostril Border. The border of the nostril is supported by dense collagenous tissue arranged in resilient, parallel, longitudinal bun-

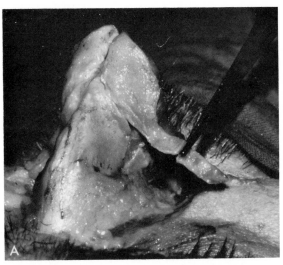

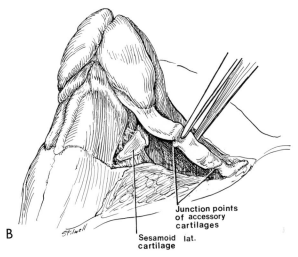

Junction points
of accessory
cartilages

Sesamoid lat.
cartilage

FIGURE 29–10. The accessory cartilages. *A*, Dissection of the nasal framework (viewed from above), demonstrating the accessory cartilages which join the lateral crus to the edge of the pyriform aperture. *B*, Drawing illustrating the accessory cartilages (three in number in this specimen) joined to each other and to the alar cartilages by the continuity of the perichondrium. (*A*, Courtesy of Dr. F. Firmin and associates.)

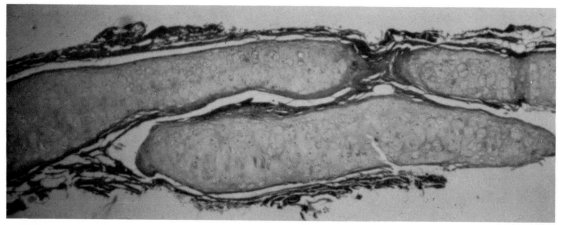

FIGURE 29–11. Photomicrograph of a histologic section showing the continuity of the perichondrium joining the accessory cartilages. (Courtesy of Dr. F. Firmin and associates.)

dles. The lateral crus is closer to the caudal margin of the external naris border in its medial third but extends away from the margin in its lateral portion. An incision along the caudal margin of the cartilage should allow for this conformation and extend farther away from the nostril border in its lateral portion. The incision should follow the curve of the caudal margin of the cartilage when dividing it into upper and lower segments to avoid excising the entire lateral portion of the cartilage.

THE SOFT TRIANGLE. The dome, point of union of the lateral and medial crura, is separated from the margin of the nostril by a triangular-shaped area known as the soft triangle (Converse, 1955) (Fig. 29–13); this consists of two juxtaposed layers of skin, the covering skin of the nose and the lining vestibular

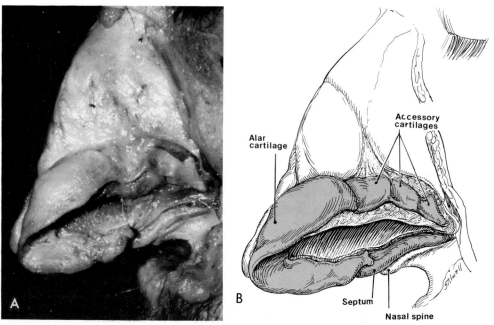

FIGURE 29–12. The narial ring formed by the alar and accessory cartilages. *A,* Dissection of the cartilages showing the alar cartilage (medial crus, dome, lateral crus, and accessory cartilages). *B,* Drawing illustrating the various structures shown in *A.* The alar cartilage and its accessory cartilages form a 3/4 circle narial ring. (*A,* Courtesy of Dr. F. Firmin and associates.)

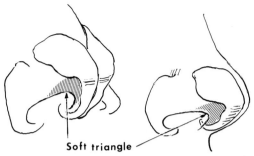

FIGURE 29–13. The soft triangle of the nose, consisting of two juxtaposed layers of skin separating the dome of the alar cartilage from the nostril border. The soft triangle is represented by the shaded area.

skin, separated by loose areolar tissue. An incision through the soft triangle should be avoided, as subsequent healing may result in a disfiguring notch. The marginal or rim incision for exposure of the alar cartilage should follow the caudal margin of the cartilage and not the margin of the nostril.

THE WEAK TRIANGLE. The lateral crura of the alar cartilages diverge in the supratip area, leaving a triangular-shaped area between them into which the septal angle is fitted. In this area in many noses, the dorsum is supported only by the septal angle (Fig. 29–14, *A*). As described earlier in the text, the alar cartilages, which overlap the lateral cartilages, are connected by aponeurotic-like tissue, which also maintains the attachment of the alar cartilages to the septal angle and acts as a suspensory ligament of the tip of the nose (Fig. 29–14, *B*).

The nose droops when the support of the septal angle is lost by injury or operative removal. This deformity may be accompanied by retraction of the columella, which may also be caused by loss of septal support.

The Columella. The columella extends from the tip of the nose to the lip, joining the lip at the upper portion of the philtrum and separating the external nares. The posterior portion of the columella is wider than the anterior portion due to the divergence of the medial crura of the alar cartilages, the lower ends of which embrace the caudal margin of the septal cartilage (see Figs. 29–9 and 29–12). The lower portion of the columella is also wider than the remainder of the columella because of the divergence of the lower portions of the medial crura; the contour of the columella depends largely upon the shape and degree of divergence of these cartilaginous structures.

THE DEPRESSOR SEPTI NASI MUSCLE. The columella is penetrated by the paired depressor septi nasi muscles which arise from the incisive fossae of the maxilla (Fig. 29–5). The muscle inserts into the caudal portion of the septum and a few fibers into the cephalic portion of the ala of the nose. Its principal function is to tense the membranous septum. In some patients it is overactive, de-

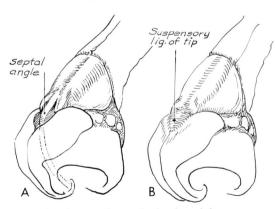

FIGURE 29–14. The weak triangle and the suspensory ligament of the nose. *A,* The soft tissues have been removed to show that the septal angle supports the area of the dorsum between and above the diverging lateral crura (the weak triangle). This area is subject to many anatomical variations. *B,* The aponeurosis joining the structures (the suspensory ligament of the nasal tip).

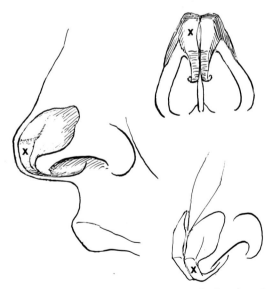

FIGURE 29–15. The tip-columella angle. Between the tip and the base of the columella there is a break in the continuity of the cephalic curve of the columella. There are numerous variations.

pressing the tip when the patient smiles or even when he speaks. In these patients, the muscle can be excised in part or in toto. The insertions of the muscle cause the mucoperichondrium of the caudal portion of the septum to be more adherent and thus more difficult to detach when the septal cartilage is being exposed, the procedure often requiring sharp dissection with the knife.

THE TIP-COLUMELLA ANGLE. The medial crura curve down from the domes, thus assuming a vertical position. At the caudal portion of the nasal tip, the cartilaginous framework (the medial crura) assumes a particular conformation. Before the crura reach their vertical and sagittal position in the lower portion of the columella, at the turning point, they form a facet, a flat surface which breaks the continuity between the tip and the columella. This area is the tip-columella angle (Fig. 29–15), flanked on each side by the soft triangles. The tip-columella angle is present in most esthetically well-shaped Occidental noses. Below the angle, the remainder of the columella shows a gentle curve with a caudal convexity.

The Vestibule. The vestibule, the antechamber of the nasal fossa (Fig. 29–16), forms the caudal portion of the floor of the nose and extends under the dome of the alar cartilage; this area is known as the recess of the vestibule. The vestibule is separated from the nasal fossa proper by the caudal border of the lateral cartilage. From a physiologic standpoint, this is the most important anatomical

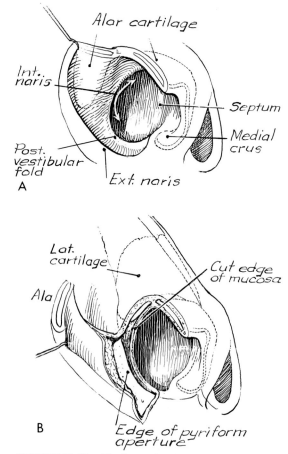

A

B

FIGURE 29–17. The internal and external nares. *A*, The internal naris (the nasal valve) is formed by the caudal border of the lateral cartilage. *B*, Dissection showing that the posterior vestibular fold extends along the border of the pyriform aperture, across the floor of the vestibule to the columella.

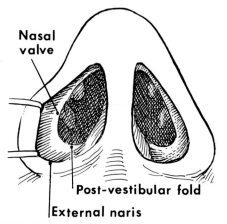

FIGURE 29–16. The nasal vestibule. The internal naris (the nasal valve), formed by the lower border of the lateral cartilage and prolonged downward along the floor of the nose by the posterior vestibular fold, constitutes the cephalic limit of the nasal vestibule.

structure of the nose. It is easily visible when one retracts the ala; the lower border of the lateral cartilage protrudes. This area was termed the "limen nasi" (the threshold of the nose) by Zuckerkandl (1892); Mink (1920) referred to it as the nasal valve. The fold formed by the protruding caudal border of the lateral cartilage is prolonged downward and medially along the crest of the pyriform aperture to form the posterior vestibular fold (Fig. 29–17). The crest with its overlying posterior vestibular fold delimits the vestibule cephalad along the floor of the nose and separates the vestibule from the nasal fossa proper.

The vestibule is delimited caudad by a medial extension of the alar border, the anterior narial fold. Thus, along the floor of the nose, the vestibule is delimited by the anterior narial fold caudad and by the posterior vestibular fold cephalad.

THE VESTIBULAR LINING AND THE NASAL MUCOUS MEMBRANE. The lining of the vestibule differs from the lining of the nasal fossa proper. The cutaneous lining of the vestibule — squamous epithelium — contains numerous hairs (the vibrissae) and sebaceous glands. The nasal valve controls the flow of air into the nasal fossa; thus the vestibule serves as an air-conditioning apparatus, warming, filtering, and moistening the inspired air.

The caudal border of the lateral cartilage is the portal of entry into the nasal fossa, which is lined by mucous membrane. The "respiratory" portion of the nasal fossa is lined by a delicate, pseudostratified, ciliated, columnar epithelium. Because of the important physiologic function of the nasal mucous membrane, its integrity must be preserved.

Over the nasal septum, the nasal mucous membrane is intimately connected to the underlying perichondrium and periosteum. When the septal framework is being exposed, these structures should be raised in unison as mucoperichondrium and mucoperiosteum.

In the cephalic portion of the nasal fossa, the mucous membrane has an olfactory function. Over the cephalic portion of the septum and the superior turbinate, the epithelium is no longer ciliated and is yellowish in color; it consists of supporting cells and olfactory cells.

The epithelial cells of the nasal mucous membrane, in association with the turbinates, play an important role in maintaining an equable temperature because they keep the surface always slightly lubricated.

The Membranous Septum. The membranous septum extends between the columella and the caudal border of the septal cartilage. Consisting of two layers of skin and intervening loose areolar tissue, the membranous septum is traversed by the paired depressor septi nasi muscles, which extend through the columella and membranous septum to insert over the caudal border and lateral aspect of the caudal portion of the septal cartilage. The loose membranous septum adds to the resiliency of the lower portion of the nose. In addition, the membranous septum plays an important part in nasal ventilation. In deep inspiration through the nose, the lips are contracted by the orbicularis oris muscle. The membranous septum and the columella are tensed by the depressor septi nasi muscles. Concomitantly, the internal nares (the nasal valves) are constricted, and the columella and membranous septum are tensed, causing the build-up of a negative intranasal pressure; dilatation of the nasal valves then controls the flow of air into the nasal fossae.

The sagittal dimension of the membranous septum varies. It is usually short in the upper portion, near the septal angle and also near the floor of the nose, and wider in its middle portion, where the columella assumes a caudad convex curve. It is subject to individual and ethnic variations, as are all of the other nasal structures.

Individual and Ethnic Anatomical Variations. Migrations of populations, invasions, and military conquests have resulted in admixtures of ethnic groups and the interaction of genetic factors. Thus there are innumerable variations of nasal structural characteristics. Wen (1921) studied the ontogeny and phylogeny of nasal cartilages in primates and in man. He noted structural differences in the nasal cartilages of white and black individuals (see Fig. 29–174). Rogers (1974) has reviewed the anthropologic literature concerning ethnic differences in nasal configuration.

From a practical clinical standpoint, among the people of the Western World, it is difficult to stereotype a patient's nose according to his ethnic origin. Usually Caucasians (the Caucasoids) have noses which vary from the short nose of the Irish, the thin, straight nose of the Scandinavians, and the longer nose of the French to the more aquiline nose of the Italians. The population of the Middle East (Armenoids) tends to have a convex dorsum, but again there are many exceptions. The sabras of Israel, for example, are quite different in appearance from Middle European or Russian Jews. There is one characteristic, however, frequently seen in Armenoids: the dislocation of the alar cartilages from the septal angle. When digital pressure is exerted over the tip of the nose, the tip is easily depressed from the septal angle, which then protrudes conspicuously under the skin in the supratip area.

A careful examination, clinical and photographic, not only of the nose but also of all the other features of the face, is essential if the plastic surgeon wishes to achieve a "natural"-appearing nose and a nose "that suits the face" and to avoid the appearance of the "surgical" nose.

The "standardized" concept of the nasal profile in the United States has been defined by Sheen (1975a): (1) the root of the nose is located at the level of the supratarsal fold; (2) the dorsum is relatively straight; (3) the tip projects more than the rest of the nasal profile; (4) the line from the tip to the base of the columella is not straight: it has a slight curve projecting caudad, and the curve is broken by the tip-columella junction; (5) the columella-labial angle is open (see Fig. 29–85, *C, D*); (6) the base of the columella should not project excessively, nor the upper lip be too short; (7) the base of the columella should have a caudal projection in relation to the base of each ala. Thus the columella-ala triangle is open (see Fig. 29–85, *A, B*).

On a frontal view the nasal configuration shows a series of curves. The nose is narrow at the root of the nose, then becomes broader, showing a gentle convexity in the region of the hump to narrow again immediately above the tip of the nose. The dorsum of the nose should be adequate in width and height to prevent a hyperteloric appearance between the eyes; the lower the dorsum, the wider apart the eyes appear. The tip of the nose should be differentiated from the remainder of the nose and be well defined. The base of the nose is in the shape of a rounded triangle, and the nares are tear-shaped.

Because of the uniqueness of the individual, noses and faces vary, and the corrective rhinoplasty must often of necessity be a compromise procedure.

The overshortened nose exhibiting its interior structures on a face with a wide bizygomatic dimension is an esthetic disaster. Prudence is required in corrective surgery in the older patient; the adolescent patient is, in most cases, the best candidate for corrective surgery.

Physiologic Considerations. In addition to being an important esthetic landmark and the site of olfaction, the nose is the main respiratory airway, the anatomy and physiology of which are often disturbed. A knowledge of respiratory rhinology is essential and should be acquired by those who intend to perform corrective nasal surgery.

The vestibules filter the air through their lining which contains mucus-secreting glands and vibrissae, entrapping foreign bodies and conditioning the temperature of the air current prior to its passage through the nasal valve. The air currents are further moistened by the secretions of the pseudostratified, ciliated, columnar epithelium of the nasal cavity. The air currents are influenced by a number of factors, including the structure and function of the cartilages of the external nose, the shape and directions

of the nasal septum, the size of the nasal turbinates, and the thickness of the nasal mucosa. Suppurative, allergic, and vasomotor diseases affecting the sinuses and nasal cavities cause swelling of the turbinates and nasal mucosa and restrict the dimensions of the nasal airway.

The most important function of the nose is to supply an adequate flow of properly conditioned air to the lungs. To achieve this the nose has other functions, including olfaction, filtration, heating and humidification of inspired air, and the ability to clean itself. Its direct communication with the paranasal sinuses results in an effect on the resonance of the voice. The average length of the nasal air passage in an adult is 10 cm. Within this distance, air of high or low moisture content, that is hot or cold, is converted to air approximately 31 to 37°C in temperature with a 75 per cent relative humidity. Exposure of inspired air to the nasal mucosa is enhanced by the anatomical arrangement of the turbinates and their relation to the nasal septum. The average width of the airway or column of air in the nose is 1 mm as it passes over, under, or beside the turbinates and septum. The air flow from the external naris passes to the internal nasal valve, where the airway narrows, increasing the velocity of flow while narrowing the column of air. From this point the flow continues along the middle meatus, between the middle turbinate and septum, and along the upper border of the middle turbinate. Larger particles of foreign material (15 microns and above) become trapped by the vibrissae or by the mucus blanket which coats the entire nasal mucosa. This is secreted by the goblet cells, present in all of the nasal mucosa except the olfactory epithelium of the cephalic portion of the nasal cavity. Here, the glands of Bowman secrete a serous fluid, whose function it is to dissolve air-borne substances into a liquid for interpretation by the bipolar olfactory cells (Smithdeal, 1975).

Lysozyme is an enzyme contained in nasal mucus and thought to be bactericidal. The nasal mucosal vascular apparatus responds like that elsewhere in the body to irritants, and submucosal vascular spaces (lakes) are responsible for engorgement or enlargement and shrinkage of the turbinates. The turbinates appear to be in a constant state of flux, one side being engorged while the contralateral side carries most of the air flow with cyclical alternations. Approximately 1 liter of water is added to inspired air daily. One third or more is recovered during nasal expiration. Thus, in cold, dry, high-altitude climates, the nose drips from secretion of more moisture than can be contained in its small volume.

The ciliary action of the pseudostratified, ciliated, columnar epithelium is continuous toward the nasopharynx. The cilia weaken and die from drying or become inactivated by strong drugs. Sinus air interchanges with nasal air pressure changes every 2 hours.

The physiology of nasal air flow appears to be highly complex, and the objective findings by various methods of measurement available at the present time are not adequate to explain many aspects of nasal ventilation. There are undoubtedly subjective factors involved in patients in whom objective findings of a satisfactory airway contrast with the complaint of nasal obstruction; other patients with obvious mechanical obstruction of the nose do not seem to be aware of it. It appears that some patients can utilize their defective structures, while others with fairly satisfactory nasal structures do not know how to use them.

Anatomical Factors Influencing Nasal Ventilation. Deviations of the septum are varied. The septum is subject to trauma as the result of a faulty position of the fetus in the uterus, as well as trauma at birth and during the postnatal period and early infancy. As mentioned previously, the caudal portion of the septal cartilage rests in a trough formed by the premaxillary wings of the premaxilla and extends to various degrees over the nasal spine, where the perichondrium surrounding the cartilage is continuous with the periosteum of the bone, providing a loose capsule which allows for a certain leeway in lateral movements of the septum.

Deviations in early childhood and septal deviations resulting from early childhood trauma show a developmental increase with growth and often cause deviation of the external nose. Septal fractures also occur as a result of injuries after nasal growth has been completed and are the usual accompaniment of nasal bone fractures.

A deviated septum is also found as a congenital malformation, sometimes showing a hereditary tendency; the lateral dislocation of the caudal portion of the septum is an example. Deviation of the septum is also a usual deformity in congenital malformations such as cleft lip and palate.

A majority of the population has some degree of septal deviation which must be carefully examined prior to a nasal operation.

Loss of support of the nasal tip resulting from an inadequate position of the septal angle will result in a drooping tip. In this type of deformity, the air currents are deviated from their normal course, a noticeable improvement in nasal breathing occurring when the tip is raised by finger pressure.

The cartilages of the nose are subjected to movements by the nasal musculature (see Fig. 29–5) and play an important role in nasal physiology. Malfunction of the external musculature and of the alar cartilages is seen in certain patients who show an indrawing and collapse of the alae during inspiration. Patients with this type of malfunction usually have elongated external nares with slitlike openings.

Nasal ventilation is dependent upon the action of the lateral and alar cartilages, the contraction of the nasal musculature, and passive movements due to variations of intranasal pressure. Malfunction of the external nose may result from injury; faulty surgical procedures, such as destruction of a part of the nasal musculature in an effort to thin the nasal structures; excessive removal of cartilage and consequently of the framework upon which the nasal musculature acts; excessive resection of cartilage and mucous membrane lining, which restricts the opening of the nasal valve; operative procedures producing rigidity in the mobile membranous septum and columella; overshortening of the septal cartilage; and excision of the membranous septum, or injudicious insertion of cartilage between the layers of the membranous septum. This procedure stiffens the mobile cartilaginous nose (the lobule) and impairs its function. *Preservation of the nasal valve by avoiding excessive resection of cartilage and mucous membrane, scarring, and stenosis is one of the most important precautions to observe in corrective rhinoplasty.*

In conclusion, the nose is not a static structure to be shaped at will in plastic surgical operations; avoidance of injury to the nasal musculature and the preservation of the dynamics of the nasal cartilages are important considerations.

CORRECTIVE SURGERY OF THE NOSE

General Considerations

As recounted in Chapter 1, the development of plastic surgery has been closely associated with the development of reconstructive rhinoplasty. Only in the present century has the technique of corrective rhinoplasty become a frequently performed operation. The operation is required to improve the shape of the nose for purely esthetic reasons; to straighten a deviated nose, thereby also establishing adequate airways; and, less frequently, to correct a depression along the dorsum.

Examination and Diagnosis

Extranasal Examination. The shape and size of the nose are readily evaluated by direct inspection: the convexity or concavity of the dorsum, the width or projection of the tip, the deviation of the nose, the shape of the columella and the thickness of the skin. The thickness of the skin is of considerable importance. Skin thickened by hypertrophic sebaceous glands is rigid and drapes inadequately over the remodeled caudal portion of the nose. The alar cartilages are readily identified in the long nose with thin skin, but their outline is more difficult to identify when the skin is thick. When a tip operation is done in a nose with thick skin, thin, nearly atrophic alar cartilages are characteristic, whereas in the nose with thin skin, the cartilages are usually well developed.

Palpation along the dorsum is helpful in detecting a curvature of the dorsal border of the septum and the position of the septal angle. Digital pressure over the tip will show the relationship of the alar cartilages and the septal angle. This test is particularly important. If the alar cartilages are dislocated caudally from the septal angle and the membranous septum is unduly elongated, resection of the caudal portion of the septum is contraindicated because the deformity would be accentuated.

Intranasal Examination. Careful intranasal examination with a speculum under adequate lighting, such as is provided by a headlight, and, if necessary, after application of a topical vasoconstrictor, such as 1 per cent Neo-Synephrine, will usually show any abnormality, including the cause of nasal obstruction. The simplest test for nasal obstruction is to occlude one nostril at a time and listen and evaluate the passage of air while the patient breathes through the opposite nasal passage.

Planning the Operation. The patient who requests an esthetic improvement may not have a functional problem. The surgeon should question the patient concerning the functional impairment, if one is present, resulting from the deformity. He should also note the patient's psychologic reaction to what may seem to be a relatively minor defect as well as to a deformity of greater magnitude. The patient's motivation to cooperate with the surgeon in achieving a satisfactory result should be evaluated.

Listening to the patient is of particular importance in esthetic surgery. Beware of autotistic patients with unrealistic expectations and particularly of patients who cannot pinpoint what they think is wrong. These patients are dangerous because they may never be satisfied.

By listening to the patient, the surgeon may detect a deep-seated psychologic disturbance, precluding the operation (see Chapters 21 and 22). The young surgeon is often anxious to operate and may undertake an operation that may not satisfy the patient: *a satisfactory result is what satisfies the patient.*

Photography is useful in determining the indications for an operation, whether corrective or reconstructive. Professional photographs (see Chapter 1) taken with standardized position, lighting, and exposure permit the patient to see himself as he really is. The photographs should include the full face, two profiles, a smiling view, which will show the caudal displacement of the tip from overactive depressor septi nasi muscles, and a basal or "worm's eye" view. "Do I really look like that?" is a remark often made.

Patients may request certain modifications of their facial structures which the surgeon may not agree upon. The surgeon is best qualified through his experience to know what can and cannot be achieved and what is best for the patient. The photograph is useful because it permits the patient first to react to his own image, second to point out to the surgeon what he thinks is wrong, and third to give the surgeon an opportunity to describe what corrective measures should and can achieve a satisfactory result. In this way an understanding is reached between the patient and the surgeon before the operation, thus avoiding a postoperative misunderstanding.

Certain modifications made on a profile matte-finished photograph are useful to show the patient how his appearance can be improved. Similar modifications can be made on a lateral cephalogram to show the change in the shape of the nose and the need for chin augmentation (Fig. 29–18). The patient thus has a preoperative concept of how he will look after the operation. The surgeon must be able to achieve what he has proposed.

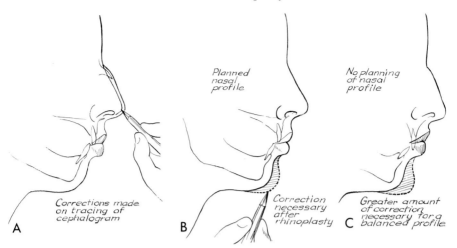

FIGURE 29–18. Nose-chin relationships; planning of a balanced profile. Such planning may be done on photographic prints prepared without a glossy finish, from tracings of photographs on transparent paper, or as shown in the illustrations from tracings of a cephalometric roentgenogram. *A*, Proposed change in the nasal profile. Note the prominence of the nose in relation to the underdeveloped chin. *B*, The nasal profile has been modified, and the outline of the chin is also traced to provide a guide for the chin augmentation. *C*, The nasal profile has not been changed, but the overall appearance is improved. A greater amount of chin augmentation is necessary to achieve an acceptable facial profile.

Misunderstandings between the patient and surgeon, some resulting in legal action, usually result from a lack of communication. Careful explanation of the possibilities and impossibilities is essential. There is a tendency to shape the nose according to preconceived standards of beauty applicable to all patients. As stated earlier in the text, this often leads to a stultified, stereotyped nose which is obviously a "surgical" nose. A "natural"-looking nose, even though less "perfect," is preferable.

In planning a nasal plastic correction, it is essential to consider the entire face. In a broad

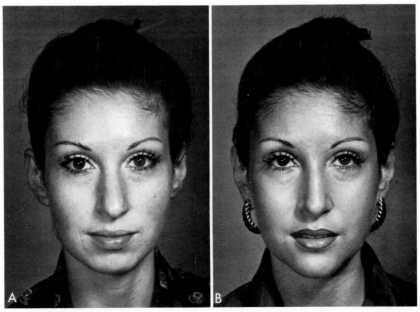

FIGURE 29–19. Corrective rhinoplasty in the long face with deficiency of the chin. *A*, Preoperative appearance. Note the broad tip, the long nose with a downward dislocated tip, and the underdeveloped chin. *B*, Postoperative appearance. The nasal length has been reduced, but sufficient length is retained to maintain harmony with the face. Chin augmentation has assisted in improving the facial appearance.

face, it would be an error to overshorten the nose. When the patient's upper lip is shortened by the impingement of the nose and septum upon this structure, shortening of the nose will provide not only a suitable nasal contour but also a more satisfactory length of the upper lip. The position and shape of the chin should also be considered, since an underdeveloped chin increases the relative prominence of the nose. In the patient shown in Figure 29–19, adequate nasal length was maintained for a harmonious face-nose relationship, while chin augmentation was indicated because of a deficiency of the mental symphysis.

Increase in the projection and augmentation of the chin by a variety of methods, which include an inorganic chin implant or horizontal advancement osteotomy (see Chapter 30), may be necessary in order to obtain facial balance (Figs. 29–20 and 29–21). Diminution of the forward projection of the chin is required in mandibular prognathism; a subsequent correc-

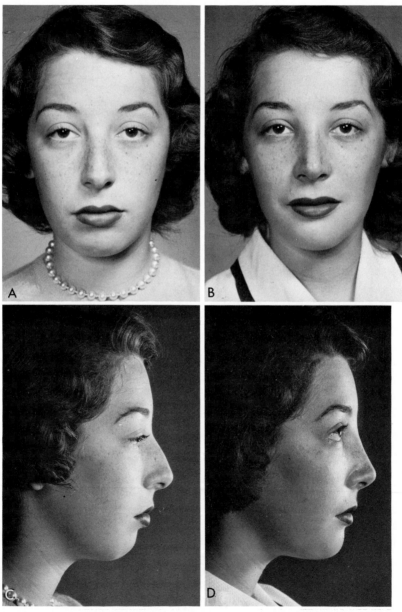

FIGURE 29–20.   Corrective rhinoplasty and chin augmentation. *A, C,* Preoperative views. *B, D,* After a corrective rhinoplasty and increase of the projection of the chin, a balanced profile is attained.

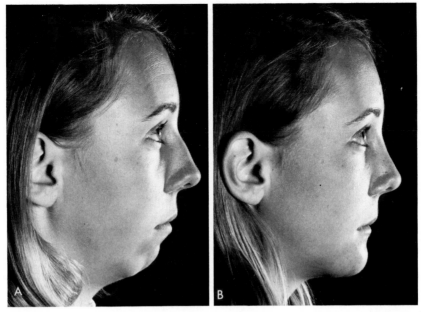

FIGURE 29–21. The importance of the chin in the facial profile. *A,* The major deformity is obviously in the mandible, yet the patient had requested only a corrective rhinoplasty. *B,* After a conservative corrective rhinoplasty and chin augmentation (for further details, see Chapter 30).

tive rhinoplasty may be necessary to improve facial appearance.

Changes in nasal shape can be visualized in the long nose with a convex dorsum by covering a portion of the dorsum with the index finger and elevating the tip.

The change in the shape of the nose should be evaluated in repose and during smiling.

The success of the operation will depend as much upon the esthetic judgment and the artistic ability of the surgeon as upon his technical skill. Aufricht (1961) has pointed out that a change in the shape of the nose is a serious undertaking equivalent to changing the entire face. A felicitous marriage of the concept of the finished masterpiece and the technical skill to achieve it is the secret of success.

Aside from considerations involving the patient's facial type, the particular anatomy of the nose in which corrective surgery is being considered should be taken into account. The long, thin nose with fine, textured skin is ideal for surgery. The broad nose with thick skin is always unfavorable.

It seems paradoxical that the long nose with thin skin frequently has overdeveloped cartilages, so that any change in their contour can be embarrassingly evident through the thin skin. On the other hand, the patient with thick skin, which hides the reductive incisions through the cartilage, frequently has thin cartilages, making changes in contour difficult and at times impossible.

Certain anatomical limitations are obvious. It is impossible to modify the points of attachment of the alae to the face without producing visible scars; an excision of tissue from the base of the nostrils assists in diminishing the flare of the nostrils and the width of the nostril floor, but it still will not modify the actual points of attachment of the alae to the face. In some cases a compromise procedure is necessary, and in very broad noses it may be advantageous to increase the projection of the dorsum and tip in order to produce a relative narrowing.

In many cases the ideal cannot be achieved. Most corrective nasal operations are a compromise. It is in establishing this compromise that the surgeon's esthetic judgment plays a major role.

Anesthesia. Local anesthesia is commonly employed for corrective nasal plastic surgery.

The importance of correct preoperative medication must be emphasized. An adequately sedated patient experiences minimal bleeding during the operation, whereas a nervous patient may bleed profusely. No direct relationship exists between the quantity of the medication administered and the resultant sedation because of the variable susceptibility of different individuals. Patients with the sleeping pill habit require larger initial doses of medication.

A subliminal type of anesthesia can be achieved by the careful selection and dosage of sedative drugs. The patient is sleeping through most of the procedure and is mostly unaware that he is undergoing an operation. An example of a preoperative medication protocol is the following:

1. A hypnotic the night before operation, Seconal (secobarbital) 100 mg per os or Dalmane (flurazepam) 30 mg per os.

2. Preoperative medication: two hours prior to surgery, Valium (diazepam) 10 to 15 mg per os; one hour prior to surgery, Pantopon (hydrochlorides of opium alkaloids) 10 to 20 mg intramuscularly, and Thorazine (chlorpromazine) 15 to 25 mg intramuscularly. An intravenous dextrose infusion is started before the operation and is used to administer small amounts of Valium (2.5 mg at a time) to maintain sedation as needed. Valium is preferred as a preoperative and intraoperative sedative because it is amnestic. Most patients are heavily sedated under this premedication protocol and do not require additional medication.

Dosage of all agents should be adjusted to meet the needs of the individual patient. Patients of light frame and build should receive reduced amounts of all agents.

Hypotensive general anesthesia administered via an intratracheal tube provides a bloodless field. This more complex technique is not advisable in the average corrective rhinoplasty. A considerable diminution in the amount of bleeding during a conventional anesthesia with intratracheal intubation (when required) can be obtained by local infiltration

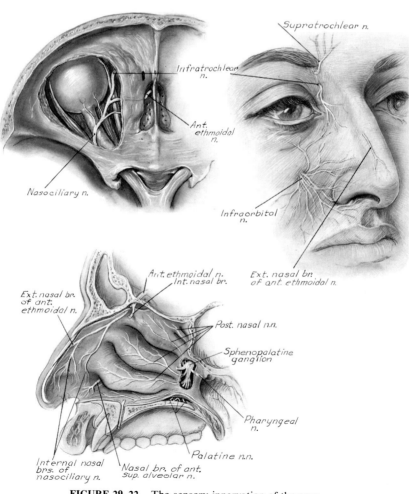

FIGURE 29–22. The sensory innervation of the nose.

of Xylocaine*-Adrenalin solution prior to induction.

Careful reassurance on the part of the surgeon is necessary at all times for the apprehensive patient; gaining the patient's confidence is an indispensable condition for satisfactory anesthesia.

TOPICAL AND INFILTRATION ANESTHESIA. Both topical and infiltration anesthesia are required in nasal plastic surgery. The sensory innervation of the nose is illustrated in Figures 29–22 and 29–23. It is derived from two main sources: the anterior ethmoidal nerve and the sphenopalatine ganglion.

Topical anesthesia precedes infiltration anesthesia. Prior to draping, a 4 per cent cocaine solution is sprayed into each nasal fossa, providing superficial topical analgesia and also vasoconstriction. After the patient has been

*Lidocaine.

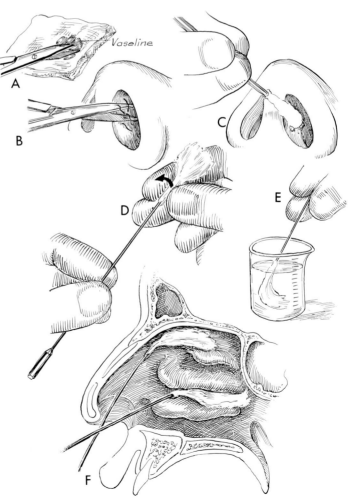

FIGURE 29–23. The sensory innervation of the nasal septum.

FIGURE 29–24. Preparation and topical anesthesia. *A*, Blunt-end scissors are smeared with petrolatum jelly. *B*, The vibrissae in the vestibule are cut and adhere to the petrolatum jelly on the scissors. *C* The vestibule is cleansed. *D*, Method of preparing cotton-tipped applicator by rotating the instrument. Applicators are made of copper and are supple. *E*, The cotton-tipped copper applicator is dipped into the solution and then squeezed dry. *F*, Position of the applicators: one is placed under the dorsum of the nose to provide anesthesia of the anterior ethmoidal nerve; the other is placed into the posterior portion of the middle meatus, where the anesthetic solution blocks the sphenopalatine ganglion. If the middle meatus cannot be entered, the applicators are placed between the middle turbinate and the septum.

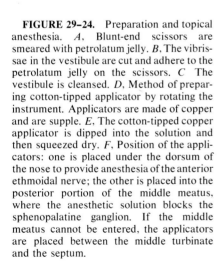

prepared and draped, cotton-tipped copper wire applicators are dipped in a solution of 5 per cent cocaine. The applicators are supple and serrated at the ends. Shredded cotton is twisted (always in one direction) and anchored to the serrations, so that the cotton will not remain in the nasal cavity when the applicator is removed. Because they are supple, the copper applicators can be introduced without causing the patient a sensation of pain or pressure (Fig. 29–24). The cotton should be squeezed to eliminate excess cocaine and thus avoid dripping of the drug into the naso-pharynx. This technique is preferable to the use of strips (or packs), which expose the patient to unnecessary larger amounts of cocaine solution.

One applicator is introduced through the nasal passage, under the dorsum to the root of the nose, where the anterior ethmoidal nerve enters the nasal cavity. The other applicator is placed, if possible, into the middle meatus situated beneath the middle turbinate and backward over the sphenopalatine ganglion, thus applying the anesthetic solution to the nerve branches from the ganglion which innervate the lateral wall. It is essential, however, to avoid any discomfort which will arouse the sedated patient. Unless the middle meatus is readily accessible, the cotton is placed between the septum and the middle turbinate. The applicators are retained in position for a few minutes.

Topical application is followed by *infiltration anesthesia* with local anesthetic solution. A solution of 1 per cent Xylocaine (or procaine) mixed with a fresh solution of 1:1000 epinephrine (Adrenalin) at a concentration of 1:50,000 is employed. A higher concentration of epinephrine may be added if a small volume of solution (3 to 5 ml) is sufficient to induce local anesthesia.

When a small volume of solution is adequate, the entire nose may be injected, blocking the branches from the supra- and infratrochlear nerves and from the infraorbital, the nasopalatine, and the external nasal nerves.

The anesthetic solution may also be injected in stages. Adverse reactions such as tachycardia, palpitations, headache, nervousness, restlessness, and anxiety are avoided; the hemostatic action of the epinephrine does not appear to be diminished by the fact that each operative stage immediately follows the injection.

The internal naris (the nasal valve) is exposed by retracting the ala. The solution is injected through a fine gauge needle into the tissues immediately above the caudal border of the lateral cartilage and directed toward the root of the nose (Fig. 29–25, *A, B*). The plane of infiltration should follow the outer surface of the cartilage and bone. Another injection is made at the junction of the lateral cartilage and septum (Fig. 29–25, *C*). A third injection is made in the region of the septal angle (Fig. 29–25, *D*). Additional solution is injected between

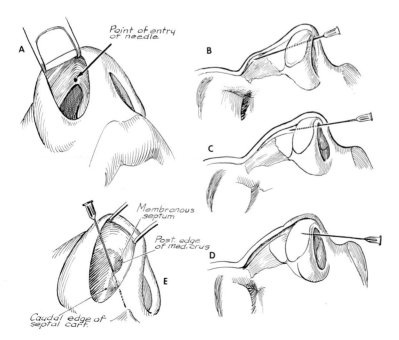

FIGURE 29–25. Corrective rhinoplasty under local anesthesia. *A*, Point of insertion of the needle. *B*, The needle is introduced between the alar and the lateral cartilages and passes over the lateral cartilage, the solution being injected at the root of the nose. *C*, An injection is then made at the junction of the lateral cartilage with the septum. *D*, The injection is continued on toward the septal angle. *E*, The anesthetic solution is infiltrated within the two layers of the membranous septum at its base.

the layers of the membranous septum to block the nasopalatine nerve (Fig. 29–25, *E*). The left ala is retracted, and an injection similar to the first one on the right side is made by placing the needle over the lateral cartilage and infiltrating toward the root of the nose. Additional injections on the left side are unnecessary, for the injections on the right side have already infiltrated the areas. The slight change of contour produced by the injection is insignificant, as only a small amount of solution is injected.

Block anesthesia is also feasible by injecting around the base of the nasal pyramid; however, in this technique the hemostatic benefits of the local infiltration of epinephrine are lost.

Adequate sedation, a high concentration of epinephrine, and careful dissection all contribute toward the control of bleeding during the operation.

In children and in the occasional patient who reacts unfavorably to local anesthesia, general anesthesia administered by tracheal intubation may be indicated.

TECHNIQUE OF CORRECTIVE RHINOPLASTY

Some Preliminary Landmarks. When the patient is on the operating table inclined at a 30° angle, the head tilted downward (Fig. 29–26), after topical anesthesia and prior to infiltration anesthesia it is essential to locate various landmarks before the first incision is made.

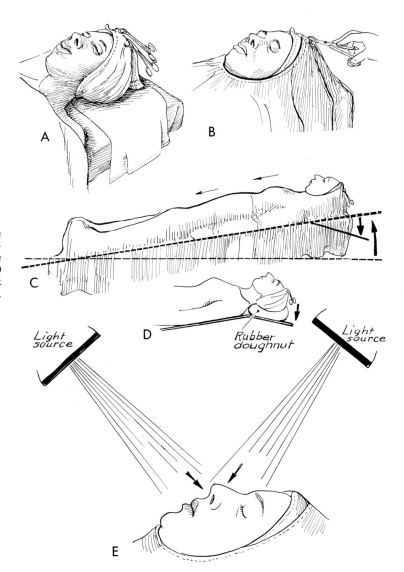

FIGURE 29–26. Position of the patient on the operating table, draping, and lighting. *A, B,* Draping the patient. *C,* Inclination of the table 30 degrees. *D,* The head is tilted back and rested on a rubber doughnut pad. *E,* Position of the operating lights.

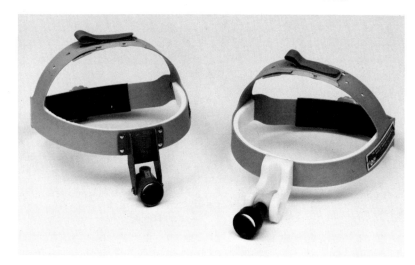

FIGURE 29-27. Two types of fiberoptic headlights that provide excellent visibility for intranasal surgery. (Designs for Vision Inc.)

Good illumination is essential. A fiberoptic headlight provides the best illumination of the intranasal structures (Fig. 29-27). A fiberoptic angulated retractor enables the surgeon to see accurately any irregularity of the structures along the dorsum (Fig. 29-28).

Palpation along the dorsum indicates the position of the septal angle. The relationship of the septal angle to the alar cartilages determines the advisability of resecting a portion of

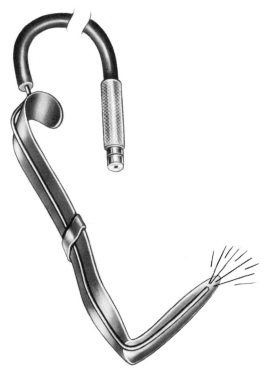

FIGURE 29-28. The rhinoscope, a fiberoptic, illuminated, angulated retractor for the examination of the skeletal dorsum of the nose (Storz).

the caudal part of the septal cartilage. If the tip is dislocated downward from the septal angle, it is no longer supported by this structure. An attempt to shorten the nose by resecting cartilage from the caudal portion of the septum would only increase the downward dislocation of the tip. The septum must not be shortened; on the contrary, it may be necessary to reattach the alar cartilages to the septal angle by the invagination procedure (see Fig. 29-81).

The degree of protrusion of the septal angle should also be considered in relation to the proposed profile line, for in the humped nose, the septal angle may be situated high in relation to the alar cartilages. The position of the septal angle may be determined by inspection and palpation, and slight downward pressure on the tip of the nose will cause it to protrude.

Aufricht (1943) described the finger test to determine the amount of shortening required (Fig. 29-29). This test, however, provides only an estimate of the amount of shortening required, as the tip of the nose assumes a new position as soon as the transfixion procedure is completed at the end of the first stage of the operation.

Surface landmarks may be indicated on the skin of the nose. Upward traction of the skin of the supratip area causes blanching of the skin at the domes of the alar cartilages, thus locating the position of these structures (Fig. 29-30). A line is drawn at the cephalic margin of each alar cartilage to outline these structures. An ink line divides the lateral crus into a cephalic and a caudal portion; the cephalic portion includes the undesirable convexity of the tip and is of variable width. Such ink landmarks are an aid during the operation.

The size and shape of the columella, its de-

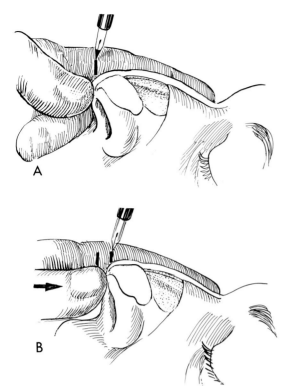

FIGURE 29–29. Finger test to determine the amount of required shortening of the nose. (After Aufricht, 1943.) *A*, The index finger is placed on the side of the dorsum, the tip of the finger resting on the root of the nose. The thumb, placed at the tip, indicates the actual length of the nose. *B*, The tip of the nose is raised by thumb pressure until the desired shortening is obtained. The distance is marked on the index finger.

gree of protrusion in relation to the base of the alae, and the angle at which it meets the lip are noted. Abnormalities or deviations of the septum or turbinates should also be noted after careful examination by means of a headlight.

The various deformities demand different approaches and procedures. An order of procedure is helpful, however, not only in teaching but also in the operative treatment of the most common nasal deformity, the nose with a dorsal hump which may be too long or too large, with varying abnormalities of the nasal tip.

Evolution of Techniques. Before describing in detail one approach to the corrective rhinoplasty, it is helpful to review the evolution of the techniques and the order of procedure arrived at by present-day surgeons.

The Joseph technique, introduced in the United States by Aufricht and Safian, has been employed as a routine procedure for rhinoplasty, minor modifications being devised by individual surgeons. The usual order of proce-

dure is to make bilateral intercartilaginous incisions, skeletonize the nose, resect the dorsal osteocartilaginous hump with a saw (Fig. 29–31), perform lateral osteotomies with a saw, a medial osteotomy and outfracture (Aufricht), and a Joseph or Safian-type tip operation (see Figs. 29–108 and 29–109).

The operation is successful in the hands of experienced surgeons. Less experienced surgeons often obtain good results in the correction of the large hump nose. Because too much hump was often resected by less experienced surgeons, it was a frequent observation that many patients showed a concave dorsum, and it became evident that teaching the beginner the art of modifying the profile of the nose with a saw was a difficult undertaking.

For these reasons, a different order of procedure was gradually developed as patients began to request the correction of less obvious defects and a safer and more prudent approach was needed.

Because of the many variations in the types and degree of nasal deformity, it would appear to oversimplify the problem to promote a "routine" order of procedure. Some believe one should correct the most obvious deformity first. There are also cases in which some of the procedures of a "routine" technique are not indicated. In the teaching of rhinoplasty, however, it is helpful to advise a sequence in the operative procedures of the corrective rhinoplasty.

Fomon (1960) and Cottle (1960) performed routine septal resection procedures as part of

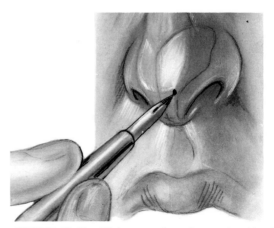

FIGURE 29–30. Slight upward traction on the skin of of the supratip area causes blanching of the skin at the domes of the alar cartilages. The position of the dome can thus be located and marked with ink. Slight pressure over the tip of the nose will also help to locate the most projecting point of the dome.

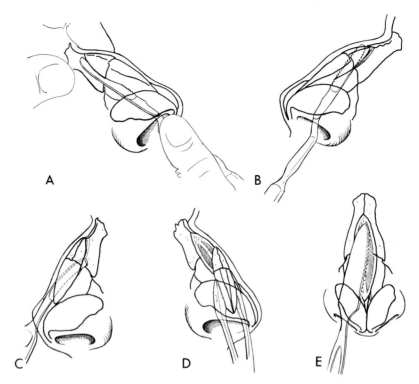

FIGURE 29–31. Resection of the dorsal hump by a saw according to the Joseph technique. *A*, A bayonet saw is placed on the right side of the hump and the resection is accomplished by a backhand technique. *B*, Completion of the hump resection from the left side. *C*, The button knife, placed beneath the hump, severs the remaining connections of the lateral and septal cartilages. *D*, The hump is removed with the hump removal forceps. *E*, Irregularities along the line of osteotomy, if present, are smoothed with a rasp. This is a satisfactory technique in experienced hands.

the nasalplasty. Aufricht performs a limited submucous resection to compensate for the narrowing of the nose. Fomon advocated complete resection of the septal framework, a technique that did not survive. Cottle used a "hemitransfixion" incision, an incision along the caudal border of the septum, as a routine approach to the septum and as a first procedure in the rhinoplasty. He was one of the first to advocate a "submucous" approach to spare the nasal valves.

Routine extensive septal operations are performed less frequently than previously. The septum is a source of the best transplant material in case the patient requires a secondary rhinoplasty; thus limited amounts of cartilage are removed if the patient requires a cartilage graft in the course of the primary operation or has nasal airway obstruction (see later section on septal surgery, p. 1131). Most patients have some degree of septal deviation, but many are symptomless.

Two principal modifications of the Joseph technique have evolved over the years: (1) the corrective surgery is begun at the caudal portion of the nose and the remainder of the nasal

skeletal framework is adapted according to the degree of projection of the tip; and (2) the bony dorsum is lowered as a first step and the cartilaginous portion is aligned to conform to the bony profile (Sheen, 1976) (see Fig. 29–94).

Whereas in the Joseph technique, after resection of the osteocartilaginous hump, the tip is approached from the undersurface of the alar cartilage (from below) (see Fig. 29–108), Sheen (1976) has advocated realigning the entire cartilaginous dorsum through a subcutaneous approach (from above), retracting the soft tissues to obtain adequate exposure of the cartilaginous vault and approaching the nasal tip cartilages through rim incisions (see Fig. 29–110). These various techniques are discussed later in the text.

RHINOPLASTY FOR THE HUMP NOSE: AN ORDER OF PROCEDURE

The operation follows an order of procedure composed of six stages. The advantage of this

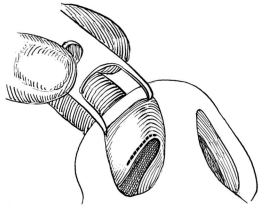

FIGURE 29–32. After retraction of the ala and eversion of the alar cartilage, the caudal border of the lateral cartilage (the nasal valve) comes into view. The incision is indicated by the line of junction between the red mucosa and the white vestibular skin. The incision can be extended laterally for a wider exposure of the nasal dorsum.

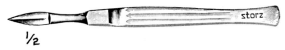

FIGURE 29–34. Modified Joseph knife.

orderly approach is the complete control maintained by the surgeon in his step by step modification of the profile.

Stage 1: Uncovering the Nasal Framework. The right ala is retracted. The ala retractor straddles the most projecting and most caudal point of the dome, previously indicated by an ink mark. The caudal border of the lateral cartilage comes into view (Fig. 29–32). The intercartilaginous incision is made between the alar and lateral cartilages. The incision should be long enough to allow adequate subsequent retraction and examination of the entire dorsum. The alar cartilage overlaps the lateral cartilage when the nose is in repose. When the ala is retracted, the overlap is accentuated and a line of mucous membrane is protracted with the alar cartilage. It is along this red line at the junction with the vestibular

lining that the intercartilaginous incision is made (Fig. 29–33, *A*). The alar cartilage is elevated by the retractor; thus it is not incised. The length of the incision, which should always extend to the midline, varies with the size of the hump to be removed and also depends upon the amount of alar cartilage to be freed during the tip surgery.

Although it is a rule to avoid resecting vestibular lining, in the case of the long nose with large vestibules, a small amount of vestibular lining is removed. The intercartilaginous incision is made a few millimeters caudad to the usual site between the lateral and alar cartilages. The excess vestibular lining is then removed when the caudal portion of the lateral cartilage is trimmed.

A double-blade Joseph knife (Fig. 29–34) is used to dissect the soft tissues from the lateral cartilage, extending the dissection to the midline (see Fig. 29–33, *B*) and slightly over the midline, the edge of the blade being used to sever the tissues over the septum and to facilitate the subsequent transfixion procedure. The plane of dissection should be as close as possible to the cartilage, thus preventing injury to the overlying musculature of the nose; little bleeding occurs, for the blood vessels of the nose are more superficial. The sharp dissection also extends over the lateral cartilage to the lower border of the nasal bones.

An incision is then made in the periosteum near the caudal border of the nasal bones with

FIGURE 29–33. The uncovering of the nasal framework. *A*, The intercartilaginous incision is of variable length, depending on the size of the hump to be resected, but always extends medially to the dorsal border of the septum. *B*, Sharp dissection over the lateral cartilage. *C*, The tip of the knife palpates the lower border of the nasal bone and incises the periosteum. A similar procedure is done on the contralateral side.

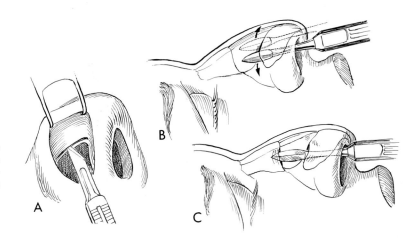

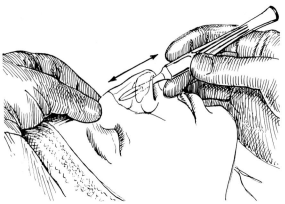

FIGURE 29–35. Position of the Joseph knife. The handle of the knife should be parallel to the dorsum of the nose to avoid perforation of the skin by the point of the knife.

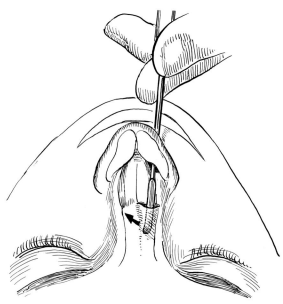

FIGURE 29–37. The periosteal elevator raising the periosteum over the bony dorsum.

the tip of the Joseph knife (see Fig. 29–33, *C*). The handle of the knife should be maintained along a plane parallel with that of the dorsum of the nose to avoid buttonholing the skin with the tip of the instrument (Fig. 29–35). A periosteal elevator is placed through the incision, and the periosteum is elevated to and over the midline (Figs. 29–36 and 29–37). Similar procedures are repeated on the left side.

Subperiosteal elevation over the nasal bones is routine, with less bleeding occurring than above the periosteal level. The elevated periosteum also serves to prevent adhesions of the overlying soft tissue to the modified nasal framework.

THE TRANSFIXION INCISION.   The next procedure is known as the transfixion incision, a technique in which the soft tissues overlying the dorsum are separated from the septum (see

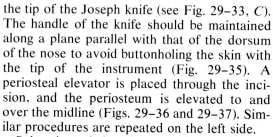

FIGURE 29–36. The periosteal elevator has been inserted through the incision in the periosteum and elevates the periosteum from the nasal bone. The periosteum is then raised on the contralateral side.

Variations in the Transfixion Incision, p. 1100). The procedure is facilitated if the surgeon moves to the head of the table and executes the maneuver from this position. A curved button knife is introduced through the intercartilaginous incision at the right internal naris into the subperiosteal pocket over the nasal bones (Fig. 29–38, *A*). An incision is made with the button knife (Fig. 29–39) along the dorsal border of the septum (Fig. 29–38, *B*) until the tip of the knife reaches the intercartilaginous incision at the internal naris of the opposite side (Fig. 29–38, *C*). The tip of the button knife, which may be palpated with the operator's left index finger as it reaches the incision at the left internal naris, protrudes into the left vestibule, and the incision is continued to the septal angle (Fig. 29–40 *A*). Prior to the incision along the caudal border of the septum, the membranous septum is tensed by a forward pull on the columella by the assistant, employing hooks, and the tip of the nose is retracted (Fig. 29–41); the button knife is then rotated approximately 90 degrees, cutting along the caudal margin of the septal cartilage towards its base (Fig. 29–40, *B*). Forward traction upon the columella ensures that the transfixion knife cuts flush against the caudal margin of the septal cartilage, leaving the membranous septum attached to the columella (Fig. 29–40, *B*). Thus, if septal cartilage is sub-

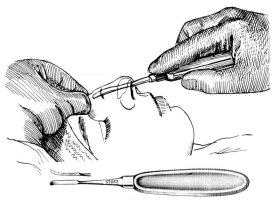

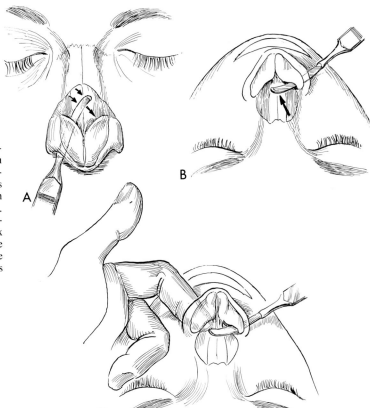

FIGURE 29–38. The transfixion incision. *A,* Position of the curved button knife which has been placed in the subperiosteal pocket over the nasal bones and which separates the structures from the dorsal border of the septal cartilage. *B,* Position of the button knife as it approaches the septal angle. *C,* The index finger of the left hand palpates inside the vestibule and feels for the tip of the knife projecting through the intercartilaginous incision.

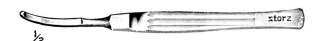

½

FIGURE 29–39. Curved button knife used for the transfixion procedure.

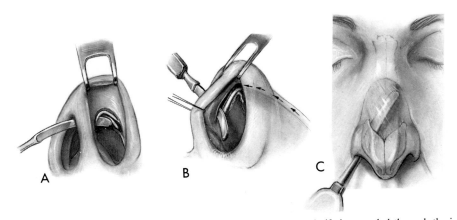

FIGURE 29–40. Completion of the transfixion procedure. *A,* The button knife is extruded through the intercartilaginous incision on the contralateral side. *B,* The incision is extended around the septal angle and downward along the caudal border of the septum. Note the upward retraction of the tip, and the forward traction on the columella by two hooks. The transfixion incision is extended to the nasal spine with a scalpel or scissors, when indicated. *C,* The Joseph periosteal elevator verifies that the skeletal structures have been separated from the covering soft tissues.

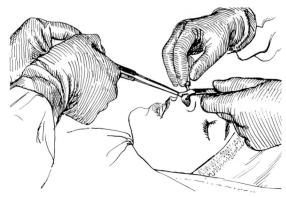

FIGURE 29–41. Completion of the transfixion incision. The operator retracts the tip upward; the assistant exerts forward traction upon the columella and the membranous septum.

sequently resected from its caudal portion, the membranous septum, which remains attached to the columella, is preserved. An exception is made when the sagittal dimension of the membranous septum is excessively increased, as in the nose with the hanging columella: the button knife incises the structure caudad to the septum, and a portion of the membranous sep-

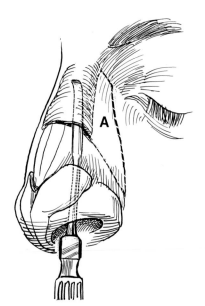

FIGURE 29–42. The outlined area delimits the area of undisturbed periosteum between the dorsal portion of the nose and the line of the lateral osteotomy, as indicated by the letter *A*. The periosteum over the dorsal portion of the nose is raised over an area sufficient to permit resection of the dorsal hump. The larger the hump, the wider will be the area of subperiosteal elevation. In the average corrective rhinoplasty, the procedure illustrated is employed; it has the advantage of leaving an area of undisturbed periosteum between the lateral osteotomy line and the dorsum of the nose.

tum is resected with the cartilaginous septum when the latter is shortened.

A #15 blade or a pair of scissors extend the transfixion toward the nasal spine if surgery upon the nasal spine and the base of the septal cartilage is required. Scissors free the tissues around the nasal spine. The periosteal elevator verifies that the exposure of the nasal framework is completed (Fig. 29–40, *C*).

In the average rhinoplasty, it is preferable to elevate the soft tissues over an area only wide enough to permit resection of the nasal dorsal hump, leaving intact the tissue on the lateral aspect of the nose (Fig. 29–42). In large noses and in older patients, the raising of soft tissues over a wide area allows for a more rapid redistribution of the skin over the reduced skeletal framework. An incision through the periosteum over the lateral aspect of the lateral wall on each side also assists in the redraping of the soft tissues in the large nose.

Stage 2: Lowering the Septal Profile; Shortening the Septum; Correcting the Nasal Tip

FREEING THE LATERAL CARTILAGES FROM THEIR ATTACHMENT TO THE SEPTUM. An angulated retractor, such as the Aufricht retractor or a modification of the retractor (Converse) (Fig. 29–43), elevates the soft tissues over the dorsum of the nose. The major portion of each lateral cartilage is now detached from the septum with a #11 (pointed) blade (Fig. 29–44, *A*). As illustrated in Figure 29–44, *B*, the mucoperichondrium has been raised, after infiltrating the anesthetic solution

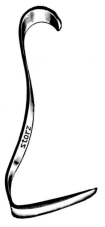

FIGURE 29–43. Angulated retractor used for examination of the dorsum and detachment of the lateral cartilages.

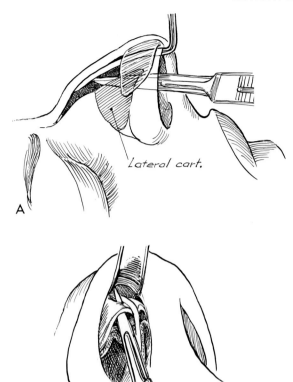

FIGURE 29-44. *A*, Severing the attachment of the lateral cartilage to the septum. *B*, As shown in the drawing, the mucoperichondrium lining the lateral cartilage has been undermined and separated from the cartilage and is not incised. The most cephalic portion of each lateral cartilage is not severed from the septum and remains attached to the nasal bone.

tures. Under direct vision with angulated scissors (Fig. 29–45), the dorsal border is trimmed, starting at the septal angle, so that the nasal tip stands free without support from the septum (Fig. 29–46). It must be emphasized that the resection of dorsal septal cartilage is done along an oblique line and does not involve the cephalic portion of the septum near the nasal bones.

The medial portions of the lateral cartilages are not trimmed at this stage; they will be adjusted to the dorsal border of the septum during the fifth stage. Thus they are trimmed only once.

At this point in the operation, the relationship between the nasal tip and the dorsum usually changes. For example, in the nose with a short columella, the tip, which has been tethered by this structure, will assume a more cephalad and projected position. The amount of shortening of the septum may then be less than originally planned. The change of position of the nasal tip is particularly noticeable in noses in which the tip, before the operation, was dislocated downward from the septal angle and in noses in which the position of the tip is influenced by overactive depressor septi muscles, an overdeveloped nasal spine, or septal cartilage protruding and invading the upper lip. Release of the tip from these contractile factors lengthens the columella and modifies the position of this important structure of the nose; often little or no cartilage resection is required from the caudal edge of the septal cartilage.

When indicated, a segment of cartilage is re-

between the mucoperichondrium and the cartilage. However, many surgeons feel that this technique is unnecessary in the large hump nose (see Submucous Approach, p. 1101). The entire length of the lateral cartilage is not detached, as *the cephalic portion of each lateral cartilage is left attached to the septum.* The stability of these structures is ensured by leaving them attached to each other.

Although separation of the lateral cartilages from the septum is necessary and inevitable when operating on the nose with a large dorsal hump, this procedure should not be regarded as routine. When the hump is minor, it is possible to shave down the cartilaginous dorsum without detaching the lateral cartilages from the septum (see The Supracartilaginous Approach, later in the text).

An angulated retractor exposes the septal angle and the dorsal border of the septal cartilage and provides exposure of the struc-

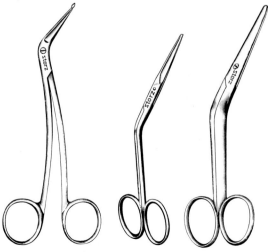

FIGURE 29-45. Three types of angulated scissors used to trim the dorsal border of the septum.

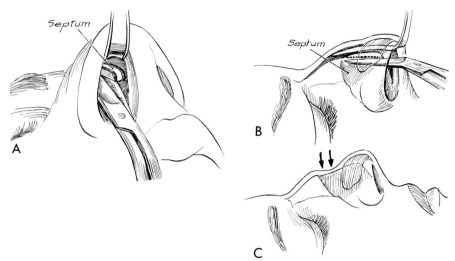

FIGURE 29–46. *A,* The angulated scissors lower the cartilaginous profile. *B,* The resection of the septal cartilage is along an oblique line. *C,* The dorsal hump is accentuated.

moved from the caudal margin of the septal cartilage. The columella is retracted to the left by the assistant, exposing the caudal margin of the septum and the septal angle (Fig. 29–47). The cartilage is steadied by grasping it with tooth forceps, and a suitable amount is excised (Fig. 29–48). It is preferable to remove the cartilage with a knife from below upward, following a curve which parallels the curve of the columella. The caudal margin of the septal cartilage should be given this type of curve and fitted to the columella.

Prudence is required in shortening the septum. Overshortening is a frequent mistake which results in a flat nasal base due to the disruption of the columella-ala triangle.

Excessive septal cartilage over the nasal spine is removed, when indicated, thus correcting an excessively wide nasolabial angle usually caused by a protrusion of the caudal margin of the septal cartilage into the lip. If the nasal spine is unduly protrusive and the upper lip is short, the nasal spine is trimmed or resected (see Fig. 29–86).

The change in the dorsal profile is evaluated by applying finger pressure over the septum; the protruding lateral cartilages are pressed down and out of the way.

At this point in the operation, the dorsal hump is accentuated and the tip appears protrusive (Fig. 29–49). The tip has also assumed a slightly more cephalic position.

The tip of the nose, now released from the remainder of the nose by the transfixion incision and the resection of a dorsal and caudal portion of the septum, assumes a new position, more cephalad and slightly more projecting. The shape of the nasal tip is now modified.

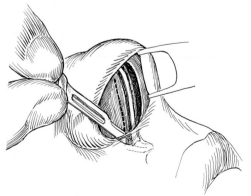

FIGURE 29–47. The retractor exposes the caudal edge of the septal cartilage; the segment to be resected is outlined.

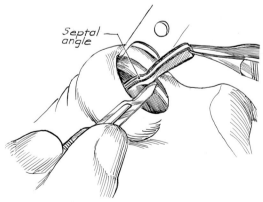

FIGURE 29–48. Shortening the septum. A segment of the caudal portion of the septum is resected.

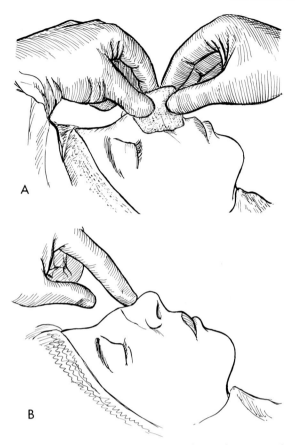

A

B

FIGURE 29–49. *A,* Gauze is placed over the nose, and blood is gently squeezed from the undermined spaces. *B,* At this point of the operation, the cartilaginous dorsum having been modified, the dorsal hump is accentuated.

sume a new position in harmony with the new profile line of the nose.

THE TIP OPERATION: A TECHNIQUE (see also Variations, p. 1105). An injection of local anesthetic solution at the base of each ala ensures completion of the block anesthesia of the tip of the nose. Prior injections have blocked branches from the external nasal and nasopalatine nerves. An injection is made into the base of the ala with a narrow-gauge short needle, thus blocking the branches of the infraorbital nerve (Fig. 29–50). A small amount of the anesthetic solution injected into the tip will reduce bleeding without distorting the tip. The immediate result of the corrective surgery can thus be observed, and the amount of hump to be removed from the remainder of the nasal dorsum can be accurately judged. This judgment is dependent upon a precise evaluation of the projection of the tip (Diamond, 1971).

After retraction of the ala, an incision is made through the vestibular lining but not through the cartilage (Fig. 29--51, *A*). The incision extends from the dome laterally. The length of the incision and its position depend upon the amount of cartilage to be resected cephalad. The extent of the cartilage to be resected varies and should not be standardized. Each nasal tip should be considered individually. Some tips require only a small amount of cartilage resection. The incision should be parallel to the cephalic border of the lateral crus and is usually located at a distance not exceeding 3 or 4 mm from the rim. The

Even when the tip of the nose appears adequate in shape and size preoperatively, surgery is required if the contour of the nasal dorsum is modified. The lateral crura of the alar cartilages are still shaped to fit the former convex dorsum. If they are not corrected, they will not fit the newly contoured dorsum, and a "pollytip" deformity will result.

A mistake occasionally made in the past was to correct the nose with a convex dorsum, leaving the nasal tip intact. Why touch the tip if it is not deformed? While it was not deformed prior to the operation, it no longer fit the modified shape of the nasal dorsum after the operation.

Two main objectives of a corrective tip operation are (1) to resect excess cartilage and thus reduce the size of the nasal tip and permit its reshaping; and (2) to weaken the cartilage between the lateral and medial crura in order that the lateral crus may "lie down" and as-

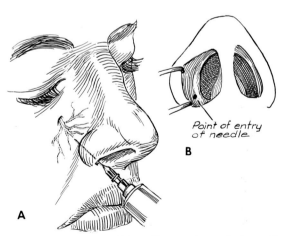

Point of entry of needle

B

A

FIGURE 29–50. *A,* The needle transpierces the base of the ala, injecting the anesthetic solution to block branches from the infraorbital nerve. *B,* The injection is made immediately in front of the inferior turbinate to block branches from the anterior-superior alveolar nerve, which innervates this area.

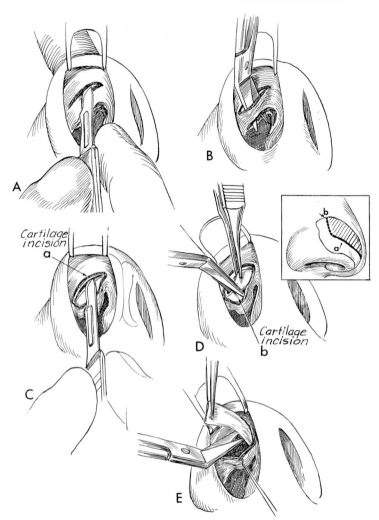

A

B

C

D

Cartilage
incisión
a

Cartilage
incision
b

E

FIGURE 29–51. The nasal tip operation: a technique. *A*, An incision is made through the vestibular lining parallel to the cephalic border of the lateral crus. *B*, The vestibular lining is raised from the cartilage. *C*, The transcartilaginous incision is made. *D*, The lateral portion of the lateral crus is divided, as indicated in the inset. The line of section is parallel to the proposed new profile of the nose. *E*, The cartilage is removed.

preservation of the continuity of the cartilage along the caudal margin of the alar cartilage prevents a displacement of the lateral edges of the sectioned cartilage, which protrude as two small "horns" under the skin of the tip of the nose postoperatively. In the broad tip, it may be necessary to transgress the caudal border of the alar cartilage, removing a sizable piece of cartilage in order to reduce the width of the nasal tip. A suture approximates the medial and lateral portions of the cartilage to close the gap left by the excision and prevents irregularities of contour of the caudal edge of the tip cartilages.

Angulated scissors (Fig. 29–52) elevate the vestibular lining from the undersurface of the cartilage (Fig. 29–51, *B*). A small amount of anesthetic solution raises the vestibular lining from the cartilage. An incision through the

cartilage is then made (Fig. 29–51, *C*), and the soft tissues overlying the cartilage are

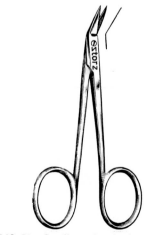

FIGURE 29–52.   Small angulated scissors for tip surgery.

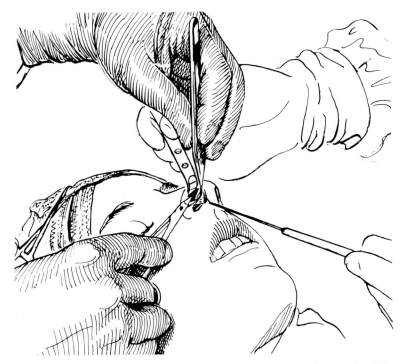

FIGURE 29–53. Position of the operator's and the assistant's hands during the tip operation. The assistant is retracting the ala and retracting the raised vestibular skin by means of a hook. The operator's hands are holding the cartilaginous segment to be excised with forceps, and the small angulated scissors are used to complete the resection.

raised; thus the cartilage is freed by subperichondrial dissection.

The transcartilaginous incision has split the cartilage into cephalic and caudal segments; the cartilage situated cephalad to the cartilage-splitting incision is resected (Fig. 29–51, *D, E*). In order to facilitate the procedure, the assistant holds the alar retractor in one hand, everting the ala with his middle finger, and a hook retracting the bipedicle flap of vestibular lining in the other hand. The operator's two hands are therefore free, and with the aid of forceps and small angulated scissors he may proceed with the resection of the required amount of alar cartilage (Fig. 29–53). The cartilage is sectioned at a suitable point and extruded. The sagittal cut through the lateral crus should be parallel to the caudal portion of the dorsum of the septum. The lateral portion of the lateral crus of the alar cartilage is usually not resected in the average case, in order to avoid postoperative constriction of the nares and a pinched appearance caused by the removal of the cartilage which supports this area. The extent of the cartilage resection is determined by the extent of the convexity of the tip, usually located medially in line with the dorsum. Excessive removal of cartilage results in a

"pinched-tip" deformity, which may not become apparent until two or three years after the operation. No vestibular lining is removed in the average rhinoplasty. Unnecessary removal of vestibular lining leaves a raw area which becomes infected, fibrosed, scarred, and contracted, resulting in stricture and a distorted

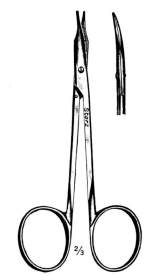

FIGURE 29–54. Blunt-tip scissors (Stevens).

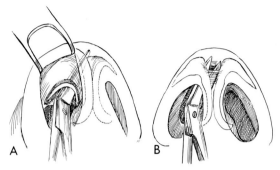

FIGURE 29–55. *A,* The small angulated scissors are placed between the medial crura and the domes. *B,* Breaking up the fibroareolar tissue between the domes. This is an effective way to approximate the domes if there is moderate bifidity of the tip.

tip. Small, blunt-tipped (Stevens) scissors (Fig. 29–54) free the skin over the supratip area. If the tip is slightly bifid, small, angulated scissors (see Fig. 29–52) are placed in a retrograde fashion between the domes, severing the fibroareolar tissue between them, thus making it possible to approximate the domes (Fig. 29–55). If the domes are adequately approximated, this area is not disturbed.

The amount of cartilage to be resected should be carefully predetermined. However, the contour may not be entirely satisfactory; additional cartilage resection may be required. The cartilage at the dome may be reshaped by *partial thickness* cuts. A short rim incision is made and the dome is exposed. A number of incisions made in the cartilage thus accentuates the angle of the dome.

In deformities of lesser degree, narrowing of the tip is obtained by resecting a measured strip of cartilage parallel to the superomedial

border of the lateral crus of the alar cartilage (Fig. 29–56). This procedure may suffice. Excision of cartilage from the medical crus will recess the tip when the latter shows an excessive amount of projection (see also section on variations, p. 1105).

Stage 3: Resecting the Bony Hump. Removal of the bony hump precedes the final correction of the profile (resection of the dorsal border of each lateral cartilage and the final trimming of the septum). An osteotome of adequate width (usually 15 mm) is placed at the caudal border of the undisturbed area of the cartilaginous dorsum, the area where the cephalic portions of the lateral cartilages and septum are continuous with the bony dorsum. The lateral cartilages are reflected laterally to allow the placing of the osteotome. The amount of bone to be removed is determined by the projection of the tip.

THE OSTEOTOME TECHNIQUE. The osteotome is held in the right hand while the operator's left hand raises the skin of the dorsum to protect it from injury. The osteotome is advanced by carefully applied blows of the mallet administered by the assistant. Before completing the separation of the hump, a narrower osteotome is used to section the upper portion (Fig. 29–57). The hump, once freed, is removed by a hump removal forceps (Fig. 29–58).

A sharp, finely honed edge is essential if the osteotome is to be effective. Any irregular bony edges are smoothed with a sharp rasp. A mirror image is helpful in estimating the change in the nasal profile (see Fig. 29–59). Various types of osteotomes are used. Some have sharp angles; others have rounded angles

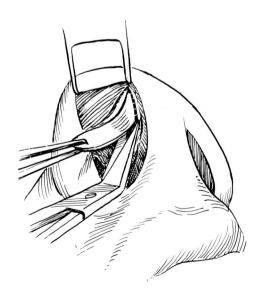

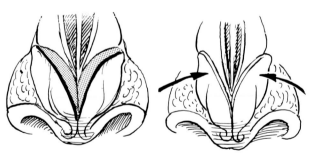

FIGURE 29–56. Minimal resection from the cephalic portion of each lateral crus when only a slight change of shape of the nasal tip is indicated.

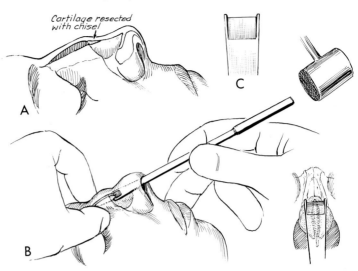

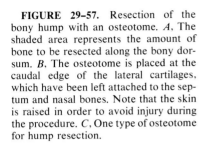

FIGURE 29–57. Resection of the bony hump with an osteotome. *A*, The shaded area represents the amount of bone to be resected along the bony dorsum. *B*, The osteotome is placed at the caudal edge of the lateral cartilages, which have been left attached to the septum and nasal bones. Note that the skin is raised in order to avoid injury during the procedure. *C*, One type of osteotome for hump resection.

or are guarded bilaterally (Fig. 29–57, *C*) in order to avoid injuring the covering soft tissues. A flat handle assists in maintaining the osteotome in a horizontal position, thus avoiding a beveled resection of the hump. A cross-osteotome was devised by Robin (1973) for this purpose (Fig. 29–60). Another variation has a concave cutting edge that resects more septum than lateral wall.

THE RASP TECHNIQUE. The rasp bevels the lateral edges of the sectioned lateral walls, thus reproducing the rounded shape of the bony dorsum (Fig. 29–61). A dull-edge curette removes the debris that results from rasping. If a sharp, back-cutting rasp is used, the rasped bone is removed by the rasp.

For the removal of all but large bony humps, the rasp is often the most efficient instrument

(see Sheen technique, p. 1100). A sharp rasp gradually reduces the bone and maintains the rounded dorsal border and the lateral convex curvatures of the bony dorsum. The rasp will not reduce cartilage unless it is exceptionally sharp and is usually not used for this purpose.

At this point in the operation, the bony dorsum and the major portion of the septal border have been lowered; the lateral cartilages and a portion of the septum still protrude (Fig. 29–62).

Stage 4: Lateral (and Medial) Osteotomies of the Lateral Walls of the Nose

LATERAL OSTEOTOMY: START LOW, FINISH HIGH. The nasal hump has been removed. The lateral walls after osteotomy must be approximated to avoid a "flat top" nasal vault.

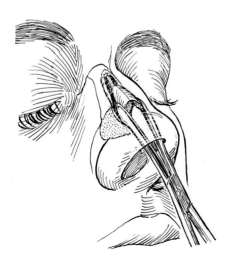

FIGURE 20–58. The bony hump is removed.

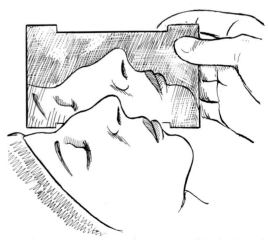

FIGURE 29–59. A stainless steel polished mirror is often useful for the reflection of the reversed image to exaggerate minor defects (profile prior to hump removal).

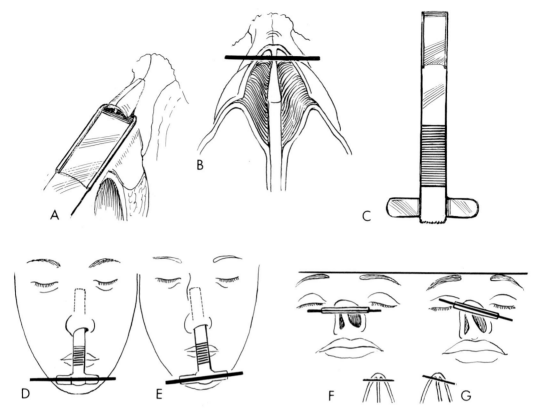

FIGURE 29–60. The cross-osteotome. *A*, The osteotome is engaged at the lower border of the nasal bones. *B*, Frontal section: the osteotome must remain horizontal. *C*, Cross-shaped osteotome assists in maintaining the osteotome in a horizontal position. *D*, *E*, The cross-bar assists in avoiding lateral deviations. *F*, *G*, Maintaining the cross-bar parallel to the level of the eyes prevents tilting of the osteotome to one side, which causes removal of more on one side than on the other. (After Robin, 1973.)

Inspection of the skeletal dorsum using an angulated retractor will show the remaining protruding dorsal septal border and the medial borders of the lateral cartilages. These structures will not be adjusted to the new profile line until after the lateral osteotomies have been performed and the bony dorsum has settled into its new lower level. The medial borders of the septum are then trimmed and adjusted to the new profile line (Stage 5).

Considerable changes in the concept of the osteotomy have arisen since the technique ad-

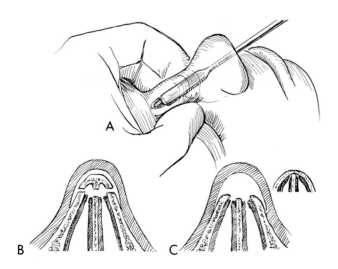

FIGURE 20–61. *A*, Rasping the bony edges after the resection of the hump. *B*, Frontal section showing the portion of the bony dorsum which has been resected. Note that the muco-periosteum is reflected downward. *C*, The bony edges are bevelled with the rasp, so that when they are approximated following the lateral osteotomy, they will reproduce the rounded shape of the bony dorsum.

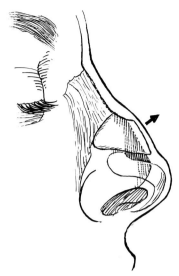

FIGURE 29–62. At this point in the operation, the nasal tip operation has been performed, and a major portion of the dorsal border of the septum has been lowered. The bone has also been resected. The lateral cartilages and a portion of the dorsal border of the septum protrude. These structures will be trimmed *after* the lateral osteotomies.

vocated by Joseph, in which an angulated saw was used to section the base of the lateral wall of the nose (the frontal process). There has been undue emphasis placed upon the need for a low osteotomy in the upper portion of the osteotomy line. It has been reported that the lacrimal sac was injured in a high proportion of osteotomies (Flowers and Anderson, 1968). This complication is caused by the penetration of the instrument behind the anterior lacrimal crest. It has become apparent to the author and to others that the lateral osteotomy should be *high* rather than *low* in the region of the root of the nose in the average corrective rhinoplasty, as emphasized by Sheen (1976). The reasons for this position include the following:

1. Attempting to narrow the root of the nose in most patients may be a mistake, because such a procedure may cause an apparent increase in the distance between the eyes.

2. If the line of osteotomy extends upward above the area of junction of eyelid and nasal skin and if this "frontier" is not transgressed, periorbital ecchymosis can be minimized or even prevented.

This stage of the corrective nasal plastic operation consists of (1) severing the base of each lateral wall of the nose in order to displace the lateral walls medially, and (2) narrowing the nose. The lateral cartilages have a broad surface of attachment on the undersur-

face of the nasal bones and frontal processes of the maxilla; the cartilages are displaced medially when the bones are infractured because of their firm attachment to the bones. There are two techniques of lateral osteotomy, extranasal and intranasal osteotomy.

ANESTHESIA. If the staged method of local anesthesia is followed, additional anesthesia is required for the osteotomy of the lateral nasal walls. A previous injection into the right vestibule, which extends through the skin of the vestibule and the base of the ala into the region of the lateral nasal fold, has blocked the terminal filaments of the infraorbital nerve.

When the *extranasal* subcutaneous osteotomy technique is employed, the ala is retracted outward, and a longer needle (5 cm) is introduced into the vestibule lateral to the border of the pyriform aperture; this is passed upward, following the contour of the bone. At the root of the nose, the needle remains above the eyelid-nose skin junction in order to minimize ecchymoses of the eyelids (Fig. 29–63); the Xylocaine-epinephrine solution blocks the branches from the infratrochlear and infraorbital nerves. A previously made injection immediately caudad to the inferior turbinate has blocked the nasal branches of the anterior-superior alveolar nerve.

When the *intranasal* osteotomy technique is employed, the edge of the pyriform aperture is located by palpation with an instrument and the needle is passed from the pyriform aperture near the floor of the nose along the *medial* aspect of the frontal process, hugging the bone; thus the needle is under the mucoperiosteum. The needle is inserted *low* and progresses to

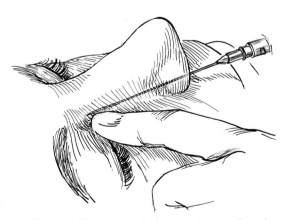

FIGURE 29–63. Stage 4: the lateral osteotomy. Branches from the infraorbital nerve have already been blocked prior to the tip operation. A long needle is inserted along the base of the lateral wall, and an anesthetic solution injection blocks the branches from the supratrochlear and infratrochlear nerves and upper branches of the infraorbital nerve.

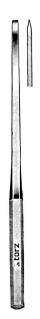

FIGURE 29–64. The 3-mm wide osteotome for lateral osteotomy.

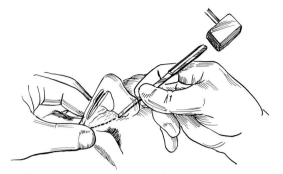

FIGURE 29–65. External lateral osteotomy with the 3-mm osteotome.

the root of the nose, where the tip of the needle is *high,* i.e., above the eyelid-nose skin junction.

THE OSTEOTOME TECHNIQUE: EXTERNAL LATERAL OSTEOTOMY. With practice, a satisfactory osteotomy is performed with a 3-mm wide osteotome or chisel (Fig. 29–64). The osteotome is placed in the vestibule at the edge

of the pyriform aperture; it pierces the lining of the vestibule and is tapped gently upward through loose subcutaneous tissue along the base of the lateral wall (Fig. 29–65). It is not necessary to elevate the periosteum along the base of the lateral wall. The osteotomy is started low at the pyriform aperture and ends high near the junction of the frontal process and the nasal bone. After bilateral osteotomy, manual pressure fractures the bone medially, first on one side, then on the other, approximating the lateral walls.

THE OSTEOTOME TECHNIQUE: INTERNAL LATERAL OSTEOTOMY. Another technique is the intranasal submucous technique of lateral osteotomy (Hilger, 1968). The blunt end of the

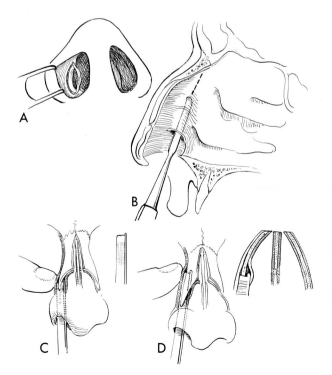

FIGURE 29–66. The internal lateral osteotomy. *A,* An incision made at the edge of the pyriform aperture. *B,* Submucoperiosteal elevation along the base of the frontal process of the maxilla. *C,* A guarded osteotome (see Fig. 29–67) is introduced. *D,* The guarded osteotome progresses along the lateral wall, being tapped upward by a mallet. Note the finger palpating the edge of the osteotome at the base of the lateral wall of the nose.

Joseph knife is used to feel the border of the pyriform aperture at its base; an incision is made through the mucoperiosteum on the edge of the pyriform aperture (Fig. 29–66, *A*). The mucoperiosteum is raised from the *medial* aspect of the lateral wall of the nose by means of the Joseph periosteal elevator (Fig. 29–66, *B*). The guarded osteotome (Fig. 29–67) is then introduced through a submucous tunnel. The osteotomy is performed from inside-out instead of from outside-in, as in the technique described above (Fig. 29–66, *C, D*). The intranasal submucous osteotomy appears to cause a lesser degree of periorbital ecchymosis than the external osteotomy; in many cases periorbital ecchymosis is totally absent.

THE INFRACTURE. Digital pressure exerted alternately over one lateral wall, then over the contralateral wall, achieves the infracture. The cephalic portion of the lateral wall is not fractured. The transverse fracture at the junction of the infractured lateral wall and the undisturbed nasal bridge may occasionally result in a step: a rasp will readily plane down the protruding cephalic bone. It is not essential in the younger patient that the lateral wall be

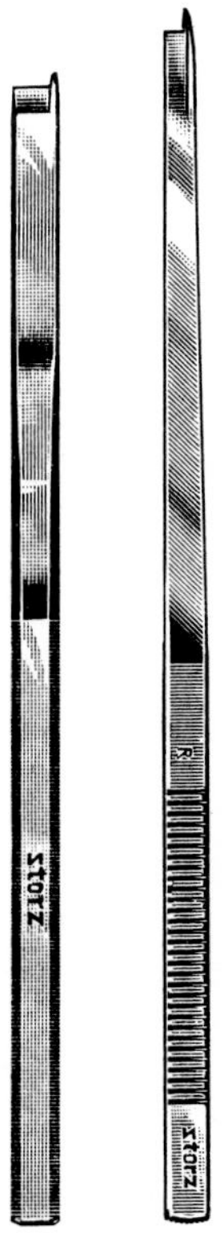

FIGURE 29-67. Guarded osteotomes for the internal lateral osteotomy; they are also used for outfracturing the lateral walls (see later in text).

sectioned along a uniform line of osteotomy; by weakening the bone by a series of cuts with the osteotome, the lateral walls can be pressed inward.

RASPING THE BONY DORSUM AFTER THE INFRACTURE. Small irregularities may be present. A small, sharp rasp is used to smooth them. The bony structures are maintained in position between the operator's left thumb and index finger while the necessary rasping is performed by his right hand.

DELIBERATE COMMINUTION OF THE LATERAL WALL. In corrective rhinoplasty for malunited fracture, convexity, or other irregularities usually resulting from a malunited fracture, it may be necessary to fragment the lateral wall in order to achieve adequate shaping. A gauze pad is placed over the area and it is struck with a mallet, thus breaking the bone into comminuted pieces. This apparently brutal technique is essential in some cases if a satisfactory result is to be obtained.

Is narrowing of the root of the nose indicated? Becker (1958) questioned the value of the medial osteotomy technique as a routine procedure, claiming on the basis of cadaver experiments that it is impossible to remove sufficient bone to obtain adequate narrowing of the upper part of the nose. He preferred to leave this area intact, allowing the infracture of the lateral wall to occur at a lower level, and, when necessary, to rasp the protruding bone of the root of the nose on each side.

The root of the nose usually does not require narrowing, and a simple infracture may be adequate without the lateral walls being mobilized by means of the outfracture technique. Excessive narrowing of the root of the nose increases the apparent intercanthal distance and may cause a drastic change in the patient's appearance. In adolescent patients, a greenstick fracture occurs, and the bones can be molded with little loss of bone continuity at the site of the osteotomy. For this reason patients of this age group often have the best results. Narrowing of the root of the nose is required in wide noses, particularly those of the traumatic type. In adults the outfracture technique not only detaches the upper portion of the lateral wall but also ensures that the osteotomy is completed.

MEDIAL OSTEOTOMY: THE OUTFRACTURING PROCEDURE AND NARROWING OF THE ROOT OF THE NOSE. These procedures have been advocated by Aufricht (1943) to fracture the remaining cephalic attachment of the lateral

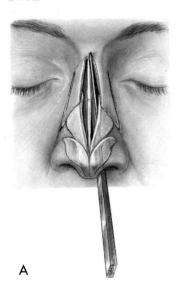

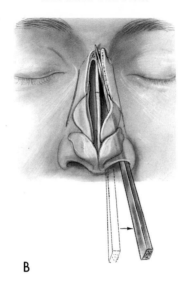

A   B

FIGURE 29-68. Medial osteotomy. Outfracturing. *A*, The button-guarded osteotome is hammered into the solid bone at the root of the nose. *B*, The osteotome is then rotated outward, outfracturing the lateral wall of the nose. Outfracturing is rarely indicated in the average corrective rhinoplasty; the technique is used in traumatic deformities and exceptionally wide noses.

nasal wall after the lateral osteotomy and to loosen the lateral wall to facilitate the infracture. A discussion of their indications will follow.

An osteotome (see Fig. 29-67) is placed in the space between the cut edge of the nasal bone and the septum to outfracture the lateral wall. A line of section upward through the remaining bone is established by the use of a mallet and osteotome (Fig. 29-68, *A*). A characteristic dull sound is heard when the osteotome penetrates the dense bone at the root of the nose. This "sign of the sound" indicates that the instrument is now solidly fixed in the bone. The osteotome is levered outward from the frontal bone, and the remaining attachment of the nasal bone and the frontal process is outfractured (Fig. 29-68, *B*).

An osteotome with a guard is employed for this procedure to protect the overlying soft tissues and skin from trauma and also to permit palpation of the tip of the instrument through the skin.

The purpose of outfracturing is threefold: (1) to disconnect the remaining upper attachment of the lateral nasal wall; (2) to ensure adequate loosening at the line of osteotomy; and (3) to establish sufficient space for the insertion of an instrument to remove the remaining bony web.

The indications for this procedure, as explained by Aufricht, involve the configuration of the upper portion of the dorsum after excision of the dorsal hump. The dorsal hump is usually situated considerably below the level of the nasofrontal angle. After removal of the

hump, a gap exists in the continuity of the dorsum in the area from which the hump has been excised, and direct examination with a retractor shows the cut surfaces of the lateral bony walls and lateral cartilages separated in their midline by the cut surface of the septum. Above this area of the hump excision, however, the nasal dorsum shows an undisturbed vault where the bones remain in continuity. Infracture of the lateral walls at this stage would result in narrowing of the nose below the level of the undisturbed bony vault. It will be recalled that the root of the nose is formed of thick bones; the upper portions of the nasal bones are narrow and thick and are further reinforced by the thick nasal spine of the frontal bone.

Removal of a wedge of bone from this area on each side of the septum is required only when the area of the root of the nose is wide. Aufricht performs the procedure with a small chisel, making two cuts—one medially along the line of the septum, and the other laterally joining the upper end of the first cut obliquely. A small triangle of bone is then removed with a hemostat.

A specially designed rongeur (Converse) (Fig. 29-69) is also employed in resection of the wedge of bone from the root of the nose. The bony wedge can be removed after completion of the resection of the bony hump (Fig. 29-70). If the rongeur cannot be introduced for lack of space, the procedure is done after the outfracture of the lateral walls. Removal of the wedge of bone provides sufficient space for

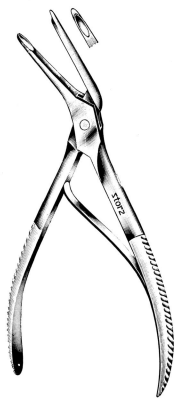

the medial displacement of the upper portion of the lateral walls of the nose. Thus the nose is adequately narrowed in its upper portion, an important feature when a large, wide nose is being reduced in size.

The lateral walls can now be infractured and displaced medially, joining each other in the midline (Fig. 29–71).

CHECKING THE LATERAL OSTEOTOMY AFTER INFRACTURE. The lateral osteotomy line should be palpated to determine whether any stepping is present. This complication may result when the osteotomy has been placed at too high a level in the lower portion of the osteotomy rather than at the base of the frontal process where it arises from the body of the maxilla. If the osteotomy is too high, a ridge lateral to the osteotomy line may result in a steplike protuberance at the base of the lateral wall. If such a complication occurs, the crest remaining at the base of the lateral wall should be fractured inwardly; a simple technique involves use of a narrow, tapered osteotome placed through the skin at the upper end of the nasolabial fold.

Stage 5: Trimming the Dorsal Border of the Septal Cartilage and the Medial Borders of the Lateral Cartilages. After the lateral osteotomies and the infracture, the bony nose has settled to a lower level. It is therefore preferable to do

FIGURE 29–69. Specially designed rongeur to resect a wedge of bone from the root of the nose when the nose is exceptionally wide (Converse).

FIGURE 29–70. Removal of bony wedge at the root of the wide nose. *A*, The bony wedge remaining on each side of the septum after resection of the hump. The bony wedge is formed by thick bone at the root of the nose, the superimposition of the nasal spine of the frontal bone, and the thick portion of the nasal bone. *B*, Special rongeur in position removing the wedge of bone. *C*, Design of the rongeur. The upper blade is guarded to avoid including soft tissue into the cutting portion of the rongeur. *D*, The nasal dorsum after removal of the bony wedge on each side. This procedure facilitates the infracture and avoids an excessive width at the upper portion of the bony dorsum.

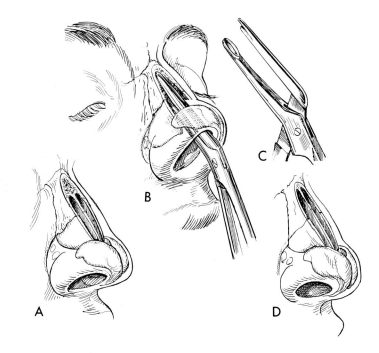

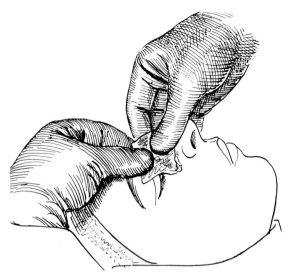

FIGURE 29–71. Infracture of the lateral walls.

the final adjustment of the profile line and to trim the medial borders of the lateral cartilages and the septum at this stage of the operation. These procedures are performed under direct inspection, using an angle retractor with good illumination and angulated scissors.

It is most important to see the structures of the dorsum. Operating room lights may provide adequate illumination, but a headlight gives superior clarity of vision. A useful instrument is the rhinoscope, an angulated retractor with a fiberoptic light source (see Fig. 29–28).

The medial border of the right lateral cartilage is trimmed and adjusted to the new profile line with the angulated scissors (Fig. 29–72). This procedure provides a good view of the septum. The dorsal septal border is trimmed. Finally, the left lateral cartilage is also ad-

justed. Final paring of the structures may be required.

The medial borders of the lateral cartilages have not been trimmed and adjusted until this stage of the operation; thus they are trimmed once, finally, and definitively.

The "final look." The esthetic result of a corrective nasal operation often depends upon careful last minute inspection and palpation. The "final look" at the dorsal skeletal structures under good illumination is most important; loose pieces of bone or cartilage and irregularities of contour of the cut edges of the bones and cartilage are removed. The dorsum of the nose is carefully palpated for irregularities. Additional correction may include rasping or the use of the osteotome in the upper portion of the dorsum; rasping the edge of the bone at the junction of the two bony lateral walls, where one edge of bone occasionally overlaps the other; and additional trimming of cartilage along the dorsal border of the septal cartilage, particularly in the region of the septal angle.

These last minute procedures are readily performed, even though the structures are separated from their attachments; the bony nose may be held between the thumb and the index finger of the operator's left hand, while a rasp gently smooths an irregular surface.

It must be emphasized that curvature or excessive thickness of the dorsal portion of the septum is the usual cause of postoperative widening of the nose following osteotomy. Measures should be taken at this stage to correct such deviations; the techniques for this purpose are described later in this chapter (see p. 1117). When an angle retractor is used with good illumination to elevate the soft tissues, an excellent opportunity is afforded to examine the shape of the septum. An excessively thick

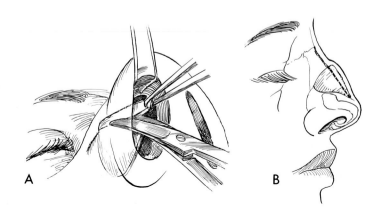

FIGURE 29–72. The final trimming of the dorsum (Stage 5). *A*, The medial edge of each lateral cartilage is trimmed with angulated scissors to the level of the cephalic portion of the dorsum of the septum, which itself has also been trimmed. *B*, The final profile of the nose is now achieved.

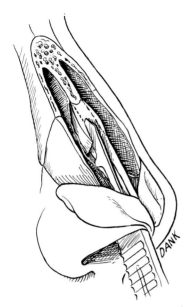

FIGURE 29–73. A thick septum as a cause for inadequate narrowing of the nose following osteotomy of the lateral nasal walls. A frequent site of a wide dorsal edge of the septum is at the junction of the septal cartilage and the ethmoid plate (the tubercle of the septum). This is also the area of the supraseptal groove (see Fig. 29–8), which causes increased thickness. Thinning of the septal cartilage is obtained by paring with a knife.

nose in patients with thick skin and large sebaceous glands. The rigid skin does not adapt to the underlying framework and maintains its round protuberance.

When a supratip protrusion due to causes number two or three (above) becomes evident in the early postoperative period, prudent injection of Kenalog (triamcinolone), 5 mg per ml, may forestall development of the deformity.

FINAL PROCEDURES. The nose is compressed upon completion of the operation; blood is squeezed from the undermined spaces by gentle finger pressure over gauze compresses. The transcartilaginous incision through the lateral crus of the alar cartilage is sutured with plain catgut. The intercartilaginous incision is usually not sutured. Catgut sutures (Fig. 29–75), transfixion sutures, or mattress sutures through the caudal septum and the columella approximate the septum and the columella. Additional support is provided by an adhesive tape or paper adhesive tape sling (see Fig. 29–77).

TRIMMING THE CAUDAL ENDS OF EACH LATERAL CARTILAGE. After the suturing is completed, the last surgical procedure of the corrective rhinoplasty is performed, if indicated. Respect for the integrity of the nasal

dorsal portion of the septum may prevent approximation of the lateral walls in the midline and require thinning (Fig. 29–73). The septum is wider at the supraseptal groove (see Figs. 29–2 and 29–8).

A polished metal reflector gives a mirror image and assists in visualizing the profile line (see Fig. 29–59).

FORESTALLING THE SUPRATIP PROTRUSION. A slight protrusion above the tip of the nose may spoil an otherwise satisfactory profile. This complication has three principal causes:

1. Inadequate reduction of the projection of the septal angle, which protrudes under the skin in the supratip area. The septal angle should be checked under direct vision. A gentle downward pressure at the columella-lip junction will cause it to blanch the skin if the angle is not sufficiently reduced.

2. Excessive removal of cartilage from the septal angle, which leaves a void between the septum and the soft tissues of the dorsum of the nose. The mucous membrane of the septum grows upward and between the two layers of the mucous membrane; fibrous tissue fills the void and causes the supratip protrusion (Fig. 29–74).

3. Excessive reduction of the dorsum of the

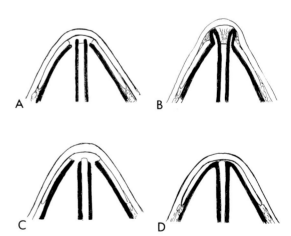

FIGURE 29–74. One of the causes of supratip protrusion: fibrous tissue between the skin and the dorsum of the septum. *A*, Frontal section through the septum near the caudal portion. Note the proximity of the septal mucous membrane to the dorsal portion of the septum. *B*, If there is a void between the dorsal skin and the dorsal border of the septum, the mucous membrane grows upward from the septal cartilage and the lateral cartilages. A fibrous tissue pad develops between the layers of the mucous membrane, causing a supratip protrusion. *C*, Excess mucous membrane should be trimmed from the dorsal border of the septum and a small strip of septal cartilage denuded of mucous membrane. *D*, Correct relationship of the dorsal skin and the septum without a supratip protrusion.

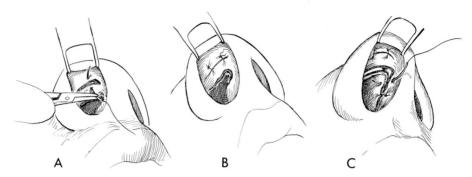

FIGURE 29–75. Suturing the transcartilaginous incision (*A* and *B*) and the transfixion incision (*C*). Transfixion sutures through the septum and columella are also employed.

valve has been emphasized earlier in the text. The purpose of such trimming is to adjust the lateral·cartilages to the new nasal length. The lateral cartilage protrudes into the vestibule in a long nose which has been shortened. Resection of an excessive amount of the caudal portion of the lateral cartilage with attached muco-perichondrium is the most frequent cause of disturbance of nasal physiology. The nasal deformity is corrected, but the patient cannot breathe through his nose. Resection of lateral cartilage, if indicated, should be done with extreme caution, as excessive resection interferes with the function of the nasal valve and stenosis of this area impairs the nasal airway. Overresection of the lateral cartilage also

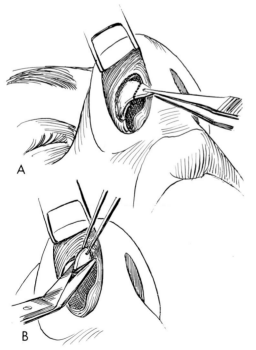

FIGURE 29–76. Resection of the protruding tip of the lateral cartilage after shortening of the nose. This procedure should be done with prudence as a last procedure without sacrificing mucous membrane.

causes postoperative retraction of the ala. The cartilage may be trimmed prudently without reseceting the mucous membrane lining (Fig. 29–76).

Except in the very long nose, excision of the cephalic portion of the lateral crus obviates the need to shorten more than a small amount of lateral cartilage. The trimming of the caudal portion of the lateral cartilage is done as a last procedure after the suturing and prior to the placing of the adhesive tape.

Vaseline gauze or other type of intranasal packing of the nasal airways may be dispensed with in the routine corrective nasal plastic operation. The patient is more comfortable, and the incidence of postoperative bleeding is diminished. Packing is not required to prevent hematoma of the septum following a procedure to straighten the septum; a horizontal incision near the floor of the nose is made through the septal mucoperiosteal flap to ensure drainage (see p. 1132).

Only occasionally is packing employed to maintain the vestibular lining reapplied to the remodeled cartilage. Nasal packing and internal splints are also needed in the deviated nose to support the realigned septum during the post-operative period (see p. 1117).

Some noses have excessive flaring at the completion of the nasal plastic operation if the nasal tip has been recessed. Resection of the base of the alae may be required to reduce the narial flare (see Fig. 29–82).

Stage 6: Splinting the Nose. The freed tip cartilages at this stage are unstable and may easily be separated by edema and blood; or they may slip into faulty positions, resulting in the formation of grooves, asymmetry, and distortion of the tip. Unlike bone, cartilage does not reestablish cartilage continuity; the cartilage fragments are joined to each other by fibrous tissue. The separated parts are therefore immobilized by splinting with regular or

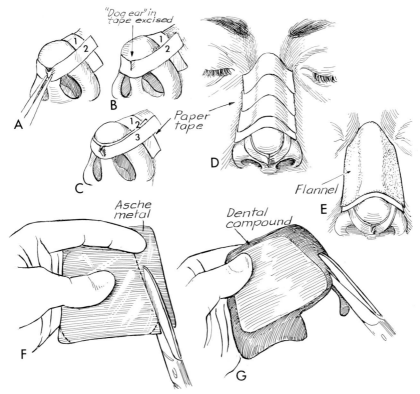

FIGURE 29–77. Stage 6: splinting the nose. *A*, One or more pieces of tape are strapped across the dorsal border of the septum in the supratip area. This important measure prevents formation of a void between the dorsal skin and the septum. *B*, A strip of paper tape is placed sling-fashion around the tip of the nose to maintain contact between the columella and the septum. *C*, Pinching the tape to take up any slack. *D*, Completion of adhesive strapping of the nose. *E*, The nose is covered by a piece of flannel. *F*, Soft Asche metal (28-gauge) is cut to shape to serve as a carrier, so that the softened dental compound is equally spread and takes an impression of the reconstructed nose. *G*, Softened dental compound has been placed over the soft metal; the excess is removed.

paper adhesive tape, which minimizes skin maceration under the tape.

A dorsal strip of adhesive tape secures the lateral crura and obliterates any dead space between the septal angle and the soft tissues and cartilages; the adhesive tape should be lined with inverted tape to allow for shrinkage of the skin. The application of the skin against the septum, as illustrated in Figure 29–77, is an important measure in order to avoid the dead space between the dorsal skin of the nose and the dorsal border of the septal cartilage. A strip of tape forms a slinglike loop which supports the tip against the septal cartilage and ensures fixation of the mobilized tip cartilages (Fig. 29–77). Additional strips are placed over the dorsum. The nose is then covered by a piece of flannel (lint) (Fig. 29–77, *E*).

The postoperative nasal splint immobilizes the tissues and maintains them against the framework, thus preventing hematoma. Dental compound (or plaster, see Fig. 29–105), employed in the splinting technique, is softened in hot water (Fig. 29–78, *A*) and molded over the nasal pyramid (Fig. 29–78, *B*). In order to avoid pressure points, the compound is spread evenly over a suitably shaped piece of soft Asche metal (28-gauge) before being applied to the nasal pyramid (see Fig. 29–77, *F*, *G*). It is hardened in situ by application of ice cold gauze. The use of a molded splint is important as the soft dental compound takes an impression of the remodeled nose and adapts to its new shape. Preference is given to dental compound (black compound, S.S. White).

The splint should not extend below the level of the cephalic borders of the remodeled alar cartilages and must not exert pressure on the tip, forcing it downward, for in most operations, cephalic elevation and projection of the tip is desired; this is an essential precaution (Fig. 29–79, *A*).

A skin varnish painted on the skin before the application of the splint not only protects the skin against irritation but also enhances the sticking quality of the adhesive tape (Fig. 29–

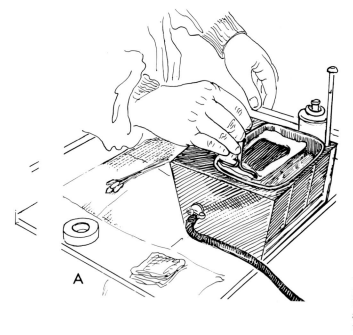

FIGURE 29–78. Splinting the nose. *A*, Dental compound heater to soften the dental compound in warm water. *B*, The compound has been placed over the Asche metal, which acts as a carrier while the compound is molded to the remodeled nose.

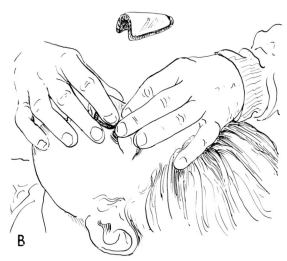

79, *B*). The splint is fastened to the face by adhesive paper tape (Steri-Strips, 2.5 cm wide) and is maintained in position for a period of five days, or longer if desired (Fig. 29–79, *C*, *D*).

A small, folded gauze compress, facetiously referred to as the "mustache," is placed across the base of the nose and fastened with adhesive strapping (Fig. 29–79, *E*); the gauze is readily renewed when saturated.

EARLY POSTOPERATIVE CARE. The patient is placed in the Fowler position upon returning to bed, the head being elevated in order to minimize postoperative oozing. Pain is controlled by medication. A soft diet is prescribed during the first two postoperative days to minimize active mastication which could cause loosening of the splint.

No intranasal treatment is required. Healing occurs faster and the incidence of postoperative bleeding is diminished if the patient is undisturbed. The routine administration of antibiotics has eliminated the occasional development of local inflammatory reaction. Postoperative edema, ecchymoses around the eyes, and occasionally subconjunctival hemorrhage are minimal when the high osteotomy technique is employed. Swelling and ecchy-

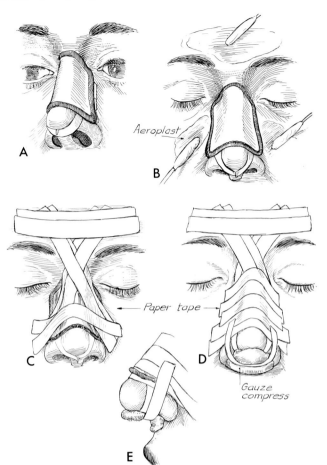

FIGURE 29–79. Splinting the nose. *A*, The dental compound mold has been hardened by the application of ice compresses. *B*, Skin varnish (Aeroplast) is painted over the forehead and cheeks. *C, D*, The splint is strapped to the face with adhesive tape. *E*, The artist has shown the sling too low; it should support the tip at the tip.columella angle.

moses, which may occur 48 hours after the operation, begin to subside on the third day. Orbital ecchymosis, if present, gradually changes from a dark bluish color to a yellowish tinge at the end of the first week. Trypsin derivatives do not lessen postoperative edema and ecchymoses. Subconjunctival hemorrhage, which disappears more gradually and may extend for a period of two to three weeks, is a rare occurrence in the average rhinoplastic operation.

Ice compresses over the eyes, although soothing for the patient, do not diminish the periocular ecchymosis or hasten its disappearance.

The nasal splint is removed after a period varying from five to seven days; the adhesive strapping, first line of defense, is left for an additional two-day period. The patient is advised against blowing his nose to avoid provoking hemorrhage or subcutaneous emphysema by the passage of air through the lines of

osteotomy. After removal of the splint, the patient is instructed to use cold cream or paraffin ointment (Vaseline) inside the nose to soften blood clots or crusts and to cleanse the nasal vestibules with cotton-tipped applicators. The patient is also informed that the nose may appear somewhat overcorrected and swollen but that the appearance will gradually improve (Fig. 29–80).

THE POSTOPERATIVE PERIOD. Postoperative manipulation by means of an apparatus such as the Joseph nasal clamp or other modifications of this instrument is not required and is contraindicated as a routine procedure. The patient should be warned against compressing the nose with his fingers.

Edema may persist over a period of months, especially in the supratip area or the root of the nose. The time period is extended in direct proportion to the amount of reduction in size of the nose and the age of the patient. Contraction of the soft tissues over the modified skele-

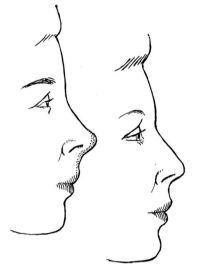

FIGURE 29–80. Change in contour after resolution of postoperative swelling. *A,* Immediate postoperative appearance. *B,* Appearance after subsidence of the postoperative swelling. (After Aufricht.)

tal framework occurs more slowly in the older patient and may require a period of from six months to a year.

The undermined skin of the tip of the nose is denervated temporarily. Sebaceous glands, which are abundant in this area, are passive and fill with secretion. During the postoperative period, frequent gentle washing with a strongly alkaline soap or a mildly detergent cream assists in the evacuation of the accumulated sebaceous secretion and facilitates the progressive contraction of the skin.

Slight irregularities may appear after the edema subsides, causing considerable anxiety to the patient. These may occur along the dorsum of the nose at the point of junction of the lateral walls; although the condition is usually not visible, the patient can feel the irregularities on palpation.

EARLY COMPLICATIONS FOLLOWING CORRECTIVE RHINOPLASTY. Many of the complications and measures to prevent them have been mentioned in the previous pages. Some of the complications are discussed below.

Hemorrhage. This is usually the result of the detachment of a scab or clot overlying a nasal area denuded of mucous membrane. Avoidance of denuded areas will minimize the danger of postoperative hemorrhage. Postoperative hemorrhage is more frequent if a septal procedure has been performed. It is usually not severe and is easily controlled by removing clots, achieving hemostasis by

the application of epinephrine or Oxycel gauze, and intranasal packing when required. Care should be exercised to avoid displacing the bony lateral walls of the nose by pressure from the packing. Occasionally, severe epistaxis may occur, requiring postnasal packing as well as packing of the anterior nasal fossae. This is fortunately a rare occurrence.

Infection. If hematoma is avoided and if small fragments of spicules of bone or cartilage are carefully removed prior to the completion of surgery, infection is rare. The usual site for an abscess, a rare occurrence, is in the upper portion of the line of osteotomy. Incision and drainage and antibiotic treatment will usually resolve this complication.

Irregularity in shape. Most complications are due to faulty planning or technique. These mistakes have been described in the previous pages of this chapter.

Progressive postoperative widening of the bony dorsum is usually caused by an undiagnosed high deviation of the septum. The following anatomical factors may impede the medial displacement of the lateral walls of the nose: excessive width of the dorsal border of the septum caused by the increase in skeletal width; hypertrophy of the mucous membrane; interposition of mucous membrane between the medially mobilized lateral nasal walls; and deviation of the dorsal portion of the septum. Such complications can be avoided by careful inspection and correction prior to completion of the operation.

Minor curvature or deviation of the cartilaginous dorsum of the nose by undetected curvatures of the septal framework can spoil an otherwise satisfactory result. Careful examination of the septum will prevent such a complication.

Irregularity in the shape of the tip. As mentioned earlier in the chapter, in patients with thin skin any irregularity of the cartilaginous structures of the tip will be conspicuous; in the patient with thicker skin in whom alar cartilages are thin, minor irregularities are usually not noticeable. More care must be taken, therefore, when the skin is thin than when the skin is thick. The removal of the entire lateral crus of the alar cartilage can be done with impunity when the skin is very thick.

Irregularities in the area of the dome and the lateral crus are the most common complications. In order to avoid an irregularity along the caudal border, the transgression of this border by surgical incision is avoided in the routine corrective rhinoplasty. If the caudal border is transgressed, which it must be in wide tips, the caudal border of the cartilage should be realigned by placing a catgut suture. Failure to realign the cartilage may result in a protrusion of the portion of the cartilage lateral to the incision. Other irregularities, such as disproportion in the shape of the domes, may occur and require secondary surgery to achieve symmetry.

Secondary corrective measures require exposure of the defective area; the Safian type of exposure (see Fig. 29–109) is an effective technique. Another technique is complete exposure of the tip cartilage after meticulous dissection through a rim incision (see Fig. 29–110).

Postoperative drooping of the tip. The tip of the nose appears to droop in the early postoperative period because swelling of the base of the columella and upper lip produces a temporary elevation of the tip; the subsidence of the swelling allows the tip to resume its position, and the patient interprets this event as a downward drooping of the tip (see Fig. 29–80). The tip of the nose will droop after a rhinoplasty if the cartilaginous lateral walls (alar cartilages) have been shortened inadequately in relation to the shortened septum. The elasticity of the cartilages will push the tip downward, the nasal tip gradually resuming its preoperative position. Ironically, overshortening of the septum may be a cause of postoperative drooping of the tip. When the tip is downwardly dislocated from the septal angle prior to surgery, shortening the septum increases the loss of contact between the structures and is a basic technical mistake to be avoided.

The supratip protrusion. A frequent postoperative complication is the supratip protrusion, which spoils a profile which is otherwise satisfactory. Various factors are responsible for this complication. These were enumerated earlier in the text (see p. 1085). The treatment of this complication is discussed later under Secondary Corrective Rhinoplasty (see p. 1152).

Excessive removal of the dorsal hump. Earlier in the text, in the description of a technique of corrective rhinoplasty (see p. 1070), the need to avoid excessive resection of the dorsal hump was emphasized. Excessive removal of bony and cartilaginous framework in the resection of the nasal hump is a complication that is difficult to correct without secondary grafting. In the nose with thick skin, it is particularly necessary to be prudent in the amount of resection along the dorsum in order to avoid the supratip protrusion.

A depressed area of the cartilaginous dorsum occurs if the septum has been removed in excess or incised along its dorsal border, particularly if the septal mucoperichondrial flaps have been badly torn, since the cicatricial contraction of the healing flap increases the tendency to depression along the dorsum (see Secondary Corrective Rhinoplasty, p. 1152).

These are a few of the early complications which occur following a corrective rhinoplasty. Later in the chapter other complications are discussed under Secondary Corrective Rhinoplasty.

Additional Corrective Procedures

The Invagination Procedure. In order to obtain a better fixation of the alar cartilages to the septal angle, the invagination procedure may be employed in those cases in which the tip is dislocated off the septal angle: the denuded septal angle is placed between the medial crura (Fig. 29–81). The structures are maintained by two transfixion sutures of 3–0 catgut and additional sutures to close the transfixion incision.

Resection of the Base of the Alae. Careful consideration should be given to resection of the alar bases. Is the procedure really necessary? The facial features should be considered in their entirety, and frequently the wide, thick alae may "fit" the broad features. The risk of a slight irregularity or asymmetry should be weighed against the minor improvement resulting from this additional procedure.

After the nose has been remodeled, the tip of the nose may have been recessed in order to align it with the new profile line. The diminution in the projection of the tip causes a flaring of the alae (Fig. 29–82, *A*). Bilateral resection of the alar base is required to eliminate the flare (Fig. 29–82, *B, C*). This procedure may also be required when the alar base is excessively wide and thick.

Weir (1892) described an operation for the correction of Negroid nostrils, consisting of the excision of a portion of the base in the area of attachment of the nostril to the cheek. Joseph (1931) and Aufricht (1943) reduced the area of excision to the base of the nostril and the floor of the vestibule. The author's technique is the following. Slight laterally applied

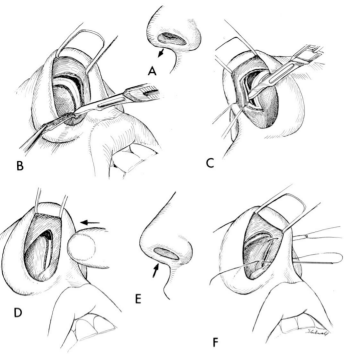

FIGURE 29–81. The invagination procedure. *A*, The tip of the nose tends to droop downward off the septal angle. *B*, The septal angle is denuded of mucous membrane. *C*, A pocket is made between the medial crura. *D*, The septal angle is invaginated between the medial crura. *E*, Suspension of the tip to the septal angle. *F*, Transfixion sutures approximate the structures. The upper transfixion suture invaginates the septal angle between the medial crura.

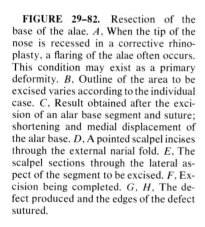

FIGURE 29–82. Resection of the base of the alae. *A*, When the tip of the nose is recessed in a corrective rhinoplasty, a flaring of the alae often occurs. This condition may exist as a primary deformity. *B*, Outline of the area to be excised varies according to the individual case. *C*, Result obtained after the excision of an alar base segment and suture; shortening and medial displacement of the alar base. *D*, A pointed scalpel incises through the external narial fold. *E*, The scalpel sections through the lateral aspect of the segment to be excised. *F*, Excision being completed. *G, H,* The defect produced and the edges of the defect sutured.

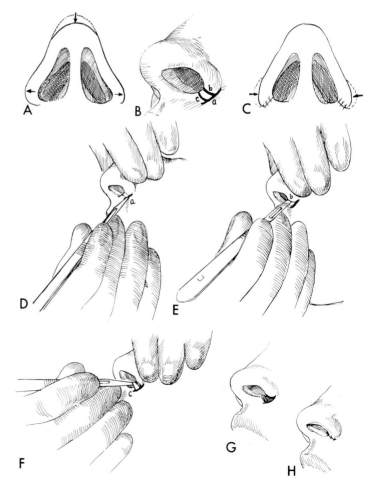

pressure is exerted on the ala; a crease appears in the anterior narial fold and the floor of the vestibule. The crease is outlined in ink. By exerting inward pressure on the ala, an evaluation can be made of the amount of excess tissue. The fold between the external naris and the upper lip is outlined (Fig. 29–82, *B*). A second line is drawn over the skin of the ala, based upon the amount of tissue to be removed (Fig. 29–82, *B*). This line rejoins the posterior extremity of the vestibular line, thus outlining a trapezoid area. Local anesthetic solution is injected. Using a sawing movement with a #11 (pointed) blade, incisions are made following the outline of the segment to be removed (Fig. 29–82, *D* to *F*). The segment is removed (Fig. 29–82, *G*), and the edges of the wound are approximated and sutured, the first suture restoring the continuity of the external nares (Fig. 29–82, *H*). Special care is taken to avoid resecting tissue from the floor of the vestibule.

Sculpturing the Alar Margin. It is rarely necessary to excise tissue from the alar margin in Occidentals. Resection of the alar base is the only procedure occasionally required.

Removal of irregularities along the alar margin is a useful procedure in secondary rhinoplasty and in the correction of the nasal deformity of cleft lip and palate (see Chapter 47).

Millard (1967b) has advocated the use of alar margin excisions to thin a bulky rim (Fig. 29–83), a modification of a procedure previously advocated by Fomon (1960), and also to elevate a drooping ala and reform its natural curve when the alar margin is more caudal than the columella.

When this procedure is combined with an alar base wedge excision, it is particularly applicable to the thinning of the alae in the Negroid nose. Spina (1966) and Boo-Chai (1964) have used this procedure in the Negroid and Oriental noses, respectively. Neither hypertrophic scarring nor keloid formation has been reported.

Correction of the Wide Columellar Base. This condition is often caused by lateral traction upon one medial crus by a deviated caudal end of the septal cartilage. One medial crus becomes separated from the other, leaving a wide gap between the cartilaginous structures. Attempts to narrow the base of the columella by means of mattress sutures through the skin

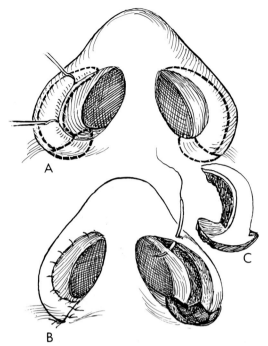

FIGURE 29–83. *A*, Outline of alar margin excisions to thin a bulky rim. *B*, The edges of the excised area have been approximated and sutured. *C*, The excised tissue. (After Millard.)

usually result in an inflammatory reaction, because the sutures cut through the skin. In order to prevent this complication, the following technique has been successfully used. An incision is made along the caudal margin of the medial crus on each side (Fig. 29–84, *A*); the overlying skin of each medial crus is then separated from the cartilage (Fig. 29–84, *B*), and the areolar tissue between the crura is resected (Fig. 29–84, *C*). When the medial crura diverge excessively from each other, a transverse incision is made in the medial crus at the point of divergence to break the spring of the cartilage (Fig. 29–84, *D*). A mattress suture of 4–0 chromic catgut approximates the medial crura (Fig. 29–84, *D, E*); the suture, placed subcutaneously, does not ulcerate through the skin (Fig. 29–84, *E*). The skin incisions are closed with 5–0 catgut sutures (Fig. 29–84, *F*).

The Columella-Ala Triangle, the Septum, and the Protrusive Nasal Spine Invading the Upper Lip. In a harmoniously shaped nose, the columella protrudes downward beyond a horizontal line drawn through the base of each ala; the columella is placed so as to form an open triangle with the alae (Fig.

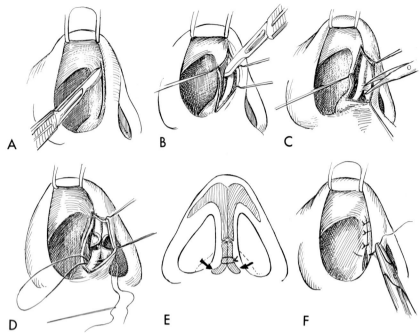

FIGURE 29–84. Narrowing the wide columella. *A,* An incision is made along the caudal margin of the medial crus. *B,* The skin is raised from the lateral surface of the medial crus. *C,* The medial crura are separated in the midline. *D,* An incision is made through each medial crus at its point of divergence. *E,* Approximation of the medial crura by a buried mattress suture of chromic catgut. *F,* The cutaneous incision is sutured with 5–0 plain catgut.

29–85, *A, B*). When the septal cartilage protrudes excessively into the upper lip, this triangle becomes more closed. Another angle formed by the columella with the upper lip, the columella-labial angle, may become

too wide (Fig. 29–85, *C*). The resection of a suitably shaped piece of cartilage from the caudal end of the septal cartilage generally corrects this deformity (Fig. 29–85, *D*). Usually, it will be noted that the septal carti-

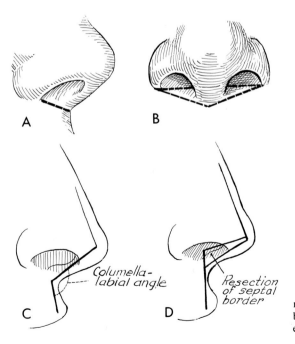

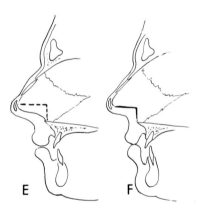

FIGURE 29–85. *A, B,* Columella-ala triangle. *C,* Columella-labial angle. *D* to *F,* The columella-labial angle may be modified by resection of the lower portion of the caudal end of the septal cartilage.

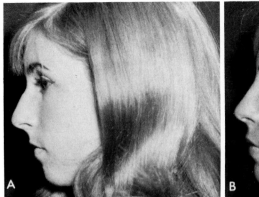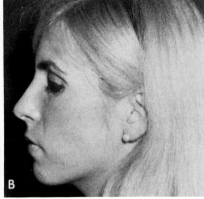

FIGURE 29–86. The protrusive nasal spine. *A*, Note the protrusion of the nasal spine under the upper lip, widening the columella-labia angle. *B*, After resection of the nasal spine. (Courtesy of Dr. H. Diamond.)

lage protrudes beyond the nasal spine, and resection of cartilage is required to correct the deformity. A suture placed through the base of the columella and through the septal cartilage "snugs" the columella base upward against the septum.

The nasal spine may also be protrusive and must be resected. The protrusive nasal spine not only causes an increased projection of the columella base (Fig. 29–86) and shortens the upper lip but also contributes to the formation of a transverse crease in the upper lip when the patient smiles.

The Hanging Columella. The anatomy of the hanging columella shows two types of deformity: (1) the medial crura have an excessive curvature, the convexity of the cartilages being caudad; (2) the membranous septum is excessively stretched, and the distance between the medial crura and the caudal border of the septal cartilages is increased.

In unusually severe cases, the medial crura must be approached and modified in shape. The procedure illustrated in Figure 29–87 is employed. An incision along the caudal border of each medial crus exposes the cartilage, which is freed of soft tissue, trimmed, or otherwise modified.

Resection of an excessively developed membranous septum may be achieved by excising the excess; an alternative is to sweep the transfixion incision caudally to the septal cartilage, then excise a segment of septal cartilage along with the excess membranous septum.

The Retruded and Retracted Columella. The columella is an esthetic landmark of the nose, a column that divides the nares and sup-

ports the tip of the nose. Any noticeable discrepancy of the columella becomes conspicuous. The columella may be retracted and the columella-labial angle acute. This deformity

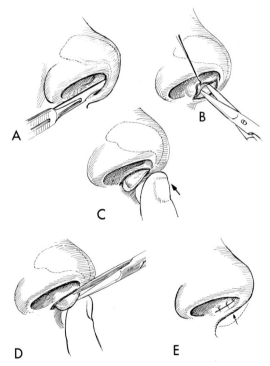

FIGURE 29–87. Correction of the hanging columella by excision of excess medial crus. *A*, Incision along the caudal margin of the medial crus. *B*, Freeing the medial crus from the overlying skin. *C*, The columella is retruded to an adequate position of correction; excess medial crus becomes evident. *D*, Trimming the medial crus. *E*, The incision along the caudal border of the medial crus is sutured with 5–0 plain catgut. This procedure can be combined with resection of the caudal portion of the septal cartilage, and nasal spine, which corrects the too-short upper lip due to invasion of the septum into the lip.

may be caused by a retraction, destruction, or resection of the caudal portion of the septal cartilage or underdevelopment of the premaxillary wings and nasal spine. A most severe retraction results from a number of causes. The columella itself may be severely scarred as a result of injury which has also affected the membranous septum; the underlying skeletal structures, the area of the nasal spine, and the anterior floor of the nose may have been fractured. All of these causes result in a retrusion and a retraction of the columella, affecting mostly its base. Many retracted columellas result from overshortening of the septum during a corrective rhinoplasty.

Careful examination is required in order to

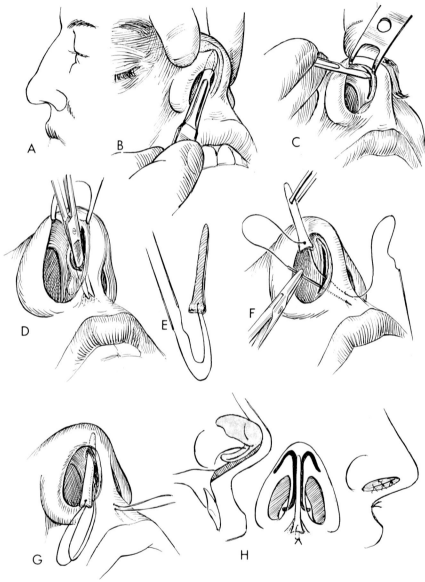

FIGURE 29–88. Increasing the projection of the retruded columella by a septal cartilage graft introduced through an anterior columellar approach. *A*, Typical appearance of patient with retruded columella and overhanging tip and ala. *B*, The tip is pinched, and the knife is placed in the recess of the vestibule along the caudal border of the dome; the incision is then extended downward along the caudal border of the medial crus. *C*, An incision along the medial crus is being completed. *D*, Scissors dissect between the medial crura anterior to the nasal spine. *E*, The septal cartilage graft with the traction sutures. *F*, The septal cartilage graft is introduced caudal to the medial crura, guided by the traction sutures. *G*, The septal cartilage graft is introduced. *H*, Position of the cartilage graft (left). The cartilage graft is maintained anterior to the nasal spine (center); the traction sutures may be brought out through the skin and tied over a piece of gauze to maintain the position of the transplant. The columella incision is sutured (right). This procedure is usually performed in conjunction with shortening of the nose to correct the overhanging tip and alae.

determine whether the columella is truly retracted or whether the retraction is relative because the lateral walls of the nose are excessively long and the alae protrude caudally in relation to the columella. In such cases, the lateral walls, in addition to the entire nose, must be shortened. This type of deformity is usually associated with the long nose with the plunging tip (see p. 1113).

Various methods have been employed to correct the retraction of the columella. A septal cartilage graft is placed through an incision in the columella, made along the caudal border of the medial crus. After the columellar skin is undermined down to the nasal spine, the lower end of the transplant rests upon, or is caudal to, the nasal spine, thus increasing the projection of the columella, and at the base of the columella improving the contour of the columella-labial angle (Fig. 29–88). A mattress suture placed through the medial crura prevents the transplanted cartilage from being displaced backward between the medial crura, thus losing its projecting function and widening the columella (see also The Round Tip, p. 1111).

To correct retrusion of the base of the columella, Aufricht (1961) employs a transverse incision through the floor of the vestibule of the nose, undermining the soft tissue over the nasal spine, and transplants septal cartilage in this area (Fig. 29–89). Resected alar and lateral cartilage may also be used for the transplant.

The retraction of the columella may be such

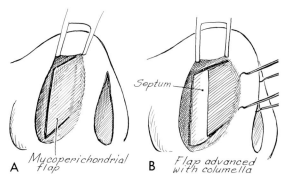

FIGURE 29–90. The sleeve procedure for the correction of columellar retrusion (Converse, 1964). *A,* Incisions are made through the mucoperichondrium and mucoperiosteum to release a flap, permitting the increase in projection of the columella as shown in *B. B,* The flap has been advanced, with the columella leaving an area of exposed cartilage which re-epithelizes spontaneously. A similar flap is designed on the contralateral side of the septum. The precaution should be made, however, to place the areas of denuded septum one in front of the other in order to avoid the possibility of a septal perforation. This procedure is effective only if it is done in conjunction with a septal columella cartilage transplant, as shown in Figure 29–88.

that the insertion of a septal cartilage graft causes blanching of the skin, making it obvious that the soft tissues must be released. The "sleeve" procedure has been successful in obtaining release of the retracted soft tissues (Converse, 1964). The procedure involves the use of bilateral vertical and horizontal incisions through the mucoperichondrium on each side of the septum, the mucoperichondrium being raised from the septal cartilage and freed as far as the caudal margin of the septal cartilage (Fig. 29–90). The columella may then be protracted, the mucoperichondrial flaps and the membranous septum following the advancement of the columella. The exposed areas of septal cartilage which result from the advancement of the mucoperichondrial flaps usually heal rapidly by secondary epithelization. In order to avoid bilateral exposed septal cartilage, the incisions through the mucoperichondrium and mucoperiosteum should be placed at different positions, one in front of the other.

The intraoral approach to the nasal spine uses a vestibular incision made on the buccal aspect of the vestibule; the nasal spine is exposed under direct vision. The graft is then placed into the base of the columella and over the nasal spine.

Nasal cartilage is usually the best material for restoring contour. Other procedures have been described to release the retracted colu-

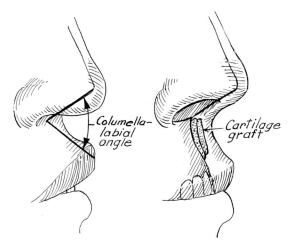

FIGURE 29–89. Opening the columella-labia angle by means of septal cartilage grafts. The cartilage grafts are introduced through an incision in the floor of the vestibule. (After Aufricht.)

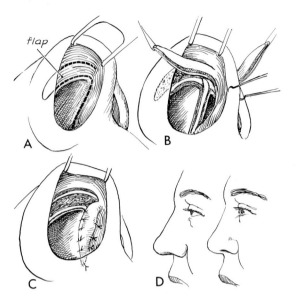

FIGURE 29–91. Increase in the projection of the columella by means of a flap of alar cartilage and vestibular lining. *A*, The flap of the cephalic portion of the alar cartilage with underlying vestibular lining is outlined. as well as the incision in the membranous septum. *B*, The alar flap is raised. *C*, The flap has been transposed. *D*, The procedure not only increases the projection of the columella but also shortens the nose, correcting the overhanging nasal tip and alae. (After Millard.)

Deepening of the Prominent Nasofrontal Angle. When the nasofrontal angle is lacking, the condition may be corrected by the following technique. A flat osteotome is placed along the line of section for the removal of the hump, and the osteotome is tapped upward to the upper portion of the root of the nose in a line which is a continuation of the new dorsal profile (Fig. 29–92, *A*). The fragment of bone is removed (Fig. 29–92, *B*) after the attachment of bone is fractured either by levering the bone with the osteotome along the line of section or by using a fine-tapered, narrow osteotome introduced through the skin at the uppermost level of the line of section. Irregularities are smoothed with a curved rasp after the wedge of bone is removed (Figs. 29–92, *C*, and 29–93).

Variations in Corrective Rhinoplastic Techniques

There is probably no area of plastic surgery that requires more judgment and careful planning than the corrective rhinoplasty. Each patient requires a different approach based on the type of nose, the ethnic background, and the facial configuration. The stilted, formalized rhinoplastic result should be avoided; the nose must fit the face. Thus many variations in the technique must be considered.

These statements appear to contradict the advocacy of the order of procedure in the earlier portion of this chapter.

mella; flaps of vestibular lining and alar cartilage (Fig. 29–91) have been used by Millard (1967b), and a composite graft of the concha of the auricle has been used by Dingman and Walter (1969) to correct the overshortened nose and retracted columella (see p. 1279).

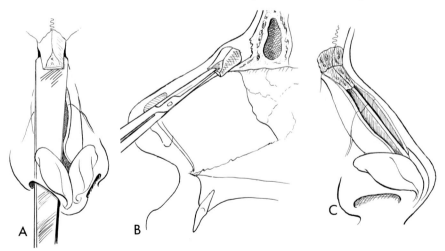

FIGURE 29–92. Deepening the nasofrontal angle. *A*, A wide osteotome, with rounded angles to avoid injury to the soft tissues, is placed along the line of resection of the dorsal hump and is tapped upward with a mallet. *B*, After the osteotome is levered upward, the upper attachment to the frontal bone is fractured (or if this is inadequate, the upper attachment to the frontal bone can be severed by sectioning with a narrow osteotome placed through the skin). The wedge of bone is removed. *C*, Deepened nasofrontal angle obtained by this procedure.

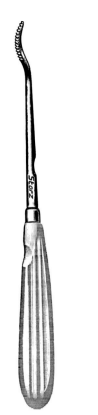

FIGURE 29–93. Curved rasp used to deepen the naso-frontal angle.

of the nose than might have been planned before the operation.

The Single Hump Operation. In this procedure, as in the Joseph technique, the saw cuts through the bony hump and the button knife is passed under the hump, sweeping caudally to resect a portion of each lateral cartilage and the dorsal border of the septum. When it is performed with great precision, the osteocartilaginous profile is modified in a single step. The technique is particularly applicable in a large nose with a prominent dorsal hump.

Robin (1969), who uses the submucous approach (see p. 1101), determines by means of measured photographs of the patient's profile at what level he wishes to resect the hump. He then cuts through the septal cartilage and the lateral cartilages at the predetermined level, introduces an osteotome, and removes the osteocartilaginous hump in one piece; also, as in the Joseph saw technique, he then modifies the nasal tip.

Both of these techniques have the disadvantage of leaving the operator with a *fait accompli:* the hump is removed, the change of the profile is definitive, and the surgeon is committed.

An order of procedure provides a precise, orderly, and prudent approach to corrective rhinoplasty. There are many variations, however, in the types of deformities, and these variations may require different techniques. In certain cases, it is not necessary to narrow the nose by lateral osteotomies; in others, the correction can be obtained without detaching the lateral cartilages from the septum. In other cases, the approach may be entirely different, as in the unusual deformity or in the deviated or depressed nose; lastly, the plastic surgeon, an individualist, may have developed his own order of procedure.

The more experienced surgeon, after careful anatomical analysis, may prefer to correct first either the most distorted portion of the nose or that part most difficult to correct.

The change in position of the nasal tip following the transfixion procedure and after judicious resection of the caudal portion of an excessively prominent nasal spine has been emphasized; the spontaneous increase in the projection of the tip resulting from the release of the downward pull of the columella is a warning to resect much less from the dorsum

The Double Hump Operation. In this procedure, the tip is adjusted to the septal angle and caudal border of the septum. The tip operation is performed, the lateral cartilages are separated from the septum, and the dorsal border of the septum is lowered to establish the cartilaginous profile as far cephalad as the caudal border of the nasal bones. The lateral cartilages are then adjusted to the dorsal border of the cartilaginous septum. The projection of the bony hump is now increased in relation to the modified cartilaginous profile. An osteotome or a rasp placed at the lower border of the nasal bones removes the hump. The cartilaginous nose is thus remodeled and the bony nose adjusted to the cartilaginous nose.

A disadvantage is a partial commitment on the part of the surgeon: he must be confident that the bony hump resection will "fit" the new profile of the cartilaginous nose. Another disadvantage of this technique is a slight irregularity which may appear at the junction of the bony and cartilaginous dorsum, usually caused by projecting cephalic portions of the lateral cartilages. Care must be taken to verify the position of these structures under direct vision at the end of the operation.

Sheen's Technique of Corrective Rhinoplasty. Although Sheen (1976) states that he does not necessarily follow a routine order of procedure in correcting the average hump nose deformity, he usually uses as his initial landmark the reduction of the bony hump. The bony nasal dorsum is reduced and shaped by means of a rasp* (Fig. 29–94). When a suitable level of reduction has been achieved, the cartilaginous nose is reduced in harmony with the bony nose under direct vision with headlight illumination and adequate retraction. A #11 (pointed) blade, the tip of the blade having been broken off, is used for this purpose. The cartilaginous dorsum is progressively shaved down until it is aligned in continuity with the bony dorsum. Sheen states that if the dorsal hump does not exceed 4 to 5 mm, it is possible to remove the cartilage in a submucous fashion through such a supracartilaginous approach without interrupting the continuity of the mucoperichondrium. In resecting larger humps, the cartilages and mucoperichondrium are removed together, thus avoiding leaving excess nasal lining. The alar cartilages are also approached in a supra-

---

*Storz rasp No. N–4554 and N–4556.

cartilaginous fashion for the tip operation. Rim incisions expose the cartilages (see Fig. 29–110). Only the required amount of cartilage is removed to achieve a satisfactory correction, a point of technique emphasized in the earlier section of this chapter. The cartilage is removed without resecting the vestibular lining. A series of partial thickness incisions accentuate the angle of the domes when required. The rim incision is sutured with fine catgut sutures.

The lateral osteotomies are done with a chisel, *starting low and ending high,* as emphasized by Sheen, and the lateral walls are infractured.

Sheen's technique provides a sound approach to the problem of the average rhinoplasty.

Variations in the Transfixion Incision. The routine transfixion incision (Fig. 29–95, *A*) is contraindicated when the nose does not require a change in the position of the tip and when only a minor dorsal removal or straightening of the nose is indicated. When additional exposure is required, the transfixion incision is extended downward around the septal angle for a short distance, sufficient to allow

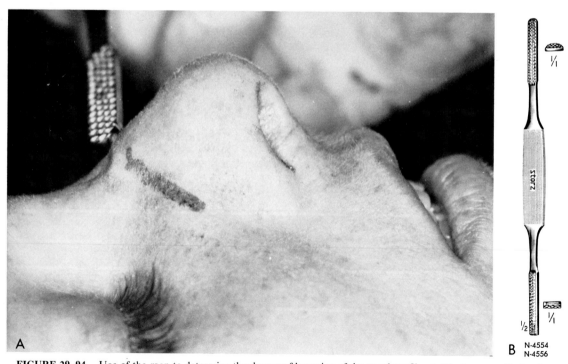

FIGURE 29–94. Use of the rasp to determine the degree of lowering of the nasal profile. *A*, The bony profile has been lowered to the desired level using the rasp illustrated in *B*. The remainder of the nasal dorsum will then be reduced to conform to the profile level established at the cephalic portion of the dorsum (Courtesy of Dr. J. Sheen). *B*, The rasp. Note the rounded surface at the upper end of the rasp and the flat surface at the lower end. (Rasp No. N–4554, fine teeth; rasp No. N–4556, coarse teeth).

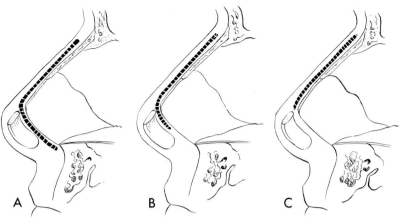

FIGURE 29–95. Complete versus interrupted transfixion. *A*, Complete transfixion. *B*, Transfixion interrupted below the septal angle. *C*, Transfixion interrupted at the septal angle.

shortening of the septal cartilage in the region of the septal angle (Fig. 29–95, *B*). Adequate exposure is thus obtained for modification of the dorsal septal profile line. The transfixion should be interrupted in the types of noses which do not require shortening; in such instances, the transfixion incision extends no further than the septal angle (Fig. 29–95, *C*).

It is also necessary to extend the incision around the septal angle to permit release of the alar cartilages from their septal attachments when complete exposure by a rim incision is required (see Fig. 29–110). In order that the dome and medial crura can be brought into view, they must not be restrained by their septal attachments. The intercartilaginous incision should be sufficiently long to permit adequate

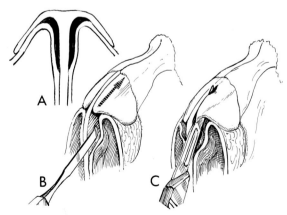

FIGURE 29–96. Submucous approach for an extramucous resection of the skeletal structures to modify the nasal profile. *A*, Frontal section through the septum and lateral cartilages; the black areas illustrate the raised areas of mucoperichondrium from the septum and the lateral cartilages. *B*, Raising the mucoperichondrium along the dorsal portion of the septum and the undersurface of the medial portion of the lateral cartilages. *C*, Severing the attachment of the lateral cartilage to the septum. (After Robin.)

mobilization of the lateral crus for exposure.

Another variation is the transcartilaginous septal transfixion made cephalad to the caudal border of the septal cartilage, a technique which is occasionally indicated in the long nose with a downward protruding tip (see Fig. 29–117).

The Submucous Approach. The septal angle serving as a landmark, the mucoperichondrium is raised bilaterally from the septal cartilage along the dorsum of the cartilage (Fig. 29–96, *A*, *B*), after subperichondrial injection of a solution of Xylocaine-Adrenalin. The mucoperichondrium is raised over an area sufficient to allow the required resection of the dorsal septal cartilage for the modification of the profile (Fig. 29–96, *B*). As the junction with the lateral cartilage is reached, the mucoperichondrial elevation is continued laterally along the undersurface of the cartilage. Thus the continuity of the mucous membrane is not interrupted between the septum and the lateral cartilage.

The lateral cartilage attachment to the septum is divided without sectioning the underlying mucous membrane (Fig. 29–96, *C*). The mucoperichondrium and mucoperiosteum are raised, using a Joseph elevator, from the undersurface of each nasal bone. The mucous membrane thus being reflected downward away from the skeletal structures which will be resected, the integrity of the highly specialized mucous membrane of the nose and its delicate, ciliated, pseudostratified, columnar epithelium is preserved, as advocated by Anderson and Rubin (1958), Cottle (1960), Anderson (1966) and Robin (1969). This technique eliminates the danger of stenosis from contracture at the critical internal naris (the nasal valve). At the end of the operation, a mattress suture of chromic catgut is placed through and through, approximating the mucous membrane flaps to the septal cartilage a few millimeters below the dorsal border of the septal cartilage.

The submucous approach, which can be performed expeditiously after some experience, is a satisfactory approach. It safeguards the integrity and preserves the physiologic mechanism of the nasal valve. The technique is contraindicated in very large noses because of the. excess of mucous membrane which remàins after the reduction of the nose. The submucous approach provides an excellent exposure of the septal framework when correction of a septal deviation is required during the rhinoplasty.

The Supracartilaginous Approach. When changes in the profile along the dorsum are minimal, this technique affords the simplest approach, with less derangement of the structures. The lateral cartilages are not detached from the septum. Minimal changes of contour of the lateral cartilages can be made by excising cartilage *from above* without penetrating the underlying mucoperichondrium in a fashion

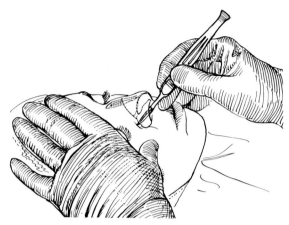

FIGURE 29–98. Position of the Joseph knife making the stab incision.

similar to the technique advocated by Sheen. The dorsal septum is trimmed. This technique is the simplest and is indicated when minimal profile change is necessary.

The Saw Techique for Lateral Osteotomy. The edge of the pyriform aperture near the floor of the nose is located with the handle end of a Joseph knife, the instrument being used to palpate the edge of the aperture (Fig. 29–97, *A*). A stab incision through the soft tissues and the periosteum is made lateral to the border of the pyriform aperture (Figs. 29–97, *B*, 29–98, 29–99, *A*). A periosteal elevator is then placed subperiosteally through the incision (Fig. 29–99, *B*). The elevator is slightly rotated upon itself as it passes up-

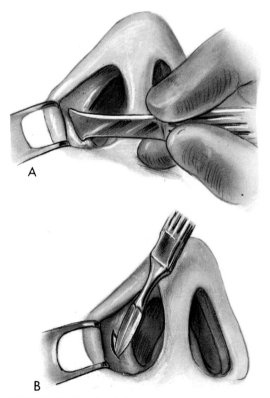

FIGURE 29–97. Lateral osteotomy (saw technique). *A*, The edge of the pyriform aperture is palpated with the blunt end of the Joseph knife. *B*, A stab incision is made at this point.

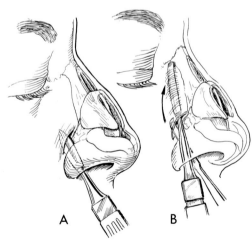

FIGURE 29–99. *A*, A stab incision is made immediately lateral to the pyriform aperture. *B*, The Joseph periosteal elevator establishes the subperiosteal tunnel along the base of the lateral wall of the nose.

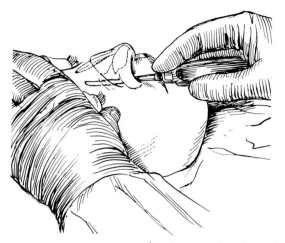

FIGURE 29–100. The Joseph elevator raises the periosteum along the line of the osteotomy.

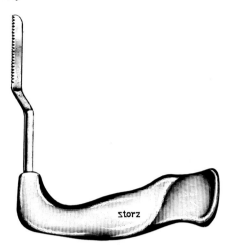

FIGURE 29–102. Saw with an anatomical handle to facilitate the procedure. Right and left angulated saws are used.

ward along the base of the lateral wall of the nose to a point anterior to the area of junction of eyelid and nasal skin (high osteotomy), establishing a subperiosteal tunnel large enough to introduce a saw blade (Fig. 29–100). A Joseph saw guide facilitates the passage of the saw (Fig. 29–101, *A, B*); the tip of the guide is directed against the bone, and traction is exerted in a downward and slightly lateral direction, thus opening the stab incision (Fig. 29–101, *B*). The osteotomy is done with a right-handed, angulated saw (Fig. 29–101, *C*). The introduction of the saw into the subperiosteal tunnel should be performed with fingertip delicacy. The instrument is held as a pen and slowly rotated into the tunnel. Friction of the saw teeth against the Joseph guide causes the blunting of the instrument; the teeth of the saw should be applied against the bone to avoid soft tissue injury. The saw cuts through the lateral wall (Fig. 29–101, *C*), and a dull-edge curette sweeps the bone dust (Fig. 29–101, *D*).

The saw (Fig. 29–102) should be directed horizontally across the lateral wall in order to

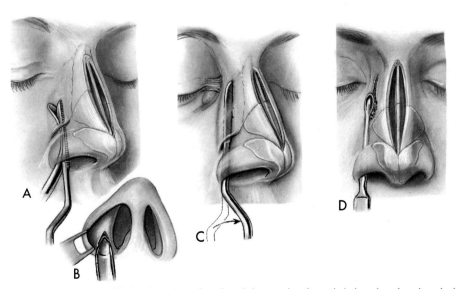

FIGURE 29–101. *A*, The saw guide has been introduced, and the angulated saw is being placed against the bone within the subperiosteal tunnel. *B*, Position of the saw guide within the intranasal incision. *C*, The saw guide after introduction is rotated and placed at an angle that will permit the saw to cut transversely through the base of the lateral wall of the nose. *D*, A smooth-edge curette sweeps the bone dust.

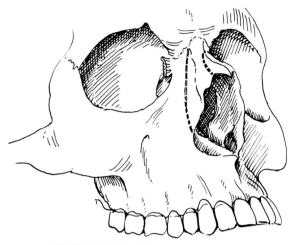

FIGURE 29–103. Line of lateral osteotomy.

cut through it (Fig. 29–103). The base of the lateral wall presents its maximal thickness at the junction with the body of the maxilla. If the saw is directed obliquely, inward, and backward, a much greater thickness of bone must be traversed, thus rendering the procedure more laborious. To facilitate the procedure, the patient's head is turned as far over to the side as possible and is immobilized by the assistant (Fig. 29–104). Only a slight amount of pressure should be exerted upon the saw in order to avoid "jamming" between the edges of the groove. The sawing is continued until the task is completed to avoid removing the instrument from its bony groove and establishing a second groove at the side of the first. The operator will be aware of a slight "give" when the saw penetrates the periosteum on the inner surface of the bone. A few remaining, lightly applied strokes of the saw complete the separation.

The lateral walls of the nose form the sides of a pyramid and are directed obliquely as they diverge toward the base of the pyriform aperture. The saw must be applied obliquely in order to be parallel to the lateral walls. Failure to place the saw correctly may result in sec-

tioning of the lower part of the lateral wall before the upper part.

The line of osteotomy is cleansed of bone dust with a dull-edge curette, the "sweeper." Each remaining minute particle of bone is potentially osteogenic, and such fragments can result in thickening along the base of the lateral wall.

Similar procedures are then undertaken on the left side, anesthesia of the lateral wall being obtained in the manner previously described.

A suitably designed, angulated saw blade with sharp teeth is a satisfactory instrument to cut through the base of the lateral wall of the nose. Saw blades should be resharpened or replaced at frequent intervals.

Choice between the saw and the osteotome techniques. The saw provides a precise line of osteotomy without radiating lines of osteotomy. It is indicated to section the lateral wall of malunited fractures when the bone is thickened and the osteotome can penetrate only with considerable force and trauma. The saw technique, however, is a more involved technique which requires more manual labor. Saws must be sharpened frequently to be efficient. In the average corrective rhinoplasty, the expedient osteotome method is a labor-saving technique.

Recession of the Nasal Dorsum. In long, thin noses which require surgical reduction in size,

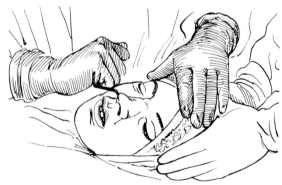

FIGURE 29–104. Positions of the patient's head and of the operator's and assistant's hands during the osteotomy with an angulated saw.

the dorsum of the nose may be delicately shaped. Surgeons have attempted to preserve this well-shaped, rounded structure.

Kazanjian, in a few patients, reduced a long nose with a well-shaped dorsum by recessing the dorsum after resecting a segment of septum and a segment from each lateral wall. This procedure was similar to that of Cottle, who advocated a "push-down" of the dorsum in order to preserve the mucous membrane, which is resected with the hump to avoid interfering with nasal physiology. The entire nasal pyramid was mobilized, and the dorsum was then pushed down. The dorsal border of the septum must be trimmed to permit this maneuver. These techniques require considerable skill to achieve the type of result expected by the patient.

Variations in Postoperative Splinting. As an alternative to the dental compound technique, the plaster splint is frequently employed. The technique is illustrated and explained in Figure 29–105.

Variations in the Technique of Tip Exposure. The *hockey-stick incision*, which was popularized by Brown and McDowell (1951), is simi-

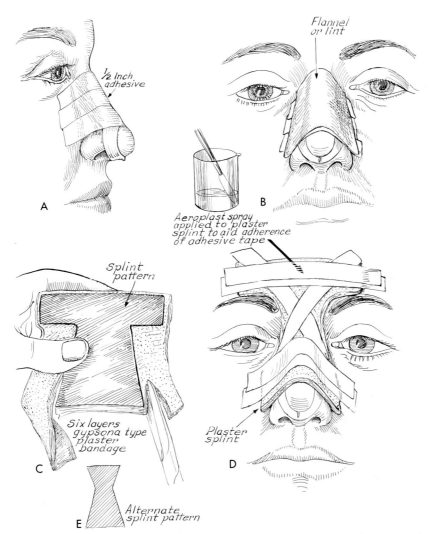

FIGURE 29–105. The plaster splint. *A*, Placing of paper adhesive strips over the remodeled nose. *B*, A piece of flannel material or lint is placed over the adhesive tape. *C*, The plaster splint is cut to fit a pattern. The splint consists of six layers of Gypsona-type plaster bandage. *D*, The splint, after being placed in water, is molded over the nose, hardened in situ, and maintained by paper adhesive strips. Aeroplast (plastic varnish) painted over the patient's face and forehead and over the splint increases the adherence of the adhesive tape. *E*, Alternate splint pattern.

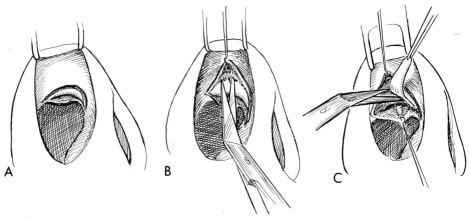

FIGURE 29–106. The retrograde technique. *A*, Intercartilaginous incision for exposure of the nasal framework. *B*, With angulated scissors, the vestibular skin has been raised; the soft tissues are elevated from the cartilage. *C*, Cartilage is resected from the cephalic portion of the lateral crus.

lar to the incision described earlier in the text which divides the lateral crus of the alar cartilage into cephalic and caudal segments. The hockey-stick incision owes its name to its shape, characterized by the curve of its medial portion which extends caudad into the dome.

The retrograde technique involves separating the overlying soft tissues and the vestibular lining from the cartilage through the intercartilaginous incision which was employed for the exposure of the nasal framework (Fig. 29–106). Excision of the required amount of cartilage from the upper portion of the lateral crus and from the region of the dome is done in a retrograde manner. The retrograde technique is convenient when only a small amount of lateral crus needs to be resected to achieve an adequate tip correction.

The eversion technique employs a posteroanterior incision which permits eversion of the lateral crus and trimming of the excess

cartilage under direct vision (Fig. 29–107). The eversion technique provides better exposure than the retrograde technique.

THE JOSEPH TIP OPERATION. The technique of nasal tip surgery developed by Joseph, with some modification, has been widely employed. Guided by preliminary landmarks traced on the skin of the tip of the nose, the lateral crus is divided by a transcartilaginous incision into upper and lower segments (Fig. 29–108, *A*). An incision is made a few millimeters cephalad to the caudal margin of the alar cartilage in the area of the dome. Scissors free the soft tissue over the cartilage by subperichondrial elevation (Fig. 29–108, *A*). At a chosen point in the region of the dome, an anteroposterior incision is made through the vestibular skin and cartilage, and a second oblique incision is made lateral to the first, delimiting a triangular or trapezoid piece of cartilage with its apex toward the margin of the nostrils (Fig. 29–108, *B*). The

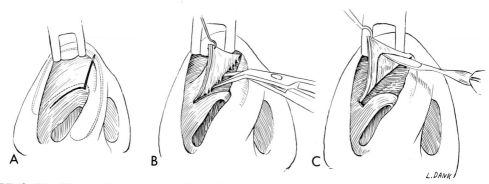

FIGURE 29–107. The eversion technique. *A*, From the medial end of the intercartilaginous incision, an additional posteroanterior incision is made. *B*, Subperichondrial separation of cartilage from the soft tissues. *C*, The cartilage is everted into an upside-down position, and necessary incisions preparatory to cartilage removal are being made.

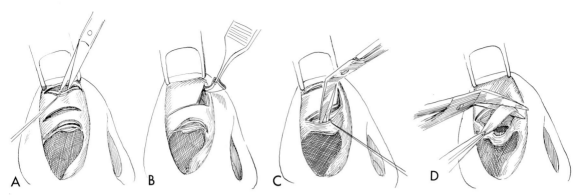

FIGURE 29-108. The Joseph tip operation (modified). *A*, The lateral crus of the alar cartilage, the dome, and a portion of the medial crus are freed from the overlying tissue. The alar cartilage has been divided into two segments by a transcartilaginous incision through the vestibular lining and cartilage. *B*, A triangular piece of cartilage and vestibular lining is resected from the dome. A quadrangular-shaped segment of cartilage is resected in a broad nasal tip. A narrow strip of caudal margin of the alar cartilage is preserved. *C*, The vestibular lining is raised from the upper segment of the lateral crus. *D*, The cephalic cartilaginous segment is resected.

segment of cartilage with its vestibular lining is removed. The continuity of the border of the cartilage should not be interrupted; a narrow strip of cartilage is preserved and not included in the triangular or trapezoid resection. The cephalic segment of the lateral crus is excised (Fig. 29-108, *C, D*). The cut surfaces of the cartilage at the dome are approximated and after a similar procedure is done on the contralateral side, the tip is examined for shape. Additional cartilage is removed if necessary.

If the caudal edge of the cartilage must be resected, a suture should approximate the me-

dial and lateral portions of the cartilaginous rim.

THE SAFIAN TIP OPERATION. The technique employed by Safian (1934) consisted of a posterior-anterior incision medial to the dome (Fig. 29-109, *A*) and a second incision separating the cartilage from the overlying soft tissues along the caudal margin of the alar cartilage (Fig. 29-109, *A, B*). The cartilage is extruded, and excess cartilage from the caudal, cephalic, or medial portions of the lateral crus and dome is excised according to the indications (Fig. 29-109, *C* to *E*). An objection to the Safian

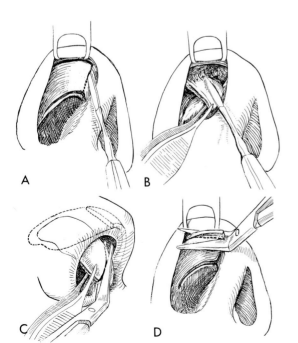

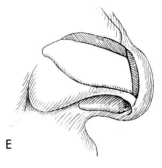

FIGURE 29-109. The Safian tip operation. *A*, The intercartilaginous incision has been made; the lateral crus is incised along its caudal margin, and an anterior-posterior incision is made medial to the dome. *B*, Subperichondrial separation of cartilage from the soft tissues. *C*, Trimming the medial border of the cartilage. *D*, Trimming the caudal border of the cartilage. *E*, The original version of the Safian operation trimmed only the caudal and medial portions of the lateral crus of the alar cartilage. A modification of the Safian procedure, as illustrated, can be employed, which involves excision of the cephalic portion of the lateral crus instead of the caudal portion.

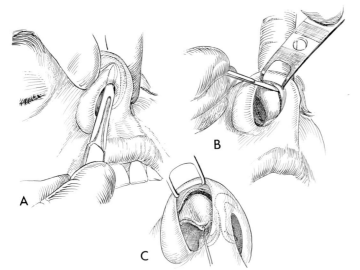

FIGURE 29–110. Complete exposure of the tip cartilages by rim incisions: degloving the tip. *A*, The tip of the knife is placed in the recess of the vestibule caudal to the dome; the tip is pinched to facilitate the procedure. *B*, The knife incises downward along the caudal margin of the medial crus. *C*, After a marginal incision along the caudal border of the lateral crus, the cartilage is separated from the overlying tissues and exposed. One or both domes can be brought into view by lateral traction with a hook.

operation is that it may sacrifice a major portion of the dome of the alar cartilage. The Safian operation is useful in secondary tip operations because of the wide exposure it provides.

TIP EXPOSURE THROUGH RIM INCISIONS; DEGLOVING THE TIP (Converse, 1940). A wider exposure of the alar cartilage may be obtained by extending the marginal incision along the caudal border of the medial crus (Fig. 29–110). The so-called rim or marginal incision should be made along the rim of the alar cartilage (Fig. 29–110, *A*, *B*) and not along the rim of the nostril. It will be recalled that the caudal margin of the alar cartilage lies considerably cephalad to the caudal margin of the nostril (see Fig. 29–13). An incision through the soft triangle which is formed only of soft tissues, being unsupported by cartilage, may result in disfiguring postoperative notching.

A subperichondrial exposure of the lateral and medial crura can be obtained by the subperichondrial elevation of the soft tissues from the cartilage by means of scissors. The cephalic border of the lateral crus is freed from the caudal border of the lateral cartilage by the intercartilaginous incision. A hook is placed under the dome, and the freed cartilage is extruded, the dome being readily accessible (Fig. 29–110, *C*). The required cartilage excisions, incisions, and remodeling can be done under direct vision. By exerting gentle lateral traction with a skin hook, both domes come into view. Thus the entire cartilaginous framework of the tip may be examined and modified.

EXTERNAL INCISIONS. The intranasal approach to rhinoplasty introduced by Roe and Joseph has been a great asset. Occasionally in corrective rhinoplasty an external incision is indicated.

Rethi (1934) described a procedure consisting of bilateral rim incisions extending along the margin of each lateral crus and downward along the caudal border of each medial crus. A transverse incision through the skin of the columella joins the two marginal incisions at the junction of the upper third with the lower two-thirds of the columella (Fig. 29–111). The soft tissues of the tip of the nose are raised from the cartilage in the manner of an elephant trunk, giving a wide exposure of both domes. Gillies described an incision similar to Rethi's, the transverse incision extending through the

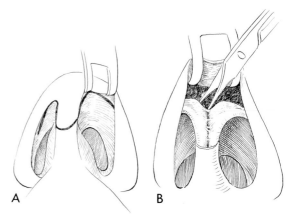

FIGURE 29–111. The Rethi exposure. *A*, Rim incisions along the caudal borders of the lateral crura, domes, and medial crura are joined by a horizontal incision across the columella. *B*, Exposure obtained. There are few indications for this type of exposure in the average corrective rhinoplasty, but it provides complete exposure of the unusually broad and bifid tip.

base of the columella. The skin of the columella is raised from the medial crura, exposing the caudal borders of both medial crura and the domes.

DeKleine (1955) advocated an approach to the tip through a midcolumellar vertical incision.

Excision of redundant skin in the supratip area may be the only means of removing thick, cardboard-like sebaceous skin (see Fig. 29–169). An ellipse of skin and subcutaneous tissue is excised and carefully sutured. Dermabrasion at a later date will usually make the scar inconspicuous.

External incisions are employed in more severe deformities but rarely in the usual corrective rhinoplasty (see later sections of this chapter).

CONSIDERATIONS ON THE VARIOUS TECHNIQUES OF NASAL TIP SURGERY. The review of methods for obtaining exposure of the tip cartilages also includes techniques for excising cartilage from the cephalic portion of the lateral crus and the dome. Such cartilaginous excisions are occasionally employed to complete the surgical correction of the long humped nose, in which the shortening and correction of the convex profile line are routine procedures. The shape and size of the alar cartilages and their relationship to the lateral and septal cartilages present a multiplicity of aspects: the cartilages are thick or thin and wide or narrow

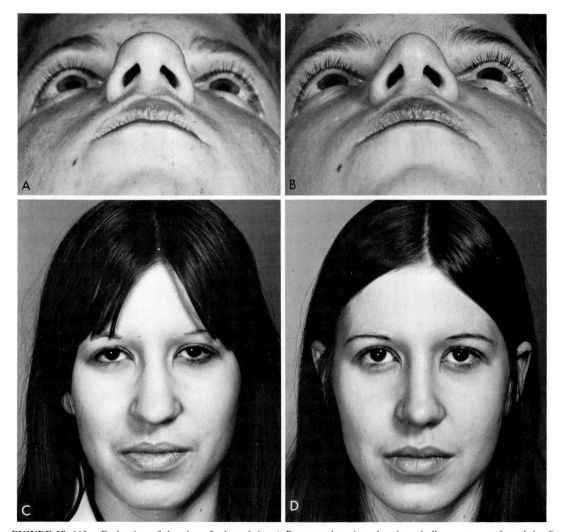

FIGURE 29–112. Reduction of the size of a broad tip. *A*, Preoperative view showing a bulbous, square-shaped tip. *B*, Result obtained after wide resection of cartilage and excision of subcutaneous tissue from the undersurface of the skin of the tip of the nose. *C*, Patient with wide tip caused by overdevelopment of the alar cartilages. *D*, After reduction of the tip.

and show a variety of shapes in the area of the dome.

Patients with thick, oily skin appear to tolerate the near-complete removal of alar cartilage with impunity (Fig. 29–112, *A, B*). It has been shown that the contour of the tip can be modified with minimal excision of cartilage (Fig. 29–113) (Converse, 1957). After complete exposure of the dome, the lateral crus, and a portion of the medial crus through a rim incision, the cartilage is incised at strategic points. The tip is molded into its new shape. The operation is hazardous when the skin of the tip of the nose is thin, as any irregularity of the cartilage will be conspicuous.

Wide-tip noses may require excision of cartilage from the dome (Fig. 29–112, *C, D*). Often it is possible to weaken the cartilage by partial thickness incisions, breaking the spring of the cartilage and maintaining the shape of the remodeled cartilage by external adhesive strapping.

Three precautions should be observed in performing surgical modifications of the shape of the alar cartilage:

1. Avoid raw areas resulting from removal of vestibular lining; the healing of such raw areas results in scar formation and distorting contracture.

2. Avoid excessive removal of cartilage, which produces a "pinched" appearance. In the region of the dome, excessive removal may leave a gap between the pieces of cartilage, resulting in an unsightly groove in the skin of the tip of the nose.

3. Sharp angles and protuberances due to overlapping cartilaginous fragments or improperly shaped cartilaginous transplants may produce external irregular prominences.

Increasing the Projection of the Tip. The caudal portion of the tip of the nose should project slightly above the profile line of the dorsum. Various procedures have been attempted to increase the projection of the tip.

Struts or "battens" have been placed into the columella to increase the projection of the tip. Various inorganic implants have been employed. Erosion of the skin of the tip is a complication. The author has removed a wide variety of such implants (glass, Silastic, metal, ivory).

Often the tip is tethered by the columella. After the transfixion procedure, and in some

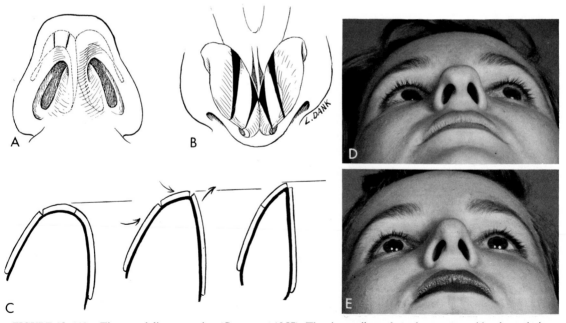

FIGURE 29–113. Tip remodeling operation (Converse, 1957). The tip cartilages have been exposed by the technique illustrated in Figure 29–110 (complete exposure of the tip of the cartilages by rim incisions). *A,* Location of the incisions through the cartilage. *B,* Another view showing the shape and size of the excised portions of cartilage. *C,* Change of shape of the alar cartilage achieved by incisions through the cartilage and suturing of the medial crura at a suitable level. *D,* Widened and slightly bifid tip. *E,* Result obtained by tip remodeling by the operation illustrated. Note the natural appearance of the tip. Partial thickness incisions are safer, as any irregularity will show under thin skin. The caudal ends of the incisions must be sutured.

cases after resection of the depressor septi nasi muscle, or in most cases release of the columella from the nasal spine, the nasal tip becomes tilted into a more cephalic and projected position.

Cartilage grafting, the graft being obtained from the septal cartilage, has been employed. A strut placed caudal to the medial crura, similar to the procedure for increasing the projection of the columella, is contraindicated as a method of increasing the projection of the nasal tip, as the transplant protrudes under the skin and may erode it.

A preferable technique using a septal cartilage transplant to increase tip projection has been advocated by Sheen (1975a). The transplant is placed between the medial crura and sutured in position to the medial crura or by the technique illustrated in Figure 29–115.

Increasing the projection of the tip by means of cartilage or bone grafts is discussed later in the chapter in the sections on bone grafting and secondary rhinoplasty.

The short columella seen in more severe deformities, such as maxillary deformities or the cleft lip nose, requires more extensive procedures (see Chapter 47).

The broad tip; the bulbous tip. The wide or broad tip, the square-shaped tip, and the bulbous tip may require extensive excision of cartilage. Complete exposure through a rim incision is indicated (see Fig. 29–110).

The domes are in close approximation and are shaped with a fairly sharp curve in tips whose contour is considered esthetically acceptable. The alar cartilages of the broad tip have a wider curve, and the domes are often separated from each other in the midline. The

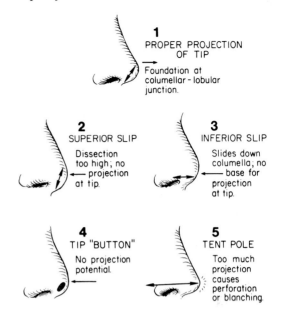

FIGURE 29–115. Correct position of cartilage graft at the tip-columella junction. (From Sheen, 1975a.)

contour of the square-shaped tip is determined by the wide, flat surface of the cartilaginous domes.

Bulbous tips are often characterized by thick soft tissues and relatively thin alar cartilages. Extensive resection of cartilage in this type of case, in contrast to the average type of nasal tip, does not appear to have dire consequences (see Fig. 29–112, *A, B*). In addition to the excision of cartilage, a careful excision of subcutaneous tissue is required, care being taken not to perforate the skin. When the incision is made through the cartilage, it is extended into the subcutaneous tissue. A layer of subcutaneous tissue is then dissected and removed with the cartilage.

Sheen (1976) has obtained good results by the lateral rotation technique (Fig. 29–114; see also Fig. 29–120 for a description of the technique).

The round tip. This type of deformity is often associated with a hanging columella. The tip can often be shaped satisfactorily by one of the more extensive tip procedures.

Sheen's technique (1975a) consists of a meticulously shaped septal cartilage graft placed at the tip-columella angle with a cephalic tilt of 35 degrees (Fig. 29–115).

Sheen makes an incision on the lateral aspect of the columella along the anterior border of the medial crus on one side. The incision is placed above the lower border of the

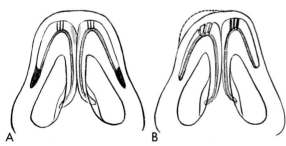

FIGURE 29–114. Technique of correction of the round tip by the lateral rotation technique. *A,* Complete exposure of the caudal portion of the alar cartilage after resection of the cephalic segment. The cartilage is dissected from its bed. A segment is resected from the lateral portion of the lateral crus. *B,* The right lateral crus is placed back into its bed and recessed. Partial thickness incisions at the area of the dome are usually required to aid the lateral rotation which is maintained by taping. (After Sheen, 1976.)

facet formed by the tip-columella junction (Fig. 29–116, *A*). A subcutaneous pocket is then formed in front of the cartilages and upward to the domes, extending into the alar rim and hugging the caudal aspect of the downward turning curve of the medial crura (Fig. 29–116, *A*). The cartilage graft is carefully shaped for the individual problem (Fig. 29–116, *B*). It is usually flat along its upper border and notched along its inferior border for better fixation, as the notch prevents rotation of the graft (Fig. 29–116, *C*). Fixation of the graft is assisted by

placing a transcutaneous 6–0 nylon suture through the graft. The incision is sutured with 5–0 plain catgut sutures. Further fixation is provided by the taping of the nose. A patient in whom a large nose with a round tip was treated by this type of septal cartilage transplant is shown in Figure 29–116.

Sheen states that the technique has been successful except in patients with very thin skin, in whom the graft revealed its presence by the blanching of the skin when the patient spoke, and in patients in whom the procedure

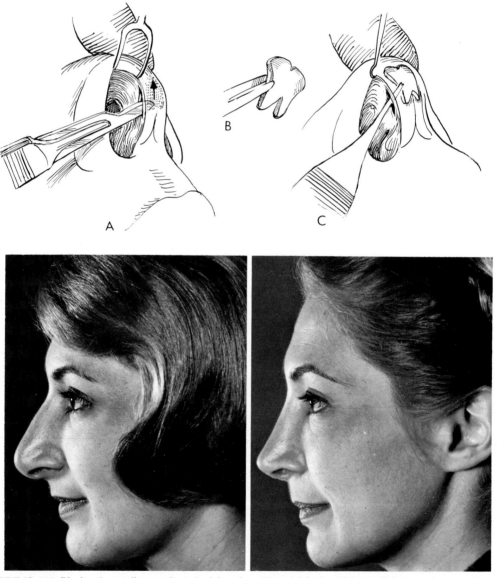

FIGURE 29–116. Placing the cartilage graft. *A*, Incision along the caudal edge of the medial crus and preparation of the subcutaneous pocket. *B*, Sculptured cartilage graft. *C*, The cartilage graft is imbedded. (After Sheen, 1975a.)
Left, Patient with large nose with round tip. Note absence of the columella-tip angle. *Right*, Result obtained after reduction of the size of the nose and imbedding of cartilage graft, as illustrated.

gave a "surgical appearance" (see also use of this technique in secondary rhinoplasty, p. 1160).

The "plunging" tip. The long nose with the "plunging" tip is a congenital condition which becomes more accentuated with aging. The anatomical characteristics of this deformity vary.

In one type, the septum is long, invading the lip, and the ligamentous attachments of the alar cartilages to the septal angle are adequate. The deformity is essentially caused by the nasal septum and lateral walls of an excessively long nose. These patients often have poorly developed alar cartilages and long, slitlike external nares.

The second type of long nose with a "plunging" tip shows, on digital palpation, a disconnection between the tip of the nose and the septal angle, the result of a loose suspensory ligament, and the nasal tip is dislocated downward from its aponeurotic attachments to the septal angle, which protrudes in the supratip area. This is also an anatomical characteristic of the Armenoid nose (see digital palpation test, Fig. 29–126).

These variations are important to consider in the treatment of traumatic deformities or noses with various congenital or ethnic characteristics. The treatment of each of the two varieties of "plunging" tip varies.

Correction of the "plunging" tip in the long nose is usually achieved satisfactorily through shortening of the septum and the lateral walls by excising an adequate amount of cartilage from the septal, lateral, and alar cartilages.

In the long nose of the first type, in which the nasal tip cartilages have an intimate connection with the septal angle, in order to avoid disruption of this relationship, the following procedure has proved effective and has given satisfactory results. Instead of the usual transfixion incision that follows the dorsal border of the septal cartilage and curves around the septal angle, thus disrupting the aponeurotic attachments of the nasal tip to the septal angle, the transfixion incision transects the septum cephalad to the septal angle (Parkes and Brennan, 1970). The incision is directed obliquely downward and forward to the mobile portion of the septal cartilage, anterior to the vomer groove, where the septal cartilage is mobile over the nasal spine (see Fig. 29–117, *A*). The caudal segment, being loosely connected in this area, may be retracted cephalad, overriding the fixed cephalic portion of the septum. In this manner the amount of shortening of the septum can be evaluated and the excess re-

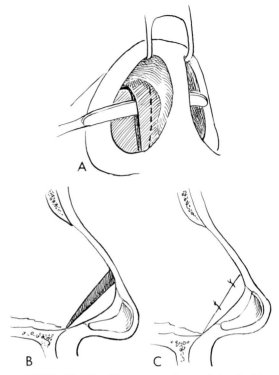

FIGURE 29–117. The transeptal transfixion incision. *A*, Transfixion posterior to the caudal border of the septal cartilage. *B*, Outline of the resected septum. *C*, The septal incision is sutured. (After Parkes and Brennan, 1970.)

moved from the fixed portion of the septum (Fig. 29–117, *B*). The caudal portions of the lateral cartilages usually must be detached from the septum and the necessary procedures done to shorten the cartilaginous nasal walls by excising a segment from each lateral crus. The transfixion incision is sutured using two through-and-through mattress catgut sutures (Fig. 29–117, *C*), and the mucoperichondrium on each side is sutured with interrupted sutures. Trimming of the dorsal border of the septal cartilage is required to align the dorsal borders of the two cartilaginous segments in order to achieve a satisfactory profile line.

In the type of "plunging" tip in which the deformity is caused by a dislocation downward of the alar cartilages from the septal angle, it would be a mistake to further shorten the septum. Instead it is essential to obtain fixation of the tip to the septal angle and, if necessary, to overlap the denuded undersurface of the alar cartilages over the lateral cartilages.

To maintain the tip, the invagination procedure (see Fig. 29–81) consists of removing the mucous membrane from the caudal end of the septal cartilage, particularly at the septal angle, and placing the septal cartilage between the medial crura, achieving an overlap of the crura over the septal cartilage. The medial crura are maintained in this position by sutures.

The plunging tip can be a difficult deformity to correct in the severe types of the deformity. An operation which is successful, despite the fact that it appears to break the basic rules of nasal physiology, is the following. After the invagination procedure in which the mucoperichonrium has been removed from the septal angle and the pocket between the medial crura, the cephalic portions of the lateral crura are denuded of their lining and are overlapped over the lateral cartilages. The surfaces of the cartilages adhere to each other after the healing process has taken place, ensuring firm fixation of the lateral walls in a cephalic position.

In the older patient, the tip of the nose tends to droop, and shortening of the nose may be indicated. The operative procedures described above are indicated. Resection of excess skin may be necessary at the root of the nose. In extreme cases, a transverse incision across the root of the nose, with bilateral vertical incisions on each side over the frontal process of the maxilla, enables the surgeon to remove the excess skin without leaving conspicuous scars because of the looseness of the skin in the aged.

The "smiling" tip; the mobile tip. In patients with mobile tips (usually the attachment to the septal angle is a loose one), the paired depressor septi nasi muscles are hyperactive. The tip undergoes a caudal droop when the patient smiles; a transverse crease is also formed occasionally at the base of the columella. In a small number of patients, the tip of the nose moves in harmony with the movement of the lips when the patient speaks. The treatment of these conditions consists in a resection of the paired depressor septi nasi muscle extending down to the nasal spine and of their attachments to the incisive fossae. Furakawa (1974) has demonstrated by means of electromyographic studies that the tip of the nose is pulled toward the columella-labial angle and also caudally by the depressor nasi muscle when the patient smiles.

Excision, partial or even complete in extreme cases, and detachment of the bony insertions of the muscle are procedures indicated in these patients.

The approach to the muscle is through the transfixion incision (Fig. 29–118), the muscle being resected from behind the columella, between the medial crura; resection of the depressor septi nasi muscle at the canine fossae can also be done through an intraoral

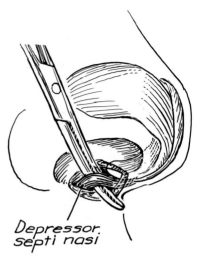

Depressor septi nasi

FIGURE 29–118. Exposure for the resection of the depressor septi muscle.

approach. Despite the resection of the depressor septi nasi muscles none of the patients has complained of nasal airway impairment. The removal of a transverse crease at the base of the columella that occurs during smiling is often caused by a short frenulum which must be lengthened by a Z-plasty. If the septal cartilage invades the lip, resection of cartilage at the caudal border is also necessary.

The projecting tip. An excessively projecting tip, the "Pinocchio nose," which also has some of the characteristics of the plunging tip, requires shortening and recession. First of all, a correct diagnosis must be made. Is the tip projected or is the dorsum recessed? In the patient shown in Figure 29–119, the dorsal profile was elevated with a septal cartilage graft, and minimal tip surgery was performed.

Lipsett (1959) described a technique for freeing the lateral crus, the dome, and the upper portion of the medial crus: an anterior-posterior transcutaneous incision is made through the skin and medial crus. The lateral cartilage is then advanced medially, and the dome and upper portion of the columellar skin and cartilage are advanced downward. Multiple incisions through the cartilage lateral to the recessed dome form a new dome, and the excess tissue (cartilage and skin) is resected from the columella. The incision is sutured. Because the technique results in the formation of a new dome on each side, it is not devoid of complications, such as irregularity in shape and position of the new domes, and thus has lost popularity.

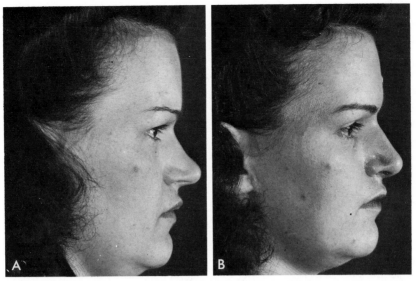

FIGURE 29–119. Correction of a projecting tip by increasing the dorsum of the nose. *A*, The tip projects because of the lack of projection of the dorsum. *B*, Result obtained by means of a septal cartilage transplant over the dorsum (see technique illustrated in Fig. 29–139).

Sheen (1976) describes his technique of lateral rotation as follows: after the usual tip operation and the resection of the cephalic segment of the lateral crus, the remaining caudal portion is everted, dissected, and freed (Fig. 29–120, *A*); its most lateral portion is amputated (Fig. 29–120, *B*). The size of the resected segment will depend upon the amount of recession required. This procedure is the reverse of the Lipsett technique. The recession is ob- tained by a lateral rotation, and what was dome becomes lateral crus, and what was medial crus becomes dome. To facilitate the formation of the new dome when the cartilage is thick, an incision partially extending through the cartilage medial to the dome will eliminate any resistance (Fig. 29–120, *C, D*). The correction may be combined with a medial crus resection. The tip is carefully taped.

The following technique is used in patients

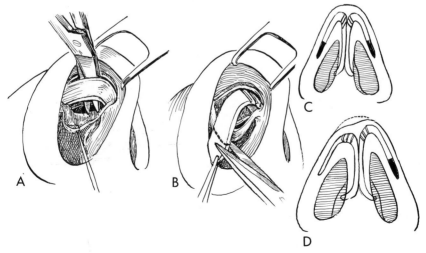

FIGURE 29–120. Correction of the projecting tip by the lateral rotation technique. *A*, After resection of the cephalic portion of the lateral crus, the cartilage is freed of its attachments. *B*, A segment is resected from the lateral end of the lateral crus. *C*, The cartilage is rotated laterally. Partial thickness incisions through the cartilage medial to the domes facilitate the formation of the new domes. *D*, The right lateral rotation has been completed; the left rotation has not, and the dome is still in the original position. (After Sheen, 1976.)

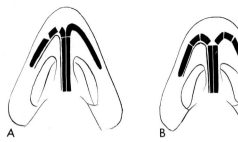

FIGURE 29–121. Correction of the excessively pointed tip. *A*, Remodeling of the shape of the tip of the nose by excision of cartilage from the dome of the right alar cartilage. *B*, The cartilage segments remain attached to the vestibular lining. (After Aufricht, 1943.) (From Kazanjan and Converse.)

with a projecting tip which needs only the usual corrective tip surgery, as the domes are well formed (Converse, 1975). The domes can therefore be preserved. Cartilage is resected from the medial crus. This can be done at various levels: the upper, middle, or lower portions of the medial crus. The medial crus is exposed by dissecting its cutaneous covering; the medial crura are separated by scissor dissection, and a measured section is removed. A measured section is also removed from the lateral portion of the lateral crus. The nasal tip is recessed. Often these patients have long, slit-shaped nares and do not require alar base resections, as the operation restores the normal flare of the nares.

The excessively pointed tip. A sharp, narrow-tipped nose is due to the anatomical configuration of the domes. The dome ordinarily forms a gently curved arch at the point where the lateral and medial crura meet; a pointed tip results if the crura meet at a sharp angle. The technique suggested by Aufricht (1943) may be used to correct this type of deformity (Fig. 29–121). The alar cartilages are exposed by the Joseph technique; the cartilages are divided at the highest point of the dome without incising the vestibular lining. A suitable segment of cartilage can then be resected; if necessary, a number of strips of cartilage are resected until a suitable curvature is obtained.

The lateral rotation technique (see Fig. 29–120) can also be used to correct the pointed tip.

The bifid tip. Approximation of the medial crura and the domes usually corrects the bifid tip deformity (Fig. 29–122). The various steps required for this procedure include exposure of the alar cartilages through rim incisions, removal of tissue between the medial crura, suitable incisions through the alar cartilages, excision of cartilage from the domes, and suturing of the medial crura. Bifidity of the columella is often best corrected by means of a small septal cartilage transplant.

The deviated nasal tip. Occasionally, the tip of the nose is severely deviated (see Fig. 29–134, *A*). In the deviated nose, the tip of the nose is often distorted. The pressure of the laterally twisted septal angle may separate the alar cartilages from one another, resulting in bifidity of the tip and asymmetry (see Fig. 29–147, *A*). Distortion of the columella by a deviated septal cartilage may displace one medial crus laterally and separate the crura, widening and distorting the columella with lateral pro-

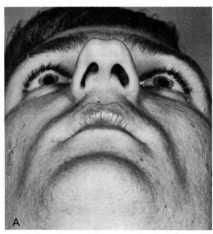
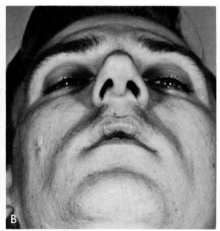

FIGURE 29–122. The bifid tip. *A*, Example of a bifid tip, characterized by a gap between the medial crura and the domes. *B*, Result obtained by bilateral rim incisions, resection of the intervening fibroareolar tissue, and approximation of the medial crura.

trusion of the lower end of one of the medial crura (see Fig. 29–147, *I, J*).

Correction of an asymptomatic septal deflection is not indicated in the average corrective rhinoplasty. The removal of an extensive amount of septal cartilage and the contraction of healing mucoperichondrial flaps may lead to loss of support. In the deviated nose, straightening the cartilaginous septum is an essential procedure. A discussion of the treatment of the deviated nose follows.

THE DEVIATED NOSE

The deviated or twisted nose is most often of traumatic origin. In the unblemished nose, the nasal dorsum lies in the mid-sagittal plane of the face (Fig. 29–123, *A*). In partial deviations, only a portion of the nose is involved. When the nasal dorsum is curved to one side (Fig. 29–123, *B*), when two portions of the dorsum are twisted in opposite directions, as in an S-shaped deformity (Fig. 29–123, *C*), or when the entire nose veers to one side, the condition is referred to as a generalized or total deviation (Fig. 29–123, *D*).

Whereas in most deviated noses the tip remains in the midline, in the last type (Fig. 29–123, *D*), the tip of the nose is also deviated.

There is also a vast number of congenital deviations of the nose caused by congenital facial clefts and other craniofacial anomalies; these will not be discussed.

Classification of Nasal Deviations. Because of infinite variations, each deviated nose must be studied individually in order to determine the surgical measures required for correction. Nasal deviations may be classified into three broad categories: congenital, acquired in childhood, and acquired in adulthood.

CONGENITAL (PRENATAL) DEVIATIONS. Some nasal deviations are caused by intrauterine injury and do not correct themselves spontaneously. A genetic component is suggested when the parents or grandparents also show a similar deformity; a familial tendency has been especially noted in cases of dislocation of the caudal portion of the septal cartilage.

DEVIATIONS ACQUIRED (POSTNATAL) IN CHILDHOOD. Deviation of the nose occurs not infrequently in the newborn following the trauma of delivery. Kirschner (1955) observed severe compression of the nose in every normal delivery. In posterior presentation, a greater amount of injury results because of more extensive rotation of the head. Some degree of deviation of the nasal pyramid to the right and of the septal cartilage, which is dislocated from the vomer groove, to the left has been observed. Most of these deviations tend to return to the midline spontaneously at the end of three months.

Injury occurring in the infant or young child as a result of a fall from the crib or while learning to walk is generally overlooked. Studies have been made of the frequency of accidents in early childhood (Kravits and associates, 1969). The battered child syndrome is another factor; the author has fortunately seen few such cases, but undoubtedly the injuries suffered by the battered child are another cause of nasal deviation.

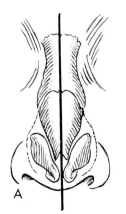 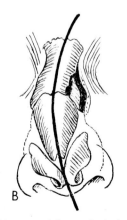 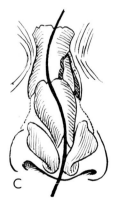 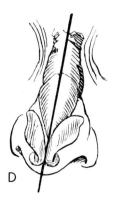

FIGURE 29–123. The straight nose and three principal types of nasal deviations. *A*, In the straight nose, the dorsum is aligned with the mid-sagittal plane of the face, which passes through nasion above and subnasale below. *B*, The C-shaped deviation. *C*, The S-shaped deviation. *D*, The generalized deviation to one side. Whereas in other types of deviation the tip of the nose is often in the midline, in the generalized deviation the tip is often also deviated.

Injuries suffered in early childhood cause deviation by fracture, hypertrophic callus, and dislocation of the bones at a time when sutures are not yet closed. Deviation may also result from the disproportionate growth caused by trauma. The deviation becomes more accentuated as the nose grows and becomes progressively more conspicuous in the adolescent. Developmental changes in the child result in greater anatomical disturbances than those which occur in the adult; this type of nasal deviation is often referred to as a developmental nasal deviation.

DEVIATIONS ACQUIRED IN ADULT LIFE. These deformities are produced by injury in adolescence or in adult life after or near the completion of nasal growth. The tip of the nose usually is in the midline, despite severe deflection of the dorsum.

It is convenient to divide the nose into upper (cephalic) and lower (caudal) portions; thus partial deviations may be designated according to the affected bony or cartilaginous portions. Such a division is arbitrary because both bony and cartilaginous portions of the nose are deviated in most cases and require straightening to obtain a satisfactory result.

Deviations of the Bony Portion of the Nose. These deviations usually show a one-sided dorsal hump, often thin-ridged and prolonged downward by a cartilaginous portion, which is formed by the septal and lateral cartilages and is particularly prominent in the developmental type of nasal deviation. The deformities are varied and include such conditions as simple deviations of the bony ridge; deviation with a dorsal hump due to hypertrophic callus or overriding fragments; widening; flattening; saddle deformity; or a combination of these deformities. The essential anatomical feature in such conditions is the disproportionate width of the lateral walls of the nose, the side of the deviation being narrower (Fig. 29–124). Deflection of the septum is a common occurrence because of the close association of the nasal bones with the lateral and septal cartilages.

Deviations of the Cartilaginous Portion of the Nose. In addition to intranasal inspection, digital palpation of the dorsum of the deviated nose from the nasal bones to the tip provides information concerning the shape and position of the dorsal border of the septal cartilage; finger pressure just above the tip of the nose discloses the position of the septal angle. The dorsal portion of the septal cartilage may be C-

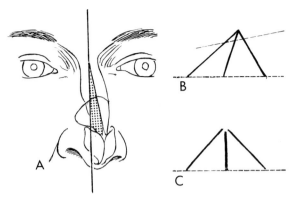

FIGURE 29–124. Disproportion between the lateral walls of the nose in nasal deviation. *A*, The shaded area represents the amount of bone and lateral cartilage excision required to equalize the lateral walls. *B*, Resection of the hump in a beveled manner equalizes the lateral walls. *C*, After correction of the disproportion between the lateral walls, the dorsum of the nose is realigned with the midsagittal plane of the face.

shaped or show an S-shaped curvature or a generalized deviation to one side. The position and shape of the septal angle and the caudal portion of the septum can be determined by placing the tip of the thumb in one vestibule and the tip of the forefinger in the other. When the nasal tip is gently elevated, the cephalic borders of the alar cartilages can also be seen protruding beneath the skin. The size, shape, and position of the alar cartilages can thus be determined.

The position and shape of the septum are confirmed by intranasal examination. Hypertrophy of the middle turbinate (and of the inferior turbinate) on the side opposite the deviation is noted in patients with severe deviation of the septum; the hypertrophy is a compensatory phenomenon to fill the void caused by the deviated septum. Spurs are also a frequent finding near the vomer–septal cartilage junction.

Because of long-standing deflection, the lateral cartilages may be asymmetrical, the cartilage on the side opposite the deviation being wider in developmental deviations (Fig. 29–125). The nasal tip feels soft to the touch and can be depressed by digital pressure when the septal angle is situated lateral to its midline position. A depression is noted just above the tip of the nose. The septal angle may protrude beneath one alar cartilage, splaying apart the alar cartilages and broadening the tip (Fig. 29–125), which is usually also asymmetrical in shape. The caudal septal border, protruding in the narial opening, causes widening and distor-

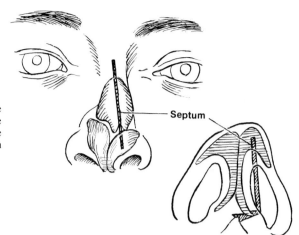

FIGURE 29–125. A severe lateral deviation of the septum; note the disproportionate size and shape of the lateral and alar cartilages resulting from a deviation of the developmental type. The septal angle, no longer being in the midline, elevates the dome of the left alar cartilage.

tion of the columella; the medial crus is separated from its counterpart, its lower portion forming a protrusion. In another less frequently encountered condition, the tip, the septum, and the entire nasal pyramid are deflected to one side (see Fig. 29–134, *A*).

When the septum has been crushed or fractured, it loses its supportive function. In such cases the tip of the nose may be pressed backward against the face without encountering the septal angle; the septum no longer supports the tip of the nose (Fig. 29–126).

Variations also occur in the angulation or curvature of the septal cartilage in the sagittal and vertical planes. The anterocaudal portion of the cartilage may be dislocated to one side of the vomer and the cephalic portion of the cartilage deviated toward the opposite side. The angulation may be such that the caudal portion of the septal cartilage lies transversely across one vestibule, with the free border of the cartilage protruding into the opposite vestibule, thus obstructing the airway.

More severe angulations occur along a line extending from the tip of the nasal bones or posteriorly at the junction with the perpendicular plate. The posterior part of the septum is often seen to be fairly straight in severe deflection of the caudal portion of the septum. The reverse condition also occurs; a septum with severe posterior deflection may be relatively straight in its anterior portion.

Deviations of the septum may be complicated by a considerable increase in the thickness of the septum and by vomer-cartilage spurs in traumatic conditions. Thickening is caused by overlapping fractured cartilaginous fragments, with lamination of the cartilage, and

by fibrous tissue thickening following hematoma of the septum. The curvature or angulation of the septal cartilage, its dislocation from the vomer groove, or a change in shape as a result of fracture may result in a decrease of the anteroposterior or vertical dimensions of the septum. The contraction following the healing of lacerated or destroyed mucous membrane can also cause a change in the position of the remaining portions of the septal cartilage after submucous resection. Charac-

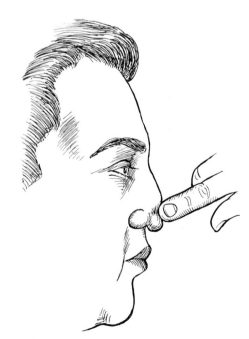

FIGURE 29–126. Digital palpation test. The septum has lost its supportive function. Digital palpation demonstrates that the tip of the nose can be depressed by digital pressure.

teristic deformities such as retraction of the columella and depression or flatness of the cartilaginous dorsum cephalad to the alar cartilages accompany these changes.

The Septum and the Deviated Nose. *The correction of septal deflection is the key to the straightening of the deviated nose.* Deviations whch occur in the cartilaginous portion of the nose can be explained by a brief review of some anatomical characteristics of the nasal septum. The component parts of the septal framework are illustrated in Figure 29–127. The septal cartilage has two areas of fixation. The first is on the undersurface of the nasal bones, where the septal cartilage has an intimate relationship with the lateral cartilages and a shallow bony groove; septal cartilage, lateral cartilages, and nasal bones are closely held together by the blending of the perichondrium and periosteum. The second area is the vomer groove; this area of fixation extends backward by means of a posterior extension of the septal cartilage into the perpendicular plate of the ethmoid (the ethmoid plate).

The caudal portion of the septal cartilage is mobile. This shock-absorbing anatomical feature protects the cartilaginous nose from trauma. The flexibility of the caudal portion of the septal cartilage is explained by the laxity of the attachments to the lateral cartilages, premaxillary wings, and anterior nasal spine.

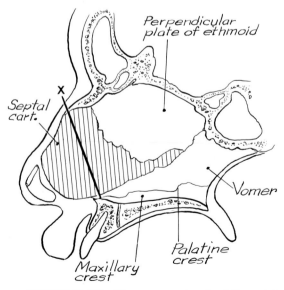

FIGURE 29–127. The component parts of the septal framework. Posterior to line X the septum is rigid.

The ethmoid plate plays a relatively unimportant role in supporting the osseous nasal vault. The area where the septal cartilage joins the perpendicular plate bone is usually thick, a resistant pillar which supports the portion of the vault formed by the lower part of the nasal bones and the lateral cartilages. This portion of the septal cartilage, the central pillar supporting the dorsal vault, must be preserved, if possible, in order to prevent the collapse of the dorsum. It is the pillar of support after the other nasal structures have been loosened from the adjacent attachments by the osteotomies in corrective rhinoplasty.

The cartilaginous septum plays a varying role in different types of noses. In the long, thin, straight nose, the border of the septal cartilage may be distinctly felt along the entire dorsum to the junction of the septal angle and alar cartilages; the septal angle is immediately subcutaneous in the area between the lateral and alar cartilages. The septal angle supports the tip if one attempts to depress the tip (see Fig. 29–126). When the septum has been fractured or when the septal support is lost by excessive submucous resection of the septal framework, the septal angle does not support the nasal tip. Septal angle support may also be absent in certain ethnic groups (Asiatic, Negroid). The alar cartilages are often dislocated from the septal angle in the Armenoid nose, a characteristic of this type of nose. The Negroid nose is more rarely subjected to deviation, its anatomy being such that the nose is more protected against trauma.

As stated earlier in the text, the septum is required as a fixed structure, a central pillar, for the stabilization of the mobilized nasal structures following corrective nasal plastic surgery. After the nasal dorsal hump is resected, the profile line modified, the nose shortened, and the lateral walls mobilized, only the septum remains as a stable structure.

Collapse of the septal skeletal framework may occur after an extensive submucous resection in conjunction with a corrective rhinoplasty if the caudal portion of the septal cartilage is removed. After the osteotomy of the lateral walls of the nose, the remaining portion of the septum remains as a cantilever at the mercy of a fracture of the perpendicular plate of the ethmoid and may collapse into the nasal cavity. When this unfortunate complication occurs, it is necessary to suspend the remaining dorsal portion of the septum and suture it to the lateral cartilages (Figs. 29–128 and 29–129).

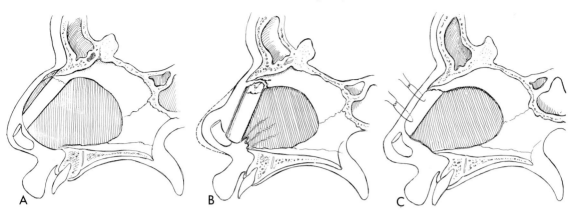

FIGURE 29–128. Collapse of the septum. *A*, Remaining portion of the septum after excision of the dorsal hump and resection of the caudal end of the septal cartilage. The remaining septal framework is supported by the perpendicular plate of the ethmoid. *B*, Fracture of the ethmoid plate, resulting in a downward displacement of the remaining septal framework. This may occur after osteotomy of the lateral nasal walls. *C*, Method for suspending the septal framework with sutures until adequate measures can be taken to maintain the fixation of the septal cartilage.

The situation is different when the continuity of the dorsal vault of the nose is undisturbed. In certain types of deviated noses following a malunited fracture of the nasal bones, when the continuity between the lateral cartilages over the dorsum of the nose is undisturbed, septal cartilage may be removed more extensively, without danger of a depression developing during the postoperative period. The

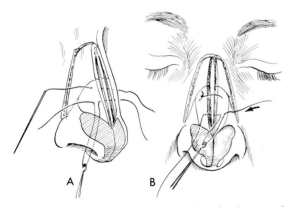

FIGURE 29–129. Technique of fixation after fracture of the septum and collapse of the nose. *A*, The septal cartilage is sutured to the lateral cartilages by transfixion sutures placed through the skin. After the sutures are exposed intranasally, each suture is drawn out by means of a hook, as shown in the drawing. *B*, The sutures are tied intranasally. An alternate technique is to obtain fixation to the lateral cartilages by means of externally placed mattress sutures tied over bolsters (small dental rolls or pieces of gauze).

present trend is to be more sparing in resecting septal cartilage.

Submucous Resection and Other Techniques to Straighten the Septum. The classic submucous resection of the nasal septum is usually a partial resection, which includes a portion of the septal framework consisting of septal cartilage, vomer, and perpendicular plate of the ethmoid (see p. 1132). The most important single operative step is to inject local anesthetic solution through a needle with a large bore and a short beveled point between the mucoperichondrium and the cartilage, thus separating the structures and facilitating the operation. Extensive resection of the septal framework is unnecessary as a therapeutic measure and endangers the stability of the nose after rhinoplasty. The operation should be done only in cases in which there are specific indications; in many cases more limited resection will give more satisfactory clinical results. A particular objection to the wide resection of the framework is the resulting flaccid septum (the "flapping flaps"). The replacement of resected septal cartilage fragments between the mucoperichondrial flaps has been advocated to avoid this complication, but this procedure is hazardous, as complications such as twisting of the transplanted cartilage may interfere with the airway.

There are also techniques for straightening the septal framework which do not require extensive resection of the septal cartilage and bone.

In straightening a deviated nose, the surgeon

has a dual objective: straightening the nasal pyramid and relieving obstruction of the nasal airways. This dual objective must be achieved by a corrective rhinoplasty without endangering the stability of the nasal structures. A submucous resection of the septum, done prior to corrective rhinoplasty, is particularly undesirable, as the preliminary sacrifice of the septal framework may leave inadequate support during the subsequent corrective operation on the external nose and the necessary secondary septal surgery is more difficult because of the residual scar tissue.

An approach to the treatment of the deviated nose and septum is to perform the septal surgery necessary to realign the septum and straighten the nose. Various conservative techniques are available and are described later in the text. If nasal obstruction is not completely relieved, a secondary conservative submucous resection a few months later will complete the treatment. This compromise approach will avoid the loss of cartilaginous vault support in most cases.

It is not always necessary to do a complete transfixion incision in operating upon a deviated nose. If the nose does not require shortening and if the dorsal profile does not require a modification, i.e., when the nose requires only straightening, the transfixion incision may be interrupted slightly beyond the septal angle. In such cases, the approach to the septum is through a hemi-transfixion incision. The tip of the nose and the columella are retracted with a double-pronged retractor in order to tense the membranous septum. An incision is then made along the caudal margin of the septal cartilage to the floor of the nose. Another horizontal incision through the mucoperiosteum along the base of the vomer ensures drainage. Nasal packing is occasionally necessary. It is important to avoid incising through the posterior vestibular fold, which delimits the floor of the vestibule from the nasal fossa proper. Failure to take this precaution may result in scar contracture and the formation of a web, which may interfere with the inflow of air currents into the nose.

When a complete transfixion procedure is performed along the caudal border of the septal cartilage, the septal framework may be approached through the transfixion incision.

If the caudal portion of the septum is straight, an L-shaped incision is made, leaving the caudal septum undisturbed and incising the mucoperichondrium posterior to the posterior vestibular fold.

Conservative Septal Procedures. After the mucoperichondrium is raised on one side, a wide exposure of the septal framework is obtained by retraction of the mucoperichondrial flap. A conservative submucous resection of the septal framework is done, removing only the most obstructive portion. The important technical point in the deviated nose is to straighten the septum while preserving the dorsal and caudal portions of the septum. The perpendicular plate of the ethmoid may be straightened by fracturing it with Bruening forceps. The vomer may be detached from the floor of the nose by means of an osteotome and replaced into the midline.

As stated earlier in the text, the turbinates, the inferior and particularly the middle, may be hypertrophied, filling the void in the nasal cav-

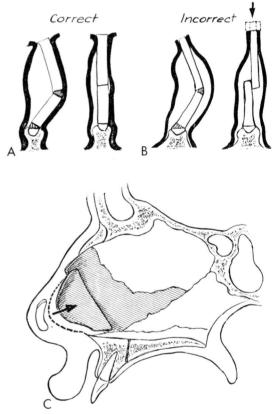

FIGURE 29–130. Principle of the mucoperichondrial splint. *A*, In an angulated deformity of the septum, a wedge is removed at the angulation; the septal cartilage is thus straightened. *B*, The mucoperichondrium left attached on one side prevents the overlapping of the fragments shown in the drawing. *C*, The same principle applies in preventing the anteroposterior overlapping following an incision through the septal cartilage. Intact mucoperichondrium on one side prevents overlap and shortening of the septal cartilage.

ity produced by the deviated septum. They may require outfracture, trimming, or electro-coagulation in order to complete the restoration of the airway after the septum has been straightened.

THE PRINCIPLE OF THE MUCOPERICHON-DRIAL SPLINT. The mucoperichondrium is elevated on one side of the remaining septal cartilage in order to obtain exposure. The mucoperichondrial elevation is limited on the contralateral side of the septum, sufficient only to permit excision of an angulated portion of the septum. When possible, the muco-perichondrium is left completely undisturbed; this ensures the continued nourishment of the septal cartilage, but, more important, the undisturbed mucoperichondrium acts as a splint, preventing overlapping of cartilage fragments after incision.

Such overlapping would result in a change in the vertical or horizontal dimensions of the septal cartilage, as well as a change in the contour of the nasal profile.

If the caudal portion of the septum is in the midline, straightening of the remaining dorsal and caudal portions of the septal cartilage may be done by means of incisions extending through the cartilage but not through the mucoperichondrium on the contralateral side (Fig. 29–130).

The septal framework is exposed by raising the mucoperichondrium and the mucoperiosteum on the side *opposite* the direction of the deviation; if the nose is deviated to the right, the septal framework is exposed on the left and vice versa. The entire framework may be exposed on one side (Fig. 29–131) and the lateral cartilage detached, as it usually must be trimmed to allow the return of the structures to the midline.

When the framework is angulated or curved,

selective incisions through the cartilage and strip excisions will straighten it (Figs. 29–130 and 29–132). The incisions may extend to the dorsal border of the septal cartilage only if the lateral cartilages have not been separated from the septum and the cartilaginous vault is intact. In most rhinoplastic operations, at this stage the cartilages have already been separated from the septum. Such incisions should be avoided in order to avoid disrupting the continuity of the dorsal border of the septum.

When both sides of the septal cartilage must be exposed, mattress sutures of chromic catgut are employed in order to prevent overlapping of cartilage fragments, and fixation is maintained by an internal splint (see Fig. 29–136).

THE SWINGING DOOR OPERATION. The swinging door operation permits straightening of the septal framework with minimal resection of the septum (Fig. 29–133). This type of operation should be reserved for septal deflections in which the caudal half (or more) of the septal cartilage or the entire nasal pyramid is angulated to one side (Fig. 29–134). The septal deflection is also characterized by a dislocation of the septal cartilage to one side of the vomer groove, with the caudal portion of the septal cartilage protruding into the vestibule. The vomer and the anterior nasal spine may be in the midline, the cartilage being dislocated from the vomer groove, or the vomer may participate in the deviation (see Fig. 29–135, *A*).

In such cases it is possible to preserve the entire septal cartilage by straightening it and replacing it in the midline. After the usual exposure of the nasal framework and the trans-fixion incision which frees the septal cartilage along its dorsal and caudal borders, the lateral cartilage attachments to the septum are severed. The mucoperichondrium and muco-periosteum are then raised from one side of the

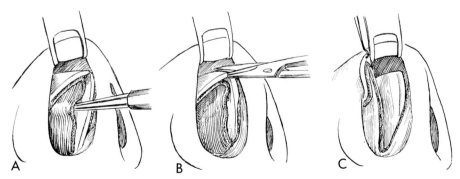

FIGURE 29–131. Complete exposure of the septal cartilage. *A,* The mucoperichondrium is being raised from the septal cartilage. *B,* The lateral cartilage is detached from the dorsal border of the septum without incising through the mucoperi-chondrium. *C,* Exposure obtained.

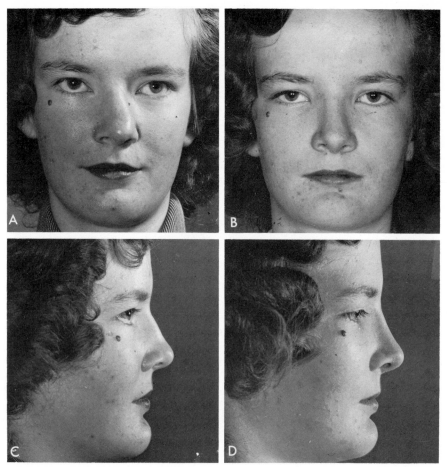

FIGURE 29–132. Developmental nasal deviation with C-shaped deformity of the dorsum. *A,* Nasal deviation as a result of trauma in infancy. Note the protrusion of the septal angle beneath the left alar cartilage. Despite the disparity in the shape of the alar cartilages, the tip is in the midline. *B,* After corrective rhinoplasty and straightening of the septum by selective incisions through the septal cartilage. *C,* Preoperative appearance. *D,* The deviation has been corrected. Adequate projection of the columella was obtained by inserting a septal cartilage transplant into the columella, according to the technique shown in Figure 29–88. (From Converse, J. M.: Corrective surgery of nasal deviations. Arch. Otolaryngol., *52*:671, 1950.)

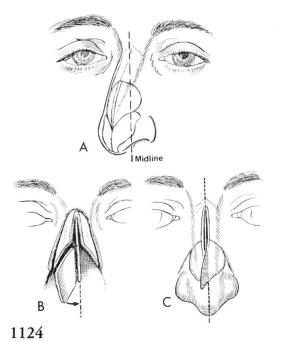

FIGURE 29–133. The swinging door operation. *A,* The entire nose is deflected to one side. *B,* A strip of septal cartilage has been resected at the point of angulation, and the caudal portion of the cartilage is swung into the midline; fixation is established in the vomer groove (see Fig. 29–135 *D*). The mucoperichondrium on the right side of the septal cartilage remains attached. *C,* Restoration of symmetry between the two lateral cartilages after replacement of the structures in the midline; a portion of the dorsal border of the overlapping lateral cartilage must be excised.

septum only (see Fig. 29–131, *A*). One should choose the side which is opposite the deviation. The purpose of this technique is to benefit from the contraction of the raised flap during the period of postoperative healing; the contraction of the healing flap assists in maintaining the septum in its corrected central position.

After the septal mucoperichondrial and mucoperiosteal flaps have been raised on one side, the mucous membrane over the septal cartilage remains intact on the contralateral side. The mucoperiosteum is raised from the vomer, however, and the mucoperiosteal elevation is extended to include the floor of the nose.

The point of angulation of the septal cartilage in the sagittal plane is cut through or resected in order to straighten the cartilage. The incisions are made through cartilage and do not extend through the mucoperichondrium on the opposite side (see Fig. 29–130).

The fibrous tissue between the dislocated septal cartilage and the vomer (Figs. 29–135, *A, B*) is incised. The septal cartilage is re-

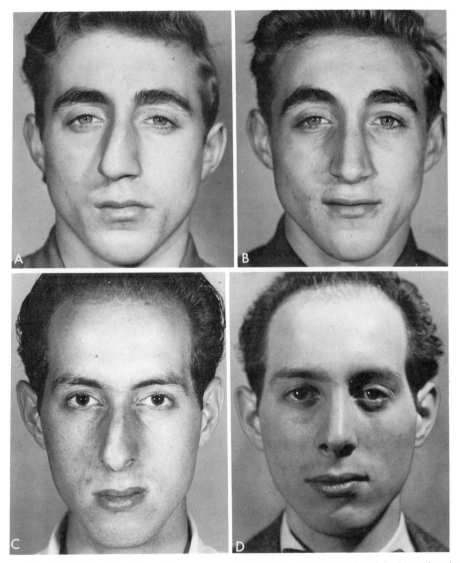

FIGURE 29–134. Generalized deviation of the nose. *A*, Deflected nose of traumatic origin. Note that the tip is also deflected in this type of deviation because of the severe angulation of the septum toward the right side. *B*, Straightening obtained following a complete corrective rhinoplasty and the swinging door operation illustrated in Figure 29–133. *C*, Another patient with developmental deviation of the nose. Note the position of the septal angle, which is highlighted under the right lateral crus. *D*, Result obtained by the swinging door operation combined with the other necessary rhinoplastic procedures.

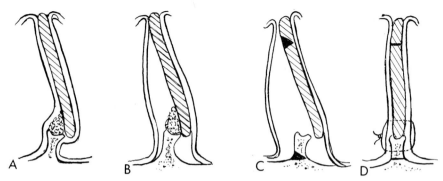

FIGURE 29–135. Straightening the caudal portion of the septal cartilage. *A*, Frontal section through the caudal portion of the septal cartilage dislocated out of the vomer groove. Fibrous tissue fills the vomer groove. *B*, The septal mucoperichondrium and mucoperiosteum over the vomer on the right side of the septum are raised. The mucoperiosteum is also raised over the left side of the vomer. The mucoperichondrium over the left side of the septal cartilage remains intact. *C*, A wedge of cartilage is resected near the dorsal portion of the septal cartilage to allow straightening. The pad of fibrous tissue in the vomer groove is removed. *D*, The cartilage is straightened, replaced in the vomer groove, and anchored in position by a suture placed through a drill hole in the premaxillary wings or the nasal spine.

tracted, an incision is made into the vomer groove, and fibrous tissue which fills the vomer groove is resected. The cartilage is separated from its vomer attachments and replaced into the groove (see Figs. 29–133, *B, C,* and 29–135, *C, D*).

The flap of septal cartilage with mucoperichondrium attached, which has been freed by incisions separating the lateral cartilages from the septum and the septal cartilage from the vomer, is swung into the midline like a door swinging on its hinges (see Fig. 29–133 *B*).

If the vomer is also deviated, it must be detached from the floor of the nose by means of an osteotome and replaced in the midline (Fig. 29–135, *C, D*). If the septal cartilage shows a curvature in the frontal plane, a wedge excision is required to replace the septal angle into the midline (Fig. 29–135, *C, D*). The structures should remain in the midline after the corrective surgery, without any tendency to fall back into their previously deviated position. It is essential to provide fixation of the septal cartilage: a hole is drilled through the nasal spine or the premaxillary wings (or both) by means of a small, round drill point activated by an air-turbine. The caudal portion is maintained in fixation with a nonabsorbable or stainless steel wire (Fig. 29–135, *D*).

Reshaping the deformed columella may require section or resection of a portion of the lower end of one or both medial crura (see Fig. 29–84).

Occasionally one may find, in severe deflections, that the mucous membrane at the base of the septum, at the junction with the floor of the nose, is under tension after the midline re-placement of the septal framework. In such cases an anteroposterior incision is made along the floor of the nose, releasing the mucoperiosteum. The resulting lateral defect in the floor of the nose is repaired by a graft of nasal mucous membrane. The graft is maintained in position for a few days by means of nasal packing and becomes revascularized rapidly.

OTHER TECHNIQUES. Fry and Robertson (1967), applying the observations made by Gibson and Davis (1958), have shown that, when the mucoperichondrium is raised from both sides of the septal cartilage and the cartilage is scored on one side, the cartilage bends to the opposite side. The authors have attempted to apply this experimental finding to the clinical problem of straightening the septum but have not found it to be as reliable as the methods described above. Actual sectioning of the cartilage is necessary in angulated deviations and curvatures. An interesting technique, mentioned earlier in the text, is that of "morselization." An instrument with jaws having protruding asperities either on one jaw only or on both jaws is employed to produce multiple incisions through the cartilage. The septal cartilage loses its resiliency and becomes membranous. The technique appears to have merit in septal cartilage deviations of lesser degree and permits straightening without resection, thus avoiding the flailed septal flaps which result from extensive resection of the framework.

THE INTERNAL SPLINT. When a number of incisions through the septal cartilage have been required, mattress sutures of chromic catgut or other slowly absorbing suture material may

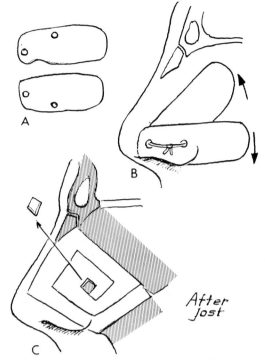

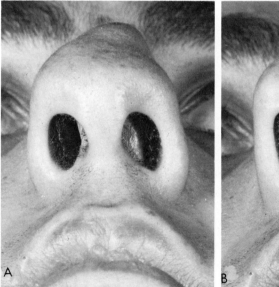

FIGURE 29–136. The internal splint. *A, B,* By placing the holes in each plate in a decussated manner, it is possible to splint the major portion of the septum when the suture is tightened. *C,* Spiral incision, which is varied according to the type of deviation, combined with removal of a small piece of septal cartilage. (After Jost.)

assist in the fixation of the fragments, in addition to the mucoperichondrial splint.

Nasal gauze packing assists in supporting the straightened septum. The packing may be inconvenient, however, when a rhinoplasty is done concomitantly because, to be effective, a considerable amount of gauze packing is required. Sheets of plastic materials, such as Teflon, polyethylene, or other substances such as X-ray film, may be cut to size, placed on each side of the septum, and joined by a *loosely* tied mattress suture. This type of internal splinting was described by Johnson (1964). The splints may be left in position for a number of weeks, and they are well tolerated.

Jost, Vergnon, and Hadjean (1973), by placing the holes through which the suture is passed in a decussated manner (Fig. 29–136, *A, B*), were able to splint the major portion of the septum. Jost uses this technique after incising the septum in a serpentine manner to prevent recurrent septal deviation (Fig. 29–136, *C*).

The Dislocated Caudal End of the Septal Cartilage

THE ANTERIOR COLUMELLAR APPROACH. Dislocation of the caudal end of the septal cartilage from its position in the vomer groove

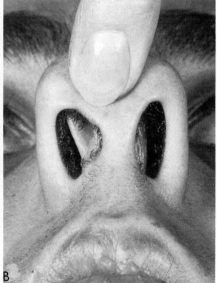

FIGURE 29–137. Dislocation of the caudal end of the septal cartilage. *A,* The caudal end of the septal cartilage protrudes into the left vestibule. *B,* Pressure over the tip demonstrates the twisted shape of the cartilage, the cartilage now protrudes into the *right* vestibule. Note the bifidity of the tip caused by the deviation of the septal angle.

causes it to protrude to one side of the columella. The protrusion itself is objectionable from an esthetic standpoint; it also obstructs the airway in some cases and nearly always distorts the columella (Fig. 29–137; see also Fig. 29–147).

The swinging door procedure can be employed to replace the cartilage in the midline without resecting the cartilage (see Fig. 29–133).

The caudal portion of the septal cartilage may be so distorted in some cases that any plan to straighten the septal framework by con-

servative surgery must be abandoned. The caudal portion of the septal cartilage is then resected; resection of the vomer spurs is often also required in order to ensure an adequate nasal airway. Retraction of the columella is prevented by embedding a strip of septal cartilage into the columella through an incision along the caudal border of the medial crus (see Fig. 29–88). The skin covering the lateral surface of the columella is raised by the injection of local anesthetic solution. A pocket is prepared beneath the skin of the caudal surface of the columella. The cartilage transplant is then

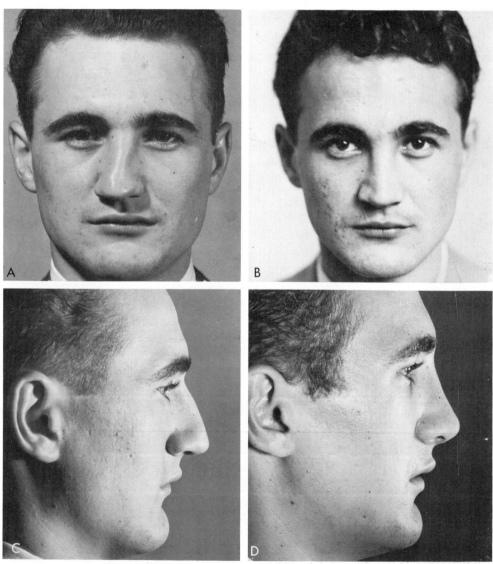

FIGURE 29–138. *A,* Traumatic nasal S-deviation with protrusion of the septal angle beneath the right alar cartilage, causing distortion of the tip. *B,* Result obtained by realignment of the structures. The septal cartilage was resected completely, and strips of cartilage were transplanted over the dorsum, as illustrated in Figure 29–139. *C,* Retraction of the columella. *D,* After corrective surgery and columellar septal transplant, as illustrated in Figure 29–88.

placed anterior to the medial crura beneath the skin extending downward over the nasal spine (see Fig. 29–88).

Total Resection and Transplantation of Septal Cartilage Over the Dorsum of the Nose. There are two types of nasal and septal deviations in which a conservative type of septal straightening cannot be done.

The first is the deviated nose in which the septal cartilage is severely twisted in the frontal plane as well as in the sagittal plane; the dorsal border of the septal cartilage shows an accentuated S-shaped curvature in both the sagittal and frontal planes (Fig. 29–138). In this type, the cartilage must be resected because it cannot be straightened. From the excised cartilage it is always possible to recover strips of straight cartilage that are used as transplants placed into the columella (see Fig. 29–88) and over the nasal dorsum (see Fig. 29–139).

A second type of deviation in which the septum must be completely resected is the flat and deviated nose often seen following repeated trauma. In this type of deformity, the septum has lost its supportive function. Septal resection is necessary because the septum is so thick that it obstructs the airway ("boxer's septum"). Complete resection of the septum does not result in any change in the shape of the nose, because the septum has already lost its role as a supporting structure. This type of nose may require reconstruction by means of cartilage (septal, costal) or bone grafts to restore the contour of the dorsum when the nose has been flattened against the face ("boxer's nose").

Technique. The dorsal hump is resected. It is usually a small pseudohump resulting from the loss of contour of the cartilaginous dorsum of the nose. The lateral cartilages are not separated from the septum; thus the continuity between the lateral cartilages and the septum is preserved. Excision of tissue from one lateral cartilage in order to equalize both, a procedure often necessary in the deviated nose, may be accomplished without cutting through the

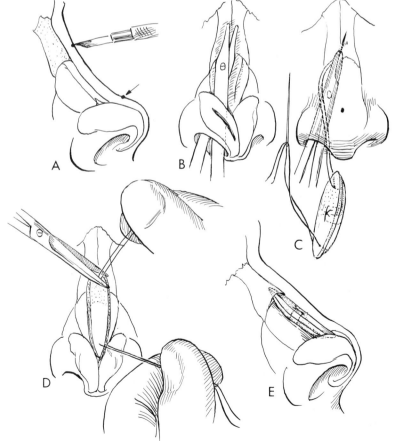

FIGURE 29–139. Technique of transplantation of septal cartilage to the dorsum of the nose. *A*, Two ink dots on the skin indicate the upper and lower limits of the transplant. *B*, Scissors undermining the area over the dorsum to be occupied by the transplant. *C*, The transplant is held by guide sutures of fine plain catgut; the upper guide suture is introduced in position by means of a straight needle, which pierces the skin through the upper ink dot. *D*, The guide suture is removed, and the plain catgut is left buried under the skin. This technique avoids displacing the graft when the suture is pulled out. The guide sutures may also be tied over bolsters. The graft may also be maintained in position by fine nylon sutures placed transcutaneously. *E*, The graft in position. The cephalic end of the graft lies under the periosteum.

mucous membrane. Thus a bed is prepared for the septal cartilage transplant.

It is possible to secure a sufficiently long, straight piece of cartilage (or cartilage plus ethmoid plate) for a suitable transplant, even in the most deviated septal cartilage. The resected cartilage is placed in a moist saline sponge until all of the other procedures of the nasal plastic operation have been completed; the cartilage transplantation is the final procedure. A single piece of cartilage or a number of superimposed pieces may be required. The cartilage should be meticulously carved, often a tedious procedure.

The cartilage graft is introduced through one of the incisions previously made to correct the tip and is placed over the lateral cartilages. The dorsal septal cartilage transplant may be placed with precision by the technique illustrated in Figure 29–139 (Converse, 1950b).

Two ink dots are made over the dorsum at points between which the cartilage is to be placed. The dots indicate the upper and lower limits of the transplantation site (Fig. 29–139, *A*), which is undermined with scissors (Fig. 29–139, *B*). Sutures of 5–0 plain catgut are threaded through the eye of a straight cutting needle, which is placed through each extremity of the cartilage transplant (Fig. 29–139, *C*). The needle carrying the cephalic traction suture is placed into the subcutaneous pocket and out through the skin (Fig. 29–139, *C*); the needle with the caudal traction sutures is also placed into the pocket and through the skin. The sutures may be tied over a small piece of gauze over the dorsum of the nose, or they may be cut and removed after the operation has been completed and before adhesive paper tape is placed over the dorsum to stabilize the transplant (Fig. 29–139, *D, E*).

The advantage of plain catgut is twofold: the buried sutures may be left to dissolve spontaneously, and the nasal splint need not be removed. Another procedure can also be employed. Instead of exerting force on the suture, which may displace the transplant, slight tension is placed on the sutures while the flat blades of the scissors are applied against the skin. The sutures are then cut close to the skin by applying pressure against the skin and upward traction on the suture (Fig. 29–139, *D*). As the tension is released, the cut ends of the suture disappear beneath the skin; these are absorbed without causing significant tissue reaction. Silk or nylon sutures occasionally break and remain under the skin, causing tissue reaction and in some cases inflammation, sup-

puration, and absorption of the graft. An alternate technique, advocated by Sheen (1975b), is to place the graft and then anchor it to the underlying tissue with transcutaneous sutures of 6–0 nylon.

One piece of cartilage may be adequate; two pieces sutured to each other may be required; occasionally three segments of septal cartilage are indicated. The cartilage is meticulously shaped with a sharp scalpel.

Straightening The Bony Nose: Equalization of The Lateral Nasal Walls. The nasal pyramid in cross section is triangular in shape. The lateral walls in the undeviated nose form equal sides of the triangle with the apex in the midline, whereas the lateral walls of the deviated nasal pyramid are of unequal length with the apex of the triangle located to one side of the midline (see Fig. 29–124). Equalization of the lateral walls is essential to straighten the nose. Because such cases usually require resection of the laterally situated hump, equalization is best achieved by resecting the hump along a beveled line; this technique is preferred to that originally advocated by Joseph, in which a triangle of bone was resected from the base of the lateral wall on the wider side.

Corrective Surgery for the Deviated Nose which Requires a Modification of the Profile Line. When the profile must be modified in the course of straightening the deviated nose, the order of procedure is similar to that followed in a typical corrective rhinoplastic operation. The septum must be straightened to avoid recurrence of the deviation by pressure of the septum against the lateral nasal wall. It is essential, however, to employ a conservative technique in order to preserve the support afforded by the septum and avoid nasal collapse.

Corrective Surgery for the Deviated Nose which Does Not Require Modification of the Profile Line

MALUNITED FRACTURES. The nasal framework is sometimes deviated from the midline in both the upper and lower portions without a change in the profile line. Malunited fractures show this pattern of deformity (Fig. 29–140). A modified corrective procedure is used in such cases.

An incision is made at the lower border of the lateral cartilage on the right side, and the soft tissues are elevated from the lateral cartilage by sharp dissection with a sharp, double-blade Joseph knife. Another incision is made

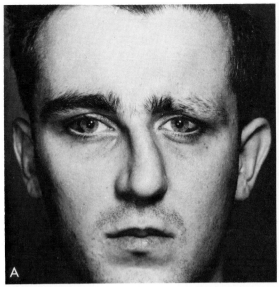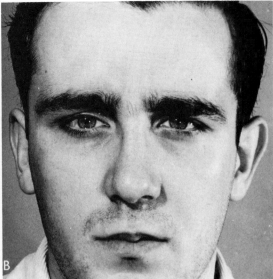

FIGURE 29–140. Corrective surgery for malunited fracture of the nasal bones. *A*, Severe deviation of the nose as a result of malunited fracture. *B*, Result maintained with the technique illustrated in Figure 29–141.

with the tip of the Joseph knife through the periosteum covering the nasal bone, and the periosteum is raised. Similar procedures are undertaken on the left side.

A submucous resection or a straightening procedure of the deviated septum is done. Osteotomy of the base of the lateral walls of the nose is performed.

A medial osteotomy is now required: a guarded, straight osteotome is placed between the mucoperichondrial flaps of the septum and is directed upward until the operator feels the lower border of the nasal bones in the midline with the tip of the instrument (Fig. 29–141). The line of osteotomy is in the midline at the junction of the nasal bones. A mallet is used to tap the osteotome upward; the bones are thus separated and can be manipulated into a realigned position because they have been completely freed from the covering periosteum and musculature.

A horizontal incision through the mucous membrane at the base of the septum prevents septal hematoma. An external nasal splint is applied; no intranasal packing is required.

Septal Surgery in Rhinoplasty. Extensive submucous resection is rarely performed in the routine corrective rhinoplasty. Conservative measures include the following:

1. Resection of only an obviously obstructive portion of the septum, or bony spur.
2. Replacing the septum into the vomer groove by incising the base of the septal cartilage.
3. Shaving areas of thick septal cartilage.

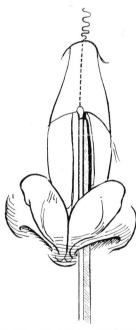

FIGURE 29–141. Technique employed in the patient shown in Figure 29–140. A button-tipped osteotome is placed beneath the septal mucoperichondrial flap on the left side to locate the lower border of the nasal bones. A midline osteotomy is then performed. This osteotomy, along with the necessary septal straightening procedures and lateral osteotomies, permits realignment of the deviated nose.

4. Straightening a curved dorsal septal border by conservative means.

5. Straightening the dislocated caudal portion of the septum.

6. If additional septal surgery is required, a judicious approach is to postpone the additional septal surgery rather than risk a nasal collapse.

The Technique of Submucous Resection of the Septum: The Radical Operation. Although the radical resection of the septal framework is rarely used except in a severely damaged nose and septum, it is a procedure that is occasionally indicated.

The technique of submucous resection of the septal framework was established in the early part of this century by the technical descriptions of Freer (1902) and Killian (1904). A wide resection of the skeletal constituents of the septum involving the major portions of the septal cartilage, perpendicular plate of the ethmoid, and vomer was advocated.

Care should be taken to expose the septal framework along a plane situated between the cartilage and mucoperichondrium. This procedure is assisted by ballooning out the mucoperichondrium and mucoperiosteum from the framework by a preliminary injection of anesthetic solution made with a large-bore needle with a short bevel; the plane of dissection is thus prepared, bleeding is eliminated, and the operation is rendered considerably easier (Fig. 29–142, *A* to *C*).

Prior to making the incision for the submucous resection of the septal framework, the surgeon should plan to leave a strip of cartilage, 1 cm or more in width, along the dorsal and caudal borders of the septal cartilage. If the caudal portion of the septum is deviated and requires straightening, the septum can be approached through the transfixion incision of

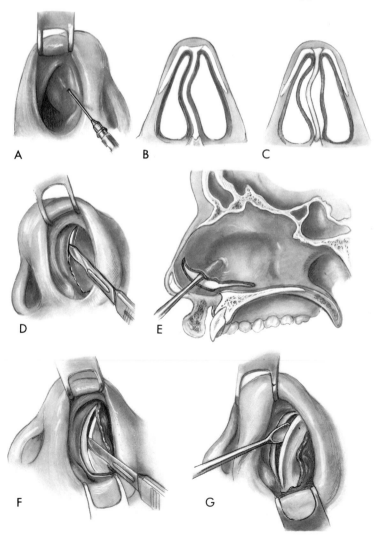

FIGURE 29–142. Submucous resection of the nasal septum. *A*, Submucoperichondrial infiltration of anesthetic solution. *B*, Sagittal section, showing the deviation of the septal framework. *C*, The mucoperichondrium and mucoperiosteum have been raised from the septal framework on each side. *D*, Beginning of the L-shaped incision of the type used when the caudal portion of the septum does not need correction. The incision is started approximately 10 to 15 mm posterior to the caudal border and extends through the mucoperichondrium to the cartilage. *E*, The incision has been made down to the floor of the nose and extends along the floor. The purpose of the incision along the floor of the nose is to provide dependent drainage. Mucoperichondrial elevation is begun. *F*, After the flap of mucoperiosteum on the left side is raised, the incision is made through the septal cartilage a few millimeters posterior to the mucous membrane incision. The incision extends through the cartilages but not through the mucoperichondrium on the opposite side. *G*, Raising the mucoperichondrium on the opposite side.

the rhinoplastic procedure or through a hemi-transfixion incision. Near the transfixion incision, the mucoperichondrium is intimately attached to the cartilage through the fibers of the depressor septi nasi muscle and often must be sharply dissected with the knife. It is essential at all times that the blue-white color of the septal cartilage be seen, a finding which indicates that the operator is in the correct plane of dissection. Failure to follow this plane of dissection will result in tearing of the mucoperichondrium, with the danger of septal perforation if the tear occurs on both sides, and a contraction of the healing mucoperichondrium, causing a depression of the nasal dorsum. A number of elevators are available for this purpose (Fig. 29–143).

When the caudal portion of the septum is not deviated, an L-shaped incision is made posteriorly to the posterior vestibular fold (see Fig. 29–142, *D*) in order to avoid the formation of a cicatricial band on the floor of the

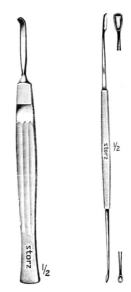

FIGURE 29–143. *Left,* The McKenty elevator. *Right,* The Converse double-end curette, convenient instruments for raising the mucoperichondrium from the septal cartilage.

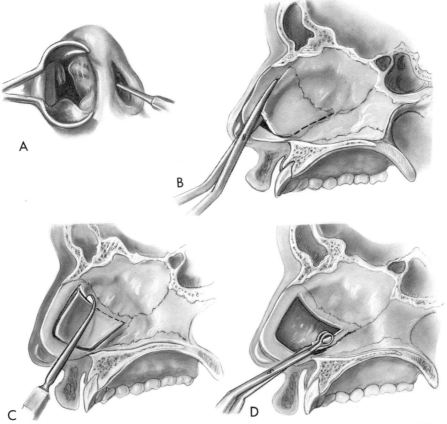

FIGURE 29–144. Submucous resection of the nasal septum. *A,* Elevation of the mucoperichondrium on the right side of the septum. *B,* Resection of the deviated septal framework with septal scissors, an adequate amount of cartilage is left along the dorsum for septal support. *C,* An angulated knife is employed to sever the septal cartilage from the perpendicular plate of the ethmoid. Cartilage, which has also been separated from the vomer, can then be removed intact and employed as a transplant when necessary. *D,* Resection of the remaining cartilage in the vomer groove. A portion of the vomer will also be resected when necessary to remove the obstructing portion of bone and spurs.

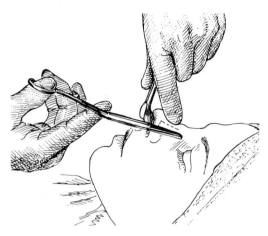

FIGURE 29–145. Position of the scissors held parallel to the nasal dorsum while the incision shown in Figure 29–144, *B* is made.

a few millimeters posterior to the mucous membrane incision (see Fig. 29–142, *F*); the mucoperichondrium and mucoperiosteum are raised from the opposite side of the septal cartilage (see Figs. 29–142, *G*, and 29–144, *A*). A medium-length nasal speculum exposes the cartilage between its blades, retracting the septal flaps, and the deviated cartilage and bone are resected. An incision cut through the septal cartilage is made, parallel to the dorsal border of the septum, by means of angulated septal scissors (see Figs. 29–144, *B*, and 29–145). The septal cartilage is then separated from the perpendicular plate of the ethmoid by cutting through the cartilage with an angulated knife (see Fig. 29–144, *C*), and the remainder of the cartilage is resected from the vomer (see Fig. 29–144, *D*). Additional septal framework is resected as required (Fig. 29–146).

Nasal packing may be dispensed with following the operation, as the incision along the floor of the nose through the mucoperiosteum provides dependent drainage. Healing is enhanced and the incidence of postoperative hemorrhage diminished. Petrolatum jelly is placed in the vestibules daily for a few days after the operation; the patient sniffs the petrolatum and lubricates the nasal fossae.

Complications Following Corrective Surgery for Nasal Deviations. In addition to the complications which occur following corrective surgery of the nose (see p. 1090), the major complication following surgery for the deviated nose is recurrence of the deviation. The most frequent cause of the recurrence is inadequate straightening of the nasal septum. The inexorable pressure exerted by a deviated septum will

vestibule. A horizontal incision which extends along the base of the septum near the floor of the nose provides dependent drainage, avoids a septal hematoma, and obviates the need for intranasal packing to prevent a collection of blood between the flaps. The incision is usually made on the left side, a convenient position for the right-handed operator. In severe traumatic septal deflection, the incision for the exposure of the septal framework is made on the concave side of the septal deflection, the mucoperichondrium on the concave side being easier to raise and less liable to be torn than that on the convex side.

After one side of the septal cartilage is exposed, an incision is made through the cartilage,

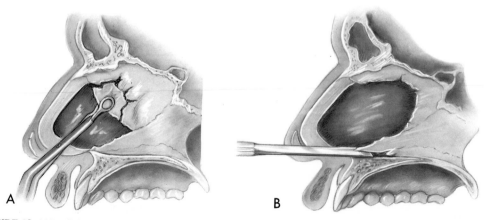

A   B

FIGURE 29–146. Submucous resection of the septum (continued). *A*, The deviated portion of the septal cartilage has been removed. The deviated portion of the perpendicular plate of the ethmoid is being resected. *B*, A portion of the vomer is resected by means of an osteotome. As a rule, only those portions of the septal framework which appear to cause obstruction are removed (see text).

press a lateral wall out of alignment, cause the recurrence of an S-shaped twist to the nose, or deviate the nasal tip and lower cartilaginous nose to one side.

A dismaying complication following a corrective rhinoplasty is a postoperative deviation in a nose that was straight preoperatively. This complication can be explained as follows: the dorsal border of the septum was straight; beneath the dorsal septal border, the septum was curved along a sagittal plane; when the dorsal border was resected, the curved portion of the septum became the new dorsal border, hence the postoperative deviation. Careful examination of the septum will suggest precautionary measures to avert such a complication. When this complication occurs, the remedy is a secondary operation to straighten the septum and realign the nasal structures.

It is advisable to leave the dental compound or plaster nasal splint in position longer than for a routine corrective rhinoplasty, but this precaution does not obviate the need to straighten the septum and external nose by adequate surgical means. A successful result requires that every portion of the nasal pyramid—the septum, the bony nose, the lateral and alar cartilages, the columella (Fig. 29–147)—be realigned and that symmetry be reestablished.

A major complication is collapse of the remaining dorsal portion of the septal framework, which, after resection of the caudal portion of the septum, remains in position as a cantilever. Fracture of the cantilever at the perpendicular plate of the ethmoid (see Fig. 29–128) causes a collapse of the remaining septal framework, a loss of contour of the nasal dorsum, and a resultant saddle-nose deformity. This complication is avoided by straightening the septum through conservative measures, thus preserving septal support.

SADDLE NOSES, NOSES WITH A DEPRESSED DORSUM, AND FLAT NOSES

Depression of the dorsum of the nose (Fig. 29–148) may occur in the bony or the cartilaginous portion of the nose; when both portions of the nose are affected, the term saddle nose is often used to designate the deformity. Foreshortening of the nose, a frequent complication following naso-orbital fractures, resulting from overlapping and telescoping of nasal

bony and cartilaginous structures which are projected into the interorbital space is a difficult deformity to correct and is discussed later in this chapter (see p. 1271). Another type of deformity seen after severe injury is the flat nose, in which all the structures of the nose including the tip are depressed.

The deformity may be further complicated by widening or deviation. Conditions arise which interfere with function; these include thickening of the septal cartilage and collapse of the lateral and alar cartilages. The septum may attain a thickness of 1 cm in cases of repeated fracture, hematoma, and fibrosis, a condition frequently observed in pugilists.

Congenital saddle nose is unusual, most deformities of this type being traumatic in origin. Saddle nose was a typical deformity resulting from syphilis before this disease was largely eradicated by modern antibiotic measures. Other diseases, such as leishmaniasis, are causes of saddle-nose deformity in countries where these diseases are prevalent. Deformities caused by syphilis, leishmaniasis, and leprosy are characterized by a loss of nasal lining, as well as of the nasal framework (see p. 1199). In these deformities it is often necessary to restore the nasal lining prior to restoring the nasal framework (see p. 1200).

A particular type of saddle-nose deformity is that caused by nasomaxillary hypoplasia. The severe type of this malformation is discussed in Chapter 30 (p. 1455).

Depression of the Cartilaginous Dorsum. Depression of the cartilaginous portion of the nose is frequently seen following excessive resection of the septal cartilage, particularly if the mucoperichondrial flaps have been torn, for, in addition to the loss of skeletal support, the contracture exerted by the healing flaps accentuates the depression of the dorsum. Cartilaginous depressions are also seen following hematoma and abscess of the septum with destruction of the cartilage; this type of complication is not infrequent in childhood.

The dorsum of the nose may show a pseudohump due to depression of the cartilaginous dorsum, frequently accompanied by widening of the bony bridge and drooping of the nasal tip. Satisfactory correction of this type of deformity can often be obtained by resecting the pseudohump, narrowing the nasal bridge by osteotomy of the lateral walls, and shortening the nose by excision of cartilage from the caudal border of the septal cartilage and from the alar cartilages. Occasionally it is possible to resect

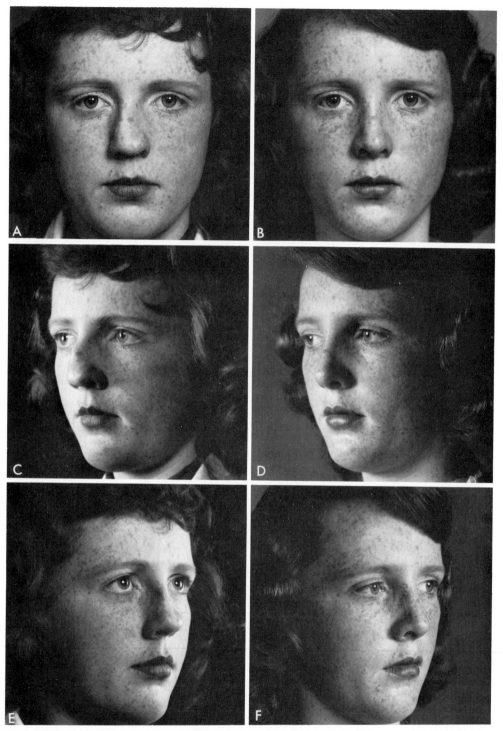

FIGURE 29–147. Straightening the deviated nose and concomitant corrective rhinoplasty. *A*, Full-face appearance shows the C-shaped deviation, widening, and bifidity of the tip. *B*, Postoperative result. *C*, Preoperative three-quarter anterior view, showing the osteocartilaginous dorsal hump. *D*, Postoperative three-quarter view. *E*, Preoperative three-quarter anterior view showing the bifidity of the tip. *F*, Postoperative view.

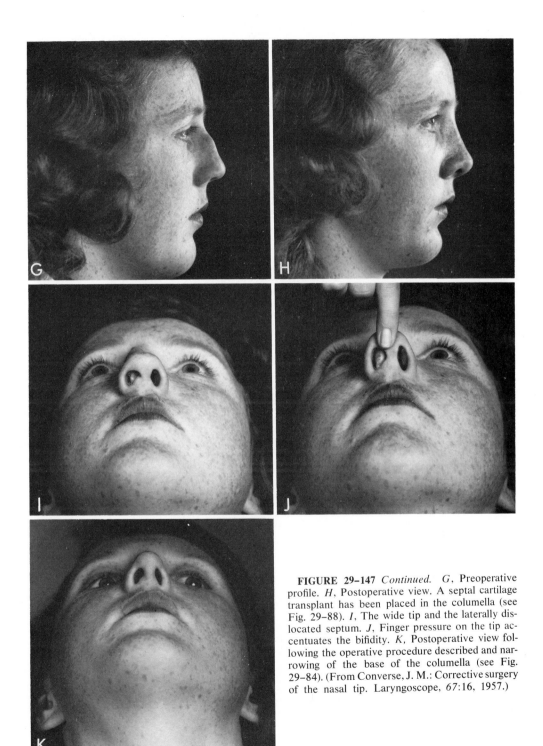

FIGURE 29–147 *Continued.* *G*, Preoperative profile. *H*, Postoperative view. A septal cartilage transplant has been placed in the columella (see Fig. 29–88). *I*, The wide tip and the laterally dislocated septum. *J*, Finger pressure on the tip accentuates the bifidity. *K*, Postoperative view following the operative procedure described and narrowing of the base of the columella (see Fig. 29–84). (From Converse, J. M.: Corrective surgery of the nasal tip. Laryngoscope, *67*:16, 1957.)

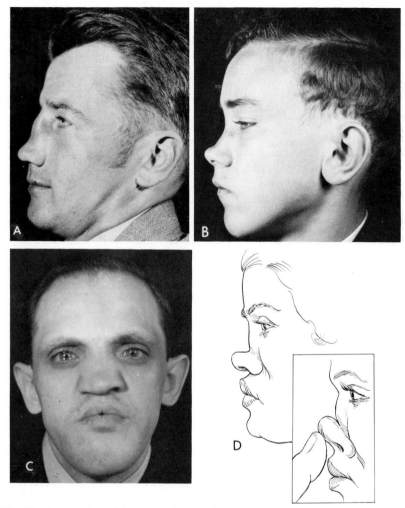

FIGURE 29–148.   The depressed nasal dorsum. *A*, Traumatic depression of the cartilaginous portion of the nose. Note the drooping of the tip and retraction of the columella. *B*, Typical saddle-nose deformity involving both the bony and cartilaginous portions. *C*, Flat nose resulting from widening of the bony dorsum and loss of septal support of the cartilaginous portion of the nose. *D*, When the cartilaginous framework is destroyed, the tip offers no resistance to digital pressure (inset).

the hump and move it caudally to fill in the depression along the dorsum.

SEPTAL CARTILAGE GRAFTS. The technique illustrated in Figure 29–139 is employed when transplantation of septal cartilage is required in more accentuated depression of the cartilaginous bridge. Two or more layers of carefully carved septal cartilage are employed to provide additional contour.

A sufficient amount of septal cartilage can be obtained, even though the cartilage has been destroyed as a result of trauma or is not available following a previous submucous resection; cartilage from the concha of the auricle is also available if it is suitable to correct the particular deformity. Costal cartilage is used when larger cartilage grafts are required.

THE FLYING WING OPERATION (KAZANJIAN). This operation is rarely performed. The type of deformity most suited to the use of this procedure is characterized by a normal bony contour associated with depression of the cartilaginous bridge, well-developed alar cartilages, and a drooping tip. The operation utilizes the lateral crura of the alar cartilages to correct the depression of the bridge, as well as to shorten, elevate, and narrow the tip of the nose.

An incision is made along the caudal margin of each alar cartilage, and the vestibular lining is raised from the cartilage (Fig. 29–149). The lateral crus is freed from the overlying skin, forming a long cartilaginous flap with a narrow pedicle attached to the dome (Fig. 29–149, *A* to *D*). Some of the fibroareolar tissue around

FIGURE 29–149. The flying wing operation (Kazanjian). *A*, Outline of the rim incision extending from the medial crus along the caudal margin of the lateral crus. *B*, The vestibular lining is raised from the cartilage. *C*, *D*, The lateral crus is freed. *E*, The lateral crura are sutured in the midline. The traction suture will be tied over a small piece of gauze. *F*, *G*, Before and after the correction of a depression of the cartilaginous nose by the procedure illustrated in *A* through *E*.

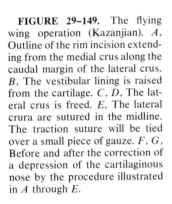

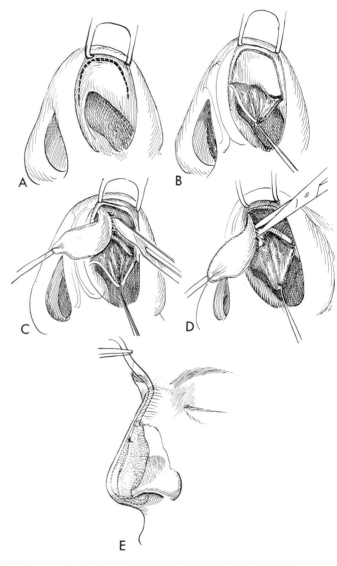

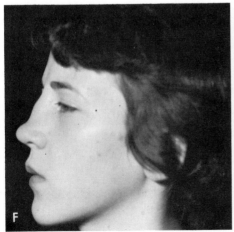

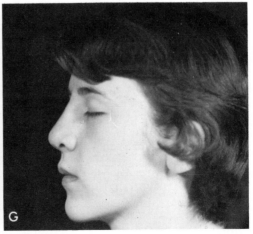

the cartilage may be included to increase the size of the flap. A similar procedure is performed on the contralateral side. The cartilages are freely manipulated, and the wings are transposed from a horizontal to a vertical position over the dorsum. The medial edges of the lateral crura are maintained with buried sutures; a mattress suture is passed through the distal end of each flap (Fig. 29–149, *E*). The free ends of the sutures are passed through the skin near the root of the nose and tied over a small piece of gauze. The two alar cartilages thus transposed from the horizontal to the vertical position are pulled upward, the tip is elevated, the alae are narrowed, and the nose is shortened.

The operation has been largely supplanted by grafting the resected portions of the alar cartilages but may have an occasional application.

OSTEOCARTILAGINOUS NASAL DEPRESSION: SADDLE NOSES AND FLAT NOSES. Nasal deformities requiring bone grafting include such depression deformities as the saddle nose, which involves the bony and cartilaginous vault, and the flat, wide nose (see Fig. 29–148).

A variety of deformities is seen in the traumatic saddle or flat nose: widening of the bony dorsum, flattening of the nasal tip, spreading apart of the alar cartilages, and an increase in the thickness of the septum. The resection of the thick, obstructive septal framework, an arduous and delicate surgical procedure, is preferably done as a preliminary procedure to improve the airway.

The collapse of the cartilaginous nose due to loss of septal support (the tip of the nose can usually be depressed by digital pressure without encountering any resistance from the deficient septum) (see Fig. 29–148, *D*) further impairs the respiratory function of the nose.

Transplants and Implants for the Repair of Saddle-Nose Deformities. Various types of transplants and implants have been employed for nasal contour restoration. A majority of plastic surgeons favor autogenous bone or cartilage, although other transplant materials have been employed. Cartilage allografts have been used extensively (Brown and McDowell, 1951). The work of Gibson, Curran, and Davis (1957) suggests the possibility of survival of fresh cartilage allografts. Fresh cartilage allografts have not been employed, because failure of maternal auricular cartilage allografts in the reconstruction of the microtic auricle has been observed. Bovine cartilage (Gillies and Kristensen, 1951) does not maintain its bulk and is progressively absorbed.

Specially prepared calf bone has been employed unsuccessfully (Haas, 1963; Bell, 1966) in saddle-nose deformities. These grafts became absorbed progressively.

Silcone rubber, acrylic, polyethylene, and other inorganic implants have also been used in the nose. It will be recalled that ivory was used as a nasal implant as late as the middle 1930's; this implant material was frequently extruded.

Although inorganic materials may be tolerated by the tissues for a varying period of time, they are often extruded because of tissue irritation around the implant, especially when they are implanted in areas of functional stress or areas which are subjected to musuclar movements or trauma. The rejected implant leaves a bed of dense fibrous tissue, complicating further reconstructive procedures. Lipschutz (1966) noted a rejection rate of 50 per cent with Silastic implants. Some of the worst "crucified" noses are those seen following the extrusion of a foreign implant accompanied by suppuration.

Some measure of success appears to have been achieved when silicone implants were employed in Asiatics in order to increase the projection of the dorsum, but their use is not indicated in the Occidental nose, except for minor deformities that can best be treated by a septal cartilage graft. All of the inorganic implants are subjected to the pull of the surrounding soft tissue scar in the course of healing and are apt to be twisted or rotated from their original position.

Allografts of sclera obtained from an eye bank, in the fresh or frozen state, have been employed for the correction of minor irregularities and depressions (Hadley, 1975). According to Hadley, Cottle used sclera in 1960, and the implant has been used in hundreds of cases and found to be useful to fill small defects. There has been no clinically observable local reaction after implantation. While gradual absorption occurs and the sclera is replaced by fibrous tissue, contour restoration appears to be maintained.

Autogenous bone grafts, when placed in contact with living bone, consolidate with the host bone and become incorporated into the bony facial framework. Bone grafting is contraindicated only if contact between the bone graft and host bone cannot be achieved.

Because bone autografts become consolidated with the underlying nasal bones, loosening or deviation of the graft is prevented. Consolidation with the nasal bones also maintains the projection of the lower part of the graft, thus achieving a cantilever effect. The bone

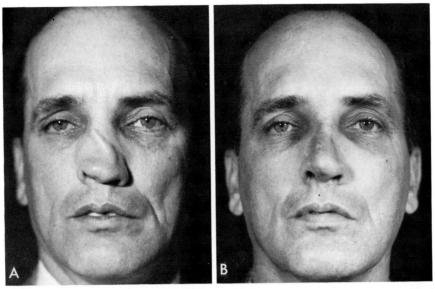

FIGURE 29–150. *A*, Example of a costal cartilage graft which has become curled and twisted out of position. The graft was not cut according to Gibson's balanced cross section principle. *B*, Result obtained by removing the cartilage graft and replacing it by an autogenous iliac bone graft.

graft may be fractured because of its rigidity, an unusual occurrence, but it usually consolidates uneventfully.

Costal cartilage autografts survive satisfactorily, do not require contact with the nasal bony framework as do bone grafts, and are specifically indicated when such contact cannot be established—for example, in cases in which the nasal bones have been destroyed (see Chapter 28, Fig. 28–169). Cartilage, however, tends to curl and bend, particularly in younger individuals (Fig. 29–150); in older patients, who have partly calcified costal cartilage, the tendency for curling is lessened. Gibson and Davis (1958) described a technique in which the cartilage is cut according to a balanced cross section; this procedure eliminates the curling of the cartilage. The technique is described in a later section devoted to costal cartilage grafts (see Fig. 29–159).

THE ILIAC BONE GRAFT FOR NASAL CONTOUR RESTORATION

Iliac Bone Graft Removal. The technique of removal of bone grafts has been described in Chapter 13. The bone graft is usually taken from the main body of the crest of the ilium. In female patients in order to avoid the visible loss of contour of the iliac crest, the graft may be taken from the medial aspect of the crest, leaving the lateral portion of the crest for contour. Another technique which may be employed, particularly in female patients in whom the iliac crest is often wide, consists of removing the bone graft from the center of the crest and infracturing the medial and lateral aspects by pressing them together, thus obliterating the site of bone graft removal. After removal of the bone graft, the periosteum and the soft tissues covering the crest of the ilium are approximated; drainage can be dispensed with if a pressure dressing obliterates the dead space between the bone and the covering soft tissues. Continuous suction drainage is indicated, however, if bleeding is profuse during the operation and if the graft is removed from the medial aspect of the crest.

Shaping the Graft. In most cases, the piece of bone removed from the crest of the ilium is boat-shaped, beveled at each end and on its undersurface. The convexity of the undersurface of the graft fits into and fills the concavity of the dorsum of the typical saddle nose; the graft should "sit" in a stable manner without any "rocking." This is an important technical detail, for it is the fit of the graft into the concavity of the saddle deformity which ensures the stability of the transplant and its ability to become consolidated to the host bone. The graft should be wider in the middle and concave transversely in order to adapt to the nasal bones and frontal processes of the maxilla.

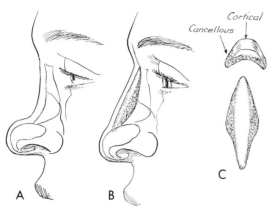

FIGURE 29-151. Shaping the bone graft. *A*, Diagram of a saddle nose. *B*, The bone graft in position. *C*, Frontal section of the bone graft (above); shape of the corticocancellous bone graft (below).

The graft should be shaped to reproduce the contour of a normal dorsum: it is narrow cephalad, wider with rounded edges, and again narrow caudad. First the graft is roughly shaped with large, double-jointed bone cutters; finally it is contoured with the aid of a Lindemann spiral burr activated by an air-turbine drill under a constant stream of sterile cold water to avoid overheating the bone (Fig. 29-151). Some of the cortex of the bone should be left on the graft for rigidity. When the graft is extended into the tip of the nose, it is shaped in the form of the prow of a ship (see Fig. 29-151, *C*).

It is helpful for the beginner to carve and shape a model of the proposed bone graft from a piece of silicone rubber. The bone graft is carved to reproduce the shape of the silicone rubber model.

Routes of Introduction of Bone Grafts. The incision for exposure should be distal to the area of the dorsum which requires the bone graft. The intercartilaginous incision can rarely be employed except for grafts placed over the bony dorsum near the root of the nose, since most grafts extend downward over the cartilaginous portion of the nose. The danger of intranasal exposure of the graft through the intercartilaginous incisions should be avoided.

A transcartilaginous incision through the alar cartilage (Fig. 29-152), extending from the medial crus medially to a predetermined point in the lateral crus laterally, the length of the incision depending upon the size of the graft, is the method of choice for all grafts over the bony dorsum extending downward toward the tip of the nose. The incision should be ex-

tended distally to the distal end of the graft in order to avoid intranasal exposure of the graft.

When the graft is to be introduced into the nasal tip, in order to avoid an external scar, an incision extends along the caudal margin of the lateral crus of the alar cartilage, around the point of junction of the lateral and medial crura, and downward along the caudal margin of the medial crus. The rim incision (Fig. 29-152), when done bilaterally, provides exposure of the nasal tip sufficient to perform the operation illustrated in Figs. 29-154 and 29-155.

Transplants over the nasal dorsum introduced through an intranasal incision are used nearly exclusively. External incisions at the tip of the nose, either the butterfly or the midcolumellar incision, both of which are preferable to Gillies' horizontal incision at the base of the columella or the Rethi incision through the upper third of the columella, are of historical interest and have only an occasional application. The vertical mid-columellar incision has proved superior to the horizontally placed butterfly or bird-in-flight incision and, in most cases, leaves a barely discernible scar. Considerable difficulty may be encountered in suturing the edges of the butterfly type of incision under tension.

External incisions placed laterally over the frontal process of the maxilla on each side of the nasal dorsum, occasionally joined by a transverse incision at the root of the nose, are

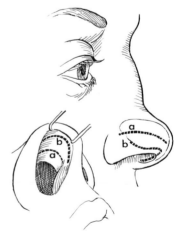

FIGURE 29-152. Intranasal incisions for the insertion of iliac or cartilage grafts. *a*, Transcartilaginous incision through the alar cartilage. *b*, The rim incision along the caudal edge of the lateral and medial crura. When the shape of the tip of the nose requires modification and excision of alar cartilage (see Fig. 29-155), the rim incisions are done bilaterally. The transcartilaginous incision may also be done bilaterally to facilitate the elevation of the soft tissues over the dorsum of the nose and the placing of the graft in the midline of the nose.

employed for the primary treatment and the secondary repair of naso-orbital fractures (see Chapters 25 and 28). Direct exposure of the dorsum is invaluable in the repair of the foreshortened nose following severe naso-orbital fractures (see p. 1274). A midline vertical incision extending from the root of the nose to the nasal tip is indicated in complicated traumatic deformities (see Fig. 29–305) and leaves a relatively inconspicuous scar when it is carefully sutured. Dermabrasion often removes the last vestiges of the scar. The presence of a preexisting traumatic scar over the dorsum necessitates the repair of the scar; the nasal pyramid can be approached through the area of scar excision.

Preparation of the Recipient Site and Introduction of the Bone Graft. The nasal dorsum is approached through one of the incisions previously described. The soft tissues over the cartilaginous portion of the nose are raised with scissors (Fig. 29–153), the plane of dissection remaining close to the cartilages. If the bone graft is of moderate or large size, it can be difficult to introduce it under the raised periosteum. As contact of the bone graft with the host bone is essential, the periosteum must be incised and reflected.

The soft tissues are dissected over the periosteum (Fig. 29–153, *A*), the lower end of the incision being joined by two horizontal incisions along the lower border of the nasal bones to an inverted T (Fig. 29–153, *B*). The periosteum is then reflected from the bone (Fig. 29–153, *C*). It is often necessary to remove bone from the

cephalic portion of the bony dorsum with an osteotome in order to flatten the host surface, reducing the projection of the host site so that the bone graft will "sit" on a flat surface and will not eliminate the nasofrontal angle. Bony irregularities are smoothed with a rasp.

In malunited comminuted fractures, it is particularly necessary to denude the bone of scar tissue in order to ensure contact between the graft and the bone. The bone graft from the ilium is shaped and introduced. The graft should rest in position without "rocking." "Rocking" is minimized by adequate shaping of the host bone, reducing the projection of the bone, smoothing irregularities caused by malunited fracture, and fitting the undersurface of the bone graft into the concavity of the dorsum. The graft consists of a cortical layer and a major portion of cancellous bone.

The Cantilever Bone Graft Wired to the Nasal Bones. In saddle-nose and flat nose deformities (Fig. 29–154, *A*), when the distal end of the bone graft extends to the nasal tip in order to increase the projection of the tip, the distal end of the graft is subjected to a downward traction, causing a "rocking" movement of the graft and a protrusion of the cephalic end of the graft at the root of the nose. A technique to prevent the downward tilting of the graft and to maintain adequate projection of the nasal tip is to wire the graft to the nasal bones. The dorsum is approached through a rim incision which extends downward to free the medial crura from their columellar soft tissue attachments (Fig. 29–154, *B*). The periosteum is

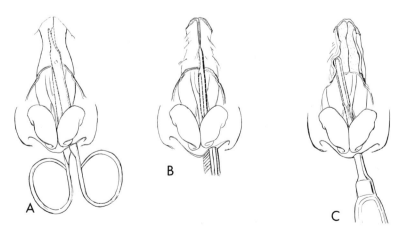

FIGURE 29–153. Preparation of the host site for an iliac bone graft to the nose. *A*, Scissors have undermined the soft tissues over the cartilages and nasal bones. *B*, A vertical incision is made through the periosteum; a horizontal incision through the periosteum is made along the lower border of the nasal bones. *C*, The periosteum is raised from the bone. (From Converse J. M.: Technique of bone grafting for contour restoration of the face. Plast. Reconstr. Surg., *14*:332, 1954. Copyright © 1954, The Williams & Wilkins Company, Baltimore.)

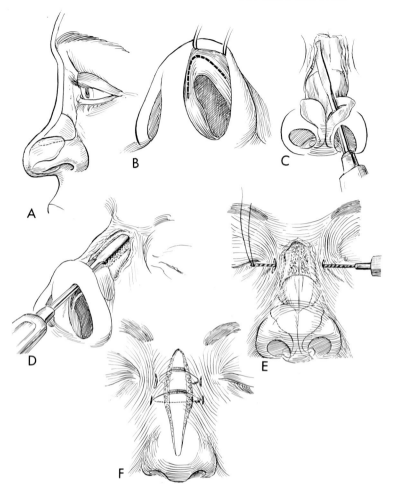

FIGURE 29–154. Technique of the cantilever bone graft. *A*, Schematic profile of a saddle nose with a flat tip. *B*, Rim incision extending along the caudal margin of the lateral and medial crura. *C*, The periosteum is reflected. *D*, Bony irregularities are rasped. *E*, A wire is drilled through the nasal bones. Short incisions are made through the skin on each side of the bony framework to expose the bone prior to drilling. *F*, Position of the wires and of the bone graft. A groove drilled over the anterior surface of the graft receives the wire. The ends of each wire are twisted and buried in the drill hole. Two wires are employed to prevent lateral twisting of the graft.

raised (Fig. 29–154, *C*), and a rasp removes any bony irregularities (Fig. 29–154, *D*). Fixation with stainless steel wire is done through small incisions made on each side of the lateral walls. A turbine-driven drill or a hand-manipulated awl (Fig. 29–154, *E*) is employed to perforate the nasal cavity from one lateral wall to the other; a stainless steel wire is passed through the nasal cavity and then looped over the bone graft (Fig. 29–154, *F*). The wire passes into a groove especially made for it on the anterior surface of the bone to avoid protrusion of the wire above the level of the graft. The wire is twisted and cut, and the remaining stump of wire is tucked into the drill hole. The edges of the skin incisions are approximated with fine sutures. Two wires placed at different levels are required to prevent lateral rotation of the graft (Fig. 29–154, *F*).

The wires maintain firm fixation of the bone graft to the host bed (Fig. 29–155, *A*). The distal portion of the graft is introduced between the medial crura immediately beneath the domes (Fig. 29–155, *B*). Tip remodeling procedures may be done in conjunction with a bone graft. Bilateral rim incisions have provided adequate exposure of the alar cartilages. If necessary, partial thickness incisions are made through the domes (Fig. 29–155, *B*) to assist in obtaining increased projection of the tip (Fig. 29–155, *C*, *D*, *E*). A nonabsorbable mattress suture joins the medial crura over the distal end of the graft, thus increasing the projection of the domes (Fig. 29–155, *C*, *D*).

Wire fixation and the cantilever bone graft technique are employed in the nose reconstructed by means of a forehead flap (see p. 1260).

The Bone Graft with a Columellar Strut. Downward tilting of the bone graft can be prevented by use of a columellar strut which maintains the projection of the caudal end of the transplant. The columella is tunneled downward toward the nasal spine, and a bony

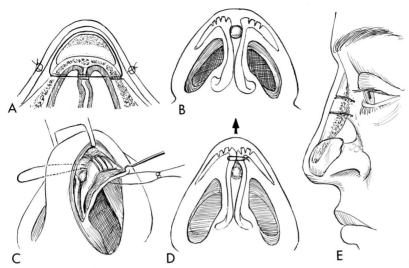

FIGURE 29–155. Technique of the cantilever bone graft (continued). *A,* Cross section showing the position of the wires and the bone graft. *B,* Position of the distal portion of the bone graft between the medial crura. In this technique, the domes and a portion of each lateral crus have been weakened by a series of partial thickness incisions; this procedure is not always necessary. *C,* A mattress suture is placed through the domes of each alar cartilage. *D,* Position of the domes over the distal end of the bone graft. The cantilever graft thus elevates the tip of the nose. *E,* The cantilever bone graft wired to the nasal bones supports the alar cartilages.

strut is placed over the nasal spine after the latter has been stripped of periosteum. It is usually necessary to excise a small, V-shaped segment of bone from the lower end of the strut in order to fit it over the nasal spine; this procedure controls the tendency of the strut to shift. The junction between the strut and the dorsal graft is best achieved by the "tent pole" technique, which prevents loss of contact between the two pieces of bone. A small hole is drilled through the caudal end of the bone graft, and the pointed end of the strut is introduced into the hole. After the desired degree of elevation of the tip is achieved, two shoulders are cut on the strut to prevent the pointed end of the strut from extending too far through the hole. The strut is often progressively absorbed, but it serves as a support until the consolidation of the graft to the nasal bones is completed.

The use of a columellar strut presupposes a columella of good quality; generally it cannot be used in the reconstructed columella. The cantilever bone graft is a preferable and more reliable technique; it does not eliminate the suppleness and flexibility of the nasal tip area, an important physiologic consideration, and the chances of fracture are less.

In patients with a depressed nasal tip accompanied by loss of septal support and a short columella, raising the tip by means of a columella strut secured to the distal end of the bone graft maintains the projected position of the tip; elongation of the columella is required to avoid excessive tension, which might cause erosion of the skin of the tip by the bone graft.

Multiple Nasal Bone Grafts. If the bone graft is not of sufficient size to provide adequate projection of the dorsum, matchstick grafts (Campbell, 1957) (small slivers of bone) are placed between the graft and the nasal bones.

Nasal Bone Grafts in Children. Bone taken from the rib (Longacre and DeStefano, 1957) has been employed in children (see Chapter 13). An incision is made parallel to one of the ribs, and the rib is resected subperiosteally. The rib is split longitudinally and placed over the dorsum after it is suitably shaped.

Iliac bone can also be used in children by employing the technique of Crockford and Converse (1972) described in Chapter 13.

Other Types of Bone Grafts. Tibial grafts were used successfully in the past but have been mostly discontinued because of the denser variety of the bone and because of possible fracture due to weakening of the tibia. In children, however, a small sliver of tibial bone from the medial aspect of the superior-anterior border can be used.

Other sources of bone grafts are the greater trochanter, the olecranon, and adjacent por-

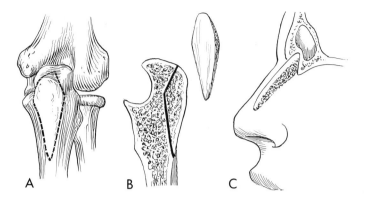

FIGURE 29–156. Bone graft removed from the olecranon. *A, B,* Site of removal of the bone graft. *C,* The bone graft is shaped and fitted into a niche in the frontal bone. (After Antia, 1974).

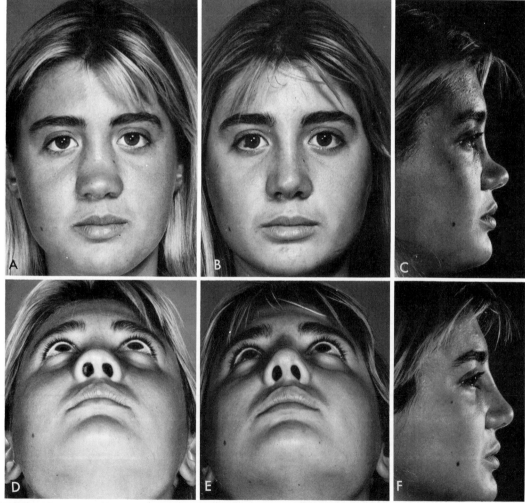

FIGURE 29–157. Saddle-nose deformity corrected by an iliac bone graft. *A,* Preoperative appearance. *B,* The bony dorsum of the nose was approached through bilateral transcartilaginous incisions through the lateral crus of each alar cartilage, which also permitted a modification of the shape of the nasal tip. A submucous resection of the septum was also done, followed by lateral osteotomies to reduce the width of the bony nose. An iliac bone graft was then shaped and placed in position. *C,* Preoperative profile view, showing the deformity resulting from a childhood injury. *D,* Preoperative shape of the nasal tip. *E,* Postoperative shape of the tip. *F,* Postoperative profile view.

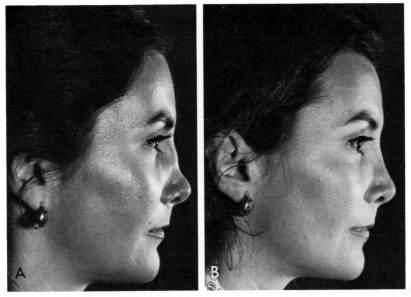

FIGURE 29–158. *A,* Saddle-nose deformity caused by excessive resection of the septum. *B,* Correction obtained by the insertion of an iliac bone graft.

tions of the subcutaneous border of the ulna (Antia, 1974). In cases of leprosy, the olecranon graft has been used as a cantilever graft introduced through an incision at the root of the nose (Fig. 29–156).

Fixation of the Bone Graft into the Frontal Bone. Another way to obtain cantilever fixation is to drill a hole into the frontal bone immediately above the root of the nose (see Fig. 29–156, *C*). The bone is reamed into the opening until it is firmly fixed. This technique is frequently employed in the course of craniofacial operations to restore the nasal dorsum (see Chapter 56).

Various Applications of Iliac Bone Grafts for the Correction of the Depressed Nasal Dorsum. Trauma in childhood was the cause of the saddle-nose deformity in the patient shown in Figure 29–157. Collapse of the nose following a rhinoplasty combined with an overzealous submucous resection of the septum was responsible for the deformity shown in Figure 29–158. In both cases a satisfactory improvement was obtained by iliac bone grafting. Bone grafting has applications in many other types of deformities: in congenital malformations, in various traumatic deformities, and in reconstruction following traumatic amputation or resection for malignancy.

COSTAL CARTILAGE GRAFTS FOR NASAL CONTOUR RESTORATION

The technique of removal of costal cartilage has been described in Chapter 12. The cartilage graft is shaped by paring it with a knife and is introduced into the nose according to techniques similar to those already described for bone grafts. Certain precautions must be taken, however, to avoid curling and warping of the transplant. The tendency to warp is particularly noted in children's cartilage; in older patients cartilage which is partly calcified does not have this characteristic. Gillies (1920) noted that the graft, when denuded of perichondrium on one side, tends to curve toward that side. Mowlem (1938), reviewing a series of 35 cartilage grafts applied to the nasal bridge, reported that 17 of these became twisted; he subsequently advocated the use of iliac bone grafts for nasal transplants. New and Erich (1941) dipped the cartilage into boiling water for a few seconds, thus eliminating the curling tendency; no follow-up concerning the ultimate fate of these grafts has been reported. Gibson and Davis (1958) showed that not only the perichondrium but also the surface layer of the cartilage played a role in the warping when it was removed on one side. They advocated a technique which applied the princi-

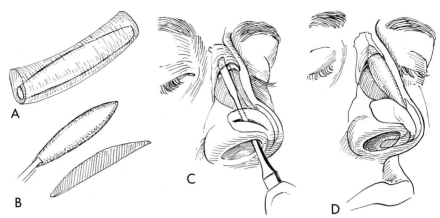

FIGURE 29–159. The costal cartilage graft. *A*, Gibson's technique (the principle of balanced cross section) to avoid warping of the cartilage graft. *B*, Shape of the graft, front and side views. The convex undersurface of the graft fits the concave surface of the nasal dorsum. *C*, Periosteal elevator, introduced through a transcartilaginous incision through the alar cartilage, raising the periosteum. *D*, The costal cartilage graft in position.

ple of balanced cross section (Fig. 29–159). All of the perichondrium surrounding a full thickness section of a rib cartilage, as well as the cortical cartilage layer, should be removed.

The one-piece, L-shaped graft that extends over the dorsum and is angulated downward into the columella as far as the nasal spine is not recommended. This type of graft produces a rigid lower nose and eliminates the natural resiliency provided by the membranous septum, thus interfering with the normal physiol-

ogy of the nose. The one-piece, L-shaped graft, when displaced from side to side, manifests its presence by a side-to-side subcutaneous protrusion under the skin of the root of the nose. The perichondrial hinge technique of Gillies gives the L-shaped graft more flexibility (Fig. 29–160).

Bone grafts have become popular for the correction of saddle-nose deformities. The costal cartilage graft also gives excellent results and has the advantage that it does not require contact with the underlying host bone for survival; a disadvantage is that the cartilage graft, because it is not consolidated with the underlying host bone, is occasionally subjected to the traction forces exerted by the soft tissues and may be pulled out of alignment.

Costal cartilage grafts are indicated in reconstructed noses in which there is insufficient remaining bone to provide a host bed for a bone graft. Satisfactory results have been obtained in these cases (see Figs. 29–276 and 29–277). Older patients in whom the costal cartilage has become partly calcified are also good candidates for costal cartilage grafts, as the partly calcified grafts have less tendency to curl or warp.

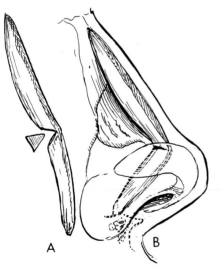

FIGURE 29–160. The hinged costal cartilage graft. (After Gillies, 1920). The hinge is provided by the perichondrium which is preserved on one side. A variant of this graft is the osteocartilaginous graft taken from the area of junction of the bony rib with the cartilaginous rib. The bony portion of the graft consolidates with the bony dorsum of the nose.

Bone and Cartilage Grafting in Conjunction with Osteotomy and Septal Framework Resection

Because many of the noses requiring restoration of contour by bone and cartilage grafts have been severely traumatized and may show, in addition to the saddle or flat appearance of the nose, widening of the bony dorsum or deviation, osteotomy of the lateral walls of the nose is required. Some severely traumatized noses have a thickened deviated septum which also requires straightening by submucous resection of the septal framework. The question arises whether these procedures can be done in a single operative stage, or whether straightening of the framework of the nose and septum should be done in a preliminary stage. Much will depend upon the magnitude of the deformity. In severely traumatized noses, septal surgery and lateral osteotomies should be done in a preliminary stage because of the tedious surgery required for a successful submucous resection of the thickened septum and adherent flaps with underlying fibrosis. After a suitable time interval, the bone or cartilage graft is performed; additional corrective nasal tip surgery can be performed in the same stage. Because of the more extensive surgery, the danger of hematoma, and the increased area of communication between the intranasal cavity and the recipient site of the graft, consideration should be given before doing septal surgery, osteotomies, and tip surgery concomitantly with a nasal dorsal transplant. The danger of wound sepsis developing after a costal cartilage graft appears to be greater than after an iliac bone graft. One explanation for this may be that the cartilage, being a nonvascularized structure, does not receive the protection of systemic antibiotic therapy, the antibiotic being perfused through the revascularized bone graft. Iliac bone grafts have been successfully performed in conjunction with lateral osteotomies to narrow the bony dorsum in carefully chosen cases.

Complications Following Bone and Cartilage Grafting to the Nose

Some of the complications which may occur following transplantation of bone or cartilage to the dorsum of the nose have already been considered. Among these are absorption, displacement, and warping of the graft. Other complications will now be considered.

Necrosis of the Skin. Necrosis of the skin results from the excessive pressure exerted by the graft. At operation, if blanching of the skin is noted, the transplant should be reduced in size in order to minimize the pressure. This complication is not uncommon in noses that have been injured by lacerations and loss of the soft tissues, or in congenital deficiency of soft tissue. If the soft tissue is inadequate to withstand the pressure of the transplant, additional soft tissue should be provided. The techniques of providing additional covering tissues to the nose are discussed later in the chapter. In the preparation of the recipient bed for the graft, the covering soft tissues of the nose should be undermined at a skeletal level. Undermining the skin too superficially impairs its blood supply. The thin layer of the skin covering the graft becomes necrotic.

When skin necrosis does occur, an advantage of the bone graft is the possibility of spontaneous epithelization over the exposed bone. The wound should receive frequent wound care, and the superficial layer of bone which usually undergoes avascular necrosis should be resected. Granulation tissue appears, and epithelization will occur progressively. Such spontaneous healing occurs in bone grafts which are revascularized and is not usually observed following exposure of the nonvascularized cartilage graft. When such exposure occurs in a cartilage graft, the transplant usually must be removed.

Intranasal Exposure of the Transplant. The bone or cartilage transplant may become exposed through the intranasal incision made for its placement or by erosion by the pressure of the graft through the intranasal lining. Intranasal examination will show the extent of this exposure. Bone grafts usually resist the deleterious effects of exposure until spontaneous regrowth of nasal lining covers the exposed area. Cartilage grafts have a lesser resistance to exposure.

Hematoma. The hematoma should be evacuated as soon as it is discovered. Hematoma is often fatal to bone grafts. Infection and suppuration of the hematoma require removal of the transplant. When a bone graft is employed, the hematoma may impair the osteogenic processes, and the bone graft will be progressively absorbed.

Inadequate Shaping of the Graft. When the transplant has been inadequately fitted to the recipient bed and all tendency to "rocking" has not been eliminated, the pressure exerted on the distal portion of the graft will cause the proximal portion to protrude at the nasofrontal angle. Secondary surgery is necessary in these cases.

Fracture of the Bone Graft.   Fracture of the nasal bone graft may occur following trauma. One of our patients, a former middleweight champion of the world, had undergone, upon retiring from his boxing career, two successful operations. The first was a laborious submucous resection of a thick, fibrotic, obstructive septum. The second operation consisted of an iliac bone graft and nasal tip corrective procedure, which provided an excellent esthetic result. About two years after these procedures, the patient was involved in a barroom brawl and received a lateral blow to the nose; when he was examined the next day, he showed a deviation of the lower portion of the nose to the right, with clinical and roentgenographic evidence of fracture of the bone graft in its midportion. Realignment of the bone and fixation by means of a splint for a period of six days permitted consolidation of the graft in a corrected position. This type of accident has occurred in a number of patients; satisfactory results were obtained when adequate treatment was provided.

When the graft becomes displaced and malunited, it must be detached from the host bed by separating it from the underlying bone with an osteotome and repositioning it correctly where it will consolidate if adequate fixation is provided. (For other applications of bone and cartilage grafts, see the section of this chapter entitled Reconstructive Rhinoplasty.)

TRAUMATIC SEPTAL-TURBINATE SYNECHIAE

In penetrating lacerations of the nasal fossae, an adhesion or synechia forms as a result of the healing of the raw areas when they are adjacent to the septal mucous membrane and one of the turbinates. Nasal obstruction is the consequence of this closure of the nasal airway. The treatment consists of cutting through the adhesion and interposing nasal packing or a sheet of plastic material, which must be left in position for a minimum of seven days in order to allow for re-epithelization of the raw areas.

If the septum is deviated to the side of the synechia, the septal cartilage should be resected prior to the incision through the adhesion between the septum and the turbinate; this procedure facilitates the incision through

the synechia and the placing of the interposed material and diminishes the chances of the adhesion recurring prior to the re-epithelization of the structures. More complicated techniques of restoring nasal lining after elimination of multiple and extensive synechiae are described in a later section of the chapter (see p. 1200).

PERFORATION OF THE SEPTUM

A through-and-through perforation of the septum may be the result of a penetrating injury with lacerations of the mucous membrane on both sides of the septum, combined with fracture or laceration through the septal cartilage. The primary repair of such septal damage will prevent a permanent septal perforation. Iatrogenic septal perforation may result from an incorrectly performed operation to straighten the deviated septum; the deviated septum caused by severe injury with consequent hematoma and fibrosis can be difficult to correct. If the septal mucoperichondrium is torn on both sides and the intervening septal cartilage has been removed, a perforation of varying size results. The edges of the mucous membrane around the perforation become epithelized, and the through-and-through septal perforation is permanent. Loss of nasal mucous membrane, whether from a large septal perforation or destruction of turbinates, results in serious impairment of nasal physiology, as the ciliated cylindrical, columnar epithelium of the nasal cavity is indispensable for nasal function. Small perforations may produce an incongruous whistling sound.

When the septal framework has been entirely removed, it is difficult to separate the septal flaps; repair of septal perforations is also a difficult procedure. In traumatic perforations, the septal framework, fortunately, is usually present. Use of a rotation flap (Fig. 29–161, *A, B*) is feasible in small and moderate-size anterior perforations. Grafts of oral mucosa, adequately thinned (Fig. 29–161, *C, D, E*), provide a covering for the raw surface of the flap. An anterior transposition flap (Fig. 29–161, *F, G*) may also be used.

In larger perforations, the only technique that has been successful, in the author's experience, has been the labial mucosal flap, raised from the labial aspect of the buccal sulcus, based at the level of the frenulum, and introduced into the nasal cavity (Fig. 29–161, *H* to *N*).

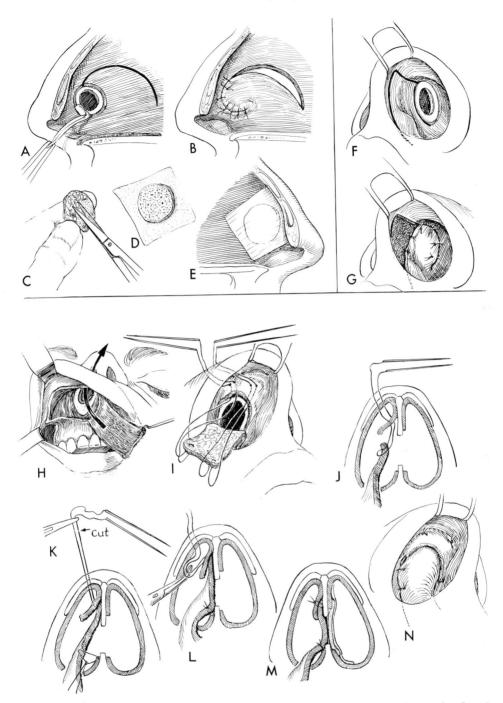

FIGURE 29–161. Techniques for the closure of septal perforations. *A*, Outline of a posterior rotation flap of muco-perichondrium. *B*, The flap is sutured in position. *C*, A mucosal graft is removed from the oral mucosa. The raw surface of the graft is trimmed, thus reducing the thickness of the graft. *D*, A mucosal graft placed on paper tape. *E*, The graft carried on the paper tape is applied to the raw surface of the rotation flap illustrated in *A* and *B* and maintained by bilateral nasal packing. *F*, *G*, Transposition flap for the closure of small perforations. *F*, A flap is outlined anteriorly from the membranous septum. *G*, The flap is transposed. *H* to *N*, In larger perforations a flap of mucosa from the upper lip is indicated. *I*, The mucosal flap from the upper lip is introduced into the nasal cavity; two catgut mattress sutures are placed through the distal end of the flap and are brought out through the raised mucoperichondrium and the cartilaginous nasal wall. *J*, Frontal section illustrating the maneuver in *I*. *K*, The sutures are cut and the needles removed. *L*, The sutures are reintroduced into the nasal cavity. *M*, The sutures are tied, providing fixation of the distal end of the flap. A graft of mucosa (*C*, *D*, *E*) is applied to the raw surface of the flap on the contralateral side of the septum. *N*, The flap is sutured.

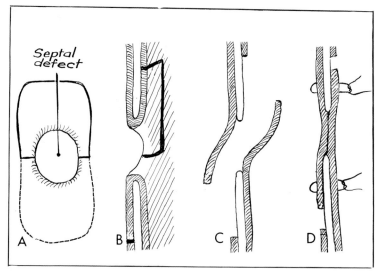

FIGURE 29–162. Another technique for closure of small perforations. *A*, Healed perforation with cicatricial edges. *B*, Outline of a hinge flap. *C*, Frontal section of bilateral, hinged, turnover flaps of mucoperichondrium. *D*, The flaps are sutured to each other with mattress sutures.

Small perforations may be closed by using two hinge flaps of mucoperichondrium, one on each side. On one side the flap is hinged on a superior pedicle; on the other side the flap is hinged on an inferior pedicle, as illustrated in Figure 29–162. Nasal packing maintains the raw surfaces of the flaps in apposition until healed.

Larger perforations may be closed by detaching the inferior turbinate from the lateral wall, leaving it attached by a posterior pedicle. The turbinate is placed into the perforation, and, after suitable incisions are made, the mucous membrane of the turbinate is sutured to the mucous membrane surrounding the perforated septum.

Large perforations, with a loss of a major portion of the septum, are intractable. Surprisingly, some patients tolerate large perforations relatively well, while the small perforation and the whistling sound may annoy the patient. All of the patients with septal perforations have crusts which must be removed, and the area of the perforation must be cleansed. The symptoms may be more severe in large perforations; loss of olfaction and nasal obstruction with atrophic rhinitis may result when mucosal changes involve the entire nasal cavity. The daily use of emollients, such as paraffin oil, sprayed to soften the crusts, and nasal irrigations with saline solution are necessary to rid the patient of the foul-smelling crusts. This extreme type of atrophic rhinitis is similar to ozena, a condition which has become rare in the United States.

The success of local flaps depends upon the condition of the surrounding tissues and the presence of septal cartilage in the vicinity of the perforation, for this cartilage can be mobilized to fill the defect between the transposed flaps.

The subject of septal perforations has been discussed in some detail by Meyer (1972), who has closed large perforations by the following technique. The cartilage is buried at the distal end of a flap of mucous membrane in the labial gingival sulcus. The flap is so designed that mucous membrane at the distal end of the flap is folded under the cartilage; thus the cartilage is enveloped by two layers of mucous membrane. After three weeks the flap is introduced into the nasal cavity, and the three-layered distal end of the flap is sutured into the septal perforation.

SECONDARY CORRECTIVE RHINOPLASTY

Because of the number and complexity of the problems requiring solutions in secondary corrective rhinoplasty, an entire volume could be written on the subject of postoperative deformities of the nose and secondary (or more) operations. The causes of unfavorable results have been touched upon in the earlier sections of this chapter; they include poor esthetic judgment on the part of the surgeon, the surgeon's inexperience, the inevitable need for a secondary operation in the difficult rhinoplasty, and many other causes.

Observations of poor results following rhinoplasty suggest that the surgeon attempted to accomplish too much rather than settle for a

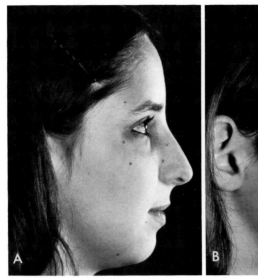

FIGURE 29–163. A corrective rhinoplasty with chin augmentation. *A*, Preoperative appearance. *B*, Sufficient length has been maintained; the slight irregularity along the dorsum avoids the long, straight appearance of the nose.

compromise which might not have achieved the "perfect" nose (whatever that is). The patient shown in Figure 29–163 is an example of a compromise. The nose is not "perfect," but it is in harmony with the remainder of the face, and a good profile balance has been achieved by the chin augmentation.

The secondary rhinoplasty is always a more difficult operation because of the presence of scar tissue following the first operation and the absence of cartilage or bone, which may have been removed in excess at the previous operation.

As more and more rhinoplasties are being performed, the number of complications and unsatisfactory results appears to increase. Relatively few publications have been presented on the subject (O'Connor and McGregor, 1955; Brown and McDowell, 1965; Pollet and Baudelot, 1967; Millard, 1969; Rogers, 1969, 1972; Rees and coworkers, 1970; Rees and Wood-Smith, 1972; Jost and Mahé, 1972; Vergnon and Jost, 1975; Sheen, 1975b). Secondary rhinoplasty was also briefly discussed in the previous edition of this book.

In the description of the technique of primary corrective plastic surgery of the nose, many of the pitfalls to be avoided were described; the indispensable step in the primary operation is a thorough examination of the remodeled skeletal framework of the nose at the end of the operation.

The Decision to Operate. The patient is often disappointed, resentful, or even angry when the surgical correction has not met his

expectations. Rogers (1972) has expressed some of his observations made during clinical examinations of patients consulting him for the advisability of a primary or a secondary corrective rhinoplasty:

> Poor rapport can lead to complications which could have been controlled if the surgeon had the proper sensitivity and perception—he must spend additional sessions with an overanxious patient, sessions which may make him decide to reject his prospective patient as psychologically "unsound" and "unfit to undergo the necessary surgery" (Steiss, 1951) or may lead to a formal psychiatric consultation. . . . The surgeon who speaks to the patient in grandiose terms about the results to be expected from either a primary or a secondary rhinoplasty is probably going to have an emotionally disturbed patient as soon as any postoperative defect makes its appearance. On the other hand, the surgeon who is too non-verbal and, worse still, too casual in his preoperative consultation may find himself confronted by an angry patient accusing him of negligence because he did not warn of the possibility of further revision.

As a matter of routine, one should not underestimate the overall results of a primary rhinoplasty performed by another surgeon (Brown and McDowell, 1965). "From the standpoint of medical ethics, humility and an understanding of the other surgeon's problems are essential (in considering a secondary rhinoplasty). Indiscreet, unnecessary, and inaccurate remarks may goad a patient to seek legal redress."

When the surgeon undertakes a secondary operation following a primary operation by another surgeon, he, along with his colleague, will be the object of resentment of the patient if the secondary operation is not, in the patient's mind, entirely successful. Third or fourth operations are rarely successful unless they are performed by expert hands, and they usually result in only minor improvements. However, some patients will be grateful for even a minor improvement.

It must be emphasized, as it was in the early part of the chapter, that a successful corrective rhinoplasty is determined by the satisfaction of the patient and not necessarily by the satisfaction of the surgeon.

Many surgeons follow the principle that the dissatisfied patient should be returned to the surgeon who performed the primary operation. However, the surgeon, in attempting to obtain an improvement, often only compounds the problem.

Secondary Rhinoplasty: Some Basic Ground Rules. Secondary rhinoplasty usually represents the last chance the patient has to obtain a satisfactory result. A secondary operation must therefore be approached only after a thorough analysis of the deformity and careful deliberation by the surgeon. Much will depend upon his judgment, ingenuity, and skill, as he is assuming a greater responsibility than in a primary procedure.

Sheen (1975b) has suggested some basic ground rules to increase the surgeon's chances for success:

1. A diagnosis of the deformity should be made. This requires that the surgeon have sufficient experience to recognize whether he is able to correct the deformity.

2. The area of surgical dissection should be limited. The surgical approach is made only to those areas directly involved in the deformity.

3. Only autografts should be employed; most often septal cartilage is the most suitable transplant. In exceptionally severe deformities, iliac bone or costal cartilage grafts must be employed.

4. A preoperative concept is necessary before any operative procedure is undertaken.

To these basic principles can be added the necessity for a sufficient delay before the secondary operation is performed. The date of the primary operation should be ascertained. A delay of six months is essential; a waiting period of as long as two years may be required in more severe deformities. Rogers (1972) has shown the remarkable improvement obtained by waiting in a patient whose soft tissue redraping took a longer period of time than it would have in an adolescent (Fig. 29–164).

Secondary Rhinoplasty: Correction of Some Basic Mistakes Made in the Primary Rhinoplasty. Infection, hemorrhage, and excessive scarring are avoidable when corrective operative procedures are performed in the primary operation. However, the surgeon may be faced with the problem of scarring and distortion following an incorrectly performed operation.

DEFECTS OF THE BONY NOSE. For the sake of simplification, bony defects are considered separately from defects of the cartilaginous nose, although the nose must always be taken into consideration in its entirety.

Minor irregularities of the bony dorsum are smoothed or contoured by means of a rasp. Aside from excessive removal of tissue from the dorsum of the nose, a problem which will be discussed later in the text, secondary deformity may be due to the inadequately performed lateral osteotomy. The correction requires secondary lateral osteotomies, generally combined with medial osteotomies and occasionally the removal of a wedge of bone near the root of the nose to facilitate the infracture when narrowing of the root of the nose is indicated.

Postoperative widening of the nose may be caused by an inadequate osteotomy or by a wide or deviated septum. Careful examination of the dorsum of the nose will show the deviation, which can be corrected. In attempting to correct postoperative widening of the nose, the fibrous tissue at the line of the previous osteotomy may prevent consolidation, and the widening recurs. In rare cases a gap is seen at the line of osteotomy after the infracture. In such cases an intraoral approach to each line of osteotomy must be made; the osteotomy area is exposed and a bone graft interposed between the base of the lateral wall and the adjacent bone to fill the gap (Converse, 1975). The postoperative splint should be left in position for a period of ten days or longer in all cases requiring secondary lateral osteotomy.

DEFECTS OF THE CARTILAGINOUS NOSE. These are most frequent. They may result from excessive removal of cartilage from the lateral crus and dome of the alar cartilage or inadequate trimming of the medial edges of the lateral cartilages, particularly at the cephalic portion of the cartilages. This omission results in irregularity of the profile line of the nose at the junction of the nasal bones and lateral cartilages. The defect requires exposure and careful trimming of the excess cartilage under direct vision.

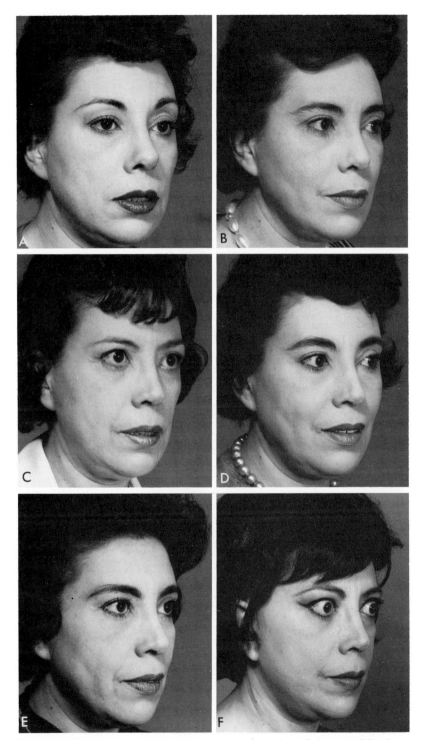

FIGURE 29–164. Progressive improvement of appearance over a period of six years following a secondary rhinoplasty. *A,* Unsatisfactory result following primary corrective operation. *B,* Ten months after secondary rhinoplasty. *C,* Twenty months following surgery. *D,* Two years. *E,* Two and a half years after secondary surgery. *F,* After six years. The patient developed thyrotoxic exophthalmos, as seen in the last photograph. (From Rogers, B. O.: Rhinoplasty. *In* Goldwyn, R. M. (Ed.): The Unfavorable Results in Plastic Surgery. Boston, Little, Brown and Company, 1972.)

A frequent cause of postoperative deviation of the nose is the following: The dorsal border of the septum is straight prior to the corrective rhinoplasty; after the modification of the profile and resection of a portion of the dorsal border of the septal cartilage, the new dorsal border may be curved. The surgeon had not observed the septal deviation and the curvature prior to the operation.

SECONDARY DEFORMITIES OF THE NASAL TIP. Recurrence of widening of the tip of the nose may be caused by an angulation of the septal angle, which splays apart the domes of the tip or causes a protrusion under the skin. The correction of some of these deformities may be extremely difficult.

Secondary correction of irregularities of the nasal tip requires adequate exposure of the remaining cartilages. The Safian technique (see Fig. 29–109) may suffice to make the necessary corrections; in more severe deformities, the entire remainder of the tip is exposed through a rim incision (see Fig. 29–110) in order to attempt some type of remodeling.

The pinched tip deformity is usually caused by removal of vestibular lining, often combined with excessive removal of alar and lateral cartilage and underlying mucoperichondrium. The treatment of this type of secondary deformity is achieved by the insertion of a thin piece of septal cartilage (in minor deformities), composite grafts from the concha, and intranasal skin grafting, which helps to restore an adequate airway and also the external contour in major secondary deformities (see Fig. 29–165). In some patients in whom for psychologic or anatomical reasons an operative procedure is risky, the use of intranasal molds combined with intranasal skin grafting may be advisable (see Fig. 29–165).

The pinched tip deformity. Excessive removal of cartilage from the dome results in a

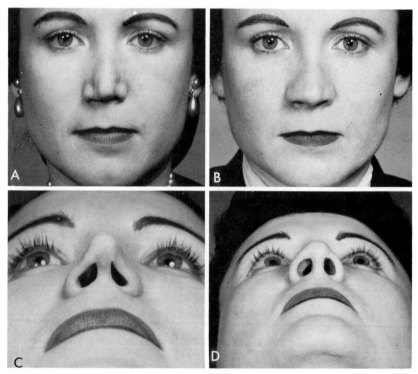

FIGURE 29–165. The pinched tip deformity caused by excessive removal of the lateral crus of the alar cartilage and vestibular lining. *A,* The patient has the typical appearance of the pinched tip deformity. Note also the inadequate lateral osteotomy, retraction of the columella, and drooping of the nasal tip. *B,* Appearance of the patient after correction obtained by a secondary lateral osteotomy, modification of the profile line, and increase in the projection of the columella by means of a septal cartilage graft (see Fig. 28–88). The scar tissue in the nasal vestibules was excised, and the deficient nasal lining was restored by skin grafting (see 'Deformities of the Inner Lining of the Nose'). After the vestibular skin graft had become revascularized, thin, pink-colored acrylic molds were employed for continuous support in order to restore the nasal airway and to correct the deformity. *C,* The deformity is well demonstrated in this view. *D,* The intravestibular molds, which can be seen in this view but which are not apparent in the full-face view. (From Converse, J. M.: Corrective surgery of the nasal tip. Laryngoscope, *67:*16, 1957.)

pointed tip, a difficult condition to correct. A pinched deformity with stenosis of the nasal airway at the internal naris usually results from excessive removal of vestibular lining and also from excessive cartilage resection from the lateral cartilage.

The pinched nose with vestibular stenosis presents a dual problem: the constriction of the airway, and the collapsed cartilaginous nasal wall resulting from excessive cartilage resection. Such cases have been treated successfully by the following procedure: intranasal scar tissue is removed and the cicatricial bands are eliminated by a Z-plasty, whenever this procedure is feasible. The remaining intranasal raw area is then covered by a thin, full-thickness skin graft, such as one removed from the upper eyelid, the posterior aspect of the auricle, or the medial aspect of the arm, or by a split-thickness graft from the oral mucosa.

Details of the technique of skin grafting inside the nasal cavity are described later in this chapter (see page 1200).

In some cases it is possible to insert a thin graft of septal cartilage to furnish skeletal support once the intranasal lining has been restored. A patient in whom this type of treatment was employed to eradicate a deformity produced by excessive removal of cartilage and vestibular skin is shown in Figure 29–165.

Most of the patients are apt to discard the intranasal molds after four or five months. Others continue to introduce them when they retire to bed in order to ensure comfortable nasal airways during sleep; other patients wear their intranasal prostheses permanently not only to guarantee the airway but also to prevent the collapse of the alae.

Composite auricular grafts. When the pinched tip is caused by excessive removal of cartilage and lining, a composite graft of auricular skin and cartilage may correct the deformity (see Fig. 29–313).

THE RETRACTED ALA. Postoperative retraction of the ala is usually caused by excessive resection of the caudal portion of the lateral cartilage and the alar cartilage as well as the vestibular lining. Correction is often difficult and, in severe retraction, may require the addition of a chondrocutaneous composite graft (see end of chapter, Fig. 29–313).

Three Most Frequent Errors in Corrective Rhinoplasty. The three major errors in primary rhinoplasty are (1) excessive reduction of the dorsum of the nose; (2) excessive resection of the caudal portion of the septum and over-

shortening of the nose; and (3) errors resulting in supratip protrusion.

1. The corrective rhinoplasty operation described earlier in the text avoids the *excessive reduction of the dorsal hump.* The step-by-step modification of the profile will prevent the concave type of dorsum which is the result of this mistake.

2. As pointed out during the description of the corrective rhinoplasty operation (see p. 1072), *excessive resection of septal cartilage from its caudal portion* results in a disruption of the columella-ala and columella-labial angles and a flat nasal base. Correction of this deformity has already been discussed (see p. 1095).

3. The causes of the *supratip protrusion* have been stated earlier in the chapter and are repeated here in order to clarify the technique of correction. In a nose with a convex dorsum, if the tip cartilages are not operated upon, a "parrot's beak" deformity will result.

The most frequent causes of supratip protrusion are:

1. Thick skin with overdeveloped sebaceous glands. In this type of nose, if the dorsum of the nose is overly reduced, the supratip protrusion will be particularly noticeable, the skin of the supratip area forming a veritable rigid carapace (see Fig. 29–171).

2. Excessive reduction of the septal angle, which allows a void between the dorsal skin and the septum. The void is filled with fibrous tissue, which is deposited between the layers of the septal mucous membrane (see Fig. 29–74).

3. Inadequate reduction of the septal angle, which protrudes under the skin of the supratip area.

CORRECTION OF THE DEFORMITY CAUSED BY EXCESSIVE REMOVAL OF BONE AND CARTILAGE FROM THE DORSUM OF THE NOSE. This is probably the most frequent secondary deformity and the one that immediately points to an inadequately performed primary rhinoplasty. The profile of the dorsum is concave, and a supratip protrusion is present. Not infrequently a "parrot's beak" deformity is also present. The deformity may also be the result of the collapse of the septum (see Fig. 29–158) caused by excessive resection of the septal framework. The deformity may be severe enough to require contour restoration by an iliac bone graft. In lesser deformities the septal framework can be used as a transplant to restore the profile line.

Septal cartilage is obtained by a submucous approach to the septum (Fig. 29–166, *A*).

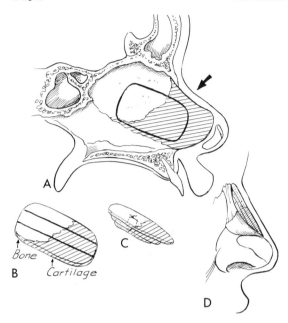

FIGURE 29–166. The septal framework as a transplant to increase the projection of the nasal dorsum. *A,* The section of septal cartilage and ethmoid plate to be removed is outlined. *B,* The transplant is divided into three parts. *C,* The three grafts are sutured by means of a mattress suture. *D,* The transplant in position. Note that the ethmoid bone is placed subperiosteally against the underlying nasal bones to provide consolidation of the graft. (After Sheen, 1975b.)

When indicated, the upper portion of the bony dorsum is flattened by removing 2 to 3 mm of bone with an osteotome or a rasp. This provides a flat seat for the graft. It is often possible to remove enough septal cartilage with the attached perpendicular plate of the ethmoid. The graft is cut in sections (Fig. 29–166, *B*) and straightened by shaving; the edges are rounded, and the bony portion of the graft is placed over the root of the nose in contact with the underlying bone. This has the advantage that the ethmoid bone consolidates with the host bone and prevents the curling up of the cephalic end of the graft. The graft is placed as illustrated in Figure 29–166, *D*. A fine-caliber nylon suture (6–0) may be placed transcutaneously through the graft, as advocated by Sheen. If necessary, two or more transplants are sutured together (Fig. 29–166, *C*). The cartilage must be meticulously carved and shaped with a sharp knife, an often tedious and time-consuming but essential task, because after the postoperative edema has subsided, any irregularity or sharp edge will become apparent (Figs. 29–166, *D*, and 29–167). Binocular loupes facilitate the shaping of the graft.

Excessive removal of the bony dorsum, combined with inadequate resection of cartilage from a bulbous tip, requires secondary tip surgery and reduction of the projecting dorsal septal cartilage over the bony dorsum.

In patients with a depressed dorsum, the tip of the nose may appear protrusive, and the temptation is to reduce the projection of the tip. In reality, careful analysis will show that increase of the projection of the dorsum is indicated.

CORRECTION OF THE DEFORMITY CAUSED BY EXCESSIVE RESECTION OF THE CAUDAL END OF THE SEPTAL CARTILAGE. Corrective procedures for the retracted columella and the resulting open columella-ala and columella-labial angles after excessive resection of the caudal end of the septal cartilage are similar to the procedures described for the deformity in the primary rhinoplasty (see p. 1095). An example of such a case is illustrated in Figure 29–168. Correction includes shortening the nose by resecting a portion of the septum near the septal angle to correct the drooping tip and reducing the dorsal hump, then embedding the septal cartilage into the base of the columella to increase its projection.

When the nose is grossly foreshortened, this can be one of the most difficult deformities to correct. The septum and the alar and lateral cartilages have been amputated to the extent

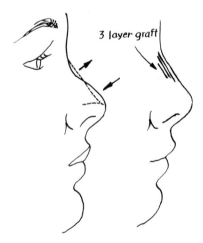

FIGURE 29–167. Correction of a nasal deformity resulting from excessive resection of the nasal dorsum in a patient with thick sebaceous skin in the supratip area. *Left,* The new profile that would be obtained by a reduction in the projection of the dorsum of the septal cartilage and the insertion of the graft shown in Figure 29–166. *Right,* The graft is in position, and the profile is modified. (After Sheen, 1975.)

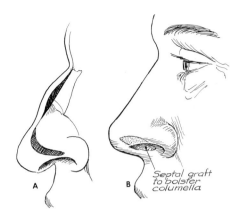

FIGURE 29–168. Secondary rhinoplasty for a plunging tip deformity resulting from overshortening of the septum. *A*, The outline indicates reduction of the hump and shortening of the septum in the area of the septal angle. *B*, Transplantation of the cartilage into the columella to correct the retraction. (From Millard, D. R., Jr.: Secondary Corrective Rhinoplasty. Plast. Reconstr. Surg., *44*:545, 1969. Copyright 1969, The Williams & Wilkins Company, Baltimore.)

that the base of the nose, the tip, and the nares show a cephalic rotation. In addition, the interior of the nares is visible. This type of deformity is no longer within the realm of corrective rhinoplasty; its correction is discussed at the end of this chapter.

CORRECTION OF THE SUPRATIP PROTRUSION. *In noses with thick skin over the tip and supratip area,* the supratip protrusion usually becomes pronounced if additional resection of the dorsum is performed, because the problem is that too much dorsum has already been resected. Attempts to resect subcutaneous tissue from the undersurface of the supratip area and to reapply the skin against the septum are only partly successful. The rigidity of the skin causes it to resume its convex form and elevate itself from the septum; more fibrous tissue is formed, which compounds the problem. In this type of problem, increase in the projection of the dorsum by means of a septal transplant

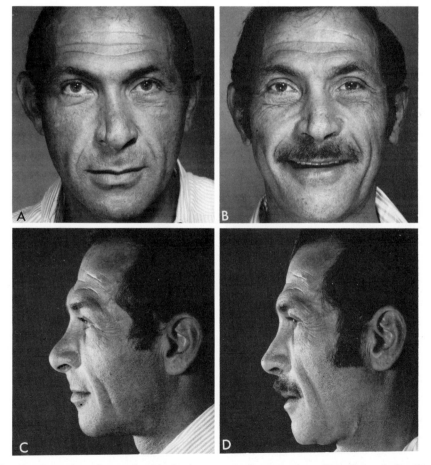

FIGURE 29–169. Resection of supratip skin in the course of a secondary rhinoplasty. *A*, Result obtained after previous unsuccessful rhinoplasty. Note the thick carapace over the supratip area. *B*, After excision of an ellipse of skin and subsequent dermabrasion. *C*, Preoperative profile view. *D*, Result obtained after secondary rhinoplasty and skin resection. (Courtesy of Dr. B. O. Rogers.)

may be indicated (Sheen, 1975b). Resection of skin from the supratip area is also indicated in some patients (Rogers, 1972) (Fig. 29–169).

In the nose in which the septal angle has been reduced excessively or in which the dorsal skin has not been reapplied against the dorsum of the septum, allowing a *fibrous pad to form between two layers of mucous membrane,* excision of the fibrous tissue is required. Removal of the fibrous tissue and careful reapplication of the skin against the septum will eliminate the void between the structures and realign the profile. A strip of Elastoplast provides continuous positive pressure, but care must be taken to avoid excessive pressure. The Elastoplast is reinforced with adhesive tape.

When the cause of the supratip protrusion is the *septal angle which has been insufficiently lowered,* secondary trimming of the septal angle reestablishes the originally planned profile, and careful reapplication of the dorsal skin against the septum eliminates the dead space between the dorsal skin and the septum. Sheen has employed his technique of embedding a carefully carved septal cartilage graft in the area of the tip-columella angle (see Fig. 29–115), in conjunction with a secondary rhino-

plasty, to reestablish the contour of the nasal profile (Fig. 29–170).

Other techniques. Dermabrasion will occasionally help to reduce the thickness of the supratip skin.

Reduction of the supratip protrusion caused by the fibrous pad by injections of steroids has been reported by Rees (1971). A nose with thick, sebaceous skin and subcutaneous tissue in the supratip area corrected by such injections is shown in Figure 29–171. According to Orentreich (1976), fibroplasia and collagen deposition in scar tissue can be resolved by the action of corticosteroids. For proper hydraulic control, a 1-ml tuberculin syringe with a 30-gauge needle is used for the intralesional administration of 0.1 ml of triamcinolone acetonide (Kenalog) at a concentration of 5 mg/ml per cubic centimeter of fibrous tissue. Because of the lag-time in tissue response, repeated treatment at monthly intervals minimizes atrophy. The concentration may be varied from 2.5 mg/ml to 10 mg/ml, depending upon the degree of fibroplasia and response to previous injections of 5 mg/ml.

The Use of Silicone Fluid for the Correction of Minor Irregularities. The prudent use of sili-

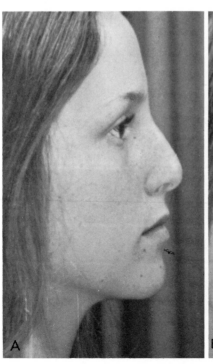
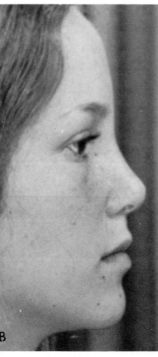

FIGURE 29–170. Loss of tip contour caused by protrusion of the septal angle and dorsal border of the septum. *A,* Downward depression of the tip and protruding septal dorsum. *B,* After secondary rhinoplasty and septal cartilage graft, according to the technique illustrated in Figure 29–115. (From Sheen, J.: Secondary rhinoplasty. Plast. Reconstr. Surg., 56:35, 1975. Copyright © 1975, The Williams & Wilkins Company, Baltimore.)

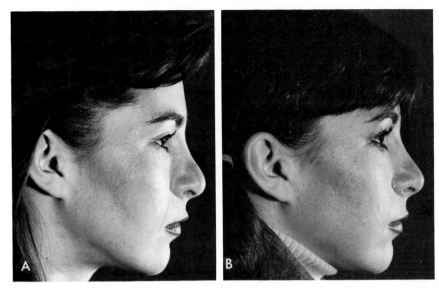

FIGURE 29–171. Example of the reduction of supratip protrusion by means of injections of triamcinolone acetonide. *A*, Supratip protrusion in a patient with thick sebaceous skin. *B*, Result obtained by secondary rhinoplasty followed by triamcinolone acetonide injections by Dr. N. Orentreich (see text).

cone liquid injections, as described in Chapter 15, is helpful in correcting minor irregularities of the nose after corrective rhinoplasty. Tragedies have occurred as a result of the excessive use of this material (Figs. 29–172 and 29–173). Liquid silicone should be used only in minor deformities, and only autogenous grafts should be employed for other than minor deformities.

According to Orentreich (1976), silicone is a safe interstitial prosthetic material that produces augmentation through controlled fibroplasia and collagen deposition. Depressed defects can be improved with injections of unadulterated 350 centistoke viscosity medical-grade polydimethylsiloxane (silicone). The administration technique that is effective and avoids complications consists of separate, discrete, subdermal injections of 0.01 to 0.05 ml at 1 cm intervals. Proper hydraulic control for injecting the viscous fluid is accomplished with a 0.25-ml tuberculin-type, three-ring held syringe with a 30-gauge needle fitted into a Luer-Lok attachment. Injections are usually given at monthly intervals to allow time for the collagen deposition to develop at the treatment sites.

Other Secondary Deformities following Corrective Rhinoplasty. Necrosis of skin, loss of an ala, and other major operative catastrophies that require reconstructive procedures are described in the last portion of the chapter.

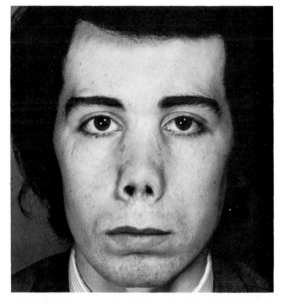

FIGURE 29–172. Nasal deformity following corrective rhinoplasties and repeated injections of liquid silicone. The patient had been in an accident and suffered a fracture of the nasal bones. A corrective operation was done for malunited fracture. Following an unsatisfactory result, a number of secondary rhinoplasties were performed, and liquid silicone was repeatedly injected. The aftermath was not only the deformity but also acute inflammation followed by suppuration through a series of fistulas. Attempts at control of the infection were unsuccessful despite intensive antibiotic therapy. The patient has undergone nasal reconstruction by means of a scalping forehead flap. The reconstructive procedures have not been completed.

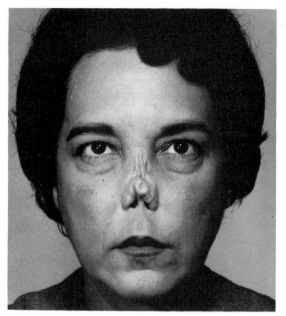

FIGURE 29–173. Appearance after a series of corrective rhinoplasties and injections of liquid silicone. After a first rhinoplasty which was not successful, a number of surgeons attempted further improvement. Liquid silicone was injected in large quantities. In addition to the nasal deformity, the skin of the nose was subjected to periodic episodes of inflammation and suppuration. Resection of the skin of the dorsum of the nose was required to replace the chronically infected skin and also to elongate the overshortened nose. This was achieved by means of a forehead scalping flap. The patient is still under treatment.

CORRECTIVE RHINOPLASTY IN NONCAUCASIANS

Considerations concerning corrective procedures on Black and Oriental patients often involve techniques described in the previous pages and the transplantation of bone or cartilage.

The population of the United States of America comprises representatives of nearly every ethnic group of the world's population. In their desire for assimilation, a considerable number of individuals from these diverse ethnic groups request the removal of distinctive ethnic traits, notably correction of the nose.

The growing desire to acquire a more Occidental appearance has manifested itself in Japan, the Philippines, and other Oriental countries in which patients request the Oriental eye operation (see Chapter 28, p. 947) and an increase in the projection of the dorsum of the nose.

Anatomical Characteristics. The noses of the Oriental and African have some features in common: the flat nasal dorsum, the short columella, the slanted external nares, and the flared nostrils. The nostril borders are usually delicately formed in the Oriental; in the Black, however, they are frequently very thick. These characteristics vary, a result of the admixture of ethnic groups.

The basic skeletal variations between the nose of the Occidental and that of the patient of African origin were studied by Wen (1921). He noted that, whereas the septal angle in the Caucasian is usually well defined, the dorsal border of the septum has a downward curve with an ill-defined septal angle in the Black patient (Fig. 29–174). Wen also described a distinct difference in the structure of the alar

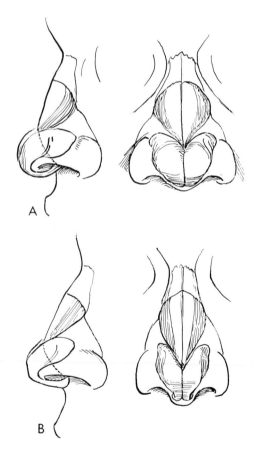

FIGURE 29–174. Anatomical relationships of the nasal cartilages in the Caucasoid and in the Negroid nose. *A*, In the Negroid nose, the septal angle is rounded and contributes no support to the tip cartilages. *B*, The cartilage in the Caucasoid nose. (After Wen, I. C.: Ontogeny and phylogeny of the nasal cartilages. Contributions to Embryology, Carnegie Institution, Washington, *414*:109, 1921.)

cartilages between the two ethnic groups. In the Black patient, the alar cartilages are often smaller and more frail, despite the external appearance of the wide flaring nares.

Corrective Rhinoplasty in Orientals. The increase in the projection of the dorsum of the nose is a frequent procedure following the Oriental eye operation. Uchida (1958) described various techniques for this purpose. Boo-Chai (1964) employed a Silastic implant over the dorsum to increase the projection. Although no longitudinal studies have been reported, the Silastic implant appears to be more successful in the Oriental nose than in the Occidental nose, where it is often contraindicated. Boo-Chai also advocated alar base wedge excisions. Furukawa (1974) elaborated upon the various techniques for rhinoplasty in the Oriental nose.

Corrective Rhinoplasty in Blacks. Rees (1969), Falces, Wesser and Gorney (1970), and Rees and Wood-Smith (1972) have described techniques for the corrective rhinoplasty in the Black patient.

The techniques include increasing the projection of the dorsum of the nose by means of an iliac bone graft, lengthening the columella, and increasing the projection of the tip by weakening the alar cartilage in the region of the domes by means of partial or full thickness incisions. The medial crura and domes are maintained by a mattress suture. These procedures are combined with wedge excisions at the base of the alae (see Fig. 29–82) and also by excision along the alar borders in selected cases (see Fig. 29–83). Although the threatening menace of keloid formation in the Black patient must be considered, it has not been reported in the papers published on this subject.

Congenital Choanal Atresia

John Marquis Converse, M.D., Donald Wood-Smith, F.R.C.S.E., and William W. Shaw, M.D.

Choanal atresia is an uncommon, yet not rare, congenital obstruction of the posterior choana which, unless treated promptly, can cause immediate postnatal asphyxia or later recurrent respiratory or feeding problems. Failure to recognize the obstruction may partially account for the alarmingly large number of unexplained infant respiratory deaths reported each year (Beinfield, 1959). In New York City, there were 729 neonatal deaths from "postnatal asphyxia" (0.45 per cent of live births), and of these, 53 per cent were infants of less than 1 day of age. In the United States there are 15,000 crib deaths a year occurring prior to 6 months of age (2 to 3 per 1000 live births) (Beinfield, 1959).

HISTORY

The entity was first described by Röderer in 1755 in Göttingen, Germany. Ronaldson (1880–1881) recorded the first classic descriptions of the syndrome, which remain accurate today. Emmert first performed surgical correction by puncturing the obstruction with a trocar in 1853. Brunk (1909) first employed the transpalatine approach for correction. Kazanjian (1942) described trans-septal and transantral corrections. Durward, Lord, and Polson (1945) gave a comprehensive review with over 300 references. Beinfield (1954, 1955, 1956, 1957, 1959) emphasized its importance in the etiology of infant mortality and popularized a technique of curetting the bony obstruction. McGovern (1953, 1961) proposed using a tube to allow gavage feeding, along with an oropharyngeal airway.

Evans and Maclachlan (1971) reported 65 cases and added another 100 references. To date, approximatley 409 cases have been reported in the English literature. Reports are also found in the Russian and French literature, as well as in the literature of other countries.

INCIDENCE

No precise data are available; however, the incidence of choanal atresia has been roughly estimated at 1 per 5000 (Parkes and Brennan, 1973; Pratt, 1974). Additional severe cases resulting in neonatal deaths and many cases of unilateral atresia or bilateral atresia with mild symptoms remain unrecognized and thus unreported. With greater awareness of the syndrome, undoubtedly, more cases will be detected. For example, Williams (1971) reported 19 cases over ten years, and ten of the cases were from the last two years. Ersner (1953), by routinely passing catheters to check the choanae in tonsillectomy patients, found five cases of unilateral choanal atresia which otherwise would have gone unreported. Parkes and Brennan (1973) reported a case of unilateral choanal atresia in a rhinoplasty candidate with presumed septal deviation.

Statistically, there is a preponderance of female over male (2:1), unilateral over bilateral (2:1), right unilateral over left (2:1), and bony obstruction over membranous (9:1) (Evans and Maclachlan, 1971). The incidence of associated anomalies is very high, 43 per cent overall and 60 per cent in bilateral atresia. There is no correlation between the severity of the associated anomaly and bilateral versus unilateral atresia.

Associated anomalies range widely from minor incidental ones to major cardiovascular, abdominal, and, most frequently, craniofacial anomalies—i.e., patent ductus, VSD (ventriculoseptal defect), vascular ring, ileal atresia, and diaphragmatic hernia (McGovern, 1953; Evans and Maclachlan, 1971; Pratt, 1974).

The associated cranofacial anomalies most frequently observed are cleft palate, Treacher-Collins syndrome, branchial cleft syndromes and craniostenosis. It should be noted that, of patients with associated anomalies, 50 per cent have multiple anomalies, with at least one being a major anomaly; 25 per cent have a single major anomaly, and only 25 per cent have a single minor anomaly (Evans and Maclachlan, 1971).

Heredity appears to play a significant role. A number of families with multiple siblings and other members with choanal atresia have been reported (Parkes and Brennan, 1973). One patient had an associated bifid thumb and an abnormal D-group chromosome (Carter, Smith, and Schindeler, 1970). Thalidomide ingestion has been implicated in a few cases.

EMBRYOLOGY AND ANATOMY

The most commonly accepted theory is that an embryonic growth arrest results in failure of breakdown of the bucconasal membrane at the posterior choana. The membrane normally ruptures at seven weeks' gestation, allowing the primitive nasal cavity to communicate with the buccal cavity and the foregut. The residual mesodermal elements account for the frequent associated bony obstruction. An embryonic inflammatory process and adhesions have been postulated, but the presence of bone, the symmetry, and the high incidence of associated anomalies make this theory untenable (Evans and Maclachlan, 1971).

Choanal atresia may occur unilaterally or bilaterally, completely or incompletely. It may be membranous, membranous with a bony rim, or completely bony, covered anteriorly with nasal mucosa and posteriorly with pharyngeal mucosa. The bony rim is frequently quite thick, making simple direct puncture hazardous and associated with a high degree of recurrence. The obstruction, usually situated just anterior to the posterior edge of the bony palate, measures 1 to 10 mm in thickness (Evans and Maclachlan, 1971; Parkes and Brennan, 1973).

CLINICAL MANIFESTATIONS

The clinical appearance varies widely from immediate postnatal cyanosis and respiratory distress to nothing more than chronic mucoid nasal discharge. The findings depend on the severity of the anatomical obstruction and the infant's ability to learn mouth breathing and to develop coordination between breathing and sucking. It is generally not appreciated that neonates are obligate nasal breathers and that oropharyngeal breathing is a voluntary and acquired function developing normally several days or weeks later (Thomson, 1937). The ability to suck and breathe simultaneously is seldom developed until 3 to 6 weeks. Infants with bilateral complete obstruction, therefore, generally manifest early severe symptoms, while those with unilateral or incomplete obstruction develop later and mostly incidental findings. Occasionally, however, they become completely obstructed when aggravated by upper respiratory infection, neonatal nasal congestion from maternal reserpine, and the prone position of the head obstructing the unaffected nasal airway. The following more specific manifestations should alert the clinician to the possibility of choanal atresia (Williams, 1971).

Asphyxia Neonatorum. Shortly after birth, after crying ceases, most infants with complete obstruction develop severe high airway obstruction. Vigorous efforts are made by the infant and severe dyspnea, sternal and intercostal retraction, and cyanosis are observed. At times, the greater the effort on the part of the infant, the tighter the mouth closes. Unless an oral airway is inserted or crying occurs, the infant may succumb to asphyxia.

Cyclic Cyanosis Relieved by Crying. Many infants who survive the initial postpartum period develop a classic pattern of cyanosis which is relieved by crying. Such infants may still succumb to eventual fatigue and thus must also be promptly treated.

Intermittent Respiratory Distress Precipitated by Feeding. A small group of infants rapidly master the technique of oral breathing but still lack the necessary coordination between breathing and feeding. The previously mild and occasional respiratory distress becomes severe during feeding. Often such infants are mistakenly studied for a tracheoesophageal fistula, vascular ring, ectopic left pulmonary artery, or esophageal stenosis.

Minor Symptoms. Most unilateral choanal atresia patients have chronic mucoid discharge from the nostrils during later infancy and childhood. The external nares and upper lip may become excoriated from the necessary constant wiping. Patients complain of never being able to blow the nose on the affected side. Anosmia, diminished taste, speech abnormality, and rarely a hearing deficit from recurrent otitis have been reported (Evans and Maclachlan, 1971). Many patients are thought to have al-

TABLE 29–1. *Symptoms in Unilateral and Bilateral Choanal Atresia*

SYMPTOM	UNILATERAL	BILATERAL	TOTAL
Nasal obstruction and/or discharge	30	6	36
Breathing difficulty	0	18	18
Feeding difficulty	1	4	5
Incidental findings	4	2	6
Total:	35	30	65

lergic rhinitis, deviated septum, and enlarged adenoids. Rarely, patients with bilateral atresia may be seen in adolescence with such symptoms.

The symptoms in Evans and Maclachlan's series (1971) are listed in Table 29–1.

DIAGNOSIS

Once suspected, the diagnosis can usually be determined without difficulty. The differential diagnosis to be considered in infants ranges from cardiac anomalies to rhinitis. In older children, tumors and acquired nasopharyngeal stricture should be considered. Acquired stenosis following tonsillectomy and adenoidectomy has been increasingly reported (McDonald and coworkers, 1973; Pratt, 1974). The surgical correction required for the acquired stenosis (e.g., tuberculosis and syphilis) is usually more difficult and quite different, as the area involved tends to be more extensive and more unpredictable. A discussion of some of the well-tested methods to confirm the diagnosis of choanal atresia follows.

Occlusion of the unaffected airway with the mouth closed should produce prompt respiratory distress and demonstrate the failure of the mucous material to bubble.

If a rubber catheter or metal probe cannot be passed more than 32 mm from the edge of the nostril in a newborn, the presumptive diagnosis of choanal atresia should be made. Normally one should be able either to pass it more than 44 mm or to see the catheter in the pharynx (Parkes and Brennan, 1973).

A lateral cephalogram or tomograms are helpful in identifying the choanal atresia and determining the thickness of the obstruction, a factor which may be important in surgical evaluation. In equivocal cases, the nasal cavity can be filled with a radiopaque dye, one nostril at a time, and lateral views taken in the supine position. Prior to the radiographic examination, the nostrils must be thoroughly suctioned and epinephrine instilled to ensure absence of mucosal congestion (Williams, 1971).

Examination under anesthesia should be done carefully under direct vision prior to commencement of surgery.

TREATMENT

Aside from general agreement on the urgency of the initial insertion of an oral airway, there is a lack of uniform opinion regarding both the timing of the definitive surgical correction and the preferred surgical approach to choanal atresia. In the past there was a great deal of enthusiasm for immediate aggressive surgery. In the last decade, however, a number of authors have proposed treating such patients by means of an oral airway and gavage feeding until 3 to 4 months of age, when the anesthesia risk is lower and the choanae much larger (McGovern, 1961; Williams, 1971). In general, when satisfactory pediatric anesthesia is available, there is little reason for delaying surgery, since delaying indefinitely increases mortality. Pneumonia due to inadequate pulmonary ventilation and aspiration are common sequelae to medical management (Evans and Maclachlan, 1971). In premature infants or infants with other more pressing congenital problems, medical management may be warranted as a temporizing measure. Ultimately, one must individualize the treatment of each case, depending on the thickness of the obstruction, the severity of symptoms, the presence of associated congenital anomalies, the availability of satisfactory pediatric anesthesia, the reliability of the nursing care, and the surgeon's own experience.

Initial Resuscitation. As soon as the diagnosis is suspected, an oral airway should be inserted and taped to the mandible. It may be necessary to trim the tube back to the level of the base of the tongue, if it provokes prolonged retching. However, with persistence, the child will usually tolerate the airway. Tracheotomy is hazardous and rarely indicated.

"Medical Management." McGovern (1961) described a large-holed nipple which allowed most infants to be trained to mouth-breathe and feed alternately with very patient nursing assistance (McGovern, 1961). A small feeding tube can also be introduced along the airway for simultaneous feeding. Such management requires superior nursing care to avoid mishaps and should be reserved for only severely premature infants or infants with other pressing major illnesses.

Surgical Correction. In general, all patients with bilateral complete obstruction should be operated on at the earliest practical moment, while unilateral cases can be treated more electively, surgery being delayed until 3 to 5 years of age. Temporary partial correction is not advisable, as it often turns out to be inadequate, tends to recur, and makes later definitive surgery more difficult. The older transantral and trans-septal approaches are rarely used today. Transnasal approaches can be performed more easily, but they are associated with a higher incidence of recurrence and occasional catastrophic injuries to the midbrain and basisphenoid which lie directly posterior (Evans and Maclachlan, 1971; Herceg and Harding, 1971). The mold required to prevent adhesions requires a great deal of care to prevent plugging. This approach should therefore be reserved for use in patients with membranous occlusion, in poor risk patients, in the very small newborn, and in the patient with a high arched palate. Whenever feasible, especially in elective cases the transpalatine approach is preferred (Owens, 1965; Cherry and Bordley, 1966).

Surgical Techniques

TRANSNASAL CORRECTION. A blind approach using trocars, Kelly clamps, dilators, and electrocoagulation is not justified in most cases (Lipshutz and Abramson, 1967; Herrmann and Klein, 1971). Singleton and Hardcastle (1968) used an operating microscope and right-angle diamond burs to remove the bone under direct vision, as practiced in middle ear surgery. This would appear to be safe and effective, but it requires specialized instruments and personnel. The method described by Beinfield (1959) involving use of a curette appears to have more universal application and is summarized here (Fig. 29–175).

A mastoid curette with markings at 3.5 and 4.5 cm from the tip is used. The curette is passed along the floor of the nose to the obstructed area and with firm pressure is rotated until the bone is perforated (Fig. 29–175, *A*, *B*). Nasal mucous membrane on the anterior aspect of the obstruction is destroyed with the bone as it is removed. However, the nasopharyngeal mucous membrane on the posterior wall of the obstruction generally remains intact (Fig. 29–175, *C*). The finger may be inserted behind the soft palate to act as a guide to the depth of curetting. The curette must not be passed beyond the 4.5 cm mark for fear of damage to the posterior pharyngeal wall and underlying spinal canal. The intact nasopharyngeal membrane is perforated. A #11 blade on a long handle is passed along the floor of the nose, and the membrane is perforated in a stellate fashion (Fig. 29–175, *D*, *E*). A #12 catheter

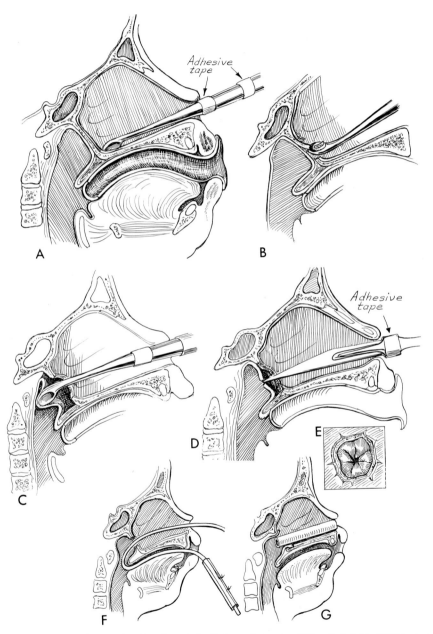

FIGURE 29–175. Transnasal operation for the relief of choanal atresia. (After Beinfield, 1959.) *A*, A curette with adhesive tape wrapped around it to indicate the depth to which the instrument penetrates is introduced along the nasal floor to the choanal obstruction. *B*, The nasal mucous membrane and obstructing choanal bony wall are resected. *C*, The pharyngonasal mucous membrane is elevated from the posterior aspect of the choanal bony wall after a sufficiently large opening has been made. *D*, A stellate incision is made through the mucous membrane. *E*, The stellate incision. *F*, A polyethylene or silicone tube is passed through the nasopharynx into the oral cavity. *G*, The tube in position, maintaining the patency of the airway.

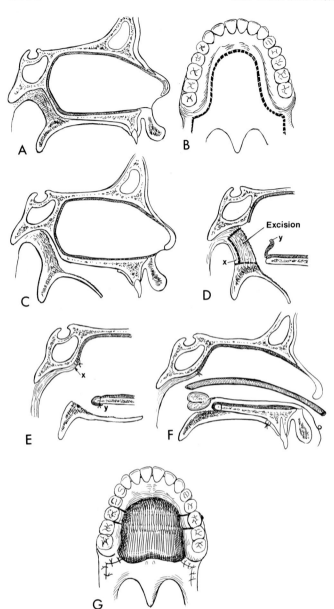

FIGURE 29–176. Transpalatal operation for the relief of choanal atresia. (After Roopenian and Stemmer.) *A*, Diagram showing choanal atresia with complete obstruction. *B*, Outline of the palatal mucoperiosteal incision. *C*, The flap is raised. *D*, The bony obstruction is resected together with the obstructing soft tissue. *E*, Mucous membrane continuity is reestablished over the sphenoid eminence. *F*, The palatal flap is reapplied against the hard palate, and a postnasal pack is introduced. *G*, Dental compound softened in warm water is applied over the palatal flap; it is held by transverse wires embedded into the compound and looped around the adjacent teeth.

is passed along the floor of the nose through the incision and withdrawn through the mouth. A silicone or polyethylene tube of a size that approximates the external nares is sutured to the oral end of the catheter and is drawn through the oral cavity and the stellate incision to the anterior naris, where it is detached from the rubber catheter (Fig. 29–175, *F, G*). Considerable force may be necessary to bring the tubing through the stellate incision in the mucous membrane, and the mucous membrane is forced forward in the form of a cuff.

A similar procedure is completed in the contralateral nasal fossa, and the two tubes are joined by a suture in front of the base of the columella. The tube is left in position for approximately four weeks. Careful postoperative suction is necessary to ensure continued patency of the tube. After removal of the tube, repeated passage of the tube through the atretic site is required every two to three days in order to guard against secondary stricture of the newly formed opening.

THE TRANSPALATAL APPROACH. In the older patient, the transpalatal approach (McGovern and Fitzhugh, 1961; Owens, 1965; Cherry and Bordley, 1966) may be utilized (Fig. 29–176). Particularly in the presence of a thick, obviously bony obstruction (Fig. 29–176, *A*), it may provide a superior approach to the atretic region.

Under general anesthesia, a large palatal flap is raised by incisions extending along the medial aspect of the alveolar border from the retromolar region on either side; the incision is extended anteriorly to the premolar region and is connected with a similar incision on the contralateral side. The mucoperiosteal flap is raised, the descending palatine vessels being preserved, and the area of the bony obstruction is exposed (Fig. 29–176, *B, C*).

The bony obstruction is removed under direct vision, and the nasal mucous membrane lying on its anterior aspect is divided (Fig. 29–176, *D*). The posterior obstruction is removed, care being taken to preserve the mucosal flap, which is rotated anteriorly to cover the raw area left by removal of the obstructing segment (Fig. 29–176, *E*). A postnasal pack and a tube are placed (Fig. 29–176, *F*). The mucoperiosteal palatal flap is replaced in its original position and is maintained in contact with the palatal bone by either softened dental compound or Xeroform gauze held in position by a wire bridge inserted between opposing molar teeth (Fig. 29–176, *G*).

Congenital Tumors of the Nose

MARK K. H. WANG, M.D., AND W. BRANDON MACOMBER, M.D.

Congenital tumors of the nose are highly diversified. They may be grouped in accordance with their embryonic origin. The neurogenic group consists of gliomas, encephaloceles, and neurofibromas. The ectodermic group consists of dermoid cysts or sinuses. The mesodermic group consists of hemangiomas.

Though benign and relatively slow-growing, these tumors, encroaching upon the bony framework of the nose, can cause disturbances of growth and subsequent deformity. Hence, early treatment is advisable. In most cases, surgery is the only effective treatment.

EMBRYOLOGY

According to Gruenwald (Brunner and Harned, 1942), the anterior wall of the external nose is cartilaginous at birth (the cartilaginous nasal capsule). Anterior and adjacent to the cartilaginous capsule the nasal and frontal bones develop. Between the frontal and nasal bones anteriorly and the cartilaginous capsule behind, the prenasal space extends downward to the tip of the nose. Within this space a teatlike projection of dura is present. During prenatal growth this projection is encircled by a bony canal, the opening of which is called the foramen cecum. In normal development the dural process is eventually sealed and the foramen completely obliterated (Fig. 29–177). Any failure in complete obliteration of this process leaves a pathway along which glial tissue may extend, hence the development of gliomas or encephaloceles. An encephalocele is an actual herniation of the brain into this potential prenasal space (Fig. 29–178, *A*), while a *glioma*, according to Schmidt (1900), is derived from an encephalocele which has been cut off from its origin (Fig. 29–178, *B*). It is not uncommon to find a fibrous stalk connecting a glioma to the base of the skull in the position of the foramen cecum. Sussenguth (1909) suggested that intranasal gliomas were the result of a portion of the olfactory process being pinched off by the closure of the frontal bone. Anglade and Phillip (1920) believed that neurogliomas surrounding the olfactory bulb were responsible for gliomas.

In the early stage of development, the nasal and frontal bones are formed by intramembranous ossification. There is a gap between

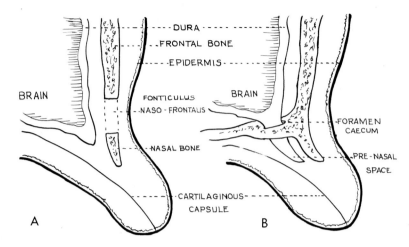

FIGURE 29–177. Sagittal section of the dorsum of the nose at birth and at a later stage of growth and development. *A,* An early stage of development. Note the presence of the membranous fonticulus nasofrontalis. *B,* A later stage of development, showing the teatlike projection of the dura through the foramen cecum.

the frontal bone above and nasal bone below. This gap, the fonticulus nasofrontalis, is filled by a membrane. At this site, the dura and the skin are therefore in contact without any intervening bony structure. Though the fonticulus nasofrontalis is eventually replaced by bone, part of the ectoderm may fail to separate from the dura and may be carried to the prenasal space. This ectopic ectoderm is the antecedent of a midline *dermoid cyst.* If it retains its connection with the skin, a *sinus* will result (Fig. 29–178, *C*).

Dermoid cysts may appear along the lateral border of the nose or beneath the ala nasi. Symmetrical occurrence has been recorded. Dermoid cysts in these localities are consid-

ered to have originated along the lines of embryonic fusion, i.e., the naso-optical furrow. They develop from the inclusion of displaced dermal cells.

Hemangiomas, either capillary or cavernous, are considered mesodermic in origin. Ribbert (1898) and many others have favored the Cohnheim theory that hemangiomas are congenital, arising through embryonic sequestration of mesodermal tissue.

CONGENITAL TUMORS OF NEUROGENIC ORIGIN

Glioma. Gliomas of the nose are rare. They may be either extranasal or intranasal. The

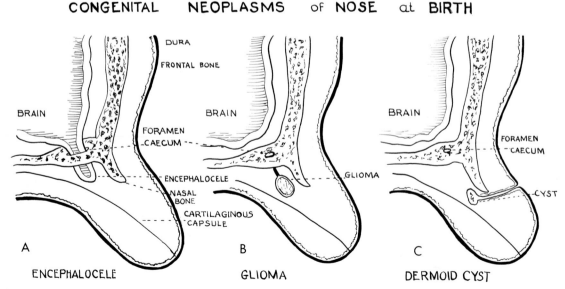

FIGURE 29–178. Diagrammatic representation of the developmental origin of the encephalocele, the glioma, and the dermoid cyst.

first case was reported by Reid (1852). The term "glioma" was first employed by Schmidt (1900). According to Rose (1966), approximately 60 per cent of the tumors are extranasal, 30 per cent are intranasal, and 10 per cent are extranasal and intranasal. The male is more often affected than the female in a proportion of roughly 3 to 2.

Extranasal gliomas are usually located at the side of the bridge of the nose. The root of the nose is often broadened, and the eyes appear more widely separated than normal. The tumor, varying from 1 to 3 cm in diameter, is rounded or dome-shaped, reddish, moderately firm, movable, and subcutaneous. There is neither pulsation nor change in size when the patient cries or strains. Usually no defect of the skull can be detected (Fig. 29–179).

The intranasal type of glioma is less common. It is situated high in the nasal fossa and is often mistaken for a polyp. The septum and nasal bones are often displaced, and the nasal passage may be blocked. Most often these tumors arise from the middle turbinate or the lateral wall of the nasal fossa. When the lacrimal duct is obstructed by the tumor, epiphora on the affected side may result.

Histologically, the glioma consists of glial and fibrous tissue in varying proportions. The glial tissue is composed largely of astrocytes and their processes. The fibrous tissue is usually predominant and forms septa between the masses of glia.

Although gliomas of the nose are clinically benign, their rate of growth varies. The typical picture of the extranasal glioma is that of a congenital mass, discovered at birth or soon after, which remains stationary in size and can be removed without recurrence. This suggests that it is essentially heterotopic. Occasionally a tumor grows more rapidly than the surrounding tissue and promptly recurs after excision. There have been five such cases recorded in the literature, as reported by Black and Smith (1950). Such tumors suggest the potentiality of autonomous growth.

TREATMENT. Gliomas can best be treated by surgical excision. In treating the extranasal type, early excision should be performed to prevent irreversible deformity of the nasal bones. If excision is complete, recurrence is rare. In the intranasal type, a biopsy may be necessary to confirm the diagnosis. A roentgenologic examination of the base of the skull is necessary to detect any defect at the site of the foramen cecum. Direct intracranial communication must be carefully ruled out before excision is attempted. When an intracranial communication is suspected, a needle aspiration obtaining cerebrospinal fluid will confirm the diagnosis. Although the intranasal approach is the most commonly employed, both external and intranasal routes are recommended to assure complete excision of large lesions. When the lesion is low in the nasal cavity, an alar incision may be sufficient for ad-

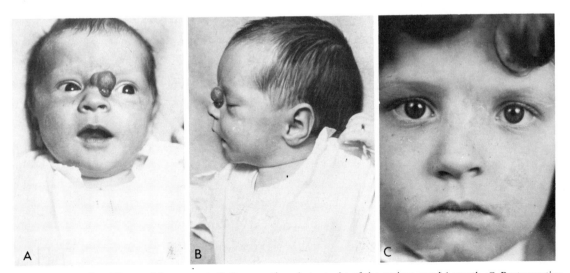

FIGURE 29–179. Glioma of the nose. *A, B,* Preoperative photographs of the patient, aged 1 month. *C,* Postoperative photograph of the same patient, aged 2½ years. Note the unilateral orbital hypertelorism of the left orbit.

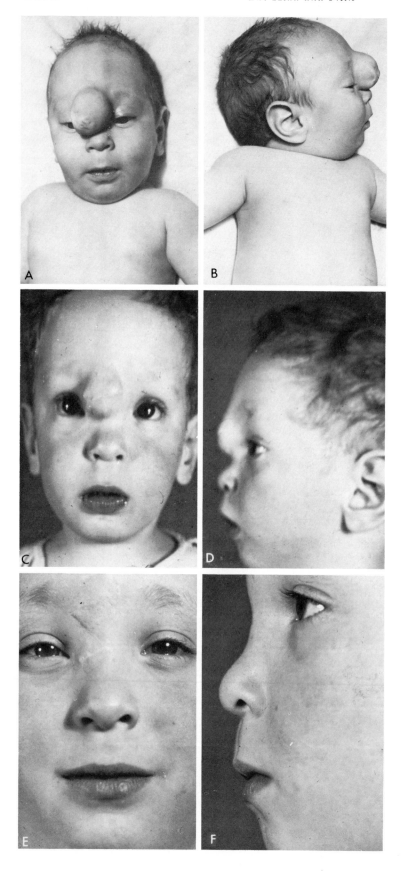

FIGURE 29–180. Frontonasal encephalocele. *A, B,* Preoperative photographs of the patient at the age of 3 months. *C, D,* Photographs taken six months after the primary excision. The residual mass is hypertrophic scar tissue. *E, F,* Photographs taken 3½ years after final surgery.

equate exposure. When the lesion is situated high, a lateral rhinotomy may be necessary. When an intracranial connection is suspected, a combined neurosurgical and nasal (craniofacial) approach is advisable (see Chapter 56).

COMPLICATIONS

Incomplete excision. This can be avoided by careful preoperative local and radiologic examination and adequate exposure during surgery. These measures are mandatory for all intranasal lesions. The presence of a fibrous cord and possible intracranial communication must be borne in mind during surgery to assure complete excision and prevent recurrence.

Dural defect. A glioma has no intracranial communication. However, a small dural tear or defect can be produced during surgery. Once

detected, such a defect must be promptly closed to prevent leakage of cerebrospinal fluid. When the defect is large, an intracranial approach may be needed for repair. Fortunately, such leakage is almost always transient and stops spontaneously without specific treatment. If the leakage is intranasal, one should avoid intranasal packing. The use of antibiotics is indicated to prevent the development of meningitis.

Hematoma. If the tumor is of a moderate size, a dead space will be created after excision, and a hematoma may form. Attempts should be made to obliterate the space by mobilizing neighboring soft tissue and removing excess skin.

Encephalocele. Encephaloceles are difficult

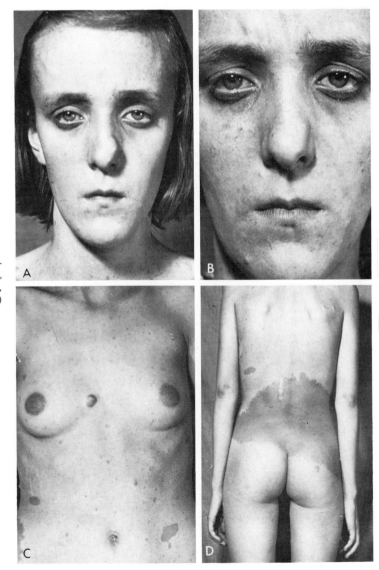

FIGURE 29–181. Neurofibroma of the nose. *A, B,* Preoperative and postoperative photographs of the nose. *C,* Multiple lesions over the chest wall. *D,* Large patch of brownish (café au lait) pigmentation over the lower trunk.

to distinguish from nasal gliomas. The two lesions are congenital in origin, are similarly located, and are of both intra- and extranasal types (Fig. 29–180). Structurally they are quite different. The encephalocele contains an ependyma-lined space, filled with cerebrospinal fluid, which communicates directly with the ventricles of the brain, while the glioma is a solid mass of glial tissue, either entirely separated from the brain or connected with it only by a fibrous stalk.

Clinically, in diagnosing an encephalocele, one must look for a defect at the base of the skull. A routine roentgenologic examination is necessary. In addition, there is pulsation of the tumor, which increases in size and tension on straining. However, it differs from vascular tumors such as hemangiomas, as an encephalo-cele is firm and unyielding, while a hemangioma is soft and compressible.

TREATMENT. The treatment of choice is excision of the encephalocele with closure of the dural defect. As a rule, a combined craniofacial and nasal approach is needed (see Chapter 56). Since the overlying skin is not involved, sufficient skin should be left behind to assure closure of the wound. After excision of the tumor, along with any irreducibly herniated portion of brain tissue, the dural defect must be closed tightly to prevent leakage of cerebrospinal fluid. If such a defect is massive, a fascia lata graft may be needed for closure. Failure to recognize the dural defect in the intranasal type may lead to meningitis after excision.

COMPLICATIONS. The common complications after excision of an encephalocele are

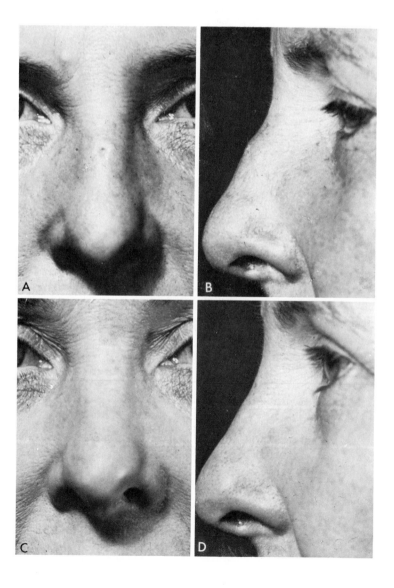

FIGURE 29–182. Dermoid cyst of the nose. *A, B,* Preoperative photographs of the nose. Note the presence of a dimpling sinus over the bridge of the nose. *C, D,* Photographs taken six months after surgery.

similar to those after excision of a glioma. Because of the larger dural defect, leakage of cerebrospinal fluid is a more common and persistent problem.

Neurofibroma. A neurofibroma of the nose is a local manifestation of generalized neurofibromatosis. According to New and Erich (1937), those on the face usually appear in the distribution of one or more branches of the trigeminal nerve. Such a tumor is subcutaneous, somewhat spongy in consistency, and rather diffuse in outline (Fig. 29–181). It can be differentiated from other tumors of the nose by its consistency, its diffuseness, the presence of multiple lesions on other parts of the body, and the coexistence of café au lait spots. The

neurofibroma is slow-growing and asymptomatic and causes no changes in bone structure. Excision is indicated only when it reaches a size sufficient to cause asymmetry of the nose.

CONGENITAL TUMORS OF ECTODERMIC ORIGIN

Dermoid Cyst or Sinus. Dermoid cysts of the nose are relatively common as compared with other congenital tumors of the nose. Midline lesions are most often encountered, while lateral ones are very rare. Dieffenbach (1829) reported the first case, and New and Erich (1937) reported 13 cases of dermoid cysts of the nose among 1495 cysts reviewed. A total

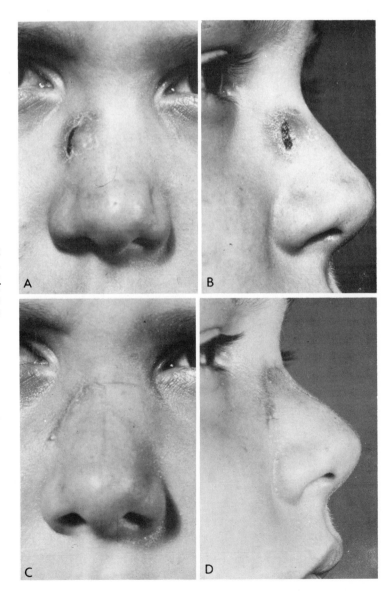

FIGURE 29–183. Dermoid cyst of the nose with discharging sinuses. *A, B,* Preoperative photographs showing draining sinus at the right side of the nose. Note the small dimple at the tip of the nose. *C, D,* Photographs taken three months after surgery.

of less than 100 cases has been recorded in the literature.

The dermoid cyst or sinus usually occurs along the midline of the nose, appearing as high as the glabella or as low as the nasal tip or the base of the columella. It is most frequently subcutaneous in location, but occasionally a tract extends underneath the frontal or nasal bone. Even more rarely, one may appear in the nasal septum.

When the lesion takes the form of a sinus, it appears externally as a dimple with or without a hair protruding from its depth. Such a dimple usually leads to a sinus tract extending upward for variable distances and depths (Fig. 29–182). Adams (1965) pointed out that penetration through the upper portion of the suture line between the nasal bones appears to be a

regular feature of the dermoid sinus. When the lesion takes the form of a cyst, it is usually globular in shape, fluctuating, and freely movable from the overlying skin. A history of recurrent infection is common in both forms. As a result of previous rupture or drainage, multiple sinus openings may be present (Fig. 29–183). Late cases may be complicated by deformity of the nasal bones as a result of direct pressure of the expanding cyst, or by osteomyelitis of neighboring bones secondary to infection. When the cyst is intranasal, it is usually in the nasal septum. Detection is difficult until the cyst has caused sufficient septal expansion to produce nasal obstruction. The cyst may erode neighboring bone.

Radiologic changes associated with dermoid cysts of the nose include bony destruction and

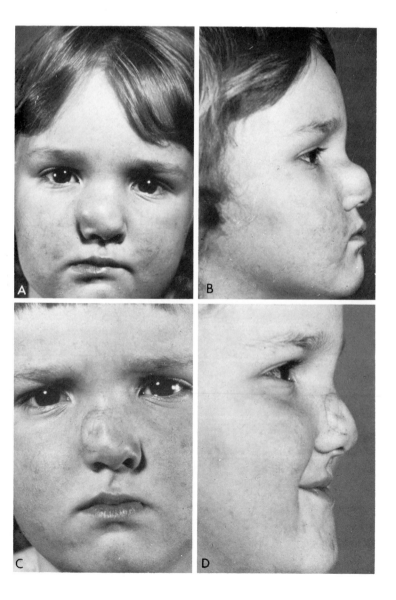

FIGURE 29–184. Cavernous hemangioma of the nose. *A, B,* Appearance of a child with hemangioma of the right side of the nose. *C, D,* After excision and full-thickness skin grafting.

separation or sparing of the nasal septum, nasofrontal angle, ethmoid, nasal dorsum or pyriform aperture. One may also find increased interethmoid-frontal sinus distance, increased interorbital distance, frontal or maxillary sinus deformity (Johnson and Weisman, 1964).

TREATMENT.   Complete excision of the entire cystic tract is the only method that ensures a cure. Prior injection of methylene blue solution into the sinus tract helps to identify the entire lesion. In uncomplicated cysts with no history of infection, dissection of the entire tumor mass with its stalk of attachment is not difficult. However, in cases with a history of previous infection, the presence of scar tissue makes the identification of the cystic tissue and its complete excision extremely difficult. If any part of the sinus is left behind, surgical excision may fail to effect a cure. The external approach is essential to provide good exposure. When the sinus extends below the nasal or frontal bone, complete excision may require the removal of part of the bony structure, resulting in a mild nasal deformity. Reconstructive surgery for such cases should be postponed until growth of the nose is complete.

COMPLICATIONS

Infection.   Any attempt to excise a subacutely or chronically infected dermoid sinus or cyst can result in an infection of the operative wound. The surgeon must postpone surgical excision until the local inflammation has subsided. A preliminary incision and drainage and antibiotic therapy are necessary to help control the local infection.

Recurrence.   Every precaution must be taken to excise the lesion completely. This is especially true for sinuses with a history of recurrent infection. After identification of the sinus tract with methylene blue, the surgeon must excise not only the tract but also all scar tissue in which some epithelial element may be trapped without direct communication with the main sinus.

CONGENITAL TUMORS OF MESODERMIC ORIGIN

Hemangiomas.   Capillary and mixed hemangiomas may be readily diagnosed by the strawberry-red skin surface of the lesion. Pure

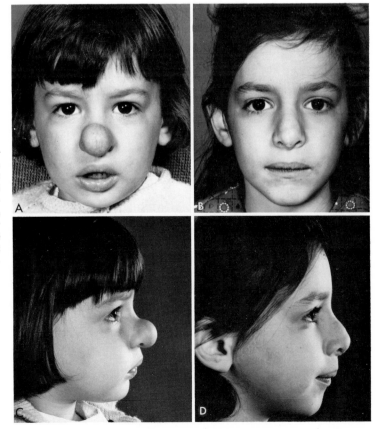

FIGURE 29–185. Cavernous hemangioma of the tip of the nose. *A,* A 5 year old girl with hemangioma of large proportions deforming the tip of the nose. *B,* Five years later, after serial excision and electrocoagulation. *C,* Preoperative profile view. *D,* Postoperative profile view. Definitive rhinoplastic surgery is postponed until nasal growth is completed. (Patient of Dr. J. M. Converse.)

cavernous lesions, distinguishable by their faint bluish tinge, soft texture, diffuse outline, and collapsibility, may also be readily diagnosed. They are, however, occasionally confused with neurofibromas because of their soft consistency and diffuseness, or mistaken for encephaloceles because of increased tension on straining. The patient with a partially fibrosed cavernous hemangioma is the most frequent victim of incorrect diagnosis, as it displays neither the bluish coloration, the softness, nor the collapsibility characteristic of the simple type (Fig. 29–184).

Most capillary hemangiomas have a tendency toward spontaneous regression, which may take many years. When completed, there is no residual scarring or deformity. No active treatment is therefore indicated.

A cavernous hemangioma may not recede spontaneously. A rapidly growing hemangioma may cause irreversible destruction of local structures. In either case, active treatment is indicated. Ligation of the contributing vessels, as advocated by Walsh and Tompkins (1956), or complete excision of the tumor may be required. After complete excision, a full-thickness skin graft is often needed to cover the residual defect.

The local injection of a sclerosing agent is effective but is occasionally followed by uncontrolable complications. Because of the tight and unyielding skin at the tip of the nose and the rich collateral circulation in that region, necrosis following injection, even with a small dose, may be widespread, involving neighboring structures such as the cheek and the lip if the patient is sensitive. Injection treatment is therefore not recommended.

In the patient shown in Figure 29–185, the large cavernous hemangioma was treated by staged resection and electrocoagulation.

Congenital Anomalies of the Nose

Mark K. H. Wang, M.D.

The Bifid Nose

The bifid nose is a rare congenital deformity. Thomas (1873) reported the first case on record. Boo-Chai (1965) found in Malaya a primitive carving of an evil spirit with a bifid nose. It is a common belief among certain aborigines of the Malayan archipelago that such a spirit can cause deformities in man similar to his own. Thus it may be inferred that this deformity did exist among early primitive peoples. Weaver and Billings (1946) found only 13 cases reported in the literature prior to the time of his report. Since then Webster and Deming (1950) reviewed their experiences with 10 cases encountered over a period of 18 years. Others have been added, particularly in the foreign literature, by Burian (1958), Wilke (1958), Sheftel (1958), and Ohmoi and co-workers (1962).

As the name implies, the malformation is characterized by a median fissure of the nose. It may vary in extent from a simple widening of the tip and columella to a complete division of the nose into separate and more or less symmetrical halves. Midline clefts of the upper lip are commonly associated with the bifid nose (see Classification of Craniofacial Clefts in Chapter 46; see also Chapter 56).

Congenital absence of the nose is an extremely rare clinical entity. Most recorded cases are associated with monstrosity, and the infant fails to survive. Those that do survive to maturity are so exceptional that very few cases have been recorded in the literature. The earliest record of this congenital deformity is an ancient Babylonian tablet (No. K 2007 at the British Museum in London, translated by Appert and Lenormant. In Items No. 18 and 19 in this tablet, absence of "tongue" and "nose" is

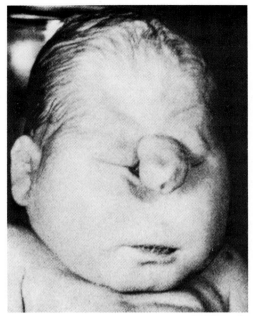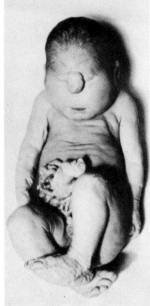

FIGURE 29–186. Cyclops. Note the single orbital fossa and the complete absence of the nose. A single proboscis appears at the midline of the eye. (From Warkany, J.: Congenital Malformation. Chicago, Year Book Medical Publishers, 1971. Used by permission.)

mentioned. In 1884, Sebenkoff described a man 34 years of age with the right half of the nose absent and replaced by a proboscis. In 1903, Wahby described a full term fetal skull (in Cambridge University Museum) with complete absence of the nasal bones; the premaxilla, nasal cavity, and maxillary sinuses were also missing. The same author described an adult Negro skull in which half of the right nasal bone was absent and the original left nasal bone and half of the right nasal bone articulated directly with the left maxilla. Davis in 1919 briefly mentioned this deformity in his classic textbook. Blair in 1931 presented the first recorded case of a complete absence of the nose, with photographs. The boy was born with no evidence of any nasal structure. There was complete absence of the nasal sinuses and passages. In the same article Blair also reported four cases of unilateral absence of the nose. Stupkaw (1938), Walker (1961), Berndorfer (1962), Berger and Martin (1969), and Gifford, Swanson and MacCollum (1972) reported six additional cases of complete absence of the nose in surviving patients.

Complete absence of the nose is often found in monsters, and the infant never survives. The monsters exhibit various forms of arhinenceph-aly, with the common feature of deficiency of olfactory lobes and nerves (see also section on Orbital Hypotelorism, Chapter 56).

Cyclops. A cyclops has a single orbital fossa, in which the global tissue may be absent, rudimentary, or doubled and the eyelids rudimentary. The nose may be absent or more often may appear as a tubular structure attached centrally above the eye. There may be a single nasal chamber not communicating with the pharynx. The nasal bones, vomer, turbinates, premaxilla, and maxillary sinuses are missing. The cerebral hemisphere is fused (Fig. 29–186).

Ethmocephaly. The two orbits and bulbi sit close together but are not united as in a cyclops. The nose is absent. In its place there is a proboscis with one or two nares. The nasal choanal openings, the nasal conchae, the nasal and lacrimal bones, and the premaxilla are absent.

Cebocephaly. Two orbits and bulbi are present but sit close together with orbital hypotelorism. The nose is rudimentary and in its normal position. There is one nasal opening

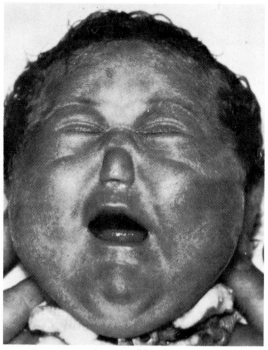

FIGURE 29–187. Cebocephaly. Note the rudimentary nose with a single nasal opening and orbital hypotelorism. (From Haworth, J. C., Medovy, H., and Lewis, A. J.: Cebocephaly with endocrine dysgenesis. J. Pediatr., *59*: 726, 1961.)

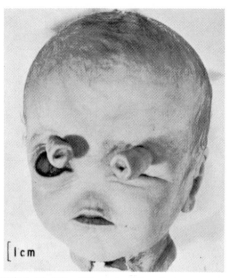

FIGURE 29–188. Bilateral proboscis. Note the complete absence of the external nose. (From Gitlin, G., and Behar, A. J.: Meningeal angeomatosis, arhinencephaly, agenesis of the corpus callosum and large hamartome of the brain with neoplasia in an infant having bilateral nasal proboscis. Acta Anat., *41*:56, 1960.)

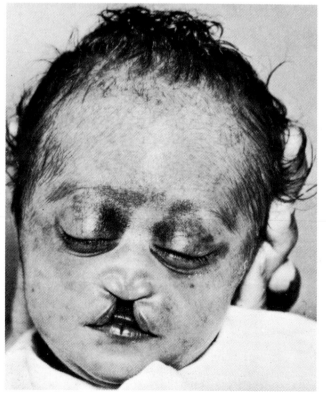

FIGURE 29–189. Median cleft of the lip with arhinencephaly. Note the absence of the philtrum, the premaxilla, and the nasal bones and septum. (From Warkany, J.: Congenital Malformations. Chicago, Year Book Medical Publishers, 1971. Used by permission.)

with one nasal cavity and underdeveloped conchae. The nasal bone, septum, and premaxilla are underdeveloped (Fig. 29–187).

Bilateral Proboscis. This is associated with complete absence of the external nose and nostrils. The proboscises are attached symmetrically to the supraorbital margins (Fig. 29–188).

Median Cleft Lip with Arhinencephaly. This deformity is more common. The infant can live for some time but never long enough to allow reconstructive work. The philtrum, the premaxilla, and the nasal bone and septum are absent, and the nose is flat. There is a single nasal cavity with hypoplastic conchae. Choanal atresia may coexist (Fig. 29–189).

Complete or Partial Congenital Absence of the Nose. This group of patients is compatible with life, and reconstructive work is of practical value.

COMPLETE ABSENCE OF THE NOSE. Complete congenital absence of the nose without monstrosity is extremely rare. Only a few such cases have been recorded in the literature. The site of the external nose is completely flat and covered by normal skin (Fig. 29–190). Occasionally a blind dimple is present at the site where the nostrils should be. There is complete bilateral bony choanal atresia and absence of the nasal cavity. The maxilla is hypoplastic, with the hard palate well formed but highly arched. The upper lip is normal. There are occasional associated orbital deformities, such as microphthalmos, coloboma of the iris, or hypertelorism. Because of complete obstruction of the nasal air passage, the infant has episodes of respiratory difficulty and cyanosis, especially during feeding. In spite of this, the infant can survive, develop normally, and even gradually adjust to oral breathing. Despite the high palatal arch, the soft palate functions well, and the patient often has adequate speech.

UNILATERAL ABSENCE OF THE NOSE. The cases reported by Sebenkoff (1884), Wahby (1903), Blair (1931), Fatin (1955), and Walker (1961) are the only ones recorded in the literature. The disorder is often associated with unilateral arhinencephaly or a unilateral proboscis, which hangs down from the medial canthus. The absent nostril opening may be represented by a blind dimple. In most cases there is a scar or a slight bony tubercle just above the inner canthus. There is usually a nasal cavity on the deformed site (Fig. 29–191) (see also discussion on Orbital Clefts in Chapter 46).

EMBRYOLOGY. At the end of the third or the beginning of the fourth week of embryonic life, as the cerebrum tilts downward in front of the oral orifice, an epithelial thickening, the nasal placode, appears on either side of the frontonasal process above the stomodeum. The placodes soon begin to sink in and form the nasal pits. The surrounding ectoderm becomes elevated by proliferation of the underlying mesoderm. The pits enlarge and deepen by burrowing into the mesodermic bed of the de-

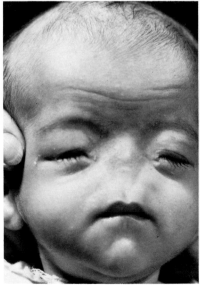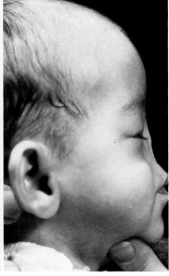

FIGURE 29–190. Complete congenital absence of the nose. (Figs. 29–190 and 29–193 from Gifford, G. H., Swanson, L., and MacCollum, D. W.: Congenital absence of the nose and anterior nasopharynx. Plast. Reconstr. Surg., *50*:5, 1972. Copyright © 1972, The Williams & Wilkins Company, Baltimore.)

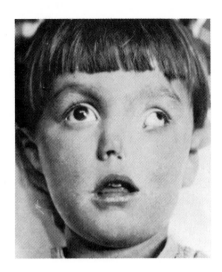

FIGURE 29–191. Unilateral absence of the nose and facial clefting. Note that the absent left side of the nose is represented by a blind dimple. (Courtesy of Annals Publishing Company, St. Louis, Mo.)

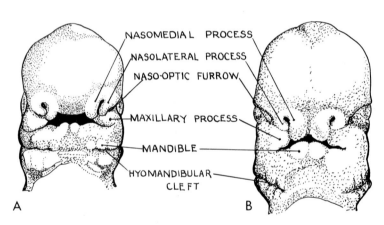

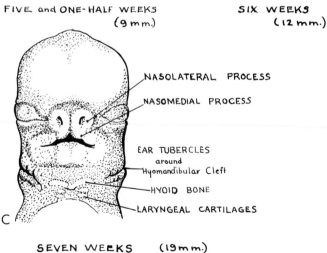

FIGURE 29–192. Frontal views of human embryos, illustrating the development of the facial structures. (After Patten.)

veloping face and extend posteriorly to the region of Rathke's pouch. The primitive nasal pouch, precursor of the nasal cavity, is thus formed. It is directly above the primitive buccal cavity. The floor of the pouch is thinned out by absorption of the intervening mesoderm. The nasal and oral cavities, however, remain separated by a thin partition, the nasobuccal membrane, until the 35th to 38th day of embryonic life, when the membrane ruptures, producing the primitive choanal openings. As the nasal pits deepen, elevations on either side become more prominent and develop into the medial and lateral nasal processes. The medial

nasal processes with the intervening frontonasal process project caudally to form the nasal tip and septum and the premaxillary process. The lateral nasal processes, combining with maxillary processes, form the lateral portion of the nose. Eventual fusion of the medial and lateral nasal processes and the maxillary processes forms the anterior nares (Fig. 29–192).

Bilateral developmental failure of the nasal placodes of the frontonasal process results in nonformation of the external nose and nasal cavity. The upper lip is normal as a result of undisturbed growth in the maxillary processes.

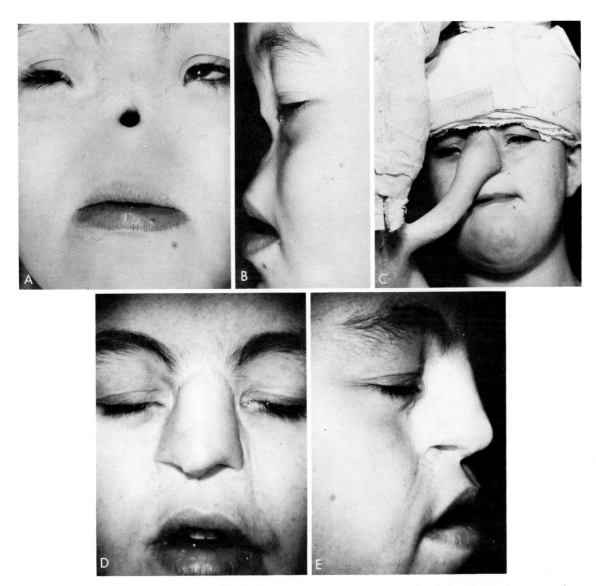

FIGURE 29–193.   Same patient as in Figure 29–190. *A, B,* Appearance of the patient before the nasal reconstruction at the age of 13 years. Note the nasal airway established at the age of 5 years. *C,* Reconstruction of the nose by a tubed flap from the arm. *D, E,* Appearance of the patient at the age of 29 years. The reconstructed nose has been completed with a cartilage graft.

In the absence of the nasal cavity and nasal septum, the palatal arch is abnormally high due to the lack of a counterbalancing downward force above the developing palate.

When failure of nasal placode development is unilateral, a unilateral absence of the nose results.

TREATMENT. The surgical treatment of complete congenital absence of the nose has two goals. First, when there is bilateral bony atresia of the choanal space, a permanent, patent air passage should be established at the normal site of the nose. Second, a totally reconstructed nose should be provided for psychologic and cosmetic reasons.

Bilateral bony choanal atresia. In spite of complete absence of the nasal air passage, the nasal obstruction rarely requires emergency treatment, such as tracheotomy. The infant usually survives to allow more definitive surgery, as in the two cases reported by Gifford, Swanson, and MacCollum (1972), for whom the surgery was performed at the ages of 5 and 6 years. The delay in surgery, which was tolerated by the patients, allows the use of a transpalatal approach, which gives direct vision of the atresia and provides more adequate scope for the repair. The detailed surgical technique is described in a previous section, Congenital Choanal Atresia (see Figs. 29–175 and 29–176).

Reconstruction of the nose in children. In congenital absence of the nose, reconstruction of the nose should be started only after a patent airway has been established at the nasal site. Although it is much easier to determine the size of the reconstructed nose after the child has reached full growth, earlier reconstruction may be needed for psychologic reasons. Penn (1967) stated that, under such conditions, the nose should be made as large as possible, since one cannot predict future growth.

Total reconstruction of the nose in a child born with congenitally absent nose was reported by Blair and Brown (1931), and reconstruction for congenital absence and acquired total loss of the nose was described by Kilner (1938), Lewin (1957, 1971), Gifford and co-workers (1972) (see also Figs. 29–190 and 29–193), Peet and Patterson (1964), and Furnas (1968).

Ortiz-Monasterio (1975) advises against reconstructing the nose in a child by means of a forehead flap, which should be reserved for the definitive reconstruction after the completion of growth.

For further details concerning reconstruction of the nose, see page 1209.

Benign Tumors
of the Nose

Most of the benign tumors of the nose are similar to those which occur in the skin of other portions of the body, and their treatment does not differ (see Tumors of the Skin, Chapter 65) except when a tissue defect requires reconstruction, the techniques of which are described in the last sections of this chapter.

Rhinophyma

BROMLEY S. FREEMAN, M.D.

Rhinophyma is an irregular, disfiguring, hypertrophic distortion of the nose varying in degree, type, and extent. Historically it has been considered the end result of acne rosacea in alcoholic men in their 50's. Although the initial disorder is that of the skin and subcutaneous tissue, the muscle, vascular elements, and even cartilage become involved in the pathologic process. The condition appears to be less prevalent than in previous times.

PATHOLOGY

Marks (1968), in a review of the pathologic material removed during surgery, observed the following histologic findings: (1) initial congestion and instability of the superficial cutaneous vascular plexus; (2) blood vessel engorgement in the upper portion of the dermis; (3) dilatation and proliferation of the superficial capillaries; (4) dermal and subcutaneous hypertrophy with consequent upheaval and irregularity of the surface epithelium.

The vascular engorgement increases the growth of the glandular elements, and finally the cartilaginous and muscular structures also become hypertrophied. The irregular surface blocks the duct openings, and retention cysts of enormous size result. Stagnation leads to chronic or subacute episodes of foreign body inflammation which, aided by additional blockage, promote chronic infection with episodes of acute infection, both multifocal and diffuse. A similar pathogenesis is responsible for areas of involvement on the cheeks, chin, forehead, and ears. Venous dilation, engorgement, hypertrophy, venous and lymphatic blockage, exudation, and fibroplasia, followed by inflammation, tumor growth, and infection, seem to be a pattern sequence in the majority of cases. The predisposing factors appear to include a hereditary diathesis, vascular sensitivity, hormonal imbalance, and a specific type of skin which overreacts to external or internal insults to form one of the five classic varieties of rhinophyma.

The emotional barrier associated with this progressive disfigurement and its social implications have been well recognized and recorded not only in the scientific literature but also in art forms and literature for many centuries. Approximately 32 terms have been used for rhinophyma (Odou, 1961).

DIAGNOSIS

A classification into five clinical types has resulted from a review of the dermatologic, pathologic, and surgical literature and the personal analysis of 60 patients seen under the general diagnosis of "rhinophyma" from 1939 to 1970: (1) early vascular (Fig. 29–194); (2) diffuse enlargement—moderate (Fig. 29–195); (3) localized tumor—early (Fig. 29–196); (4) diffuse enlargement—extensive (Fig. 29–197); (5) diffuse enlargement—extensive with localized tumor (Fig. 29–198). Of these patients, 10 were female and 50 male (Table 29–2). In contrast to most reports (Odou and Odou, 1961; Anderson and Dykes, 1962; Matton and coworkers, 1962), 14 of these patients had grandparents or parents with similar nasal disfigurement. Twenty patients had had an alcoholic history—prolonged imbibition of alcohol or wine. Two were specific about the onset of the lesion after prolonged steroid therapy. Some individuals complained of flushing or prolonged nasal tip engorgement after even a modest imbibition of wine and brandy, yet none after drinking neutral spirits, whiskey, or beer. Some had never had an alcoholic drink. In patients who reacted to steroid or androgen medication by a frank, if relatively modest, appearance of rhinophyma of the vascular type, the nasal swelling and discoloration subsided completely after medication was stopped. In susceptible individuals, sustained exposure to sunlight, cold, and wind caused swelling, persistent discoloration, and enlargement of the nose. In many there were associated changes in the chin, cheeks, and ears. In six cases carcinoma in situ was found in the specimen. Recurrent basal cell epithelioma was the result of multifocal lesions in only two patients. The rather low incidence of carcinoma in situ undoubtedly would have been higher if multiple sections

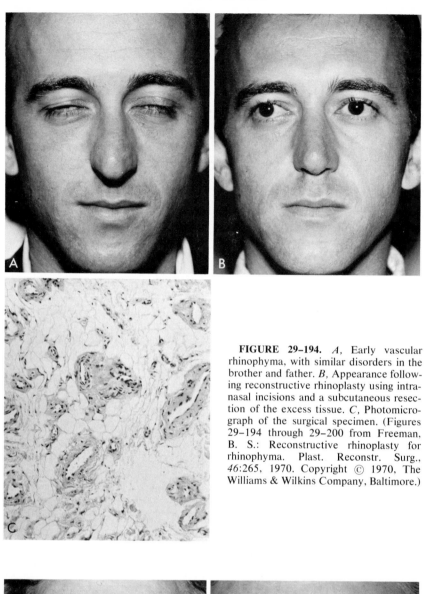

FIGURE 29–194. *A*, Early vascular rhinophyma, with similar disorders in the brother and father. *B*, Appearance following reconstructive rhinoplasty using intranasal incisions and a subcutaneous resection of the excess tissue. *C*, Photomicrograph of the surgical specimen. (Figures 29–194 through 29–200 from Freeman, B. S.: Reconstructive rhinoplasty for rhinophyma. Plast. Reconstr. Surg., *46*:265, 1970. Copyright © 1970, The Williams & Wilkins Company, Baltimore.)

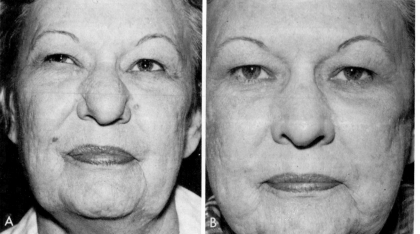

FIGURE 29–195. *A*, Diffuse enlargment—moderate size rhinophyma. *B*, Treated by subcutaneous resection and a corrective rhinoplasty, including remodeling of the cartilages.

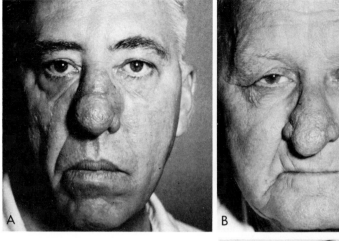

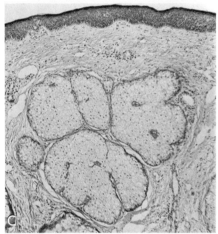

FIGURE 29–196. *A, B,* Two patients with localized tumor—early type of rhinophyma. *C,* Photomicrograph of typical sebaceous adenomatous formation seen in most rhinophymatous tissue. Inclusion cysts may also be found deep in the dermis.

had been made of the surgical specimen in each case (McDowell, 1969). Two patients had extensive squamous cell epithelioma in association with rhinophyma.

TYPES OF OPERATIONS

The operations employed for the correction of rhinophyma have been divided into several main categories (Friedrich, 1967) and have included:

1. Reconstruction of the skin surface by planing, paring, excision, or "decortication"; wire-brushing; electrocoagulation; carbon dioxide slush; and resection by the coagulating wire loop.

2. En bloc resection of skin and subcutaneous tissue and coaptation (Dieffenbach, 1845; Grattan, 1925).

3. Subcutaneous resection of soft tissue through external incisions with elevation of flaps, or through intranasal incisions without elevation of flaps.

In some cases, all of the above measures have been combined. Early "vascular" lesions and relatively early diffuse and diffusely enlarged lesions have been treated by a corrective rhinoplastic procedure, using either a gull-wing tip incision or intranasal incisions with a subcutaneous resection of the excess soft tissue. This has been followed, when necessary, by planing at a later date (see Figs. 29–194 and 29–195).

For patients in the other groups (Table 29–2), planing, open excision, cartilaginous reconstruction, and flap closure were used. Staged procedures, modified from patient to patient, have given satisfactory results with relatively minor complications.

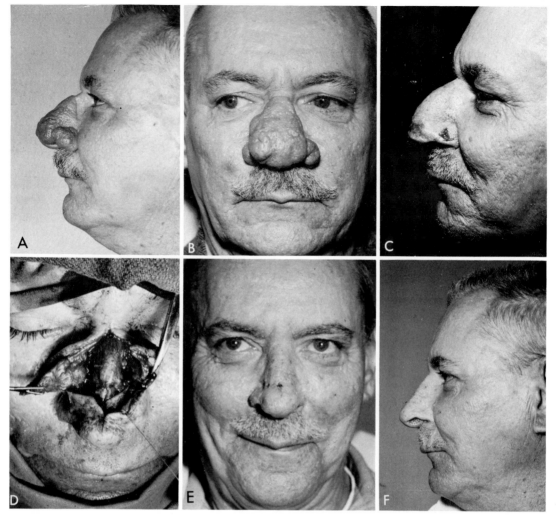

FIGURE 29–197. *A, B,* Diffuse enlargment—extensive type. *C,* After first decortication. *D,* Second operation, with exposure of the nasal bones and cartilages and elevation of skin flaps. *E, F,* Eary result.

PLANNING THE OPERATION

A study of the sketch, photographs, and cast of an extensive rhinophyma often shows how inadequate will be the changes produced by simple decortication or planing, particularly if the objective is to restore a nose of shape and size harmonious with the rest of the face (see Fig. 29–198).

Preliminary Preparation. A preliminary period (varying from one week to one month) of intensive cleansing of the skin, plus administration of systemic antibiotics, is initiated in all patients. The antibiotic coverage is continued until healing is complete.

OPERATIVE TECHNIQUE

Planing. A Castroviejo or similar small dermatome (even a potato peeler) is used to shave the entire nose—dorsum to tip, alae, and rim—using shims of approximately 1 mm in thickness. This is continued until the surface of the misshapen nose is relatively smooth. Suitably large sections of the skin strips are saved for possible covering of surface defects that may occur as a result of the operative defects (see Fig. 29–198) or are stored for later use in case of slow healing. Hemostasis is obtained by pinpoint electrocoagulation; large vessels are sutured or ligated; capillary oozing is controlled by sustained pressure.

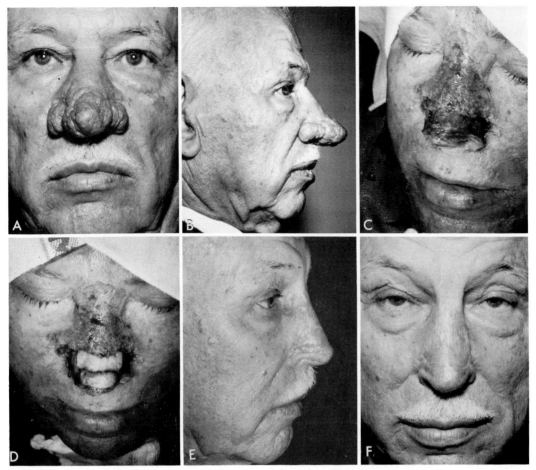

FIGURE 29–198. *A, B,* Diffuse enlargement—extensive localized tumor type. *C,* Immediately after planing, excision, cartilaginous reconstruction, and closure of flaps. *D,* A few minutes later, after application of the skin grafts removed from the nose during the decortication. *E, F,* Result one year later.

Outlining and Raising Dermoepidermal Flaps. When possible, an incision close to the tumor-free portion of the tip (but sometimes through diseased tissue) is made across the dorsum; another is made vertically in the midline. These incisions permit elevation of flaps. Hinged on the rims and tip of the nose, similar

flaps are raised distally (see Fig. 29–197, *D*). Despite the increase in vascularity of the diseased tissue, relatively thick flaps should be elevated.

Resecting Diseased Tissue and Sculpturing. En bloc excision under the flap removes the excess subcutaneous tissue and muscle, exposing the cartilaginous framework of the lower nose. The cartilages—curved, looped, and irregular—can then be reconstructed according to the preoperative plan or modeled as in a routine rhinoplasty. The alar cartilages are trimmed, and the lateral cartilages are shortened and narrowed to restore a nasal shape harmonious with the face (see Fig. 29–198). The resection of wedges from the alae is frequently necessary because of elongation of the nose as a result of the disease; thick alae are thinned by oval or elliptical excision of skin and subcu-

TABLE 29–2. *Survey of 60 patients with rhinophyma*

	FEMALE	MALE
Early vascular	2	5
Diffuse enlargement—moderate	6	12
Localized tumor—early	—	9
Diffuse enlargement—extensive	—	10
Diffuse enlargement—extensive with localized tumor	2	14

taneous tissue (occasionally in continuity with a resection of a portion of the base of the nostrils, and the floor of the nose). *Caution is necessary to avoid interrupting the blood supply of the inferiorly based flaps.* Many patients also require septal resection and trimming of the septal mucous membrane.

When the nose has been shortened and narrowed and the tip elevated to an adequate position, the flaps are tailored to size. Buried sutures (nonabsorable) aided by subcuticular sutures coapt the flaps (Fig. 29–199). Intranasal packing and an external splint (lined with nonadherent gauze) provide the mild counter-

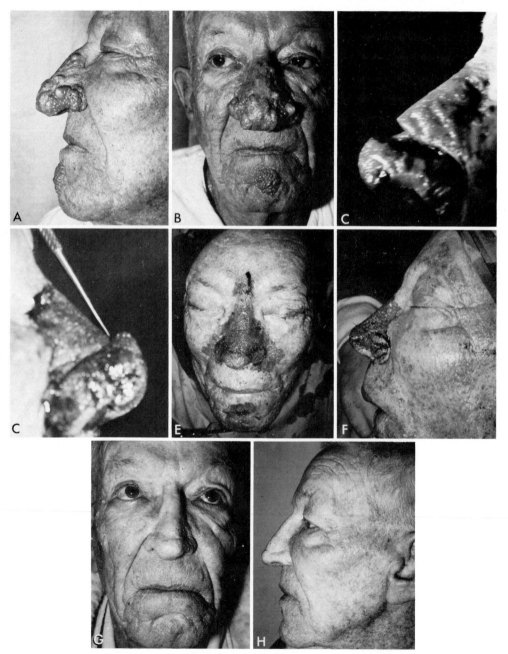

FIGURE 29–199. *A, B,* Extensive acute and chronic diffuse rhinophyma. *C,* Full thickness excision to shorten the nose. *D,* The shortening; the hook raises the tip. *E, F,* After suture of the defect and decortication. *G, H,* Final appearance.

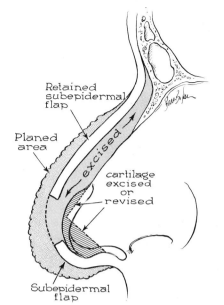

FIGURE 29–200. Schema of the technique of reconstructive rhinoplasty for rhinophyma.

pressure essential for hemostasis and prevention of edema. The schema of the operation is shown in Figure 29–200.

SECONDARY PROCEDURES

Timidity in removing cartilaginous or bony protuberances has necessitated secondary cartilaginous reconstruction in 12 patients (see Fig. 29–197). Others undoubtedly underwent secondary surgery elsewhere. All of our patients were offered, and most received, later surface improvement by various modalities, such as the application of trichloroacetic acid, wire-brushing, surgical abrasion, shaving with the dermatome, abrasion with sandpaper, use of the diamond wheel, or chemical "peel."

Dermabrasion. Surgical abrasion (see Chapter 17) with the aid of a fluoroethyl spray is used for the correction of superficial irregularities at a primary or secondary stage. The abrader, diamond wheel, wire brush, or "macerator" is chosen to suit the type and depth of the skin changes. The freezing spray and a wire brush are advisable for gross surface irregularities but can produce uneven grooves. Corrugated, nodular protuberances require a dermatome; the small Castroviejo dermatome

and the Brown dermatome are suitable. The latter, properly adjusted, is an excellent instrument for deep removal but may be too broad and clumsy for the small lesion. Initial scalpel or razor shaving is rapid and can be supplemented by any of the foregoing. Hemostasis is readily established by pressure, electrocoagulation, ligation, or suturing.

Overgrafting. Multiple scars and surface irregularities may result after the various treatments. In order to correct color changes and residual surface irregularities, overgrafting as a primary or secondary procedure has been employed. Preparation of the recipient site by surgical abrasion using the freezing technique and a diamond wheel, or even by a delicate excision of the scarred epidermis with the dermatome, provides a base which can be resurfaced by a lateral cervical split-thickness skin graft or a postauricular or supraclavicular full-thickness skin graft. The stabilizing matured scar does not interfere with the vascularization of the dermal or scar base, and a thin but soft graft of satisfactory color match usually results. When overgrafting is employed, early inspection for the evacuation of hematomas and seromas is essential on the first postoperative day. Thereafter, the graft is left exposed or immobilized by net fixation. Skin grafting may also be delayed for 24 hours.

COMPLICATIONS

As would be expected in an area of chronic infection and abnormal vascularity, especially if distally based flaps are used, wound healing may be delayed. Although complications have been many and varied, they have always been minor. Severe hemorrhage occurred in none of the patients. If healing by first intention did not occur, at least a satisfactory end result was obtained without the need for a secondary operation in the majority of cases. There have been no sloughs of flaps and no evidence of chondritis. According to Maliniac (1930), exposure of the bare cartilage by removal of the perichondrium without a viable flap covering resulted in necrosis requiring flap closure. This has not occurred in the author's series. Low grade infections have subsided under antibiotic therapy (topical and systemic). Although frequent wet dressings to the nose may be annoying to the patient, several grafts have been saved by this technique.

Secondary procedures are best deferred until the operated area is soft and the scars have matured. However, some patients have undergone additional surgery as soon as three weeks after the initial procedure; others have waited five years. Necrosis of the edge of the flaps or loss of skin grafts required the immediate application of skin grafts taken from either the postauricular or supraclavicular area.

Recurrence, noted on the distal aspect of the flaps and other areas, should be dealt with. It is essential that the nares be opened, and secondary subcutaneous excision or remodeling via the usual intranasal incisions may be required. Scarred nodules should be excised and resurfaced. The few patients who had immediate grafting of epidermis from the diseased or rhinophymatous nose healed rapidly with considerable surface irregularity but with satisfactory color match. Conspicuous scars have occurred, and late narial contracture and septal thickening have impaired the airway and also required additional treatment. The end results after secondary surgical procedures, although not always satisfactory from the surgeon's viewpoint, have been satisfying to the patients.

Malignant Tumors of the Nose

John Marquis Converse, M.D., and Phillip R. Casson, F.R.C.S.

Fear of disfigurement has been a principal cause of recurrence in the treatment of cancer of the nose. Fear of the resulting nasal defect has often resulted in the lesion being undertreated. Thus it is obvious that reconstruction of the defect, i.e., restoring acceptable contour, is an integral part of the treatment of the patient (Converse and Casson, 1969).

Fortunately, with modern methods of reconstruction, the patient can be assured, in most cases, that a satisfactory reconstruction can be achieved. In those patients in whom reconstruction may be contraindicated because of the age of the patient or medical problems, a generally satisfactory prosthetic nose can be worn by the patient; it is admittedly a makeshift substitute for a nose constructed with autogenous tissues.

The common tumors of the nose are the basal cell and squamous cell carcinomas of the skin. Sweat gland tumors, malignant melanomas, sarcomas, and malignant neurilemomas occur less frequently (Conley, 1966). Because of their conspicuous position, such lesions tend to be small when first seen; extensive tumors requiring radical and therefore disfiguring surgery or high dose radiation for their treatment are fortunately becoming rare (Kazanjian and Roopenian, 1963). When such tumors occur, they are most often the result of neglect on the part of the patient or of unsuccessful treatment.

In the management of any tumor of the nose, cure of the disease is the first consideration, and the advantage of early resection should not be lost in attempts to avoid disfigurement by a sparing resection with narrow margins of safety, by the avoidance of full-thickness excision, by inadequate irradiation, or by other insufficient modalities of treatment. For the more advanced lesions, treatment planning must include some form of replacement of the nose so that the patient may resume a relatively normal life.

BASAL CELL EPITHELIOMA

Basal cell epithelioma is by far the commonest tumor of the nose. In the series reported by Conley (1966), 87 per cent were basal cell lesions. These lesions occur classically in the fair-skinned individual with a long history of exposure to the sun. Although basal cell epithelioma is a disease affecting older age groups, young adults and even children are not immune (Murray and Cannon, 1960). Another predisposing factor of importance is previously administered radiation for the treatment of acne or hirsutism (see Chapters 20 and 65).

In appearance, a basal cell epithelioma may mimic a variety of skin conditions, including simple cysts, pigmented nevi, freckles, warts, and psoriasis. When the slightest doubt exists as to the diagnosis of any such lesion, a biopsy is indicated, as the incidence of error on clinical grounds alone is as high as 30 per cent even in experienced hands (Monvalliu, 1968). On histologic examination there is considerable variation in the microscopic picture, and from it some indication of the clinical behavior of the tumor may be obtained (see Chapter 65). Metastases are extremely rare, but it should be remembered that they do occur; the authors have personal experience of metastases in two cases.

As with any tumor, the best opportunity to cure basal cell epithelioma is at the time of initial therapy. The surgeon may choose from several equally effective modalities. A detailed discussion is beyond the scope of this chapter, but a brief review of these modalities follows.

Techniques of Treatment of Basal Cell Epithelioma. In lesions 2 cm or less in size, desiccation and curettage, radiation, and surgical excision when applied with equal skill all give a cure rate of around 90 per cent (Freeman and coworkers, 1964). Tumors over 2 cm in diameter, in which some spread in depth may be anticipated, are best treated by radiation or surgery. The selection of treatment is determined by the site of the tumor, its histologic appearance, the general condition of the patient, and the modalities of therapy available (see Chapter 65). Surgery does have the advantage that a specimen is available for pathologic examination, either at the operating table by frozen section or by routine paraffin section.

Another technique being used with more frequency is that of chemosurgical excision as developed by Mohs (1956a) (see Chapter 65). In brief, it consists of removal of the tumor after fixation of the tissue by the application of zinc chloride paste; it is then excised in layers, each of which is examined histologically until a tumor-free plane is reached. It results in a high cure rate, even of recurrent lesions, but has the disadvantage of being time-consuming and costly. Moreover, the technique is available only in a few centers.

Recurrent basal cell lesions are much more difficult to treat. They often receive inadequate treatment because the surgeon fails to appreciate the true extent of the invasion and extension into adjacent skin and, for the sake of preserving the cosmetic appearance of the patient, fails to resect sufficient tissue. Recurrence is a danger signal and is an indication for aggressive treatment to eradicate the disease and to avert the onset of a series of recurrences and excisions which may eventually lead to the death of the patient.

In the treatment of recurrent lesions, Mohs' chemosurgical excision has an impressive cure rate of 97.5 per cent (Robins, 1975); if available, this method would seem to be the treatment of choice, preserving as it does the maximum amount of tissue.

SQUAMOUS CELL CARCINOMA

Squamous cell carcinoma of the nose may affect the skin or, more rarely, the squamous epithelium of the vestibule. It is the second most common tumor of the region, comprising 9 per cent of the series reported by Conley (1966) and 18 per cent of 338 cases, treated exclusively by radiation, reported by Stoll, Milgrom, and Traenkle (1964). The problems in management are similar to those of basal cell carcinoma, and according to Freeman, Knox, and Heaton (1964), similar results are obtained with squamous cell carcinoma of the skin if treatment is by any of the three common techniques: desiccation and curettage, radiation, or surgical excision. Stoll, Milgrom, and Traenkle, using radiation in a group of 62 histologically proved squamous cancers of the nose, reported a five-year cure rate of 94.5 per cent. This figure would be difficult to improve upon by any other means.

Metastases occur in this disease but are not as common as with squamous cell carcinoma elsewhere. Metastasis was detected only once in the series reported by Stoll and his associates.

Other rare tumors that may occur on the nose are malignant melanoma, sweat gland carcinoma, fibrous sarcoma, and malignant schwannoma. Case reports of these lesions are few, but available data indicate that the prognosis is poor. Such lesions should be treated by wide excision as they are elsewhere in the body. Neck dissection is reserved for those patients who develop clinically palpable nodes.

CHOICE OF METHODS OF REPAIR

The method of repair depends upon the type of defect resulting from the eradication of the malignant lesion. The defect may involve the skin only in superficial lesions, and a satisfactory immediate repair may be effected by means of a skin graft, preferably a full-thickness skin graft taken from the retroauricular or supraclavicular areas. These donor areas are chosen because of the excellent color match with the skin of the nose. A split-thickness graft taken from another area of the body, admittedly to provide only temporary resurfacing, is indicated if there is doubt as to whether the tumor was adequately excised. Local flaps are readily available from adjacent tissues in patients of the older age group in whom the relaxed soft tissues make more tissue available. A flap from the nasolabial area is a particular favorite in older patients.

It is appropriate to emphasize that when reconstruction by means of a skin flap is required, the forehead flap (see p. 1210) is the most practical of the available techniques in the cancer patient, especially a patient in the older age group. Patients in this age group do not readily tolerate the necessary acrobatic positions imposed by such methods as the Tagliacotian arm flap. The color and texture match of the forehead skin results in a harmonious blending with the remainder of the skin of the face. With the exception of the Tagliacotian flap, this is not generally true of flaps migrated from other positions of the body. When the forehead is not available as a donor area for a flap, a tube flap can be migrated from a distant donor site or from neighboring areas, such as the lower cervical area or the acromiopectoral area. Full thickness defects of the nose, varying in size from the loss of an ala to total destruction of the nose, require restoration not only of the covering soft tissues but also of lining and skeletal supportive tissues.

TIMING OF THE RECONSTRUCTION

Immediate reconstruction is satisfactory in well-defined lesions excised with an adequate margin of safety. In lesions involving skin only, immediate replacement by a full-thickness retroauricular or supraclavicular graft gives excellent results. After adequate excision of an alar lesion, immediate reconstruction by a composite auricular graft can give a dramatic result.

In lesions whose extension is doubtful, as in multicentric lesions, and in those conditions designated by Conley (1966) as "field cancerization," the ultimate extension of the malignant process is in doubt. In such cases, reconstruction should be postponed. The authors have not found that frozen sections always give sufficient information to be entirely reliable. The lesion is frequently more widespread than its clinical manifestations would suggest. In such cases, Mohs' chemosurgery (1956b) with its careful histologic verification and its ability to ferret out snakelike extensions is the treatment of choice. Mohs' chemosurgery technique is also employed when histologic verfication of the excised specimen shows inadequate excision.

Immediate Versus Delayed Reconstruction. Immediate forehead flap reconstruction is generally contraindicated in malignant disease, although one of our patients (see Fig. 29–288) underwent an immediate reconstruction following excision and has survived for 20 years. The procedure is not advisable for two reasons: (1) the resected specimen should undergo careful histologic examination to verify that the lesion has been excised with a safe margin; and (2) the patient should realize the magnitude of his deformity. Amputation of the nose is always a traumatic experience. Experience has shown that the patient will be more grateful and satisfied with the reconstructed nose (which is never as satisfactory as hoped for) if he has been obliged to live with the amputated nose for a period of months. The reconstruction should not be undertaken until the patient is free of cancer and the delay allows the tissues of the residual stump to soften and become well vascularized.

A flap may mask progressively developing underlying disease. It is preferable to suture the skin to the nasal mucous membrane along the edges of the excisional defect and to add a split-thickness graft if a surface defect is also present. In the case of a composite graft, the prohibition of immediate reconstruction is not so drastic, as additional auricular donor areas are available and the composite graft may be repeated after re-excision and histologic verification.

Generally speaking, after subtotal resection of the nose for cancer, a period of 6 months to a year should be allowed for confirmation of the cure. Additional verification by biopsies can be obtained during this period.

A delay of four to six months is required following Mohs' chemosurgery. The sclerotic process extends into the neighboring tissues, and sufficient time should be allowed for the tissues to soften and become adequately revascularized.

During the waiting period prior to reconstruction, the patient can be provided with a transitional prosthesis that will provide temporary esthetic restoration of either the major portion or a smaller portion of the nose.

Deformities of the Skin of the Nose

John Marquis Converse, M.D.

Cutaneous Scars. Scars of the skin of the nose, when linear and smooth, are barely visible; scars resulting from poorly sutured wounds, however, are conspicuous, particularly when they cause notching of the alar border or distortion of the nasal tip. Approximation of the borders following excision of scars usually results in a fine linear scar. Such a line is more easily attained in the upper half of the nose, for in this area the skin is loosely attached over the bony framework. Scars traversing the horizontal skin folds of the upper portion of the nose may require a Z-plasty after excision in order to change their direction. A W-plasty may often be indicated in troublesome scars that have been sutured in a linear fashion at the primary operation. Over the tip and alae of the nose the skin is thicker and contains many sebaceous glands; it is firmly attached to the underlying cartilaginous structures. At the alar border a linear scar may produce notching of the alar border and require a tongue and groove or a Z-plasty procedure. Superficial scars near the root of the nose, requiring the excision of an appreciable area, can generally be satisfactorily repaired by direct advancement of the adjacent skin; a W-plasty is usually indicated (see Chapter 1). At the tip and alae of the nose, even small defects are difficult to close without distortion (Fig. 29–201). In Figure 29–202 a technique is shown to correct alar notching by the Z-plasty technique.

Irregularities of the surface of the scar and

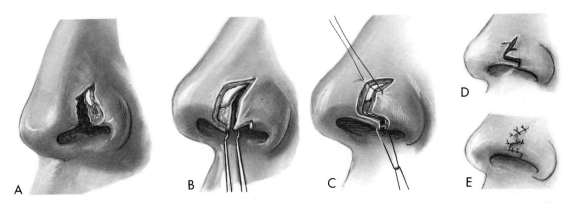

FIGURE 29–201. Restoration of the continuity of the alar border. *A,* Irregular defect of the nostril border. *B, C,* Use of the halving and stepping techniques to avoid postoperative notching of the nostril border. *D, E,* A Z-plasty may also be employed in conjunction with the stepping method.

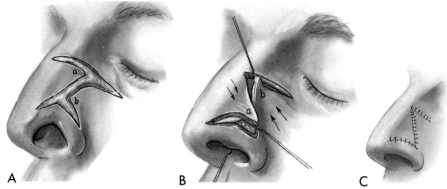

FIGURE 29–202. Stellate scar retracting the nostril and its correction. *A*, Drawing of the scar showing the retraction. The letters *a* and *b* indicate the tips of the flap to be transposed. *B*, Transposition of the flaps and lowering of the nostril border. *C*, After interpolation of the flaps as in a Z-plasty, the lateral wall of the nose has been elongated, correcting the alar retraction.

differences of level between the scar and the surrounding skin can be considerably improved by surgical dermabrasion.

Loss of a considerable amount of skin, as in burns, and the resulting contracture cause a telescoping of the alar cartilages over the lateral cartilages and a foreshortening of the nose. The alar borders, which may be partly destroyed, are also everted, exposing the vibrissae of the vestibule, and the columella, relatively fixed by the cartilaginous septum, appears to protrude downward. Resection of the cutaneous scar permits the return of the cartilages to their original position, thus disclosing the true extent of the defect. Such distortions may result from simple loss of skin without concomitant injury to the underlying framework.

Choice of Method of Repair in Cutaneous Defects of the Nose. As in other defects of the skin of the face, the choice lies between the use of local tissue, skin grafts, tissue from the forehead, and rarely a flap from a distance, such as a Tagliacotian arm flap. The procedures are simpler in defects with loss of only skin and subcutaneous tissue than in full-thickness defects of the nose, which will be considered later in this chapter.

Generally speaking, moderate-sized defects of the upper portion of the nose may be closed by local flaps; in the lower nose, skin grafts from the retroauricular or supraclavicular areas give excellent results. Over the dorsum of the nose, when some of the deeper structures have also been destroyed, a skin graft, even of full

thickness, will not compensate for the loss of tissue in depth; in some cases it is possible to overgraft the first graft after dermabrading it.

Various types of flaps are available for this type of defect. Satisfactory esthetic results are obtained in such defects by the use of an island forehead flap, a technique that will be described later in this chapter (see Fig. 29–245).

Defects Repaired by Local Flaps. Local flaps of skin are usually employed in the repair of small defects of the looser tissue covering the upper portion of the nose. The Z-plasty technique will give good results if scar contractures occur.

When defects extend deeper than the skin, skin grafts will not provide a satisfactory repair, for example, over bare bone or cartilage. In such cases a local skin flap is essential.

The soft tissues in the area of the base of the lateral wall of the nose are loose. This characteristic makes it possible to transpose a skin flap from the upper portion of the nose to the lower when the area to be resurfaced is not amenable to a full-thickness skin graft. In defects of the lower portion of the nose, a flap may be shifted from the upper to the lower portion of the nose, and a skin graft or flap is applied to the secondary defect. Local flaps of nasal tissue can be used for repair of small defects of the upper part of the nose. Local flaps from the lower part of the nose, however, should not be used, as they may result in distortion of the tip or alae of the nose.

In some instances, if the bony and cartilaginous structures of the nose are reduced in size, thereby increasing the amount of available skin, the defect can be closed by local flaps sutured without tension.

In suitable cases, especially in elderly patients, skin can be borrowed from the surrounding area of the face without producing conspicuous additional scars.

THE NASOLABIAL FLAP. The nasolabial flap (Fig. 29–203) is useful to provide skin replacement for the nose in older individuals in whom the looseness of the soft tissue permits closure of the donor site of the flap and a minimal resulting scar. This mode of repair is not advocated in the younger patient, who may form a hypertrophic scar at the donor site and in whom the tendency for the flap to contract will result in a puckered repaired area. Although the flap is designed in a retrograde fashion in relation to the blood supply, the vascularization of the area is adequate to provide a satisfactory flap blood supply.

The nasolabial fold is the area of junction between the tightly bound skin of the lip and the loosely bound skin of the cheek. In males it also delimits the hair-bearing area of the lip from the non–hair-bearing portion of the cheek. When a defect of the nose is being repaired, the flap should be taken from above the nasolabial fold in the non–hair-bearing area. The nasolabial flap may also be designed with a subcutaneous pedicle which provides greater mobility. After the nasolabial flap is raised, the secondary defect is closed by direct approximation; the approximation is done without difficulty because of the looseness of the cheek tissues, especially in older individuals. Closure of the donor site of the flap brings the base of the flap closer to the nose; the flap thus assumes a position which facilitates its placement over the nasal defect without tension. For further details concerning the technique of the nasolabial flap, see page 1218.

THE CHEEK ADVANCEMENT FLAP. Skin defects of the lateral aspect of the dorsum of the nose may be covered by direct advancement of the skin of the cheek (Fig. 29–204). The looseness of the cheek tissues facilitates this advancement in older individuals, and the cheek skin may be advanced over the dorsum of the nose. A straight advancement flap is outlined by making an incision in the nasolabial fold and another through one of the lower folds of the lower eyelid. The skin outlined in the flap is raised from the underlying subcutaneous tissue and is advanced over the nasal defect. If necessary, in a second stage three weeks after the first, the flap is incised at the base of the lateral wall of the nose, and the defect resulting from the relaxation of the medial and lateral tissues is covered by a full-thickness retroauricular or supraclavicular skin graft. The second procedure releases the tension of the advancement flap and restores the angle between the base of the lateral wall and the cheek. As in the case of the nasolabial flap, this mode of repair is not advocated in the young patient.

Defects Repaired by Skin Grafts. Skin grafting of the nose is a relatively simple procedure

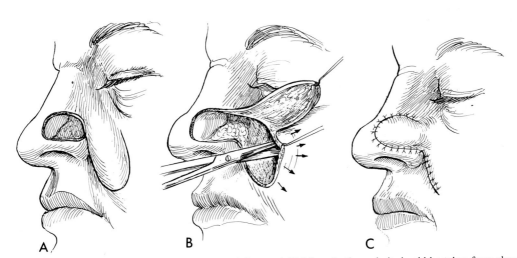

FIGURE 29–203. The nasolabial flap. *A*, Design of the nasolabial flap. In the male it should be taken from above the bearded area of the face. *B*, Undermining the donor area of the cheek to facilitate closure. *C*, The flap has been transferred and the donor area of the flap closed by direct approximation.

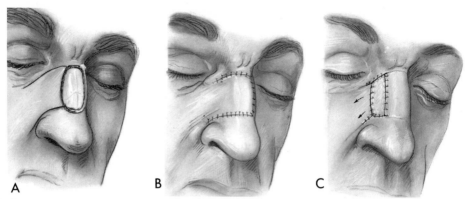

FIGURE 29–204. The 1–2 flap (Converse, 1964). *A,* Defect over the dorsum of the nose; a cheek advancement flap has been designed. *B,* The flap is advanced to cover the nasal dorsal defect. This type of flap is particularly indicated in older individuals in whom tissues are loose. *C,* If necessary, in a second stage an incision is made near the base of the lateral wall of the nose, and a full-thickness skin graft taken from the retroauricular area is placed in the resulting defect.

and is generally successful under favorable conditions. As is true of local flaps, the length of time involved in hospitalization and convalescence is considerably shortened as compared with that required for the transfer of distant flaps. Satisfactory results are obtained by the use of full-thickness retroauricular grafts; skin may be obtained from the supraclavicular areas in males. The entire retroauricular area from the rim of the helix to the hairline is removed; the resulting retroauricular defect is covered by a split-thickness skin graft. Sufficient skin may be obtained to cover the entire nose. If necessary, both retroauricular areas may be used as donor sites. The greater part of the outer covering of the nose can be resurfaced in one operation (Fig. 29–205, *A*). When skin from these areas is not available, the graft is taken from more distant sites—for example, the inner aspect of the arm—but the color match is often poor.

Difficulties are encountered in maintaining adequate pressure over the skin graft because of the shape and resiliency of the lower part of the nose. The open method of skin grafting (see Chapter 6) is preferable when the patient

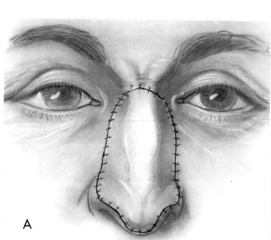
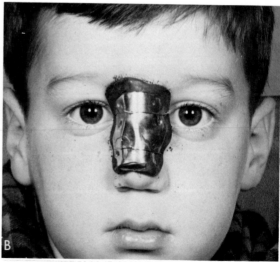

FIGURE 29–205. Resurfacing the dorsum of the nose by a skin graft. *A,* The graft has been sutured to the edge of the defect. In the adult, the open method is often the preferable technique. *B,* In the child, a splint consisting of dental compound carried on a piece of Asche metal and maintained by through-and-through wires traversing the skeletal structures of the nose is a useful device.

is an adult and the operation can be done under local anesthesia.

In children a pressure dressing is usually necessary to avoid disturbance of the graft. The nasal vestibules are firmly packed to prevent depression of the cartilages, and uniform pressure is applied to the nasal pyramid. A satisfactory method of obtaining uniform pressure in the child is the dental compound splint maintained by transosseous wiring (Fig. 29–205, *B*).

After the skin graft is sutured to the edges of the defect, it is covered by a layer of nonadherent dressing material. A thin layer of absorbent cotton or Acrilan moistened with saline solution is placed over the graft and maintained by the splint; the cotton dries and hardens, forming a solid covering. The cotton is again moistened at the first dressing in order to facilitate its removal.

A difficult area to skin graft is the lateral wall of the nose near the medial canthus. Transosseous wiring (see Chapter 28, Fig. 28–158) placed through both bony lateral walls permits the application of adequate pressure over the graft. Acrylic buttons lined with softened dental compound and maintained by the twisted transosseous wires ensure fixation of the pressure dressing.

Defects Repaired by Forehead Flaps and Distant Flaps. Distant flaps are indicated when local tissue for flaps is not available, when the recipient bed is unsuitable for a skin graft, or when the nature of the defect requires subcutaneous tissue as well as skin. The donor areas of skin flaps in the order of their preference are the forehead, arm, neck, chest, and abdominal wall.

Forehead flaps are preferred to distant flaps for the correction of nasal defects in most cases because the skin of the forehead harmonizes in color and texture with that of the nose and the rest of the face; moreover, the forehead flap requires fewer operative steps.

Additional details concerning the technique of forehead flaps and distant flaps can be found later in the chapter (see p. 1209). When a large area is to be resurfaced, a scalping flap is satisfactory (see Fig. 29–252); a median flap (see Fig. 29–240) can be employed for smaller defects. An excellent technique which provides one-stage repair of a surface defect of the nose is the island flap technique (see Fig. 29–245). Of the other types of distant flaps, the Tagliacotian brachial flap is often preferred because of the thinness and suppleness of the skin of the medial aspect of the arm.

Deformities of the Lining of the Nose

John Marquis Converse, M.D.

Contraction following loss of the lining of the nose through injury, infection, radiation, or disease results in contracture or stenosis of the nasal vestibule or fossa and in some cases collapse of the nasal dorsum. The condition is more complicated when the supporting framework of the nose has been fractured or partially destroyed. The external contour of the nose is not usually altered by adhesions of moderate degree within the nose; extensive loss of nasal lining, however, especially when complicated by infection, may alter the contour of the lower part of the nose.

The surgical treatment of nasal stenosis depends upon the extent and location of the obstruction, the condition of the surrounding lining, and the degree of external deformity.

Z-plasty for Linear Scar Contracture. When the loss of vestibular skin is not extensive and the air passage is obstructed by a linear ring of scar tissue, the repair is accomplished by Z-plasty transposition flaps. These procedures are indicated when the web is limited to the vestibule, where incisions for the transposition of flaps are feasible.

The two layers of the ring of the stenosed area are separated by an incision along the border of the constriction. A vertical incision is made through the caudal portion of the vestibular lining, beginning at the roof of the nostril close to the septum and extending down to the edge of the ring (Fig. 29–206, *A*). Another flap is formed on the cephalic lining of the stenosing ring by an incision along the lateral wall (Fig. 29–206, *B, C*). The contracture is relieved by transposing a triangular flap from each side of the constricted ring (Fig. 29–206, *D, E*). Petrolatum gauze packing is maintained in the vestibule for a few days. If contraction leading to recurrence of the contracture is feared, an impression of the vestibule is taken with softened dental compound, and an acrylic mold is fabricated and worn by the patient for a period of time. This is routine if intranasal skin grafting is indicated.

Skin Grafting Within the Nose. Earlier in this chapter (see Fig. 29–165), intranasal skin grafting for relief of stenosis caused by faulty surgical procedures in the course of a corrective rhinoplasty was described. Penetrating injuries, lacerations, faulty readjustment of the intransal tissues following partial avulsion of

the nose, loss of nasal lining mucous membrane by destruction or avulsion—these are some of the causes of constricting scars which produce stenosis of the nasal airway. The most severe case was that of a young man who was admitted to the Institute of Reconstructive Plastic Surgery one week after sulfuric acid had been poured, as an act of vengeance, into his left nasal fossa while he was asleep. Extensive destruction had resulted in sloughing of intranasal tissue and complete obliteration of the left nasal fossa to the nasopharynx. The fabrication of a mold carrying a split-thickness skin graft was required to reline the nasal fossa from the vestibule to the choana after the septum and the lateral nasal wall had been separated. A submucous resection of the septal framework was done to facilitate the procedure. In more moderate types of intranasal stenosis involving the nasal vestibule and the nasal valve, the scars are excised and the lateral wall is freed from the septum. A full-thickness retroauricular graft or a graft removed from the medial aspect of the arm, or a split-thickness graft of oral mucosa, is employed, depending on the size of

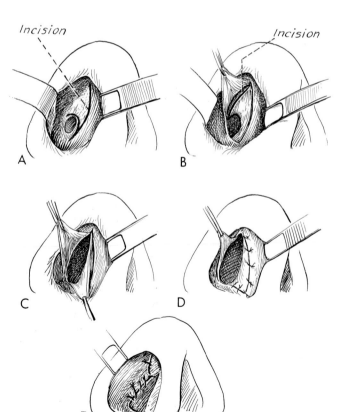

FIGURE 29–206. Correction of nasal stenosis. *A,* Incision through the septal mucoperichondrium is extended around the opening of the stenosed area. *B,* The flap is carefully dissected from a posterior flap, which is outlined. *C,* The posterior flap is raised. *D,* The posterior flap covers the defect on the septum. *E,* The anterior flap covers the raw area over the lateral wall.

the intranasal defect. Provision is also made for fixation of the skin graft within the nose. A temporary mold of dental compound serves as the carrier for the graft. The compound is softened and molded into an oval cone, then is cooled and hardened. The outer layer is covered with petrolatum and flamed; the inner part of the compound is not softened. The cone is then reintroduced into the nasal cavity, molded against the lateral wall, and removed (Fig. 29–207, *A*). It is necessary to overexpand the raw area by making the mold larger than necessary without risking excessive tension on the soft tissues of the nose. An excess of skin graft can thus be introduced, and the tight fit of the mold ensures coaptation of the graft to the raw area. The graft is wrapped around the mold, dermal surface outward; it is then inserted into the nasal cavity (Fig. 29–207, *B, C*). A similar procedure is done on the contralateral side in a separate stage, if the stenosis is bilateral.

Two sets of dental compound molds are made. The first compound mold is used immediately to serve as a graft carrier and to maintain the stenotic area in a state of dilatation. The second set is sent to the laboratory, where it is duplicated in acrylic.

The mold is retained for five to seven days. When the temporary compound mold is removed, the thin, hollowed acrylic mold is introduced into the nostril. Shrinkage and constriction of the graft are thus minimized. The postoperative mold is retained for several months until the tendency for contraction of the skin graft has been overcome.

When stenosis is the result of excessive removal of lateral and alar cartilage as well as nasal lining (see Fig. 29–165), the prosthesis supports the deficient cartilaginous structures and may be retained permanently to assure patency of the airway and support of the alae. The advantage of the mold technique, despite the inconvenience to the patient of wearing an intranasal prosthesis, albeit not visible to the onlooker, is that the shape of the nose is modified by changing the design of the mold.

Mucosal grafts removed from the oral mucous membrane may be employed for the intranasal grafts; mucosa does not tend to crust or produce a fetid odor as does skin.

The Nasomaxillary Skin Graft Inlay. A severe deformity results when the nasal bones and the middle portion of the maxilla have been destroyed or are underdeveloped due to trauma in childhood. The condition has been referred to as a "dish-face deformity." Gillies (1923) developed a technique which frees the nose and the adjacent soft tissues from the atrophied or underdeveloped skeletal structures and lines the cavity with a skin graft and a prosthetic appliance. The technique was applied to the treatment of the syphilitic nasomaxillary deformity, a rare condition at the present time. Antia (1974) has reported excellent results in correcting the saddle-nose deformity of leprosy by the nasomaxillary skin graft technique. The nasal lining is progressively necrosed in leprosy, and the necrotic process spreads to the cartilages and bones of

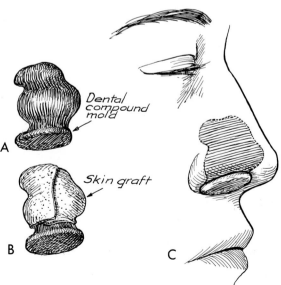

FIGURE 29–207. Skin grafting inlay technique for the correction of intranasal stenosis. *A*, A dental compound mold has been made from an impression of the nasal airway after resection of the scar tissue causing the intranasal contracture. A skin graft is wrapped around the mold. A duplicate mold is also made and sent to the laboratory for the preparation of the definitive acrylic mold. *B*, The mold covered by the skin graft. *C*, The position of the mold inside the nasal cavity is outlined.

the nose. The nasomaxillary area thus freed from its constricted state is supported by a prosthesis.

The technique, which has the inconvenience that the patient must continuously wear, cleanse, and replace the appliance, is best suited for the edentulous patient as the prosthe-

tic support for the nose is an extension of the denture.

The nasal skin graft inlay technique is illustrated in Figure 29–208. A typical example of a patient requiring such reconstruction is shown in Figure 29–209. The patient was injured by a bomb fragment which entered the face in front

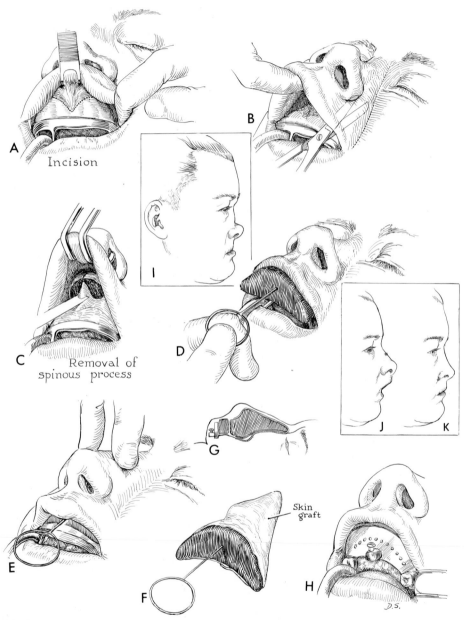

FIGURE 29–208. Technique of the nasomaxillary skin graft inlay. *A*, Outline of the intraoral incision. *B*, The nasal cavity is entered through the mouth. *C*, The nasal spine is resected. *D*, A dental compound mold is fitted to the nasomaxillary cavity. *E*, The softened dental compound is molded to the nasomaxillary cavity by external digital pressure. *F*, The mold is covered with a split-thickness skin graft, raw surface outward. *G*, The mold carrying the skin graft is placed inside the maxillary cavity. It is held in position by a splint anchored to the upper molar teeth. In this patient, the remainder of the maxillary teeth are absent. *H*, The dental appliance maintaining the mold in the nasomaxillary cavity. *I, J, K*, Appearance of the patient before, during, and after the skin graft inlay procedure.

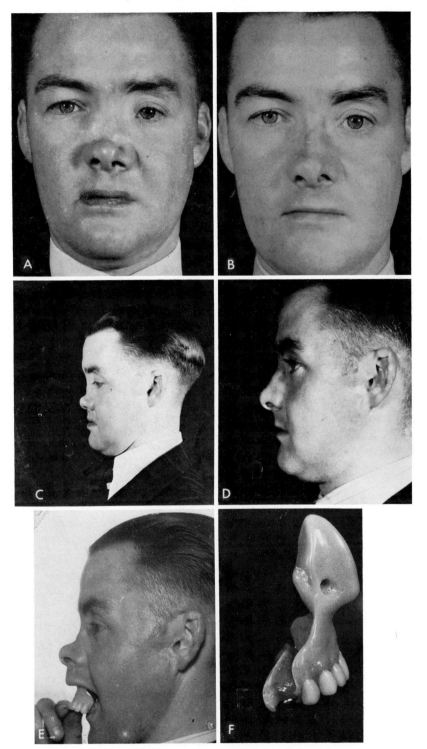

FIGURE 29–209. Contour restoration of the nasomaxillary area by the skin graft inlay technique. *A*, The deformity of the nasomaxillary area caused by a bombing injury, which resulted in destruction of bone (nasal bone, superior alveolar process, and adjacent maxillary bone), nasal septum and nasal lining. Note the deepened nasolabial folds and the retrusion of the midface. *B*, Result obtained by the nasomaxillary skin graft inlay technique illustrated in Figure 29–208. Note the change in contour of the midface and upper lip. *C*, Profile view of the patient before the operation. *D*, Restoration of contour obtained by the nasomaxillary skin graft technique. *E*, The patient introducing the prosthesis. *F*, Photographs of the appliance. The denture is prolonged upward by an extension forming the nasal support. Holes are provided in the appliance to provide nasal airways.

1204

The Head and Neck

of the left ear. The missile traversed the upper part of the maxillary sinus, penetrated the lateral wall of the nose, continued across the nasal cavity, and made its exit on the right side of the nose. Most of the supporting nasal structures were destroyed; the skin, however, except for the scars remaining in the wake of the bomb fragment, remained intact.

A description of the operative procedure follows. Under oroendotracheal anesthesia, an incision is made in the upper buccal sulcus (Fig. 29–208, *A*); the nasal fossa is entered from within the sulcus (Fig. 29–208, *B*), and the nasal structures are freed of adhesions; an extensive raw area results. The nasal spine is removed (Fig. 29–208, *C*). A dental compound mold is constructed to fit the pyramidal cavity (Fig. 29–208, *D*) with the apex pointing upward

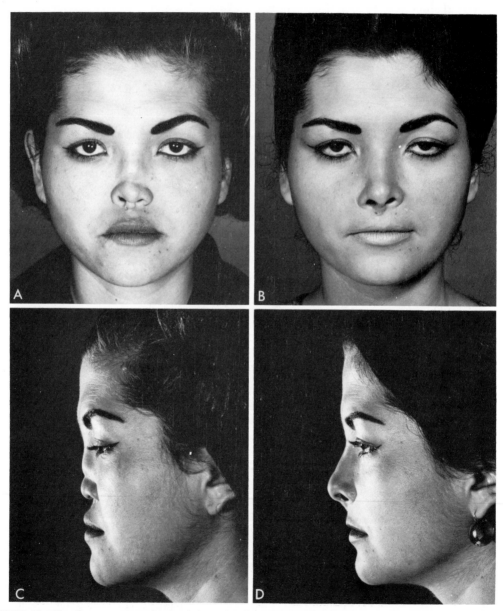

FIGURE 29–210. Contour restoration by the nasomaxillary skin graft technique. *A*, Appearance of the patient with complete loss of nasal lining and nasal obstruction resulting from the application of radon seeds at the age of 8 years for the treatment of epistaxis. *B*, Result obtained by the nasomaxillary skin graft inlay technique. *C*, Preoperative profile view showing nasomaxillary retrusion. *D*, Postoperative result.

in order that the mold can be inserted and removed easily. The mold is duplicated to construct a permanent acrylic prosthesis. (The permanent prosthesis may be prepared in the operating room using quick-curing acrylic.) A split-thickness skin graft from a nonhairy donor area is spread over the mold, raw surface outward, and is inserted into the nasal cavity (Fig. 29–208, *E* to *G*). The skin graft–carrying mold is maintained by a splint attached to the molar teeth (Fig. 29–208, *H*). The preoperative contour of the patient is shown in Figure 29–208, *I*. The tissues should be distended by the compound mold in order to ensure close coaptation of the graft with the soft tissues and to counteract possible subsequent contraction of the graft (Fig. 29–208, *J*); the mold is removed after two weeks and the cavity examined and cleansed. At intervals during subsequent weeks, the size of the mold is diminished. After a period of many weeks, a permanent acrylic prosthesis maintains the contour of the final nose (Figs. 29–208, *K* and 29–209). When the patient is edentulous, the prosthesis is an upper extension of the denture (Fig. 29–209, *F*).

The nasomaxillary skin graft inlay technique is indicated, as a last resort, in certain types of nasomaxillary deformity when no other solution can be found. It has also been employed in patients who received radiation early in life and in whom the nose failed to develop (Fig. 29–210). One of our patients with a severe nasomaxillary deformity resulting from an automobile accident sought corrective treatment after ten previous surgical attempts had failed and has worn such a prosthesis for over 25 years. In certain types of "dish-face" nasomaxillary deformities, correction can be achieved by the LeFort II or the naso-orbitomaxillary advancement osteotomy, which is described in Chapter 30 (see p. 1455).

Nasolabial Flaps for Relining the Nose. One method of repairing the collapsed nose consists of restoring the lining by turning two flaps of skin inward from the nasolabial region (Kazanjian, 1948). This technique is applicable in the older patient in whom the abundant tissue of the nasolabial area is available without causing undue scarring or distortion. An incision is made around the alar margins extending to the base of the columella, and the tip and alae of the nose are retracted upward. The nasal lining is freed from the scar tissue and dissected freely over the entire nose, including the region of the bony bridge. A flap is prepared on each side within and parallel to the nasolabial folds (Fig. 29–211, *A*). The flaps are raised, turned inward, crossed over one another, and sutured in place to form a new lining for the nasal cavity. No attempt is made to suture the bases of the alae at this time (Fig. 29–211, *B*). The pedicles of the flaps forming the inner lining of the nose are divided two weeks later; some of the excess tissue is excised, and the bases of the alae are replaced and sutured (Fig. 29–211, *C*).

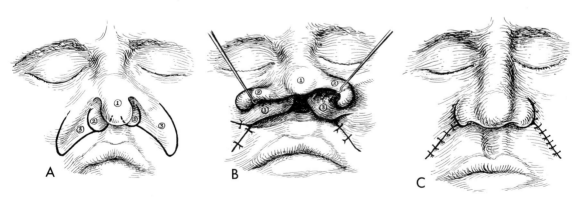

FIGURE 29–211. Restoration of nasal lining by nasolabial flaps. *A*, Outline of incisions for nasolabial flaps. The incisions extend around the base of the alae and the columella. *B*, The alae and the nasal tip are retracted upward; the scar tissue inside the nasal fossa is resected, and the nasolabial flaps are turned into the nasal cavity. *C*, In a second stage, the pedicle of the nasolabial flaps is severed, the alae are replaced, and the donor areas of the nasolabial flaps are closed by direct approximation. (From Kazanjian, V. H.: Plastic repair of deformities about the lower part of the nose resulting from loss of tissue. Trans. Am. Acad. Ophthalmol. Otolaryngol., *43*:338, 1937.)

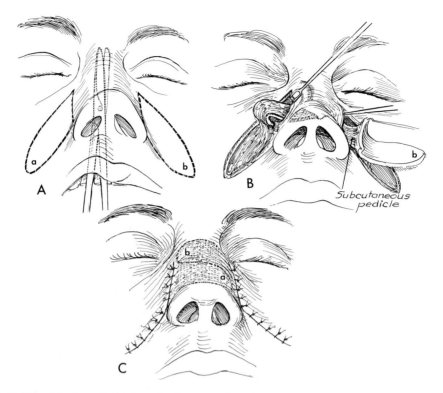

FIGURE 29–212. Island nasolabial flaps for the restoration of the lining of the nose. *A,* Outline of island nasolabial flaps. The scar tissue inside the nose is resected through an intraoral approach. *B,* The nasolabial flaps have been raised on a subcutaneous pedicle and are introduced into the nasal cavity. *C,* Position of the nasolabial flaps one above the other. The donor areas have been closed by direct approximation. (After Antia, 1974.)

Antia (1974) has been able to raise large flaps in patients with leprosy who have loose tissue in the nasolabial areas without detaching the alae by hinging the flaps on the nasal mucoperiosteum (Fig. 29–212).

Median Forehead Flap for Relining the Nose (Kazanjian, 1948). The median forehead flap technique for relining the nose is shown in Figure 29–213, and a patient in whom the technique was employed is shown in Figure 29–214, *A, B.*

The following are the stages of the relining procedure:

1. A transverse full-thickness incision is made through the cartilaginous nose, and the nasal cavity is entered. The incision releases the lower portion of the nose, permitting it to resume its anatomical position (Fig. 29–213, *A*).

2. The true defect which becomes manifest when traction is exerted on the tip of the nose is lined by a median forehead flap, which is turned down, skin surface facing the nasal cavity; the edges of the flap are sutured to the edges of the remaining nasal lining (Figs. 29–213, *B*).

3. The raw surface of the pedicle of the flap is covered by a thin split-thickness skin graft, which serves as a temporary skin dressing (Figs. 29–213, *C* and 29–214, *C*).

4. The pedicle of the flap is severed a few weeks later; the temporary skin graft is removed; and the upper portion of the flap is split and introduced into the nasal cavity, thus supplying additional nasal lining (Fig. 29–213, *D*).

5. The covering skin is sutured (Fig. 29–214, *D*). In a subsequent procedure, the contour is improved by an iliac bone graft (Fig. 29–214, *E, F*).

Variations. In conditions such as leishmaniasis and leprosy, rarely encountered in the United States, the loose external soft tissues permit two modifications of the technique. The first is to use a median island flap (see Fig. 29–245), which makes possible a one-stage introduction of forehead skin into the nose. The

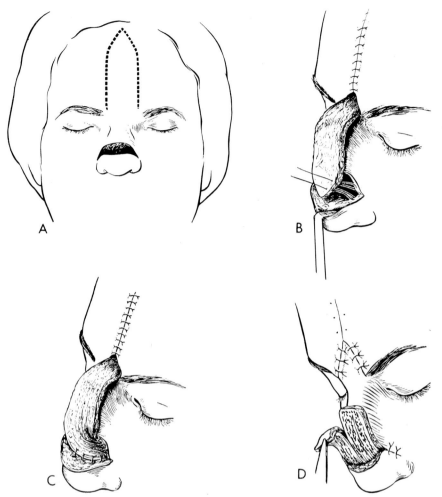

FIGURE 29–213. Restoration of nasal lining by a median forehead flap. *A*, Outline of median forehead flap. A full thickness transverse incision has been made through the cartilaginous portion of the nose. The nasal cavity is entered. The incision releases the lower portion of the nose. *B*, The median flap is introduced into the nasal cavity, skin surface toward the nasal cavity. The edges of the flap are sutured to the nasal lining. *C*, The raw surface of the flap is covered by a split-thickness skin graft. *D*, At a later stage, the pedicle of the flap is severed, the skin graft is removed, the flap is split, and each half is introduced into the nasal cavity, thus supplying additional nasal lining.

second is to de-epithelize the pedicle; the pedicle is thus more supple and may be introduced subcutaneously under the skin over the nasal bones instead of being skin-grafted and exposed to fibrosis.

Composite grafts from the auricle have also been employed with good results to provide additional lining in the foreshortened nose. The reader is referred to the last section of the chapter, which deals with techniques of length-ening the foreshortened nose and provides additional information on methods of reconstructing the lining of the nose. However, the nasomaxillary deformity is more than a nasal deformity characterized by shortening of the nose. The central maxillary area is hypoplastic and retruded, and dental malocclusion is often present. Maxillary osteotomies combined with lengthening of the nose are discussed in Chapter 30.

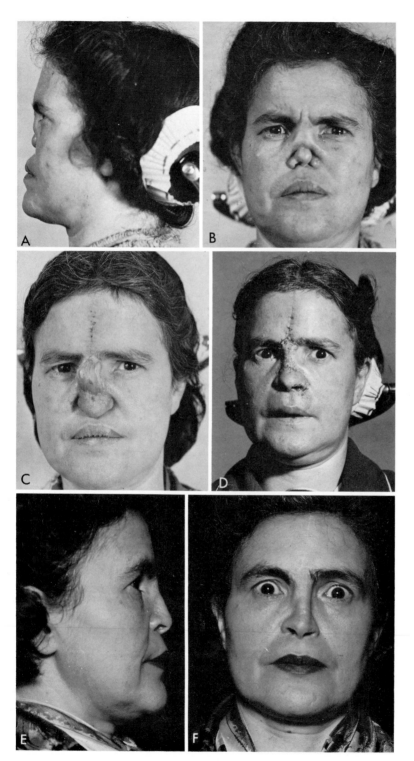

FIGURE 29–214. Stages in the reconstruction of the nose according to the technique illustrated in Figure 29–213. *A, B,* The deformity resulting from loss of nasal lining and nasal cartilages. *C,* The median forehead flap has been introduced into the nasal cavity. The raw surface is temporarily covered with a split-thickness graft. *D,* Second stage. The pedicle of the median flap has been severed, and the remainder of the flap has been introduced into the nasal cavity according to Figure 29–213, *E, F,* Appearance of the patient after the restoration of the nasal lining and subsequent restoration of contour by an iliac bone graft. (From Kazanjian and Converse.)

Full–thickness Loss
of Nasal Tissue

Defects which involve the full thickness of the nose may be relatively small, involving the loss of the ala only, a portion of the tip of the nose, or the caudal or cephalic portions of the nose. If the defect is extensive with subtotal loss of the nose, only a stump of the nasal bones remains. Loss of the entire nose is unusual in traumatic injuries but occurs following radical resection for malignant disease.

Reconstructive procedures required for full-thickness defects of the nose include restoration of the outer covering, the inner lining, and the supporting framework.

HISTORICAL BACKGROUND

The development of plastic surgery is so intimately associated with that of reconstructive rhinoplasty that a summary of the history of the art of reconstructing the nose assists one in understanding the development of newer techniques.

In ancient times amputation of the nose was considered a justifiable punishment for a variety of crimes ranging from robbery to adultery. There were episodes in ancient India during which conquered peoples were marked by amputation of the nose. In India during Vedic times (2000 B.C. to 500 B.C.), the prevailing punishment for adultery was amputation of the nose. The amputation of Lady Surpunakha's nose by Lord Rama's younger brother in Ancient India is the first recorded case of such punishment, as reported by Almast in 1967. This custom provided Indian practitioners with ample opportunity to reconstruct a missing nose. The use of the forehead flap in nasal reconstruction bears the name of "the Indian method." Blandin (1836) reported:

Baronio relates that in 1769 A.D. the city of Kirtitoor in the island of Ceylon was besieged by the Ghoorka King Pritwinarizan, and that the city was taken by treason after a long resistance. The victor, irritated by the resistance, ordered the death of the most illustrious citizens and the cutting of the nose and lips of all the inhabitants except those who knew how to play a wind instrument. The order was executed without pity for the vanquished, and the victor, to add a cruel irony to his barbarous resolve, decided that the city would from thence on carry the name Nescatapoor, which means "city of the cut noses."

Self-mutilation by cutting off the nose was also practiced by women who wished to protect their honor by disfiguring themselves. According to Rousset, as related by Nélaton and Ombrédanne (1904), this occurred during the Danish invasions of England, and when the Saracens stormed Marseilles, the Mother Superior of a convent and 40 nuns inflicted this disfigurement upon themselves.

Even in our present era, in certain regions of India and Pakistan avulsion of the nose by a sharp cutting instrument is dealt out as punishment to adulterous wives (Blocksma and Innis, 1955).

The Koomas of ancient India, members of the caste of potters, had developed the art of reconstructing the destroyed nose by means of a forehead flap, a method often referred to as the Indian method and described in the writings of Susruta (circa 800 B.C.).

In Europe during the fifteenth century, Branca and his son developed a successful rhinoplasty technique, as related by Ranzano in 1442. The elder Branca practiced the method of repair described by Susruta. Arabian scholars during the eighth century had made Arabic translations of the works of Susruta; Sicily was a center of Arabian, Greek, and Occidental learning in the eleventh and twelfth centuries. Such facts suggest that knowledge of the ancient Indian operation may have reached Branca (Gnudi and Webster, 1950).

During the sixteenth century, Tagliacozzi, eminent anatomist and surgeon of Bologna, was the first to practice reconstruction of the nose by means of a direct delayed flap from the arm. His skillful technique became known as the "Italian" or Tagliacotian method and is described in detail in his book (1597).

Reconstructive rhinoplasty appears to have been neglected during the subsequent two centuries and even to have fallen into disrepute. The period of doubt began during the sixteenth century when no less an authority than Ambroise Paré, writing in 1575, after scoffing at the concept that a severed and detached portion of the nose could ever be successfully replanted, expressed an unfavorable opinion concerning nose reconstruction (see Chapter 1, p. 5).

During the seventeenth and eighteenth centuries Tagliacozzi's work and the subject of nose reconstruction came to be symbols of the ridiculous, and tales arose of "sympathetic slaves" and "sympathetic noses." Stories were told of slaves who gained their freedom by donating portions of the buttock to furnish the tissue for the reconstruction of a gentleman's missing nose.

In Butler's *Hudibras* the long-suffering slave or porter is no longer credited with sacrificing merely a portion of his arm or his own nose but rather that part which has eternal comic appeal to mankind, his *derrière:*

> So learned Taliacotius from
> The brawny part of Porter's bum
> Cut supplemental Noses, which
> Would last as long as Parent breech:
> But when the last Date of Nock was out
> Off dropt the Sympathetick Snout.

Such a choice morsel as this could not be allowed to languish. Voltaire seized upon it, giving a free translation of Butler's lines, with a final macabre twist of his own.*

Interest in the Indian rhinoplasty was revived through the case of an ox driver named Cowasjee who worked for the British Army in India; the story was told in the *Hiracrrha* or gazette of Madras in 1793. This man had been captured by Typo-Sahib, who ordered that his nose be cut off to punish him for his treachery. Cowasjee's nose was later restored by a forehead flap operation performed upon him by members of the initiated caste. The publication of this case prompted English surgeons to attempt the operation, and in 1816 Carpue published the successful results of the operation in two patients (see Chapter 1, p. 8).

Von Graefe (1818) performed a nasal reconstruction in Berlin using the method of Tagliacozzi, and the following year he employed the Indian method. In Munich Reiner, after a voyage to England where he had seen Carpue operate, also employed the Indian method (Jobert, 1849). In France, the Indian rhinoplastic operation was practiced by Delpech in Montpellier in 1823 and within the next few years by Lisfranc (1827) and Labat (1833, 1834).

Dieffenbach, as early as 1829, began to classify procedures and improvements in the technique of forehead flap rhinoplasty and described them in 1845; his book is a major contribution to the literature of plastic surgery.

One can only marvel at the dexterity of the surgeons and the courage of both patients and operators in those pioneer preaseptic days before the development of anesthesia. The following episode told by Labat (1833) is illustrative of an operation for reconstructing the nose performed by him in the year 1827. Labat's patient, named Lannelongue, was a former solider in the Napoleonic armies; he had lost his nose as a result of frostbite during the retreat from Moscow. The patient, maintained by two aides, was seated in a chair:

> ... when I lengthened the incision toward the root of the nose, the patient suffered such intense pain that he struggled from the firm grasp of the aides and ran toward the door to avoid submitting himself to the remainder of the surgical procedure. At this moment Lannelongue presented a frightful aspect: his forehead showed a gaping wound, the edges of which were further retracted by pain, his face, neck, and clothing were inundated with blood; but the most horrible sight of all was the flap of palpitating flesh which flopped first over one cheek and then the other with every movement he made. Judging that my exhortations would be useless because persuasion could no longer have any effect on the mind of Lannelongue, exasperated by the pain, I ran after him and locked the door of the apartment, putting the key in my pocket. In the authoritative tone required by the peculiar position in which I found myself, I ordered him to return to the place I had assigned to him for the operation, under the threat of the use of force. Lannelongue, realizing that further resistance was useless, sat down on the chair and withstood the remainder of the operation without even being required to be held by the aides.

THE EVOLUTION OF THE FOREHEAD FLAP

The subject of reconstructive rhinoplasty during the nineteenth century received considerable attention. Amputation of the nose in battle and the prevalence of "scrofulous" disease, syphilis, noma, and cancer explain this interest. Keegan, whose book published in 1900 is a culminating point of this abundant literature, states that in 1897 at least 152 reconstructive

---

*Ainsi Taliacotius grand Esculape d'Etrurie répara tous les nez perdus par une nouvelle industrie; il vous prenait adroitement un morceau du cul d'un pauvre homme, l'appliquait au nez proprement; enfin il arrivait qu'en somme, tout juste à la mort du prêteur, tombait le nez du l'emprunteur, et souvent dans la même bière, par justice et bon accord, on remettait au gré du mort le nez auprès de son derrière (Voltaire, 1785).

rhinoplastic operations had been reported in Europe. His book also gives an account of his personal experience of 100 rhinoplastic operations during his five-year stay in India. The outstanding reviews on the subject include those of Carpue (1816), von Graefe (1818), Delpech (1824), Labat (1834), Blandin (1836), Dieffenbach (1829–1834, 1845–1848), Liston (1837), Zeis (1838), Malgaigne (1838), Velpeau (1839), Serre (1842), von Ammon and Baumgarten (1842), and Jobert (1849). The first reconstructive rhinoplasty in America appears to have been performed by Warren in 1837. The American translation in 1852 of Velpeau's textbook included a report on the work of Pancoast and Mutter of Philadelphia and that of Mott, Post, and Buck of New York (Gnudi and Webster, 1950). Published in the latter part of the nineteenth century, the works of von Szymanowski (1870) and of Verneuil (1877) are outstanding.

The nineteenth century literature was compiled and classified by Nélaton and Ombrédanne (1904) in a book in which the authors illustrated with drawings the various techniques previously described. The comprehensive treatise by Nélaton and Ombrédanne remains one of the most reliable sources of reference for the surgeon. Joseph (1931) reviewed the subject and described his technique in two patients.

The historical reviews of Davis (1919 and 1941) and Fomon (1939) and the erudite treatise by Gnudi and Webster (1950) are more recent valued contributions in the English language.

In the early operations the median Indian flap was used exclusively. That some difficulty with vascularization of the flap was encountered is illustrated by the opinion of Dieffenbach, who, impressed by the fact that inadequately vascularized flaps became blue, advocated ligating some of the nutrient vessels, a precept violently opposed by many of his contemporaries, including Blandin and Serre. Leeches were also employed to assist in decongesting the blue flap due to venous embarrassment.

The twisting of the base of the pedicle of the forehead flap, attaining an angle of 190 degrees, frequently resulted in vascular congestion and produced a kink at the root of the nose. Surgeons hesitated to remove this kink by severing the pedicle in a second stage operation for fear of depriving the new nose of its vascular supply and also of imposing an additional operation upon the patient, a painful

ordeal before the discovery of anesthesia. Some surgeons also felt that the reconstructed nose would collapse after the pedicle was sectioned (Fig. 29–215). It is of interest that Millard (1974) has advocated preservation of the neurovascular bundle when the pedicle is severed to enhance the vitality of the flap.

The disadvantage of the kink was alleviated by modifications introduced in the incisions outlining the base of the pedicle. Lisfranc in 1827 extended one incision lower than the other, and Dieffenbach lengthened one incision until it reached the defect (Fig. 29–216), thus reducing the twisting of the base of the pedicle and the resultant deprivation of blood supply. The immediate results of these operations appeared satisfactory. Considerable shrinkage occurred in the postoperative period, however, and the narial openings of the reconstructed nose became constricted. Larrey observed the late results of Blandin's and Lisfranc's reconstructions and found them "horrible." Dupuytren was also liberal with his sarcastic remarks at the meetings of the Surgical Society. Later in the nineteenth century Denonvilliers was to comment disdainfully that all surgery accomplished was to "replace a disgusting deformity by a ridiculous one." Most surgeons, however, were in accord with Dieffenbach in attempting to relieve the sufferer laboring under such an affliction, "at the sight of whom all men turn in disgust and abhorence, and at whose presence children cry and dogs bark."

The Raw Area Under the Flap; the Lining. The danger of a raw area under the flap, open to suppuration, fibrosis, and contraction, came to be realized. The understanding of the necessity for providing a lining was the next advance in the development of the technique of forehead flap rhinoplasty. In their early operations Carpue, von Graefe, Delpech, Labat, Blandin,

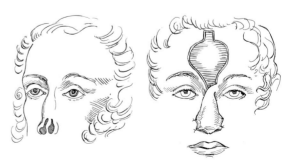

FIGURE 29–215. Design of an early 19th century rhinoplasty, showing the narrow pedicle of the median Indian-type rhinoplasty.

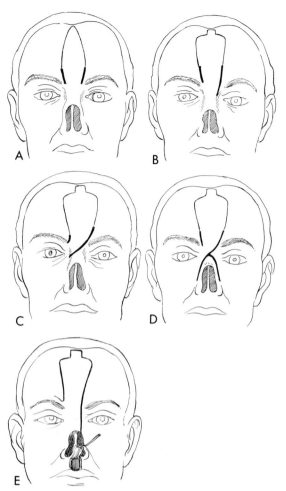

FIGURE 29–216. Evolution of the incisions to diminish the twist of the base of the forehead flap. (After Nélaton and Ombrédanne, 1904.) *A*, Incisions employed in the Indian rhinoplasty. *B*, Lisfranc's modification. *C*, *D*, Labat's modifications. *E*, Dieffenbach's modification.

traction of the tip of the reconstructed nose to the presence of a raw surface on the posterior aspect of the new columella that became adherent to the raw surface under the remainder of the flap; he advocated raising the flap from the upper lip to line the new columella.

To eliminate the raw area on the deep surface of the forehead flap, surgeons began to utilize the integument of the remaining portions of the nose, turned down as a lining flap, as advocated by Volkmann (1874); flaps from the adjacent facial area (Thiersch, 1879); or split-thickness skin grafts (Lössen, 1898).

The preliminary lining of the flap by a split-thickness or a full-thickness skin graft has been attempted in subtotal reconstructive rhinoplasty by a number of surgeons during the present century. The flap, however, is rigid and does not adapt to the rounded shape of the dorsum, and a line of cleavage between flap and graft cannot be developed for the placing of a skeletal framework.

The publication by Blair (1925) gave the final consecration to use of the forehead flap for subtotal and total reconstruction; the distal end was folded upon itself to provide the columella, the tip, and the lining of the alae and was lined with adjacent flaps. Later developments included the use of an auricular chondrocutaneous graft to line the ala (Gillies, 1943), of a septal chondromucosal graft for the same purpose (Converse, 1956), of nasolabial flaps for the lining of the alae in preference to the infolded distal end of the flap (Millard, 1966, 1974), and of the forehead island flap when a larger amount of lining was required (Converse, 1969).

The Length of the Flap. Additional problems confronting surgeons included obtaining a flap of sufficient length to permit folding the end of the flap upon itself and providing a columella of adequate length, which often could not be achieved with the Indian median flap (Fig. 29–217, *A*). Most of the reconstructed noses showed a short columella and downwardly retracted tip. According to Verneuil (1877), Auvert, a French surgeon practicing in Moscow prior to 1850, designed a flap slanting across the forehead at an angle of 45 degrees in order to obtain a longer flap (Fig. 29–217, *B*). Ward described a similar oblique forehead flap in 1856. The oblique flap appears to have come into general use in the latter part of the nineteenth century, and most of the flaps described by the German surgeons in this period assume an even more horizontal posi-

and Dieffenbach appear to have folded the distal end of the forehead to form the columella. The alar portions do not appear, however, to have been lined; an attempt was made to maintain the narial openings by rubber tubing. Serre in 1842 stated, "by folding the end of the flap, placing the deep surface in contact with itself, it would be easier to preserve the shape of the nose." According to Calderini (1842), Petrali was the first to emphasize the folding of the distal end of the flap upon itself in order to form the tip, the alae, and the columella and to eliminate raw areas in the lower part of the reconstructed nose.

Sédillot (1856) attributed postoperative re-

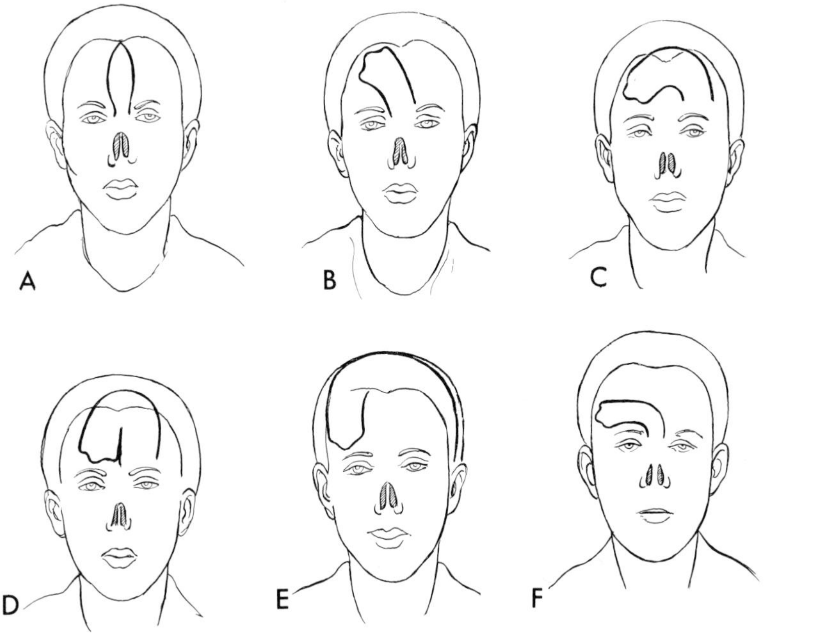

FIGURE 29–217. Various types of forehead flaps. *A,* The Indian forehead flap. *B,* The oblique flap. *C,* Gillies' up-and-down flap. *D,* Gillies' modification of the up-and-down flap. *E,* The scalping flap. *F,* The supraorbital flap. (From Converse, J. M.: Reconstruction of the nose by the scalping flap technique. Surg. Clin. North Am., *39:*335, 1959.)

tion, with a wider base which includes the blood supply from the supraorbital vessels on one side. Millard (1966), in order to achieve adequate length and width, used a horizontal flap which included a major portion of the forehead for total nasal reconstruction (See Fig. 29–291).

In 1935 Gillies described a radical departure from the oblique forehead flap which had come into general use; he used a flap which ascended into the hair-bearing scalp and then descended down into the forehead, a technique to which he gave the name "up-and-down" flap (Fig. 29–217, *C, D*). This procedure permitted obtaining greater flap length while utilizing a flap of sufficient width to ensure blood supply. The scalping flap (Converse, 1942) is a further extension of the "up-and-down" forehead flap technique (Fig. 29–217, *E*). Schmid (1952) employed horizontal supraorbital flaps for piecemeal subtotal nasal reconstruction.

Importance of a Long Columella. Increase in the length of the forehead flap provides adequate projection of the tip of the reconstructed nose which depends upon a columella of adequate length (see Fig. 29–258). The new columella must be reinforced by lining its posterior surface with a hinge flap from the recipient site. Millard (1966) has used a flap of labial mucosa brought up through a buttonhole in the lip for this purpose, a useful method if the re-

cipient site of the columella is scarred and poorly vascularized.

The Skeletal Framework. A further advance was made when the reconstructed nose was provided with a skeletal framework. Ollier in 1861 suggested including the periosteum of the frontal bone in the forehead flap in the hope that bone would regenerate from the transplanted periosteum. In 1864 he attempted to include a strip of frontal bone under the forehead flap; these attempts proved unsuccessful. König (1886) added a strip of bone in the forehead flap, and Israel (1896) employed a tibial bone graft for support. After von Mangold (1899) employed costal cartilage for the repair of a saddle-nose deformity, Nélaton (1902) embedded costal cartilage under the forehead flap prior to the transfer of the flap to the defective nasal area, a procedure which Gillies (1920) considered unsound, reaffirming this opinion in his book (Gillies and Millard, 1957).

Gillies advocated the use of the remaining portion of the septum, swinging it forward on an inferior pedicle, at the time of the reconstruction of the nose to support the tip. Millard (1974) modified this concept, advancing the remnants of the septum on a superior pedicle by means of an L-shaped incision (see Fig. 29–282).

Millard (1966) has succeeded in furnishing a

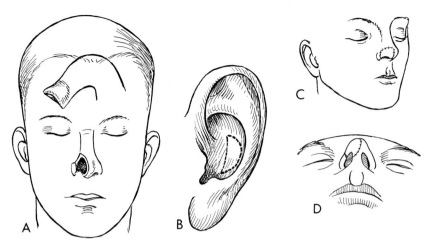

FIGURE 29–218. Use of a conchal composite flap in conjunction with an up-and-down forehead flap. *A,* Up-and-down forehead flap with a conchal composite graft imbedded under its distal end. *B,* Outline of conchal composite graft. *C, D,* The reconstruction of a defect involving the tip and the ala resulting from a dog bite. (After Gillies, 1943.)

cantilever bone graft to the reconstructed nose during the primary operation.

If the columella is of sufficient length to maintain the projection of the reconstructed nasal tip, the placing of the framework, whether bone or cartilage (the latter when the nasal bones are destroyed), can be the final step in the reconstructive procedure, providing the "final touch" to the reconstructed nose. This is a simpler. although less spectacular approach, and the risk of failure is diminished.

Further experience is required to reach a conclusion concerning the respective merits of furnishing the framework during the primary stage or during a later stage.

The Composite Graft. Mention must be made of the development of the composite graft by König in 1887. This technique simplified the reconstruction of small and moderate-sized defects and, as mentioned earlier in the text, was later employed in conjunction with a forehead flap (Gillies, 1943) (Fig. 29–218).

SMALL TO MODERATE-SIZED FULL–THICKNESS DEFECTS OF THE LOWER PORTION OF THE NOSE

Repeatedly, the need for eclecticism has been emphasized in this text, the choice of the method of repair being made according to the clinical situation at hand. In addition, the age of the patient and the presence of preexisting traumatic, postoperative, burn or radiation scars

are factors to be considered in the selection of a suitable technique. Some of the techniques are applicable irrespective of the patient's age; others, such as the nasolabial flap technique (see Fig. 29–228), are indicated in older patients whose loose tissues permit borrowing of tissue without distortion or conspicuous scarring. Older patients may be satisfied with an esthetic result which might be considered inadequate in the younger patient. More sophisticated procedures may be required in the younger patient, particularly in female patients, such as composite grafts combined with flaps in larger defects in order to satisfy esthetic requirements.

Reconstruction with Adjacent Tissue. Local tissue is used effectively for small defects of the ala. The composite auricular graft is employed more frequently than in the past and will be described later in the text.

The border of the defect forms an acceptable alar rim in suitable cases, if an adequate nasal lining can be provided. A curved incision through only the skin is made approximately 0.5 cm posterior to the margin of the defect (Fig. 29–219, *A*). The skin of the edge of the ala is rolled downward to form the new alar border. The deficiency of the nasal lining tends to retain the alar border in its upward retracted position. In order to obviate this complication, one may mobilize additional nasal lining from the mucoperiosteum under the nasal skeleton (see Fig. 29–219, *B*). A full-thickness retroauricular skin graft remedies the deficiency of skin (Fig. 29–219, *C*).

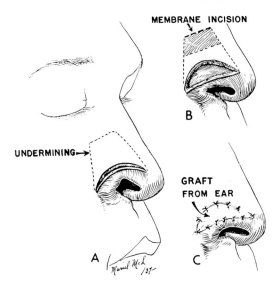

FIGURE 29–219. Correction of a retracted ala by releasing the lining and adding a full-thickness skin graft. *A,* An incision is made above the retracted ala. The nasal lining is raised from the undersurface of the lateral cartilage and nasal skeleton, where it is released by a transverse incision. A flap of mucoperiosteum and nasal mucous membrane can then be outlined. *B,* The released nasal lining leaves an area of exposed bone on the undersurface of the nasal skeleton which will undergo spontaneous reepithelization. The ala is rolled down. A skin defect persists. *C,* The skin defect is covered with a full-thickness graft from behind the ear.

In defects involving the ala satisfactory results have been obtained by releasing the deficient inner lining by mobilizing the mucoperiosteum from the undersurface of the nasal bones (Figs. 29–219 to 29–223).

Two procedures (Figs. 29–224 and 29–225) attributed to Denonvilliers by Verneuil (1877),

with an added modification using the Z-plasty technique, have also been employed with satisfactory results in victims of trauma and in older patients. The flaps extend through the full thickness of the cartilaginous nose.

RECONSTRUCTION BY THE SEPTAL FLAP TECHNIQUE. De Quervain (1902) employed this technique for correction of defects of the lateral wall of the nose. It was adapted by Kazanjian (1937) for the reconstruction of defects involving the ala. The procedure includes three stages. The first stage consists of raising a rectangular septal flap through the entire thickness of the septum at the level of the defect (Fig. 29–226, *A, B*); the base of the flap is at the dorsal border of the septum, transferred on a superior mucoperichondrial flap. The flap of cartilage, covered on both sides by mucoperichondrium, is sutured to the borders of the alar defect and is supported by a mold of dental compound or by nasal packing (Fig. 29–226, *C, D*). The remaining attachment of the septal flap to the septum is separated in the second stage; this upper border is sutured to the edge of the defect along the bridge of the nose (Fig. 29–226, *E*). In a third stage, the exposed mucous membrane of the flap is carefully dissected from the perichondrium and covered by a skin graft or flap placed over the perichondrium of the cartilage (Fig. 29–226, *F*). The septal flap should be designed in such a manner that sufficient septal cartilage remains along the dorsum of the nose to provide support. The result of this procedure is quite satisfactory, as the border of the reconstructed ala is suitable in thickness and harmonizes with the unaffected ala.

The septal flap technique is most useful in

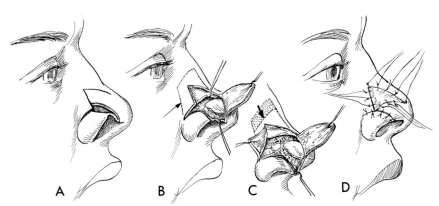

FIGURE 29–220. Repair of a defect of the ala by local flaps. *A,* Local flaps are outlined and released. *B,* The lateral cartilage is exposed, and the underlying mucous membrane is undermined; the undermining extends under the nasal bones. *C,* The shortness of lining is remedied by a technique similar to that shown in Figure 29–219. *D,* The ala has been restored. A cutaneous defect is covered by a full-thickness skin graft from behind the ear.

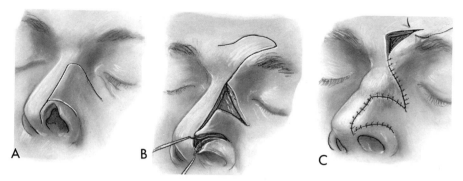

FIGURE 29–221. Repair of a defect of the ala by means of local flaps. *A*, Outline of incisions. *B*, The position of the ala is restored. Additional lining is obtained from the undersurface of the nasal bones, as shown in Figure 29–219. *C*, The operation is being completed; the cutaneous defect is closed by a forehead flap. The donor area of the forehead flap is closed by direct approximation. In this type of deformity, a composite auricular graft can be considered as an alternative method of treatment.

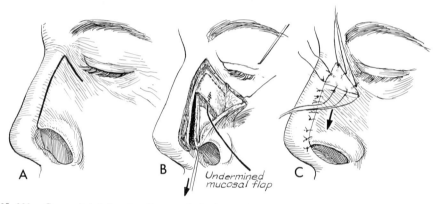

FIGURE 29–222. Congenital deformity. Retracted ala due to short lateral nasal wall. *A*, Outline of incisions. *B*, The lateral cartilage is exposed. The mucoperiosteum is elevated from the undersurface of the nasal framework in order to gain additional lining. *C*, The ala is in position. The cutaneous defect over the nasal bones is covered with a full thickness retroauricular skin graft.

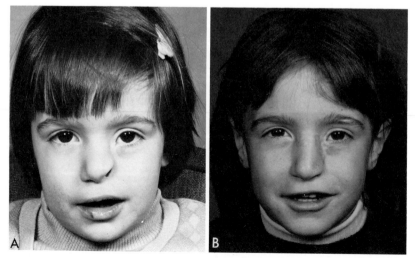

FIGURE 29–223. Defect of the ala due to a facial cleft. *A*, Appearance of the child at the age of 5 years. *B*, Three years later, after correction according to a variation of the technique shown in Figure 29–222.

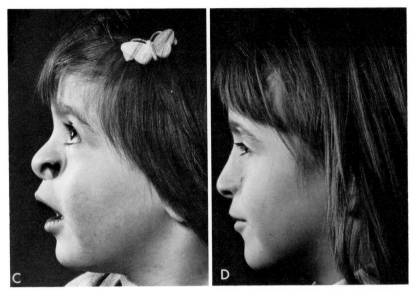

FIGURE 29–223 *Continued.   C,* Preoperative appearance. *D,* Postoperative appearance. The skin-grafted area will be covered at a later date by an island forehead flap.

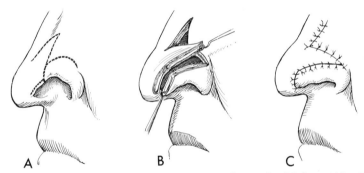

FIGURE 29–224.   Local flaps to lower the border of the ala for repair of defects. (After Denonvilliers.)

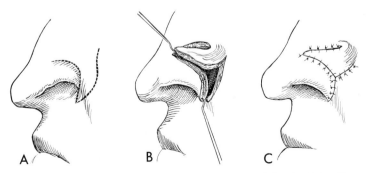

FIGURE 29–225.   Another variety of local flaps to lower the border of the ala. (After Denonvilliers, 1863.)

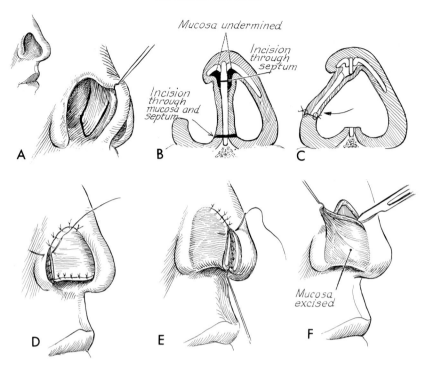

FIGURE 29–226. Repair of a full-thickness defect of the lower portion of the nose by the septal flap technique. *A, B,* Outline of the septal flap. *C,* The septal flap has been transferred into the defect and sutured to the lower border of the defect. *D,* Suture of the septal flap to the border of the base of the ala. *E,* In a second stage, the remaining connection of the septal flap to the septum is severed, and the edge of the flap is sutured to the edge of the defect. *F,* In a third stage, the mucosa is removed from the perichondrium of the septal flap, and the resultant defect is covered with a full thickness retroauricular or supraclavicular skin graft over the perichondrium. (From Kazanjian and Converse.)

the repair of larger defects of the lateral wall of the nose; a forehead flap provides the outer covering. A variant of this technique is to resect a septal cartilage graft covered on one side with mucoperichondrium. The septal cartilage and mucoperichondrium on one side is separated from the mucoperichondrium on the opposite side. The mucoperchondrial raw surface becomes reepithelized spontaneously; thus the entire thickness of the septum is not excised. The chondrocutaneous graft obtained from the septum is placed under a forehead flap, with the mucoperichondrial side of the graft against the host bed; in a later stage the septal composite graft provides the lining of the forehead flap for reconstruction of the defect (see Figs. 29–268 and 29–269).

RECONSTRUCTION WITH A NASOLABIAL FLAP. The principle of utilizing a flap from the cheek, reversed upon itself as a hinge flap, was attributed to Dupuytren by Labat (1833). Dieffenbach (1845) modified the technique by taking the flap from the nasolabial area, thus minimizing the secondary scarring. Dieffenbach folded the flap longitudinally to restore both the outer covering and the inner lining of

the ala (Fig. 29–227). This method is similar to that used to obtain a nasolabial flap to cover the skin of the nose. In male patients, the flap may include skin from below the nasolabial fold, for hair follicles in the portion of the flap employed to restore the inner lining of the ala replace the nasal vibrissae of the nasal vestibule. Use of the nasolabial flap is an expeditous technique in the older patient with a defect resulting from the excision of a carcinoma.

A small alar base defect is closed with a vertically oriented flap. The flap is based superiorly, the anterior edge being the posterior margin of the defect. The width of the flap is approximately 80 per cent that of the defect, but this will vary with the skin turgor and is a matter of individual judgment. The length of the flap should be 2½ times the vertical dimension of the defect to allow for shrinkage and production of a rolled edge.

When the alar margin has been retracted as a result of the healing of a lateral nasal defect, it is released and replaced in its anatomical position. The resultant lateral wall defect is repaired by a nasolabial flap (Fig. 29–228), which

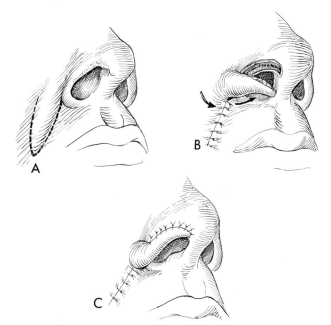

FIGURE 29–227. Nasolabial flap for the restoration of the alar border. (After Dieffenbach.) *A*, Design of the nasolabial flap. *B*, The donor area of the flap is closed by direct approximation, a procedure which tends to approximate the base of the flap to the base of the alar defect. *C*, The nasolabial flap is sutured to the border of the alar defect (see also Figure 29–228). (From Kazanjian and Converse.)

is raised together with approximately 2 mm of subcutaneous tissue. The tip and lateral border of the flap are sutured into the defect with 4–0 or 5–0 absorbable sutures, the knots of which are placed on the nasal cavity aspect. It is easier to leave the sutures untied until the majority are placed into position. A skin hook is placed to tense the skin and equalize the margins, removing the dog-ear effect. Repair of the skin edges is completed with nonabsorbable 4–0 or 5–0 sutures. Note that the subcutaneous tissues

mimic the nasal border roll and that the flap should appear a little overcorrected in size to allow for postoperative shrinkage.

The defect is closed, and the donor site edges are approximated with nonabsorbable sutures. It should rarely be necessary to undermine the margins for more than a few millimeters in the older patient; however, if tension is evident, the superolateral margin may be undermined for 1 cm. It is important that the inferomedial margins not be undermined for

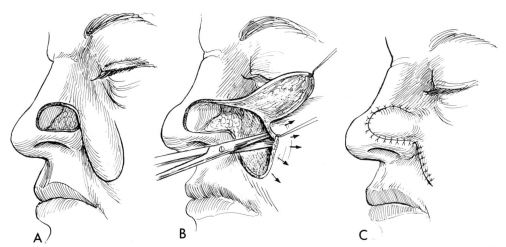

FIGURE 29–228. The nasolabial flap. *A*, Design of the nasolabial flap. In the male, it should be taken from above the bearded area of the face. *B*, Undermining the donor area of the cheek to facilitate closure. *C*, The flap has been transferred and the donor area of the flap closed by direct approximation.

more than 1 to 2 mm, as distortion of the ver-
million border may readily result. The sutures
are removed from the donor area in six to eight
days and from the nose in ten days.

For the repair of a defect resulting from a
lesion requiring excision of a larger area of alar
margin, the flap will constitute the major portion of the alar rim. The length should be 10 to
15 per cent longer than the defect and should
be measured from the lateral portion of the flap
base. The width should approximate three
times the vertical dimension when this constitutes less than 50 per cent of the ala, and 2½
times when it is greater than 50 per cent.

A notch will develop between the remaining
ala and the flap, no matter how careful the
closure, and will require later repair (see Triangular Flap Technique, Fig. 29–269).

Composite Grafts of Skin and Cartilage.
The use of composite grafts removed from the
auricle, consisting of a segment of auricular
cartilage covered on both sides by skin, to restore the alar defects was reported by König
(1887). The method does not appear to have
been utilized to any extent until interest was
revived by Gillies (1943), who reported a case
in which he had employed a composite graft
consisting of a segment of auricular cartilage
with the attached conchal cartilage (see Fig.
29–218). The graft provided the lining and
cartilaginous support for a destroyed ala and a
portion of the tip of the nose, reconstructed by
Gillies' up-and-down forehead flap technique.
An excellent result was obtained. The composite graft is transplanted in a preliminary stage
under the part of the forehead flap which is to
form the ala. Brown and Cannon (1946) renewed interest in the König type of composite
graft to restore alar margins and defects which
involved portions of the ala.

Technique of the Composite Auricular
Graft. Excision of scar tissue along the
margin of the ala is a prerequisite for obtaining
a recipient bed of well-vascularized tissue.
Hemostasis is essential, for postoperative
bleeding may prevent accurate apposition of
the graft. The dimensions of the defect are
measured, and the composite graft is removed
from the auricle.

A favorite donor site of König was the posterosuperior portion of the auricle (Fig. 29–
229). The posteroinferior area immediately
above the antitragus and the anterosuperior
area have also been employed. The secondary
defect of the ear is usually repaired by direct
approximation; notching of the helix border is

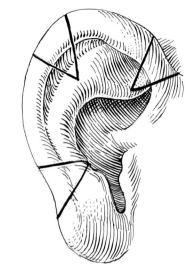

FIGURE 29–229. Donor sites for composite grafts
from the auricle.

avoided by the tongue-in-groove or Z-plasty
technique.

The graft is sutured to the edges of the
defect; the inner layer of skin is approximated
to the nasal lining with catgut sutures; the
outer layer is sutured to the skin border of the
defect with fine nylon sutures (Fig. 29–230).
Vestibular packing with moist cotton pledgets
provides a satisfactory internal splint. Composite grafts heal satisfactorily without an external dressing (Fig. 29–231).

Vascularization of Composite Grafts.
Since König (1887) first employed a piece of
auricular scapha to restore an alar defect, composite grafts of skin and cartilage, skin and fat,
and skin, fat, and cartilage have become popular in the repair of small and moderate-sized
defects of the lower portion of the nose.
Whereas a skin graft becomes vascularized
from vessels over the entire surface as well as
from the edge of the recipient site (see Chapter
6), composite grafts must depend for their
revascularization upon a much smaller surface
of contact situated along the edge of the graft.

A considerable amount of experimental data
has accumulated on the mode of revascularization of composite grafts. An experimental
model was set up by Ballantyne and Converse
(1958). A composite graft consisting of cartilage from the rabbit's ear with skin attached on
one side was placed over the chorioallantois of
the chick embryo, and the revascularization of
the composite graft was studied by histologic
examination of sections removed on the fourth

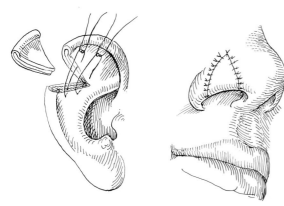

FIGURE 29-230. Technique of a composite auricular graft to repair an alar defect. *A,* The composite graft removed from the auricle. *B,* The composite graft is inserted into the nasal defect and sutured in two layers.

and fifth days after transplantation. The difference in structure between the avian nucleated erythrocytes and the non-nucleated erythrocytes facilitated the study. The avian vessels, unable to penetrate the cartilage portion of the graft, were seen to extend along the undersurface of the cartilage until the dermis of the attached skin was reached; at this point the vessels penetrated the dermis of the composite graft.

Studies have shown that the revascularization process of skin grafts is particularly active

at the junction of the graft with the edge of the skin of the recipient site (Ballantyne, Uhlschmid and Converse, 1969). Revascularization appears to be more active in this area than in the bed of the graft in the experimental animal chosen—namely the rat.

Present concepts to explain the surprising success of composite grafts can be summarized as follows. Highly vascularized tissues, such as the nose and the auricle, contain a proportionally denser network of endothelial channels than other tissues. This characteristic facilitates the imbibition of fluids from the recipient tissues, which maintain the moisture of the graft until vascular connections and vascular ingrowth from the host establish the final revascularization of the graft. As in skin grafts, stereomicroscopic observations in man (see Chapter 6) show that after a period of 48 hours, vascular flow can be observed in composite grafts (Rees, Wood-Smith, Converse and Guy, 1963). Stereomicroscopic observations have shown that the blood flow is established in the area adjacent to the area of junction with the host bed; active flow is gradually propagated toward the graft during subsequent days.

It may be concluded, therefore, that the wider the surface of contact between a composite graft and the host, the more rapid the revascularization of the graft. The success or failure of a composite graft depends not only

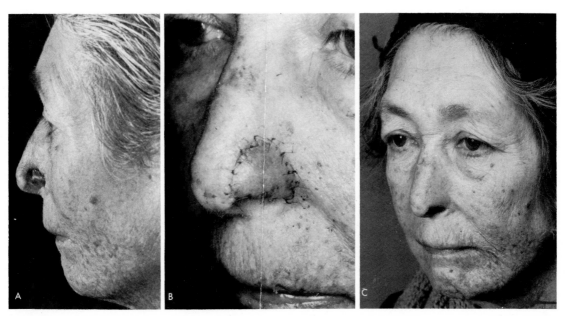

FIGURE 29-231. Composite graft for the repair of an alar defect. *A,* Large alar defect. *B,* Composite graft sutured to the edges of the defect. *C,* Result obtained following transplantation of the composite graft taken from the postero-superior portion of the auricle.

upon the surface of contact with the host bed but also upon the size of the graft. In larger grafts, the survival of the transplant is dependent upon the rate of revascularization versus the rate of the destructive processes. The graft, which is at first dead-white, subsequently becomes blue; areas of pink coloration progressively appear and spread throughout the graft, turning it to a cherry-red color (McLaughlin, 1954).

When performing large composite grafts, one should attempt to increase, as much as possible, the raw surface available for revascularization. An excess of skin over cartilage is one

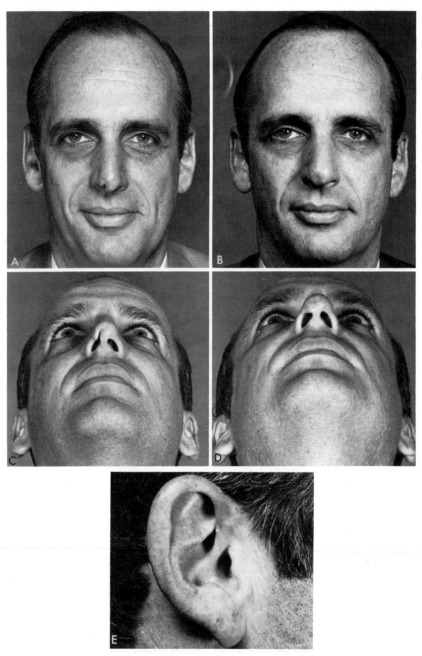

FIGURE 29–232. Composite graft for the repair of a defect of the nasal tip. *A,* A nasal defect which involves the tip of the nose. *B,* Result obtained following a composite graft taken from the anterior portion of the auricle (see *E*). *C,* View from below, showing that the defect is larger than is obvious on the full-face photograph. *D,* The composite graft has reconstructed the area of the soft triangle, the dome, and the medial portion of the lateral crus of the tip of the nose. Note the equalization of both sides of the tip. *E,* Inconspicuous scar remaining after direct approximation of the defect produced by removal of the composite graft from the anterior portion of the helix.

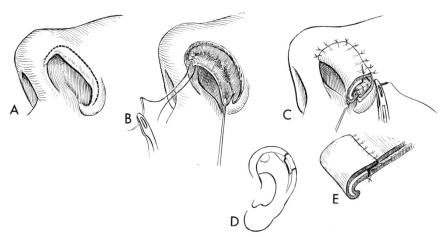

FIGURE 29–233. Hinge flap employed to increase the surface of contact between the composite graft and the recipient site. *A*, Outline of the incision for the hinge flap. *B*, The hinge flap turned down. *C*, Application of the composite graft to the recipient site. *D*, The auricular donor site of the composite graft. *E*, Suture of the composite graft to the recipient site. (From Kazanjian and Converse.)

way of achieving this. In this manner, the area of contact between graft and host is not merely an edge-to-edge contact but is increased by the overlapping as the numerous vascular anastomoses in the dermis aid in transmitting blood flow (the bridging phenomenon).

It has become customary to apply gauze compresses, refrigerated by contact with ice cubes, over the composite graft. The advisability of this modality of treatment has a purely empirical basis. Medawar (1942) hypothesized that lowering the temperature of a transplant would lower metabolic activity in the graft, thus reducing destructive processes occurring during the period of vascular deprivation. Conley and von Fraenkel (1956) first advocated this procedure on a clinical basis.

The size of the composite graft is still a matter of conjecture. Usually a width of 1 cm is considered compatible with survival; survival of composite auricular grafts of dimensions attaining 2.5 cm have been observed, however.

One might presume that the chances of survival are greater in the young patient, but successful large grafts have also been observed in older patients.

The auricular composite graft is particularly useful in defects of the nasal tip. It is possible to restore the missing portion of the tip by fashioning the composite graft to reproduce the missing part (Fig. 29–232).

The contact surface area may be enlarged by turning down a hinged flap from the skin at the edge of the defect, provided that the tissue is well-vascularized (Fig. 29–233). The composite graft should be placed over a host raw surface of increased size to produce a desirable overlap and to enlarge the area of apposition of the graft and host.

A modification of the König procedure consists of incising the alar border above its margin. The full thickness of the ala is incised. The alar border is retracted downward, and the composite auricular graft is sutured into the

FIGURE 29–234. Another method of utilizing a composite graft. *A*, Outline of incision to mobilize the alar border downward. *B*, The alar border has been mobilized downward. *C*, Auricular composite graft in position, repairing the secondary defect. (From Kazanjian and Converse.)

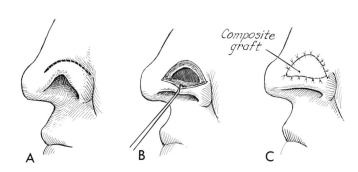

secondary defect and thus receives nourishment from the entire circumference of the graft (Fig. 29–234).

In order to avoid notching at the junction of the composite graft and the alar border, a tongue-and-groove junction is helpful. The edge of the defect is incised and angulated, a triangle is excised from the edge of the graft, and the triangular graft edge is fitted into the host triangular recipient bed. A smooth alar border is thus achieved.

THE WEDGE COMPOSITE AURICULAR GRAFT FOR DEFECTS OF THE BASE OF THE ALA AND ADJACENT NASOLABIAL AREA. This technique, which has been employed to reconstruct the nasolabial area after excision for carcinoma (Fig. 29–235, *A*) (Converse, 1950a), is also applicable in the repair of defects resulting from injury. A strip of skin 0.5 cm wide is excised along the edge of the alar defect. The graft thus has a wider surface of contact with the edges of the defect than by edge-to-edge approximation, and revascularization is facilitated (Fig. 29–235, *B*).

A pattern of the defect is made, and the alar fold is indicated on the pattern by an ink line;

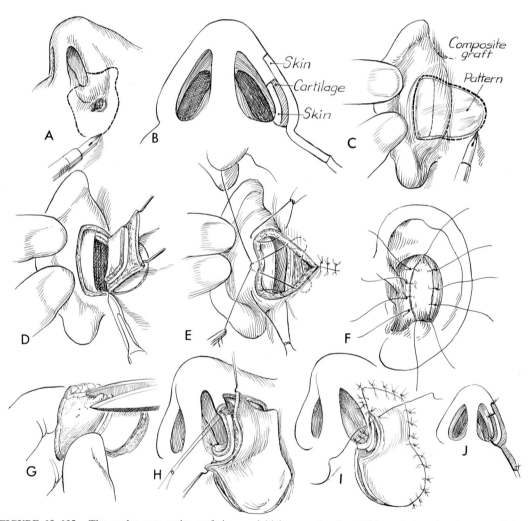

FIGURE 29–235. The wedge composite graft in nasolabial reconstruction. This technique has been used for the repair of defects resulting from resection for malignancy. *A*, Outline of defect which will result from excision of the malignancy. *B*, The plan of the repair. A composite graft will be employed which contains covering skin, supporting cartilage, and lining skin. *C*, Area from which the composite graft is removed (the retroauricular groove will reproduce the lateral nasal groove). *D*, The graft contains conchal cartilage and conchal skin. *E*, Closure of the auricular defect. *F*, Full thickness postauricular graft to repair the conchal defect. *G*, Fat is resected from the undersurface of the graft. *H*, The wedge composite graft in position. *I*, Suturing is being completed. *J*, Schema of the completed procedure. (From Converse, J. M.: Reconstruction of the nasolabial area by composite graft from the concha. Plast. Reconstr. Surg., 5:247, 1950. Copyright © 1950, The Williams & Wilkins Company, Baltimore.)

the pattern is then applied to the retroauricular area on the same side and placed so that the ink line lies over the retroauricular fold (Fig. 29–235, *C*). An incision is made through the auricular skin; the skin is raised from the cartilage for a distance of 0.5 cm, and the conchal cartilage and skin are sectioned (Fig. 29–235, *D*). The required area of retroauricular skin is removed with the composite graft, which comprises the full thickness of the concha.

The postauricular defect can usually be closed by direct approximation (Fig. 29–235, *E*), and a full-thickness graft from the upper portion of the postauricular area is sutured into position to cover the conchal defect (Fig. 29–235, *F*).

The composite graft, after fat is trimmed from the base of the dermis (Fig. 29–235, *G*), is carefully sutured to the edge of the defect; the conchal skin is sutured to the vestibular skin with 4–0 plain catgut, and the graft is sutured to the edge of the defect (Fig. 29–235, *H*). The conchal skin is sutured to the postauricular skin along the anterior border of the nostril (Fig. 29–235, *I, J*). Narrow-strip gauze or cotton pledgets moistened in saline are carefully packed into the vestibule to provide an internal support for the graft.

The extent of shrinkage depends upon the size of the graft and the rapidity with which it becomes revascularized. The color match is usually good, and restoration of the full thickness of the ala and nasolabial area is achieved.

COMPOSITE GRAFTS OF SKIN AND ADIPOSE TISSUE. Retroauricular grafts with a thin layer of fat, purposely left attached to the deep surface of the dermis, are transplanted to the area of the nasal tip. Excision of the scarred skin exposes the perichondrium of the alar cartilage. The skin-fat graft is employed to avoid a depression in the grafted area. The survival of such grafts is accounted for by the rich vascular supply of both donor and recipient sites and by revascularization from the edges of the defect (see Chapter 6, Revascularization of Skin Grafts).

Grafts of skin and fat removed from the lobe of the ear (Dupertuis, 1946) are employed for the repair of small defects of the nasal tip, the medial portion of the ala, and the columella. The postoperative shrinkage of skin-fat grafts must be considered when the reconstructive procedure is being planned.

A graft consisting of the base of the ala is

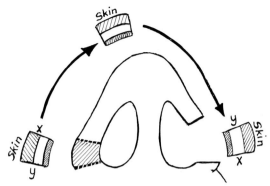

FIGURE 29–236. A wedge of tissue from the base of the ala can be transplanted to the defective contralateral ala.

readily transplanted to repair a defect on the contralateral side (Fig. 29–236).

REPEATED COMPOSITE OVERGRAFTING. In the reconstruction of nasal defects in children, serial composite grafts have given excellent results. After a first composite graft has been successfully transplanted, a time interval of a few months is allowed. A second composite graft may be transplanted over the previous one after the epidermis of the recipient graft is removed by dermabrasion. Alar and columella defects in children have been repaired by successive composite overgrafts.

COMPOSITE GRAFTS IN CHILDREN: THE GROWTH OF THE GRAFTS. Observations made over a period of ten years have shown that composite grafts in young children grow in proportion to the remainder of the nose; thus the symmetry of the two alae is maintained (Fig. 29–237).

RECONSTRUCTIVE RHINOPLASTY FOR LARGE FULL-THICKNESS DEFECTS OF THE NOSE

The complexities of reconstruction vary. When the tip has been preserved and can be used in restoring the nose, the problem of furnishing tissue for the lining, the skeletal framework, and the covering of the dorsum of the nose is less difficult than when the tip of the nose has been amputated. The achievement of a nasal tip and alae of satisfactory appearance and of

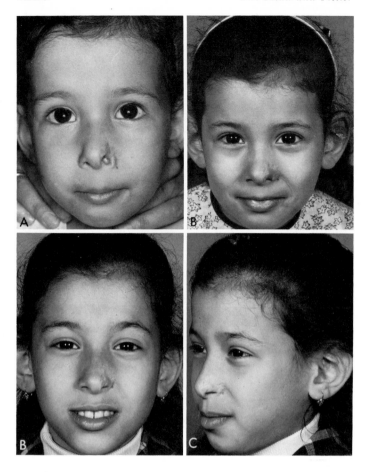

FIGURE 29–237. Growth of composite grafts in children. *A,* A 5 year old girl with the left ala destroyed by radiation for the treatment of a hemangioma. Repair by composite graft. *B,* Result two years after composite graft reconstruction. *C, D,* Appearance ten years later.

an adequate nasal airway has always been a challenge to the skill of the plastic surgeon.

It is paradoxical that loss of the tip of the nose and some of the adjacent tissue may be as complex a problem of reconstruction as a subtotal reconstruction of the nose; reconstruction of the tip is a difficult procedure, and the new structure must blend into the remainder of the nose. Similarly, loss of one ala and a portion of the lateral cartilage presents the challenge of replicating the contralateral side.

Forehead Flaps for Nasal Reconstruction

The types of forehead flaps which are commonly employed are the median flap (see Fig. 29–217, *A*), the oblique flap (see Fig. 29–217, *B*), the up-and-down flap (see Fig. 29–217, *C, D*), the scalping flap (see Fig. 29–217, *E*), the horizontal supraorbital flap (see Fig. 29–217, *F*), the sickle flap (Fig. 29–238), and a horizontal forehead flap using the major portion of the forehead (see Fig. 29–291).

The median, oblique, and scalping flaps are the types of forehead flaps most frequently employed; these flaps provide adequate forehead tissue for the repair of nasal defects of varying sizes. Median and oblique flaps may be of adequate length in bald patients or in patients with a high forehead.

New's sickle flap (1945) (see Fig. 29–238) has three disadvantages: (1) the pedicle of the flap is long, requiring one or two preliminary delay operations; (2) the base of the flap is kinked or twisted after transfer, a factor which tends to interfere with the blood supply of the flap; and (3) the flap tends to lie over the patient's eye and cause discomfort.

Horizontal forehead flaps are indicated when a large flap is required.

Washio (1969) has used a retroauricular temporal flap for the reconstruction of an alar defect. The method is somewhat unwieldy, and considerable temporary venous congestion occurs after the transfer of the flap. Washio (1972) warned that use of the retroauricular temporal flap is not advised in elderly individuals.

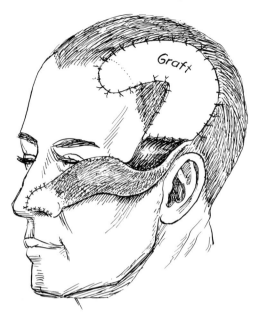

FIGURE 29–238. Sickle flap. (After New, 1945.)

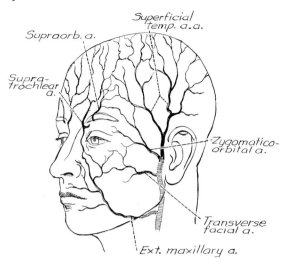

FIGURE 29–239. Blood supply of the forehead. A simple test to assist in locating the vessels is the "elastic test." A rubber band is placed around the patient's head. The veins become dilated and indicate the position of the arteries.

Orticochea (1971) had used two delayed retroauricular temporal flaps for nasal reconstruction.

The forehead flap is the method of choice in defects of the nose too large to be repaired either by composite auricular grafts or by flaps of adjacent tissue. A forehead flap may also be required for defects of the nasal dorsum which are inhospitable to a skin graft because of exposure of bone or cartilage or radiation changes in the recipient bed. When forehead tissue is available, reconstructing the nose with a forehead flap is indicated because the skin of the forehead is adjacent to the nose, it is similar in color and texture, and it has a good blood supply (Fig. 29–239).

An additional advantage of the forehead flap is that the patient does not experience discomfort as he does with the Tagliacotian flap or other distant flaps. For these reasons, the forehead flap is preferred as a source of skin for reconstructing the nose.

The main objection to the procedure is the secondary scarring of the forehead. This can be minimized by various techniques, however:

1. Using a flap removed from the midline area of the forehead similar to the Indian flap which was popularized in our era by Kazanjian (1946). If the amount of tissue required is moderate and does not exceed 5 to 6 cm, the procedure usually permits closure by direct approximation, leaving only a linear scar, without injury to the frontalis muscles, as the flap is removed from an intervening area devoid of musculature.

2. Placing the defect on the side of the forehead, rendering it less visible in the full-face view. In female patients, the defect can be hidden by the hair. To avoid scars on the forehead, the incisions outlining the flap are placed behind the hairline, with the exception of the skin grafted area on the lateral aspect of the forehead (the scalping flap technique. Converse, 1942).

3. Covering the secondary forehead defect with well-matched full-thickness skin, preferably from the retroauricular or supraclavicular regions.

4. Avoiding damage to the frontalis muscle. A conspicuous deformity following a forehead flap technique is the absence of expressive movements of the forehead resulting from the removal of a section of the frontalis muscle.

5. A variety of transposition and rotation flaps are available to close the defect on the forehead, thus leaving a linear scar which, in the older patient particularly, becomes inconspicuous.

Timing of the Reconstruction. If the nose has been amputated in an accident, the skin edges should be sutured to the nasal mucous membrane to eliminate any raw area. Split-thickness skin grafting may be employed to cover the remaining raw areas.

Cancers of the nose, if eradicated by wide

excisional surgery, do not generally recur. As the most common nasal cancer is basal cell epithelioma, lymphatic spread and metastases are rare, and the prognosis is generally favorable.

The resected specimen is then carefully examined, and histologic verification of complete eradication can be made. It is unwise to reconstruct the nose immediately, as careful histologic examination of the resected specimen is the best guarantee of complete eradication.

Whether the loss of the nose is the result of trauma, amputation, radiation, or chemosurgery for malignant disease, a waiting period of many months should elapse before reconstruction is undertaken. Two principal reasons justify this delay. The first is that the tissues must be revascularized and softened; the second reason is psychologic: the patient will be more appreciative of the surgeon's efforts and of the result obtained if he has had to endure a period of waiting with the deformity.

Delay of Forehead Flaps: The Outline Delay. Satisfactorily designed forehead flaps rarely require preliminary delay, for the blood supply is adequate, thus ensuring the survival of the tissues. Flap delay done in the usual manner, by raising the flap and replacing it in its original bed in a preliminary stage, is contrain-dicated. Unless the flap is transferred within ten days, this type of delay results in a stiffening of the flap, and the lack of suppleness makes it more difficult to adapt the flap to the defect and very difficult to infold the distal portion of the flap for the reconstruction of the nasal tip, columella, and alae. If flap delay is necessary, the delay technique consists of a simple incision outlining the flap. The outline delay technique suffices, as the blood supply to the area is derived from blood vessels that enter the circumference and not from perforating vessels. Outline delay is reserved for older patients with arteriosclerosis, for patients in whom preexisting scars may impede the vascularization of the flap, and for patients in whom the forehead has previously been irradiated or burned. The blood supply of scalping flaps (see Fig. 29–239) is so abundant that forehead tissue which had been previously covered by split-thickness skin grafts (following deep burns) can be transplanted for total reconstruction of the nose after an outline delay.

Technique of the Median Forehead Flap. The median forehead flap (Kazanjian, 1946) is a vertical flap from the median section of the forehead, a modification of the flap employed in the ancient Indian rhinoplasty (Fig. 29–240). It may be employed in various types of

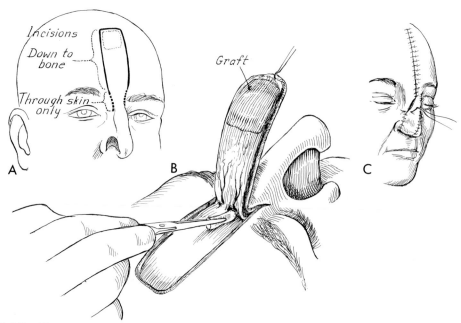

FIGURE 29–240. The median forehead flap. *A*, The median flap. Dotted lines at the base of the flap emphasize that incisions extend through skin only. *B*, Blunt dissection at the base of the flap to avoid injury of the supratrochlear vessels. A septal composite graft has been added to the distal part of the flap for alar reconstruction. *C*, Flap being sutured to defect. (After Kazanjian, 1946.)

nasal defects and in full thickness defects of varying size resulting from loss of the entire lower portion of the nose.

Two parallel incisions over the forehead extending from the hairline to the root of the nose are joined at the hairline by a transverse incision (Fig. 29–240, *A*). The incisions are extended through the soft tissues and the periosteum; the incisions are made in the midline of the forehead between the frontalis muscles, which leave between the incisions an interstice devoid of muscle. Thus there is no interference with the forehead musculature of expression, a distinct advantage of the technique.

The median forehead flap receives its blood supply from the paired supratrochlear arteries.

The manner in which the incisions are made is important in order to obtain a flap of adequate length and to ensure the flexibility of the base of the pedicle, without endangering the blood supply. The incisions extend from the hairline to a point immediately above the nasofrontal angle and penetrate through the periosteum covering the frontal bone; from this point downward the lines of the incision are extended through the skin only, medial to the eyebrow, to a point lateral to the root of the nose. Elevation by blunt dissection only is

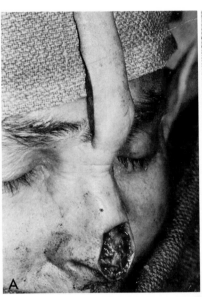

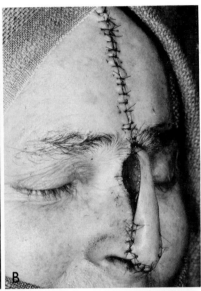

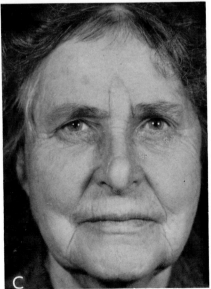

FIGURE 29–241. Repair of a defect of the nasal tip with a median forehead flap. *A*, Defect of the tip of the nose. The flap is raised. Note that the base of the flap extends to the root of the nose. *B*, The median flap is sutured into the defect, and the forehead defect is closed by direct approximation. *C*, Final result obtained. (After Kazanjian, 1946.)

done in the lower portion of the flap at the junction of the forehead and the root of the nose (Fig. 29–240, *B*). This precaution and the fact that the incisions outlining the lower portion of the flap are made through the skin only prevent injury to the supratrochlear vessels. The soft tissues over the lower portion of the forehead in the midline and the root of the nose show a peculiar laxity which permits the action of the frowning muscles. This characteristic facilitates the twisting and downward mobilization of the base of the pedicle and provides sufficient length to the flap, thus making it possible to reach the tip of the nose (Fig. 29–241) and to restore the columella (see Fig. 29–301).

The median flap can be used in conjunction with a septal composite graft to reconstruct a nasal defect involving the ala, as shown in Figure 29–240, *C,* or to resurface the dorsum of the nose.

CLOSURE OF THE FOREHEAD DONOR SITE. After raising the median flap, the secondary defect in the midline of the forehead is closed by direct approximation, and the flap is turned downward and sutured to the edges of the nasal defect. The pedicle of the flap is severed 18 to 21 days later; the lower portion of the nonutilized pedicle of the flap is then reinserted into the lower portion of the forehead suture line. After direct approximation of the edges of the forhead defect, puckering may tend to bring the medial ends of the eyebrows together; such tension may be relieved in a second stage procedure, in which the pedicle of the flap is severed and the base of the median flap is replaced in the lower portion of the defect.

The resulting vertical scar line is inconspicuous, particularly in patients of the older age group. Although forehead skin is not as elastic as tissues of other parts of the face, moderately large defects can be closed by approximation after the forehead tissues on both sides are undermined. If the defect covers a wider area, the tissues are freely undermined on each side, and one or two incisions are made on the undersurface parallel to the incised edges, thus splitting the fibers of the frontalis muscle on each side without penetrating through the subcutaneous fat into the skin (Fig. 29–242, *A*). This procedure tends to loosen the skin of the forehead and permits approximation of the borders of the wound without undue tension.

In more extensive defects (exceeding 5 to 7 cm), closure by direct approximation may be difficult. Closure is made possible by two advancement flaps of the remaining forehead skin (Fig. 29–242, *B*). Curved incisions, one along the hairline and the other above the eyebrows, are extended, if necessary, as far as the temporal region; the flaps are undermined and brought together to close the gap. The resulting forehead scar line is conspicuous in some cases, but the scar can be excised at a later date and the wound resutured.

Swinging rotation flaps extending into the scalp may also be employed to close a defect resulting from a wide flap (Fig. 29–243) (Schimmelbusch, 1895). The closure of a defect by rotation flaps is shown in Figure 29–244.

VARIATIONS OF THE MEDIAN FOREHEAD FLAP. The design of the median forehead flap varies according to the demand of the nasal de-

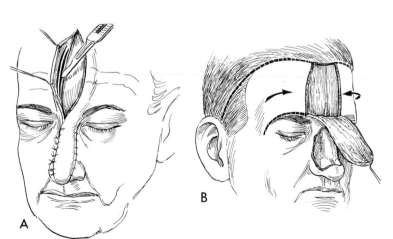

A

B

FIGURE 29–242. Two techniques for closure of the donor area of a median forehead flap. *A,* The pericranium and frontalis muscle on each side of the defect are incised vertically to assist in the closure. *B,* Bilateral advancement flaps can be used for larger defects.

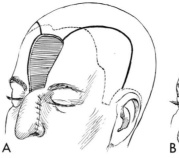
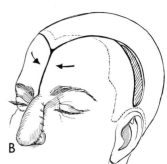

FIGURE 29-243. Technique of closure of the median defect of the forehead with large rotation flaps. (After Schimmelbusch, 1895.)

formity. Millard (1974) has designed a gull-shaped flap that outlines the columella and alae of the nose and also facilitates the closure of the secondary defect (see Fig. 29-283).

In order to ease the downward twist of the flap, the pedicle can be based on the supratrochlear vessels on one side instead of on the paired supratrochlear vessels, as in Kazanjian's technique (Fig. 29-240). An outline delay,

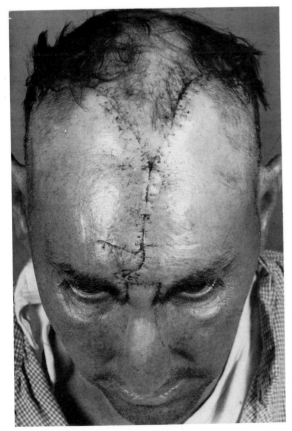

FIGURE 29-244. Donor area of a median forehead flap for reconstruction of the nose closed by mobilization of rotation flaps, as illustrated in Figure 29-243.

which is not necessary in the classic median forehead flap, is a prudent precaution prior to transfer of the gull-shaped flap.

The Island Forehead Flap with a Subcutaneous Tissue Pedicle. The island forehead flap with a subcutaneous pedicle differs from the ordinary Indian type of flap by the absence of the usual pedicle of skin (Fig. 29-245). An island of skin of predetermined size is completely detached from the surrounding skin, but the subcutaneous tissue of the skin island is continuous within a subcutaneous pedicle which contains the supratrochlear vessels. Heanley (1955), Barron (1959), Kubaček (1960), Kernahan and Littlewood (1961), Converse and Wood-Smith (1963), and Barron and Emmett (1965) have reported the use of similar flaps.

In the repair of large defects of the dorsum of the nose, the island forehead flap is preferable to a full-thickness retroauricular or supraclavicular graft, since despite a good color match, such grafts may leave a depressed area with inadequate contour restoration.

ADVANTAGES. The island flap with subcutaneous pedicle provides greater mobility than other types of forehead flaps because the subcutaneous pedicle is more readily twisted, and the skin flap is more easily adjusted into the recipient site. Because a flap with a skin pedicle is less pliable, the twisting of the pedicle and the kinking of the skin tend to cut off the blood supply to the flap. A second appreciable advantage of the island flap is that only one stage is required, the island flap being raised and placed immediately into the entire defect; the secondary defect is closed and the operative procedure completed in one stage. The preparation of the subcutaneous pedicle is technically easier than the minute dissection required to isolate the vascular pedicle in the artery island type of flap (Monks, 1898; Esser, 1917). A third advantage of the island flap with

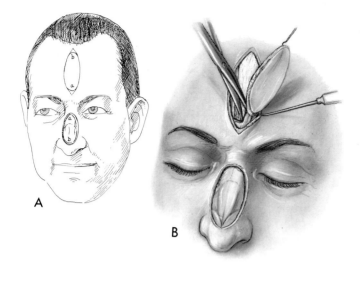

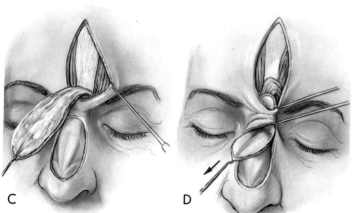

FIGURE 29–245. Island forehead flap with a subcutaneous pedicle. *A,* Nasal defect and proposed island flap in the midline of the forehead. *B,* A subcutaneous pedicle is being raised. *C,* Island flap with subcutaneous pedicle prior to transfer. *D,* The skin between the donor area of the flap and the host bed is undermined, and the island flap is threaded through the subcutaneous tunnel.

a subcutaneous pedicle is that the venous and lymphatic return flow from the flap is not interrupted, and the flap remains smooth and flat in its new recipient site.

DISADVANTAGES. The principal disadvantage encountered with the island flap is the protrusion which may remain at the root of the nose as a result of the presence of the subcutaneous pedicle. The protrusion may require secondary excision, although regression of the protrusion occurs over a period of three to six months. The considerable degree of venous congestion observed in the flap during the first 48 hours after transplantation is always a subject of concern, particularly if the surgeon is performing this operation for the first time. The color changes of the flap resemble those displayed by composite grafts.

TECHNIQUE. A flap of appropriate length is outlined over the median aspect of the forehead skin supplied by the supratrochlear vessels (Fig. 29–245, *A*). The full thickness of the skin is incised around the inverted pattern of the defect.

A V-shaped segment of skin is excised superficially from the area immediately below the island flap in order to facilitate subsequent closure of the forehead defect; a similar inverted V is removed from the area immediately above the island flap (Fig. 29–245, *A*). The skin of the forehead is then superficially undermined downward over the glabella and the dorsum of the nose as far as the nasal defect. The undermining of the skin is extended laterally toward the vascular pedicles in the supratrochlear region. The subcutaneous

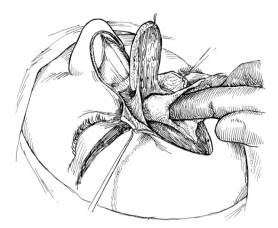

FIGURE 29-246. Gauze dissection raises the periosteum near the root of the nose to preserve the blood supply to the subcutaneous pedicle originating from the supratrochlear vessels.

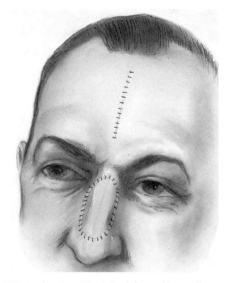

FIGURE 29-247. The island flap with a subcutaneous pedicle has been transferred. The flap is sutured in position, and the forehead defect is closed by direct approximation.

pedicle is prepared by raising the subcutaneous tissue from the frontal bone (Fig. 29-245, *B*), and the vessels are thus included in the pedicle (Fig. 29-245, *C*). Gauze dissection protects the vessels from injury (Fig. 29-246). The island flap and subcutaneous pedicle are now mobilized and rotated 180 degrees through the subcutaneous channel to the defect (see Fig. 29-245, *D*).

The skin edges of the island flap are sutured to the edges of the defect with fine interrupted sutures (Fig. 29-247). Undermining of the margins of the forehead defect facilitates direct approximation of the edges of the secondary defect.

An alternative procedure to the tunneling technique is the preparation of the subcutaneous pedicle under direct vision by means of an incision extending from the island of skin to

the defect (Fig. 29-248). The skin incision is superficial in order to leave the subcutaneous tissue intact, and the skin is separated from the subcutaneous tissue over the area destined to become the subcutaneous pedicle.

Clinical Applications of the Median and Island Forehead Flaps. The median and island forehead flaps are employed in a variety of nasal defects and also in combination with other flaps or grafts:

1. They provide a satisfactory skin covering in defects unsuitable for skin grafting, such as defects with exposure of the nasal bones (Fig. 29-249) or deeply scarred radiated areas.

FIGURE 29-248. Variation of the median island forehead flap with a subcutaneous pedicle: donor and recipient areas are joined by a cutaneous incision. *A*, The island flap prior to transfer. *B*, Sutured flap and donor area.

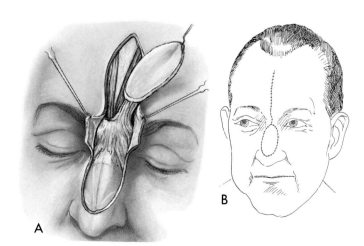

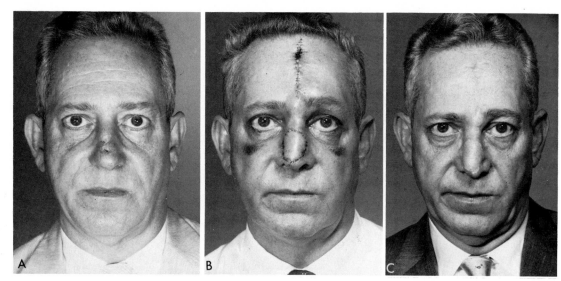

FIGURE 29–249. The median island forehead flap. *A*, Recurrent radiated basal cell carcinoma extending into the nasal cartilages and the underlying mucous membrane. *B*, Appearance after wide excision of cutaneous, cartilaginous, and mucosal tissues and reconstitution of a lining by the approximation of adjacent tissues. The island flap is in position. The forehead defect is closed by direct approximation. Five days postoperative. *C*, Four weeks following transfer of the median island forehead flap (see technique illustrated in Figs. 29–245 to 29–247). (Figs. 29–245 to 29–247 from Converse, J. M., and Wood-Smith, D.: Experience with the forehead island flap with a subcutaneous pedicle. Plast. Reconstr. Surg., *31*:521, 1963. Copyright © 1963, The Williams & Wilkins Company, Baltimore.)

2. The median flap is an excellent method for the replacement of a deficient nasal lining. In saddle noses with shortening due to damage to the nasal framework and scarring of the nasal lining, the median flap is introduced into the nasal cavity through a transverse incision across the cartilaginous portion of the nose (see Fig. 29–213). The end of the flap is su-

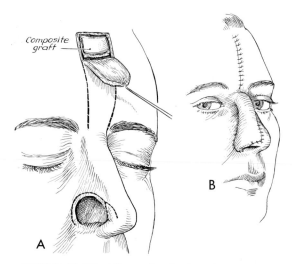

FIGURE 29–250. The median forehead flap lined with a septal composite graft lining. *A*, In a first stage, a septal composite graft is placed under the distal portion of the median flap. *B*, After a period of six weeks, the flap is transferred. The septal composite graft furnishes the lining and cartilaginous support of the new ala (see Fig. 29–269 for technique of joining the alar portion of the flap with the tissues of the nasal tip).

tured; the skin surface is turned inward to form the nasal lining; and the edges of the flap are sutured to the edges of the severed nasal lining. The island flap combined with a scalping flap provides the lining tissue in a full-thickness defect of the nasal dorsum (see Fig. 29–275).

3. In full-thickness defects of the nose, the median flap may be lined in a preliminary procedure by a septal composite graft (Figs. 29–250 and 29–251).

4. The median flap may be employed for the repair of defects of the tip and the columella. The tissues at the base of the flap are loosened by blunt dissection to obtain a flap of sufficient length to reach the tip of the nose or the base of the columella (see Figs. 29–246 and 29–301).

5. When the forehead is adequate in its vertical dimension, particularly in older patients with a recessed hairline, the median forehead flap also provides adequate tissue for subtotal reconstruction.

The Scalping Flap

The scalping flap (Figs. 29–252 and 29–253) has proved a valuable and reliable technique for subtotal nasal reconstruction since it was first employed (Converse, 1942).

The scalping flap technique presents six specific advantages:

1. The first and most important advantage is the fact that the scalping flap can be loosened from the cranium until adequate length is ob-

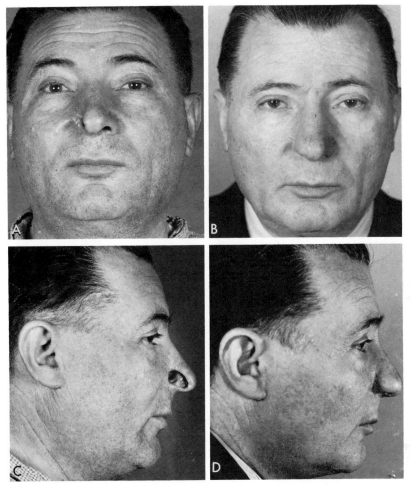

FIGURE 29–251. Reconstruction of the ala and lateral nasal wall by a median forehead flap lined with a septal composite graft. *A, C,* Defect resulting from resection of a recurrent radiated basal cell carcinoma. *B, D,* Result obtained by the technique illustrated in Figure 29–250.

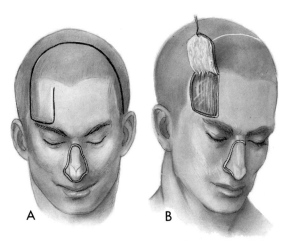

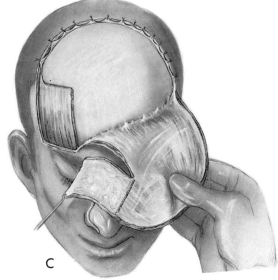

FIGURE 29–252. The scalping flap. *A,* Nasal defect and proposed scalping flap. *B,* The flap has been raised from the frontalis muscle. *C,* Above the area where the frontalis muscle blends into the galea aponeurotica, the remainder of the flap is raised from the pericranium (see continuation in Fig. 29–253).

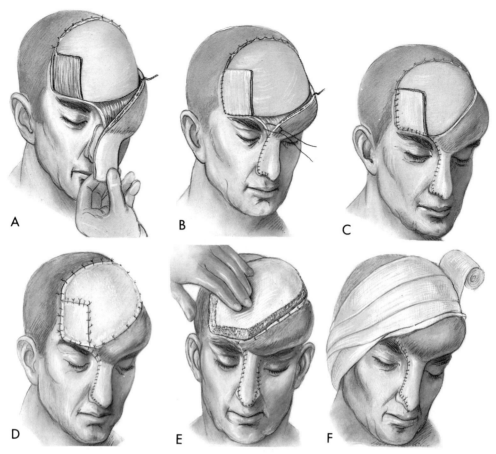

FIGURE 29–253. The scalping flap (continued). *A,* The scalping flap has reached sufficient length to permit its transfer. *B,* A full-thickness retroauricular graft has been placed over the area of the permanent defect situated over the frontalis muscle. The scalping flap is sutured over the nasal defect. *C,* The scalping flap has been tubed to itself, thus eliminating any raw area. *D,* Telfa serves as a temporary dressing. *E, F,* A pressure dressing is applied over the area of the temporary defect.

tained, thus permitting the infolding of the distal portion of the flap for the construction of the columella.

2. Most of the incisions outlining the flap are placed behind the hairline of the scalp, and the resulting scars are thus mostly hidden.

3. The skin grafted area of the permanent defect is placed over the lateral aspect of the forehead, where it is less conspicuous. In female patients the skin grafted area is readily hidden by the patient's hair by a simple change in hair style.

4. The large size of the flap permits it to be rolled on itself and tubed, thus greatly diminishing the area of exposed raw tissue.

5. The scalping flap technique makes possible the reconstruction of the nose in patients with narrow foreheads and a low hairline. Brown and McDowell (1951) stated that the oblique forehead flap cannot be used if the pa-

tient has a small forehead; they gave the minimal dimensions of the forehead for the oblique flap. Such limitations have rarely been encountered in the scalping flap. Should additional tissue be needed, some of the scalp can be included over the upper portion of the nose and depilated at a later date.

6. The scalping flap can be used bilaterally on both sides of the forehead in two separate stages. If the first operation for nasal reconstruction is unsuccessful, the contralateral side of the forehead can be used for the second and presumably successful attempt.

The scalping flap, as well as all other forehead flaps, in addition to providing a reconstructed nose which has a satisfactory color and texture match with the skin of the face, offers the advantage of avoiding the discomfort to the patient of the Tagliacotian brachial flap or other distant flaps.

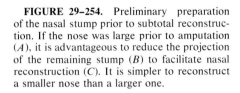
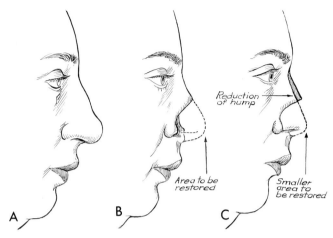

FIGURE 29–254. Preliminary preparation of the nasal stump prior to subtotal reconstruction. If the nose was large prior to amputation (*A*), it is advantageous to reduce the projection of the remaining stump (*B*) to facilitate nasal reconstruction (*C*). It is simpler to reconstruct a smaller nose than a larger one.

The scalping flap is provided with an abundant blood supply from the superficial temporal artery, as well as from the branches of the frontal, supraorbital, and supratrochlear arteries. The venous return is assured by the branches of the superficial temporal vein, which unites with the internal maxillary vein to form the posterior facial vein, and the supraorbital and frontal veins, which drain into the angular vein, which in turn, drains into the anterior facial vein.

The scalping flap has a number of other applications, including restoration of the roof of the orbit, the eyebrow, or the cheek.

Preliminary Rhinoplastic Reduction. When nasal reconstruction is planned after subtotal loss of the nose, it may be advisable to reduce the projection and the width of the remaining bony portion of the nose. It is easier to reconstruct a smaller nose than a larger one, and the reduction of the projection of the nasal stump simplifies the problem of obtaining an adequate projection of the reconstructed nasal tip (Fig. 29–254).

Planning and Design of the Forehead Flap. Correct planning and design of the forehead flap are essential. A piece of cloth can be used to simulate the flap. A rehearsal of the flap transfer procedure, using a cloth pattern material, should always precede the actual operation. In subtotal nose reconstruction, particularly when the distal end of the flap must be folded upon itself to form the tip, columella, and alae of the new nose (Fig. 29–255), the pattern is folded in the same manner and is thus essential in determining the required dimensions. The pattern is made slightly larger

than the nasal defect to allow for the slight contraction of the forehead skin after the flap is raised. The pattern is sterilized and made available for use during the operation.

Technique of the Scalping Flap

OUTLINING THE FLAP. Careful preoperative measurements and the preparation of the pattern determine the size and shape of the portion of the forehead skin to be utilized for the reconstruction. The area is outlined slightly wider and longer than the pattern and incised. The incision line delimiting the lateral bound-

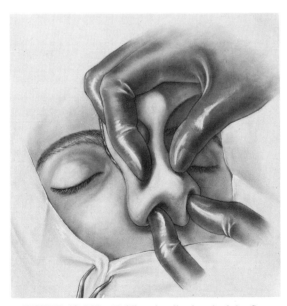

FIGURE 29–255. Folding the distal end of the flap to form the tip, alae, and columella. The forehead flap is folded in the manner illustrated, and the bases of the new alae and columella are then sutured to the prepared sites.

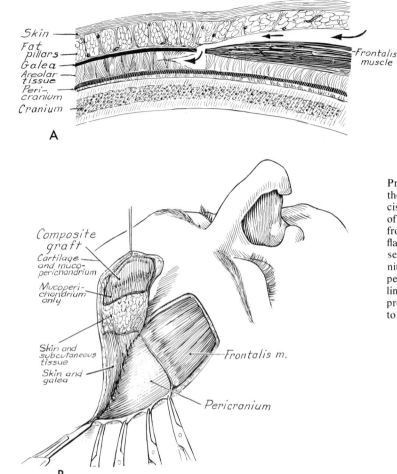

Skin
Fat
pillars
Galea
Areolar
tissue
Peri-
cranium
Cranium

Frontalis
muscle

A

Composite
graft
Cartilage
and muco-
perichondrium

Mucoperi-
chondrium
only

Skin and
subcutaneous
tissue
Skin and
galea

Frontalis m.

Pericranium

B

FIGURE 29–256. The scalping flap. Preservation of the frontalis muscle in the area of the permanent defect. *A,* Incision through the galea above the area of the permanent defect covered by the frontalis muscle. Raising of the scalping flap is done within the areolar layer separating the galea from the pericranium. *B,* The frontalis muscle over the permanent defect. The scalping flap, lined with a septal composite graft in a preliminary stage, is raised for transfer to a lateral nasal wall defect.

ary of the defect is extended upward toward the vertex of the cranium, until it reaches approximately the level of a transverse line extending through the upper tips of the auricles; the incision then curves medially across the midline and downward over the contralateral auricle, curving as far forward as possible but not extending through the frontal branch of the superficial temporal artery (see Fig. 29–252, *A*).

TECHNICAL DETAILS. It is not necessary to shave the hair. The scalp hair should be closely clipped rather than shaved. The hairline remains visible, an indispensible landmark, and the patient's hair will be restored more rapidly. In female patients only that portion of the scalp which is part of the flap is clipped; the patient can have a hairpiece made from the removed hair to wear during the period of hair regrowth. The operation is usually done under oral endotracheal anesthesia; controlled hypotension is not necessary. Bleeding during the

operation is diminished when the patient is placed in an inclined position with the head elevated above the remainder of the body. Bleeding is also diminished and dissection facilitated by infiltration and hydraulic dissection between the pericranium and the galea aponeurotica with a dilute solution of local anesthetic. The operation can also be performed under local anesthesia (infiltration and regional block anesthesia).

The area over the frontalis muscle should not be injected with the local anesthetic solution in order to facilitate the identification of the frontalis muscle fibers and sharp dissection of the forehead skin from the muscle. An injection in this area blanches the muscle and makes the identification of the muscle fibers more difficult.

The operation is begun by outlining the area of the permanent defect on the forehead (see Fig. 29–252, *A*). Careful sharp dissection separates the cutaneous layer from the frontalis muscle fibers (see Fig. 29–252, *B*). It is essential to preserve the frontalis muscle in the area of the permanent defect, thus also preserving the expressive movements of the forehead under the skin graft which resurfaces the area. The nerve supply to the frontalis musculature (originating from the temporofacial division of the facial nerve) is undisturbed.

The dissection of the skin from the frontalis muscle fibers is extended over the entire vertical length of the frontalis muscle until the galea aponeurotica is reached. The dissection is continued over the galea for another 1 or 2 cm; the galea is then sectioned transversely. Subsequent raising of the scalping flap is accomplished within the loose areolar layer separating the galea from the pericranium (Fig. 29–256). The galea is thus raised with the flap, as well as the remainder of the frontalis muscle, with the exception of the portion of the muscle in the area of the permanent defect (see Figs. 29–252, *C* and 29–253, *A*).

After the portion of the flap to be used for nasal reconstruction is in position, the remainder of the pedicle of the scalping flap is folded upon itself to eliminate any exposed raw area in the flap (see Fig. 29–253, *B*, *C*). The distal portion of the scalping flap can be used in various ways, depending on the defect to be repaired, and is often folded to form the alae, tip, and columella of the nose. Technical details concerning the various applications of the scalping flap are described later in the chapter.

Subtotal Rhinoplasty: Four Basic Principles. 1. ADEQUATE FLAP LENGTH. In subtotal rhinoplasty, it is essential to obtain a flap of sufficient length to provide a columella also of adequate length. A long columella provides the new nose with an adequately projecting tip (Fig. 29–257) and thus avoids the typical appearance of most reconstructed noses, which show a downward curve of the lower portion. The reconstruction of a columella of adequate length and of an adequate projecting tip also makes possible the addition of a skeletal framework either primarily or secondarily (see p. 1256), a technique which maintains the projection of the tip. The scalping flap (or a long median or oblique flap) should be mobilized until the distal portion of the flap extends downward beyond the patient's upper lip (Fig. 29–258). When only the upper portion of the forehead is used to provide tissue for a nasal defect and when the flap is used in the bald patient, further lengthening can be obtained by an incision extending downward toward the eyebrow (Fig. 29–259).

The importance of adequate columellar length is well-illustrated in Figure 29–260, which shows a 74 year old patient (Fig. 29–260, *A*, *C*) who underwent nasal reconstruction by means of an oblique forehead flap; adequate flap length could not be obtained. The full-face appearance of the patient after surgery is shown in Figure 29–260, *B*. The patient refused further refinement of the recon-

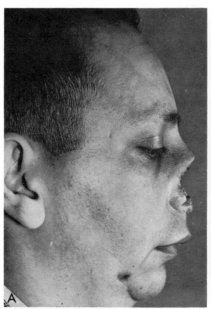
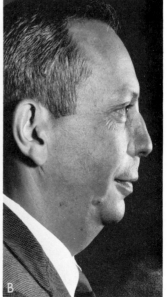

FIGURE 29–257. Reconstruction of the nose by scalping flap. *A*, Appearance of patient following amputation. Note the large projecting stump. *B*, Profile obtained following a preliminary reduction in the size and projection of the stump (see Fig. 29–254). Note the adequate projection of the tip provided by the long columella and the mobilization of the scalping flap as far down as the lower lip (see Fig. 29–258).

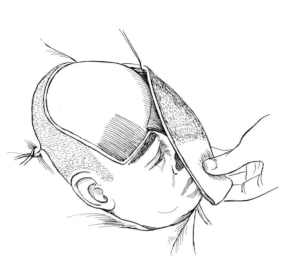

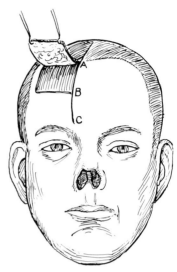

FIGURE 29–258. In order to reconstruct the tip of the nose, the columella, and the alae, the flap must be sufficiently long to reach the lower lip.

FIGURE 29–259. When only the upper portion of the forehead is required for the reconstruction, particularly in balding patients with a recessed hairline, additional lengthening of the flap is obtained by an incision extending downward (*A, B, C*) toward the eyebrow. The entire portion of the forehead composed of the flap can thus be loosened for greater mobility.

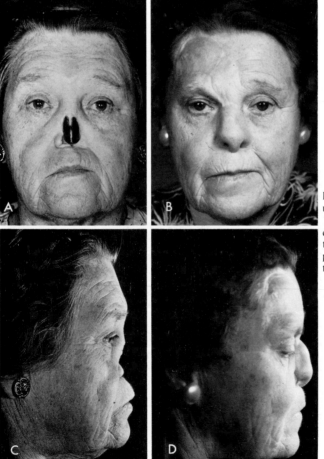

FIGURE 29–260. Nasal reconstruction by oblique forehead flap. *A,* A 74 year old patient who underwent amputation of the nose for carcinoma 15 years earlier. *B,* Following reconstructive rhinoplasty with an oblique forehead flap. *C,* Preoperative profile view. *D,* Postoperative view of the profile. Note the retraction of the tip caused by the short columella.

structed nose. The postoperative profile (Fig. 29–260, *D*) shows the inadequacy of the length of the columella and of the projection of the nasal tip.

2. AVOIDING TENSION. Tension is the main cause of failure, as it interrupts the blood flow to and from the flap. Adequate length avoids tension. Tension is also influenced by the choice of the side of the forehead which will serve as the donor area of the flap. Many amputated noses have a portion of the lower nose present. The major defect is therefore on the contralateral side. The flap should be designed so as to use the skin of the forehead situated on the same side of the face as the major defect (see Fig. 29–261).

3. PROVIDING A BASE FOR THE NEW NOSE. If adjacent tissue has been resected and the defect includes adjacent cheek skin and bone from the pyriform aperture, a base must be established before undertaking a subtotal or total rhinoplasty. A median flap (Fig. 29–261) and a cheek advancement flap (see Fig. 29–276) have been employed for this purpose.

4. ESTABLISHING ONE-PIECE CONTINUITY. The flap must blend into the remainder of the nose. A piecemeal reconstruction should be avoided (Fig. 29–262). This technique also

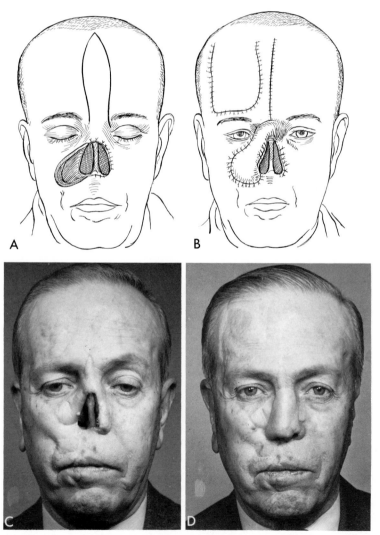

FIGURE 29–261. Consecutive use of a median forehead flap and a scalping flap. *A*, Large defect involving the nose and the medial portion of the cheek. *B*, In a first stage, the cheek defect is covered by means of a median forehead flap. *C*, Following application of the median flap. *D*, Appearance following nasal reconstruction by the scalping flap technique.

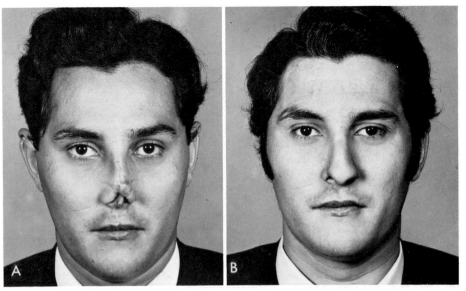

FIGURE 29–262. Reconstruction of the nose by the scalping flap technique. *A,* Loss of the lower portion of the nose as a result of amputation by a knife. *B,* Reconstruction obtained by the scalping flap technique.

provides a larger host bed for the revascularization of the transplanted flap (see The Scalping Flap in Subtotal Nasal Reconstruction: Technical Details, p. 1244).

REPAIR OF THE PERMANENT FOREHEAD DEFECT: IMMEDIATE, DELAYED, OR SECONDARY. In the repair of moderate-sized defects, the required forehead skin can be taken from the upper and lateral portion of the forehead near the hairline, thus further minimizing the secondary defect. The defect on the forehead is repaired primarily by means of a full-thickness retroauricular or supraclavicular skin graft (see Fig. 29–253); these types of skin grafts are chosen because of their excellent color match.

It may be preferable to delay the repair of the permanent defect and apply the skin graft during the second stage when the pedicle of the scalping flap is severed and returned to its original site. The delay does not seem to interfere with the vascularization of the graft, and the delayed grafting on a dry bed eliminates subjacent hematomas.

The skin situated between the helical border of the auricle and the hairline behind the mastoid process is usually adequate in surface area to repair the permanent defect of the forehead. After removal of the full-thickness retroauricular skin graft, the helical border is sutured to the posterior margin of the defect, thus completely obliterating the retroauricular fold. At a later date, the skin deficiency behind the auricle can be repaired by means of a split-thickness graft from another area of the body. The auricle is released from its pinned back position. Occasionally, if the forehead defect is large, additional skin is required to repair the forehead defect and is obtained from the contralateral retroauricular area. When retroauricular skin is not available, supraclavicular skin, if available, is preferable. In severely burned patients a split-thickness graft is used if the above-mentioned donor areas are unavailable.

The skin grafted donor area on the forehead improves spontaneously with the passage of time. Occasionally it is necessary to improve the junction line between the graft and the surrounding forehead skin by dermabrasion (see Chapter 17). The color match, when suitable full-thickness skin grafts are employed, is generally satisfactory, and the patient's appearance is enhanced by the presence of frontalis muscle activity under the graft.

In a partially or more extensively bald patient, a rotation or transposition flap from the scalp repairs the forehead defect; the secondary scalp defect is skin grafted (see Fig. 29–243). A hairpiece will camouflage the skin-grafted area.

CARE OF THE TEMPORARY SCALP DEFECT. One of the objections to the scalping flap has been the large temporary defect and the wide area of pericranium exposed during the time interval between the transfer of the flap and its replacement in a second stage. In the first patients who underwent a scalping flap reconstruction of the nose, the temporary defect was covered by a split-thickness graft generally removed from the patient's abdomen, thigh, or buttocks. Skin autografts were later replaced by a variety of temporary resurfacing agents, such as skin allografts, embryonic calf skin (Rogers and Converse, 1958), and a variety of prosthetic skin substitutes. A simple method of treatment is successfully employed at present. After the area of the permanent defect has been covered by the full-thickness graft and the flap transferred to the nasal defect, the temporary raw area is covered by a layer of Telfa, a readily available commercial dressing (see Fig. 29–253, *E, F*). A pressure dressing is usually applied for a period of 24 hours. The dressings are then removed, and the Telfa-covered wound is exposed to the air and remains in a dry state, which eliminates wound sepsis.

Porcine skin xenografts also furnish an excellent temporary means of resurfacing the raw area.

THE SECOND STAGE: RETURN OF THE PEDICLE. The severance of the pedicle of the flap and the return of the remainder of the flap to its original donor site are usually performed between the fourteenth and eighteenth days (Fig. 29–263). Further delay results in some difficulty in replacing the flap because of fibrosis and shrinkage. A curved hemostat is passed under the pedicle of the flap immediately above the portion of the flap that will serve for the reconstruction; an incision is then made through the flap down to the hemostat. Excess subcutaneous tissue is removed from the upper

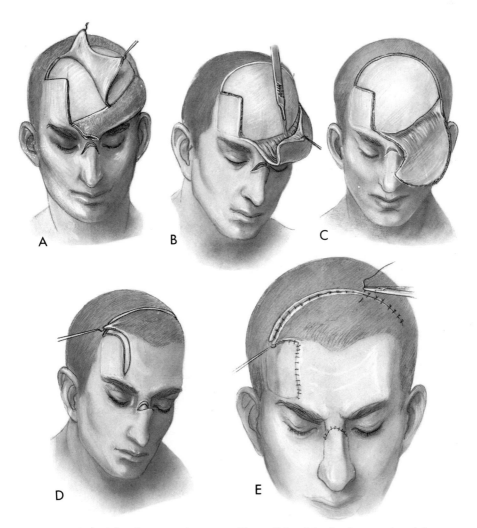

FIGURE 29–263. The scalping flap: second stage. *A*, The pedicle of the flap is severed, and the temporary dressing is removed. *B, C*, The tubed portion of the flap is unfurled. *D, E*, The flap is returned to its original site and sutured in position.

portion of the flap remaining on the nose, the edges of the nasal defect are freshened, and the flap is fitted into the nasal host bed. The remainder of the scalping flap is then unfurled and returned to its original position.

The Scalping Flap in Subtotal Nasal Reconstruction: Technical Details. One of the most frequent nasal defects is that which involves a major portion of the cartilaginous nose. The de-

fect involves the tip, alae, and columella and the cartilaginous nose. A stump of the bony portion of the nose is usually present; the skin of the area can be used for lining. The remaining stumps of the alae and columella are often present.

As previously mentioned, the flaps should be of sufficient length to form a columella of adequate length, which is essential to provide adequate projection of the nasal tip and a harmoni-

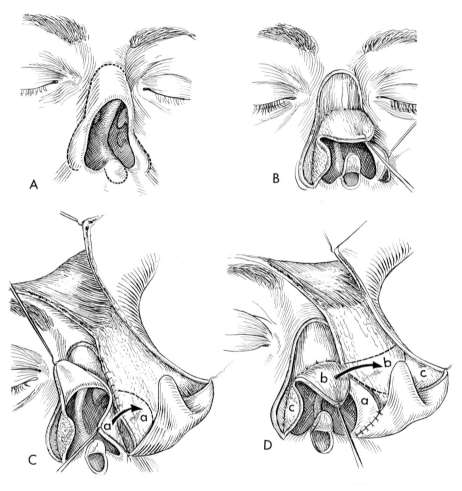

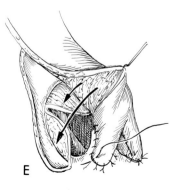

FIGURE 29–264. Local lining flaps in nasal reconstruction. *A,* The dorsal flap from the nasal stump, the turned-in hinge flaps from the bases of the alae, and a flap from the median portion of the lip are outlined. *B,* The various flaps are turned in for lining. *C,* The arrow indicates a triangular area on each side which is not covered by the flap from the nasal dorsal stump. These areas are covered by hinge flaps from the alar stumps. *D,* The arrow indicates the position that the flap from the nasal dorsal stump will occupy. The left hinge flap from the alar stump has been sutured into position. *E,* Suturing of the lining flaps being completed.

ous profile line (see Figs. 29–254 and 29–258). The profile can be further improved, in a later stage, by the addition of a skeletal framework. Skin covering the stump of the nose is usually turned down as a flap, thus providing lining (Fig. 29–264). Additional skin may be excised in order to establish a wide surface for the revascularization of the transplanted flap and to provide a one-piece continuity to the dorsum, avoiding a transverse break at the junction of the transplanted flap and the dorsal skin of the nose. Overlap between the flap and the alar stump is also necessary for a better blood supply and more rapid healing, as well as for an improved esthetic effect. It is essential that the distal end of the flap, which forms the columella, heals *per primum* at its point of insertion.

A trapdoor flap is raised, the base of the flap being toward the nasal cavity, either from the stump of the columella, if present, or from the area of insertion of the new columella. If the area is deficient in blood supply, the mucosal flap from the inner aspect of the upper lip, as used by Millard (1966), can be brought up

through an opening to be used as a backing for the transplanted columella and to reinforce its blood supply. The flap is then sutured to the posterior edges of the new folded columella, and the distal portion of the new columella is sutured into the defect.

The distal portion of the scalping flap is folded upon itself, and the infolding is maintained by catgut sutures (Fig. 29–265). In order to obtain some refinement in the shape of the tip, alae, and columella, careful thinning of the distal portion of the forehead flap can be done by excising some of the subcutaneous tissue with sharp scissors. Demjén (1967) has performed this procedure for many years without endangering the vitality of the flap. A bolstered mattress suture is placed through the flap in the supratip area in order to eliminate dead space and to prevent hematoma formation (Fig. 29–266).

CONSECUTIVE OR COMBINED USE OF THE SCALPING AND MEDIAN FOREHEAD FLAPS. When the defect extends beyond the area of the nose, involving a portion of the cheek, the median forehead flap can be used to repair the

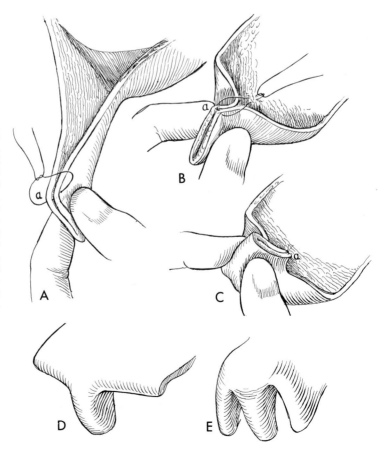

FIGURE 29–265. Infolding the distal end of the flap to reproduce the tip, columella, and alae. *A,* A chromic catgut suture placed to maintain the flaps in apposition *(a)*. *B,* The distal part of the flap is infolded to form the columella. The suture maintains the infolding by approximating point *a* to the undersurface of the flap. The degree of infolding determines the length of the new columella. *C,* The infolding is completed. *D, E,* The nasal tip, columella, and alae formed by the folded flap. (From Converse, J. M.: Reconstruction of the nose by the scalping flap technique. Surg. Clin. North Am., *39*:335, 1959.)

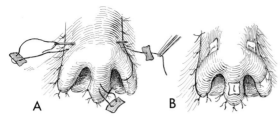

FIGURE 29–266. Mattress sutures are used to eliminate the dead space between the lining flaps and the scalping flap; these sutures should be used with caution.

defect in a preliminary stage (see Fig. 29–261, *A, B*). After a suitable interval, the nose is reconstructed by means of a scalping flap (see Fig. 29–261, *C, D*). The median flap or the island forehead flap can also be used in combi-nation with the scalping flap, the former flaps serving to furnish a lining for the nose when required (see Fig. 29–261).

RECONSTRUCTION OF LARGE UNILATERAL ALAR AND LATERAL WALL DEFECTS. It is often more difficult to obtain a satisfactory esthetic result in unilateral defects involving half of the tip of the nose because of the problem of achieving symmetry with the unaffected contralateral half of the tip. Figure 29–267 shows the successful repair of a defect involving the tip, ala, and lateral wall of the nose by means of a scalping forehead flap lined with a septal composite graft. When the defect is a smaller one, a median flap lined with a septal composite graft is indicated (see Figs. 29–250 and 29–251).

Defects of the lateral wall of the nose and

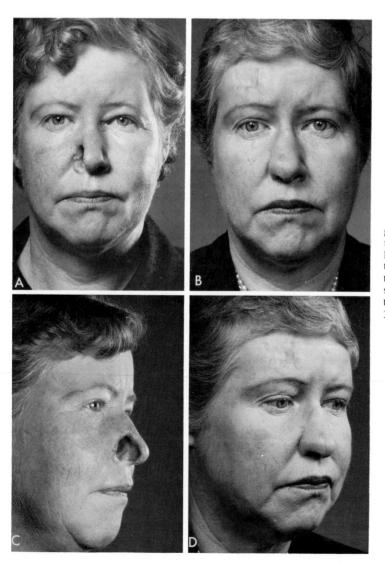

FIGURE 29–267. Septal composite graft and forehead flap for reconstruction of the nose. *A, C,* Defect of lower half of nose. *B, D,* Result obtained by techniques illustrated in Figures 29–268 to 270. (From Converse, J. M.: Reconstruction of the nose by the scalping flap technique. Surg. Clin. North Am., *39:* 335, 1959.)

ala are adequately reconstructed by the scalping flap method. A septal composite graft provides the skeletal support and lining of the new ala (Fig. 29–268, *A*) (Converse, 1956). A suitable portion of the cartilaginous septum is usually found to be slightly curved. A graft of suitable size is chosen in the area where the septal cartilage has the appropriate curvature to reproduce the curvature of the ala (Fig. 29–268, *A*, *B*); cartilage with mucoperichondrium attached is removed. The mucoperichondrium on the contralateral side of the septum is preserved in order to avoid a perforation of the septum; the raw area over the mucoperichondrium heals rapidly by secondary epithelization. When a large graft is required, care should be taken to leave sufficient dorsal support, as well as an anterior buttress of cartilage,

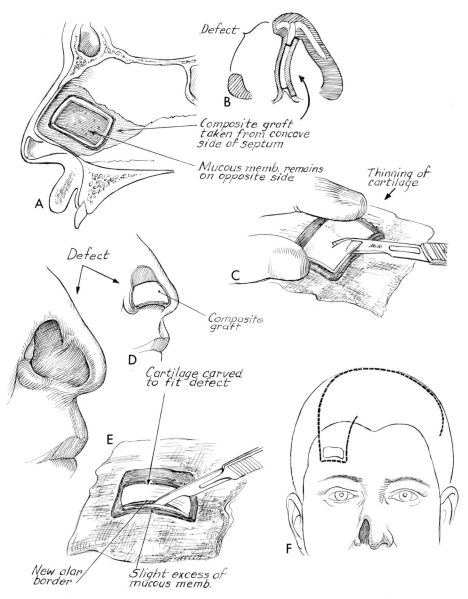

FIGURE 29–268.   Reconstruction of a lateral nasal-alar defect by means of a septal composite graft and scalping flap. *A*, *B*, Area of the septum from which the composite graft is removed. *C*, Thinning of the cartilage by shaving off slices of cartilage. *D*, The defect of the lateral wall of the nose and the size of the composite graft required. *E*, Trimming the distal border of the cartilage graft to reproduce the curve of the alar border. *F*, Position of the septal composite graft under the scalping flap (see Fig. 29–269). (From Converse, J. M.: Composite graft from the septum in nasal reconstruction. Trans. Lat. Am. Congr. Plast. Surg., *8*:281, 1956.)

to prevent depression along the dorsum of the nose and retraction of the columella. The outlining incisions are extended backward toward the perpendicular plate of the ethmoid. The cartilage of the composite graft may be too thick; slices of cartilage are removed if necessary (Fig. 29–268, *C*). The reconstruction has been planned using an Asche metal pattern (Fig. 29–268, *D*). Additional cartilage may require resection so that there is an excess of

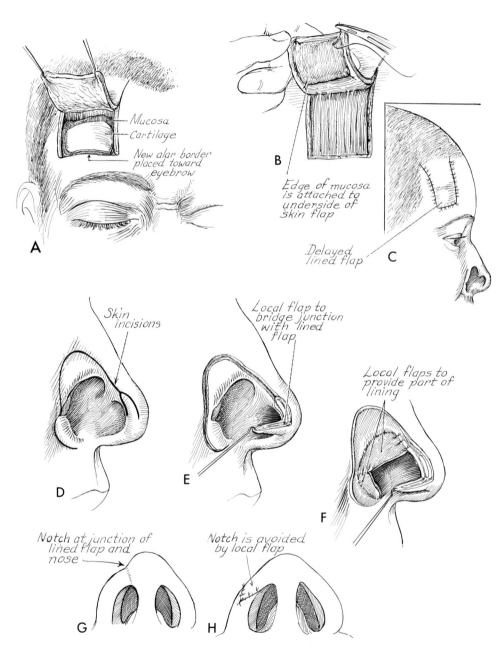

FIGURE 29–269. Reconstruction of a lateral nasal-alar defect (continued). *A*, Position of the septal composite graft on the forehead. *B*, The septal composite graft is sutured to the undersurface of the forehead flap. *C*, The forehead flap is sutured back into position. *D*, Incisions for the lining hinge flaps and the medial triangular flap. *E*, The medial triangular flap is mobilized. *F*, The hinge flaps are turned in to provide a portion of the lining of the defect; the medial triangular flap is in position. *G*, Notching occurs when the triangular flap technique (*E*) is not employed. *H*, The medial triangular flap prevents notching at the area of junction between the forehead flap and the tip of the nose. (From Converse, J. M.: Reconstruction of the nose by the scalping flap technique. Surg. Clin. North Am., *39*:335, 1959.)

mucoperichondrium (Fig. 29–268, *E*). The composite graft is then placed under the distal portion of the scalping flap (Fig. 29–268, *F*).

In a preliminary stage after the outline of the portion of the forehead to be used in the reconstruction, the flap is raised and the composite graft is placed under the distal portion of the flap, mucosal surface facing the frontalis muscle (Fig. 29–269, *A*). The graft is sutured to the undersurface of the flap (Fig. 29–269, *B*). The flap is sutured (Fig. 29–269, *C*). An outline delay of the scalping flap may be performed at this stage. The size of the composite graft need

not be very large, as the major portion of the lining can usually be obtained from the skin situated above the defect, which is rotated downward as a hinge flap.

One of the problems facing the reconstructive surgeon in restoring a missing ala of the nose is avoiding a notch between the reconstructed part and the tip of the nose. A triangular flap consisting of skin and cartilage is outlined and incised (Fig. 29–269, *D*) and is transferred on a cutaneous pedicle (Fig. 29–269, *E*). The lining hinge flaps are turned in (Fig. 29–269, *F*), and the recipient area is

FIGURE 29–270. Reconstruction of a lateral nasal-alar defect (completed). *A*, The scalping flap lined with the septal composite graft is ready to be sutured into position. Note the triangular flap (see Fig. 29–269, *E*) and the local hinge flaps serving as lining. *B*, The triangular flap is joined to the edge of the scalping flap. *C*, Suture of the lining is being completed. *D*, Detail of the suturing of the triangular flap into the border of the scalping flap. *E*, Position of the septal composite graft, which provides alar support. *F*, The intranasal suturing is being completed. Note the respective positions of the new alar border with the triangular flap.

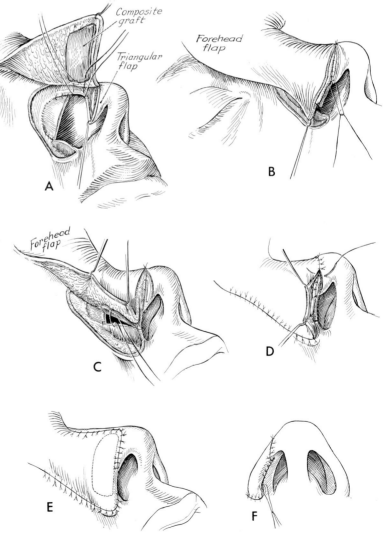

prepared for the forehead flap. Figure 29–269 *G* and *H* illustrates how the triangular flap prevents notching.

Details of the insertion of the new ala and the final suturing to the lining flaps and the edges of the defect are illustrated in Figure 29–270. The triangular flap (Fig. 29–270, *A*) is inserted into the border of the new ala between the skin and the mucoperichondrium of the composite graft; the inner layers are sutured first (Fig. 29–270, *B*, *C*); the skin edges are then sutured (Fig. 29–270, *D*). The operation is completed (Fig. 29–270, *E*, *F*).

The advantages of the septal composite graft in reconstruction of defects involving the alar border are threefold: (1) the length of the forehead flap is diminished, because the infolding of the distal end of the flap is not a requirement, the lining being provided by the composite graft; (2) the risks involved in the folding of the distal end of the flap, with its attendant

diminution of the blood supply, are eliminated; (3) the border of the ala is thin, in contrast with the thicker alar border formed by the infolding of the distal end of the forehead flap.

If septal cartilage is not available or is not of adequate shape, a composite graft is obtained from the auricular concha (see Fig. 29–218) (Gillies, 1943).

Immediate transplantation of the septal composite graft has been attempted to restore the lining at the time of the forehead flap transfer. The rich vascularization of the scalping flap may lead to the assumption that such a graft will be successful. In our experience, however, shrinkage and contraction cause a disappointing distortion of the alar border.

THE SCALPING AND MEDIAN FOREHEAD FLAPS IN LATERAL NASAL DEFECTS. The septal composite graft, utilizing both septal cartilage and the perpendicular plate of the ethmoid, is embedded under the forehead flap in a

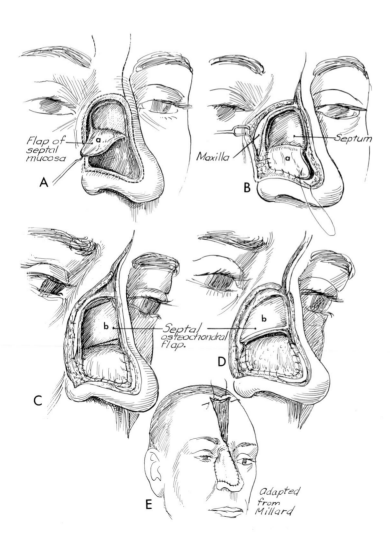

FIGURE 29–271. Lateral nasal wall defect repaired by a median forehead flap and the septal framework and lining. *A,* The septal mucous membrane *(a)* is raised from the remaining septum and turned down to furnish the lining of the lower part of the lateral nasal wall. *B,* The flap is sutured in position. *C,* After completion of the suturing. *D,* The remaining portion of the septum is transferred, hinged on a mucous membrane flap near the dorsum of the nose, and rests on the maxilla (see Fig. 29–272). *E,* A median forehead flap provides cutaneous coverage. (After Millard, 1967, 1967a.)

preliminary stage. At a later date, the flap is transferred to the defect. This technique, as well as the septal flap technique illustrated in Figure 29–226, is an excellent method for restoring the lateral nasal wall.

Millard (1967a) has employed a modification of the septal flap technique (see Fig. 29–226) for a lateral wall defect involving the bony as well as the cartilaginous framework of the nose (Fig. 29–271). The mucoperiosteum is raised from the perpendicular plate of the ethmoid, freed from its cephalic, lateral and medial attachments, folded down to form the lining of the lower portion of the defect (Fig. 29–271, *A, B*), and sutured to the edges of the defect. The perpendicular plate of the ethmoid and some of the cartilaginous septum are freed by cutting through three sides of the structures, leaving the septal flap hinged on the dorsal border of the septum. The septal flap is transferred laterally, where it rests on the maxilla and is fixed by a suture (Figs. 29–271, *C, D* and 29–272). A median forehead flap covers the reconstructed nasal lining (Figs. 29–271, *E* and 29–273).

THE SCALPING FLAP FOR RECONSTRUCTION FOLLOWING CHEMOSURGICAL TREATMENT. The patient shown in Figure 29–274, *A* had undergone Mohs' chemosurgical treatment (see Chapter 65) for a multicentric basal cell

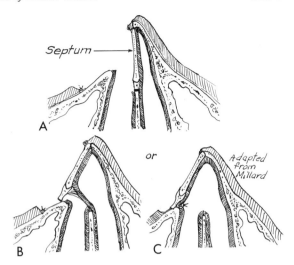

FIGURE 29–272. The septum used for framework and lining in a lateral nasal defect. *A*, The septum and the defect. *B*, The base of the vomer is sectioned; the mucous membrane on the contralateral side remains attached; the septum rests on the maxilla, where it is anchored by a suture. *C*, An alternative procedure. (After Millard, 1967a.)

carcinoma which had extended over the skin of the dorsum. Reconstruction was achieved by resurfacing the dorsum of the nose with a scalping flap and was completed in a later stage by a costal cartilage graft (Fig. 29–274).

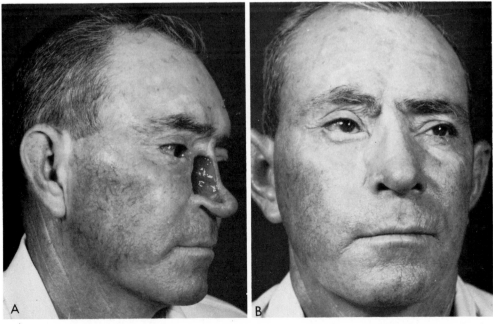

FIGURE 29–273. Repair of lateral nasal wall defect. *A*, Defect resulting from resection of recurrent basal cell carcinoma. *B*, Result obtained by the technique illustrated in Figures 29–271 and 29–272. (From Millard, D. R., Jr.: Hemirhinoplasty. Plast. Reconstr. Surg., *40*:440. 1967. Copyright © 1967, The Williams & Wilkins Company, Baltimore.)

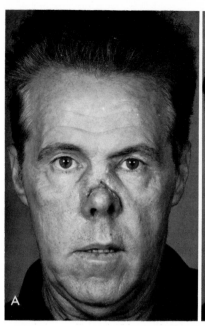

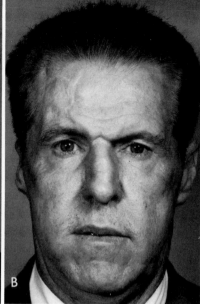

FIGURE 29–274. Resurfacing the nose by a scalping flap after chemosurgery. *A,* Deformity resulting from Mohs' chemosurgical treatment for the eradication of a multicentric, recurrent basal cell carcinoma. *B,* After excision of the scar, elongation of the nose, and resurfacing with a scalping flap.

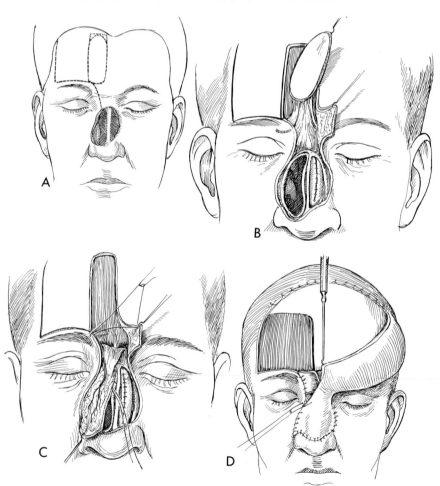

FIGURE 29–275. Reconstruction of a full-thickness defect of the nose by a combination of a scalping flap and an island forehead flap. *A,* Respective positions of the forehead flaps, which will provide the covering and the lining tissue. *B,* The island flap is raised on a subcutaneous pedicle. Mucous membrane from the septum provides lining tissue over the left nasal fossa. *C,* The island flap furnishes the lining for the remainder of the defect. *D,* The scalping flap transfer is being completed. (From Converse, J. M.: Clinical applications of the scalping flap in reconstruction of the nose. Plast. Reconstr. Surg., *43*:247, 1969. Copyright © 1969. The Williams & Wilkins Company, Baltimore.)

THE SCALPING FLAP IN FULL-THICKNESS DORSAL NASAL DEFECTS. Use of an island flap with a subcutaneous tissue pedicle has proved to be an excellent technique when employed in conjunction with a scalping flap in reconstructing full-thickness defects of the dorsum (Fig. 29–275, *A*). A cloth pattern of the required lining is measured and placed upside down at the suitable level of the forehead to ensure a flap of adequate length to reach the defect. After the island flap with its subcutaneous pedicle and its supratrochlear blood supply is mobilized (Fig. 29–275, *B*), the island of skin is placed, cutaneous surface downward, into the defect (Fig. 29–275, *C*). A scalping flap of suitable size furnishes the covering skin (Fig. 29–275, *D*).

The use of two superimposed flaps is superior to the employment of a skin graft placed in a preliminary stage under the scalping flap. As previously stated, a skin graft lining renders the placing of a subsequent skeletal framework very difficult, if not impossible. In contrast, when two superimposed flaps are employed, a cleavage plane is readily found into which supporting bone or cartilage can be introduced. In the patient shown in Figure 29–276 (*A* and *C*), a costal cartilage graft was later employed, as the nasal bones had been resected and there was no bony recipient site for a bone graft (Fig. 29–276, *B*, *D*).

The island flap technique is particularly suited to the repair of defects of the nasal lining; the subcutaneous pedicle may be cut

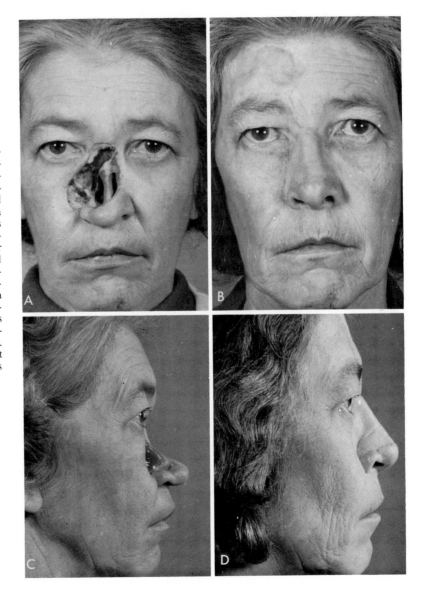

FIGURE 29–276. Reconstruction of the nose by combined scalping and island forehead flaps. *A, C,* Large, full-thickness defect of the nose and adjacent area of the cheek. In a first stage, the cheek tissue was advanced to cover the defect lateral to the nose. *B, D,* After reconstruction by combined scalping and island flaps, as illustrated in Figure 29–275. Structural support was provided by a costal cartilage graft. (From Converse, J. M.: Clinical applications of the scalping flap in reconstruction of the nose. Plast. Reconstr. Surg., *43*:247, 1969. Copyright © 1969. The Williams & Wilkins Company, Baltimore.)

rather narrow as the flap falls into place, skin surface downward, without the accompanying twist required when the flap is employed for the repair of surface defects.

The island flap method does not require a separation of the pedicle and thus is a one-stage procedure. If the subcutaneous pedicle is too wide, an objectionable bulge may be noted at the root of the nose. Subsequent subcutaneous excision of the excess tissue may be required.

RECONSTRUCTION OF THE NOSE FOLLOWING EXTENSIVE RADIATION. Because ra-

diated skin showing signs of skin damage and telangiectases is potentially malignant and also has a poor blood supply, the skin of the stump of the nose cannot be employed as a turnover flap to provide the necessary lining. A forehead island flap with a subcutaneous pedicle furnishes the lining.

Following radiation of tumors of the upper portion of the nose, the medial canthal areas may also show radiation damage.

If the septum is not involved, sufficient lining tissue may be obtained from the septal mucous membrane, as less tissue is needed to line a de-

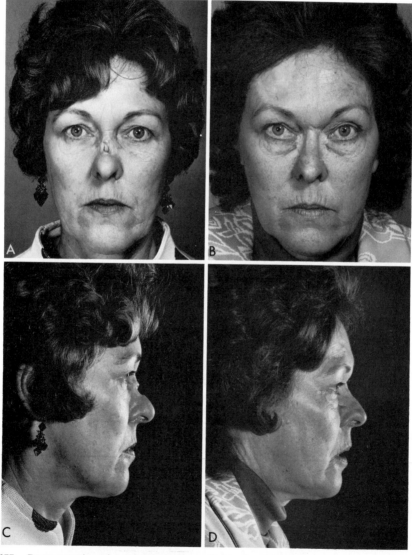

FIGURE 29–277. Reconstruction of nasal defect after radiation for the treatment of basal cell carcinoma. *A,* A full thickness defect is surrounded by an area of radiated skin extending laterally to each medial canthus. *B,* After reconstruction. Sufficient lining was obtained from the mucous membrane of the septum and lateral wall of the nose. A scalping flap resurfaced the entire radiated area. A costal cartilage graft was introduced at a later date for skeletal support. *C, D,* Before and after profile views. Hair styling will hide the donor site of the scalping flap.

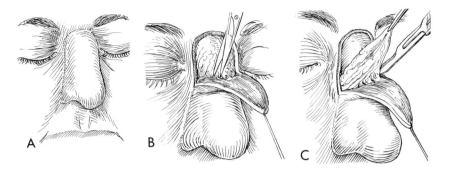

FIGURE 29–278. Reduction in bulk and defatting of the reconstructed nose. *A*, Immediately following the reconstruction. *B*, A flap is raised from the upper half of the nose, and the underlying subcutaneous tissue is exposed. *C*, The excess fat is resected.

fect in this narrower upper portion of the nose. The skin of the scalping flap may also be required to resurface the canthal areas after excision of the damaged skin (Fig. 29–277).

"RETOUCHING" PROCEDURES. Elderly patients may be satisfied with the result of the two initial procedures, but as a rule the best possible result is desired by most patients.

Retouching operations are required at suitable intervals starting not earlier than four months following the completion of the reconstruction. Retouching procedures include the resection of excessive subcutaneous tissue, the thinning of the alar margins and columella, and

occasionally the adjustment of the edges of the flap to the adjacent tissues.

The upper half of the flap is raised, and excess subcutaneous tissue is excised (Fig. 29–278). A dental compound nasal splint is applied after the flap is sutured back into position to prevent hematoma formation. A carefully molded dental compound splint (see Fig. 29–77) does not endanger the viability of the undermined flap.

In a second stage, the lateral aspects of the lower half of the flap are raised in the area of the alar groove (Fig. 29–279). In the normal nose, this is the area that overlies the nasal

FIGURE 29–279. Postoperative defatting of the reconstructed nose. *A*, The reconstructed nose with excessive bulk. *B*, After the upper half of the nose has been operated upon (see Fig. 29–278), flaps are raised on each side to expose the underlying subcutaneous tissue. *C*, Excess subcutaneous tissue and fat are resected. A similar procedure is done on the opposite side. *D*, Appearance following defatting procedure.

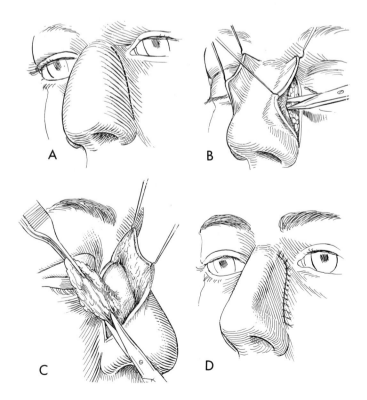

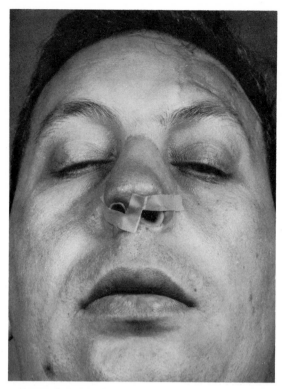

FIGURE 29–280. Intranasal molds have been made from dental compound impressions. Molds are made of thin acrylic and are worn by the patient for a period of time after retouching procedures on the tip of the nose have been completed.

valve, the area of junction between the alar and lateral cartilages. The redundancy of the reconstructed ala is thus decreased. Again a carefully molded dental compound splint is applied as a dressing.

The alae may require thinning, and the tendency for constriction and stenosis of the new vestibule of the reconstructed nose is counteracted by the insertion of acrylic molds made from dental compound impressions (Fig. 29–280).

Restoration of the Skeletal Framework. Providing a skeletal framework for the reconstructed nose has been of concern to surgeons performing reconstructive rhinoplasty. Ollier (1861) attempted to provide support by means of a flap of periosteum included in a forehead flap, hoping that the periosteum would regenerate bone. König (1886) included a piece of bone in the forehead flap. Neláton (1902) embedded costal cartilage under the forehead flap prior to the transfer of the flap. Gillies (1920) considered this procedure unsound and

advocated using the remaining septum instead to provide skeletal support at the time of the reconstructive rhinoplasty.

In subtotal rhinoplasty much of the septum is preserved; Millard (1974) has modified Gillies' concept (Fig. 29–281) in the following manner (Fig. 29–282). The septum is cut in an L-shaped manner (Fig. 29–282, *A*), is separated from the vomer groove, and is advanced forward on a superior pedicle (Fig. 29–282, *B*); the base of the L-shaped segment of septum is then set and fixed on the nasal spine (Fig. 29–282, *C*). The size and shape of the septal flap are planned in advance by means of a paper model (see Fig. 29–283).

THE GULL-SHAPED MEDIAN FLAP (MILLARD, 1974). In patients with a recessed hairline, a frequent occurrence in older patients, the median flap may be extended upward, thus pro-

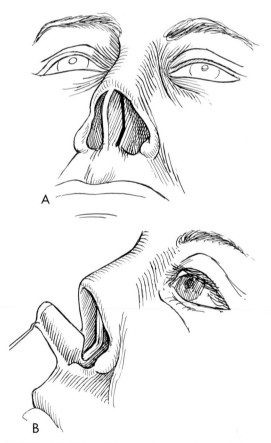

FIGURE 29–281. Gillies' technique of using the septum for skeletal support of the lower portion of the nose. *A*, Outline of incision through the septum. *B*, The septum is transferred on an inferior pedicle.

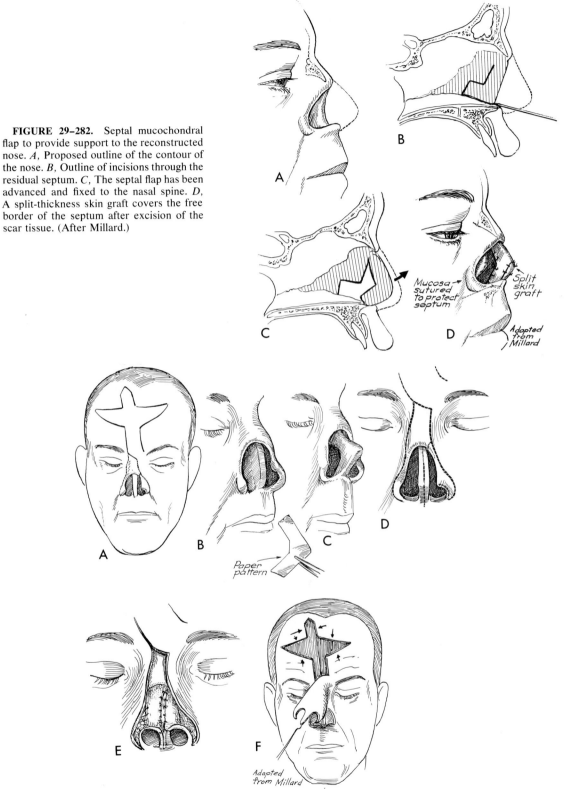

FIGURE 29–282. Septal mucochondral flap to provide support to the reconstructed nose. *A,* Proposed outline of the contour of the nose. *B,* Outline of incisions through the residual septum. *C,* The septal flap has been advanced and fixed to the nasal spine. *D,* A split-thickness skin graft covers the free border of the septum after excision of the scar tissue. (After Millard.)

FIGURE 29–283. The gull-shaped median forehead flap. *A,* Outline of the flap. In order to reconstruct the defect shown in Figure 29–284, a composite auricular chondrocutaneous graft was placed under the future right ala. A small cartilage graft was placed under the future tip. Note the design of the pedicle of the flap. The flap was delayed. *B,* The defect. *C,* The septal mucochondral flap (see Fig. 29–282) for support. *D,* Outline of turnover lining flaps. *E,* The lining flaps sutured. The defect of the right ala will be restored by the composite graft carried by the median flap (see *A*). *F,* The flap is transferred. The arrows indicate the direction of the closure of the forehead defect. (After Millard.)

viding extra length. Among the many variations in the shape of the median flap is the
gull-shaped flap (Fig. 29–283, *A*), which has
the advantage of facilitating closure of the
forehead defect in two directions (see Fig. 29–
285, *D*). When sufficient alar tissue is not
available to furnish adequate lining (Fig. 29–
284), a composite graft is embedded under the
flap, which is delayed in a preliminary stage
and transferred two months later. In the patient shown in Figure 29–284, a chondrocutaneous auricular graft was placed under the fu-

ture right alar border in the preliminary stage.

When no tip tissue is available, Millard has
employed nasolabial flaps for lining; the tips of
the nasolabial flaps embrace each other to form
the columella (Fig. 29–285).

In order to facilitate the transfer of the flap,
the design shown in Figure 29–283, *A* is used.
Millard leaves the pedicle of the flap undivided
until all of the secondary surgery required to refine the reconstructed nose is completed. Two
months later he partially divides the pedicle,
preserving a subcutaneous pedicle containing

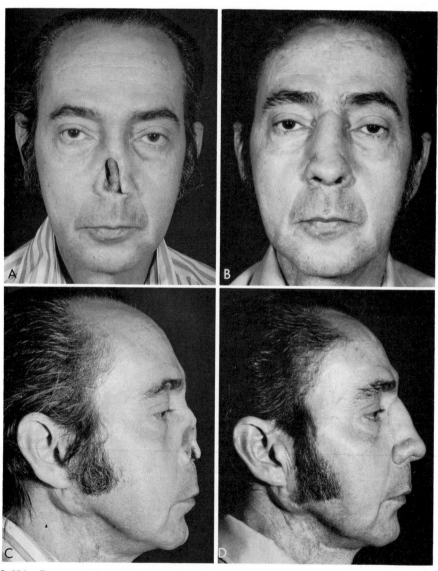

FIGURE 29–284.   Reconstruction of the lower half of the nose. *A*, Defect resulting from resection of squamous cell carcinoma. *B*, Result obtained by technique illustrated in Figures 29–282 and 29–283. *C*, Preoperative profile appearance. *D*, Postoperative appearance. (From Millard, D. R., Jr.: Reconstructive rhinoplasty for the lower half of a nose. Plast. Reconstr. Surg., *53*:133, 1974. Copyright © 1974, The Williams & Wilkins Company, Baltimore.)

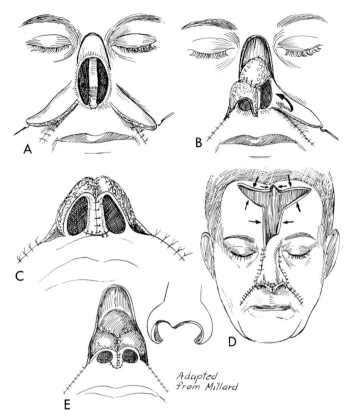

FIGURE 29–285. Reconstruction of the lower half of the nose. Use of nasolabial flaps for lining. *A*, Outline of turnover hinge flap from the nasal stump for lining. Two nasolabial flaps have been raised. *B*, The right nasolabial flap and the turned-down flap are sutured. *C*, The nasolabial flaps furnish the lining of the tip and alae and join to form the columella. *D*, The gull-shaped flap furnishes the cover. The arrows indicate the direction of the closure of the forehead defect. *E*, The donor areas of the nasolabial flaps are closed. The gull-shaped flap is ready to be applied over the lining flaps.

the nourishing blood vessels and lymphatic drainage and thus avoiding the edema which follows complete severance of the pedicle.

SECONDARY GRAFTING OF A SKELETAL FRAMEWORK IN SUBTOTAL RHINOPLASTY. A supportive framework is provided after the completion of the soft tissue reconstruction, but not until the tissues are softened and well-vascularized. If a sufficient area of the nasal bones has been preserved, the area of junction of the flap with the nasal stump is incised and raised (Fig. 29–286, *A*, *B*). The skin and subcutaneous tissues are raised and undermined downward to the tip (Fig. 29–286, *C*), and a cantilever bone graft provides adequate skeletal support (Converse, 1964). A plane of dissection is found between the inner lining and the outer covering flap and is extended down to the tip of the nose.

The bone is exposed and a trough is made in the midline of the bony dorsum by means of an air turbine-driven bur (Fig. 29–286, *D*, *E*, *F*). Stainless steel wires are passed through the bony tunnels (Fig. 29–286, *G*). A suitably shaped bone graft, usually removed from the iliac crest (a split rib graft in a child), is inlayed into the bony trough and extends downward into the subcutaneous pocket to the tip of the reconstructed nose (Fig. 29–286, *H*, *I*). The wires are then looped over the bone graft, firmly anchoring it into the bony trough. The wires are twisted and the ends of the wire buried in the drill holes (Figs. 29–287 and 29–288).

When only a small portion of the nasal bones remains after the resection or destruction of the remainder of the nose, fixation and adequate angulation of the bone graft are more difficult. A hole is drilled into the frontal bone at the nasofrontal angle; the proximal end of the bone graft, once wedged into the hole, is anchored. The angulation suitable for the nasal profile is controlled by a wedge-shaped piece of bone placed under the bone graft and the bony stump of the nose. Millard (1966), using the technique illustrated in Figure 29–286, *J* with costal bone, has calculated that the graft is capable of supporting 9.95 pounds.

A costal cartilage graft is usually preferable as a means of skeletal support (see Figs. 29–276, 29–277, and 29–289) when the nasal

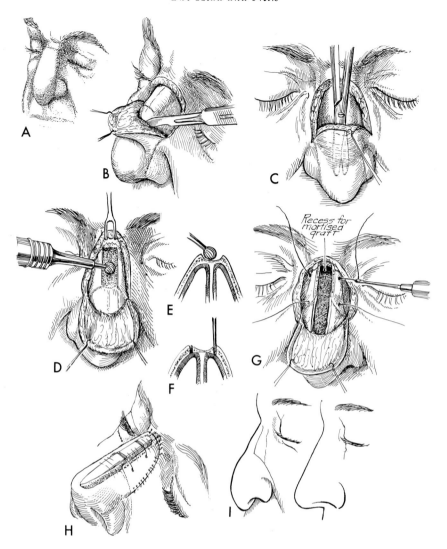

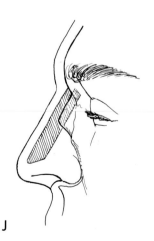

FIGURE 29–286. Provision of a skeletal framework for the reconstructed nose. *A,* Reconstructed nose with a tendency toward drooping of tip owing to lack of skeletal support. *B,* Exposure of bony stump of nose. *C,* Undermining of soft tissue down toward the tip of the nose. *D,* Establishment of a groove in the bony stump. *E,* The groove. *F,* If necessary, the entire thickness of bone may be removed. *G,* Wires are passed through the nasal bones for fixation of the inset bone graft. *H,* Cantilever inset bone graft maintained by wire fixation to bony stump. *I,* Manner by which skeletal framework maintains contour of the reconstructed nose. When sufficient bone is not available because of more extensive resection and cannot provide a satisfactory host bed bone graft, a costal cartilage graft is preferable (Fig. 29–276). *J,* Millard's technique using a costal bone graft wedged into the frontal bone. (*A* to *I* from Converse, J. M.: Clinical applications of the scalping flap in reconstructive surgery of the nose. Plast. Reconstr. Surg., *43:*247, 1967. *J* after Millard, 1966.)

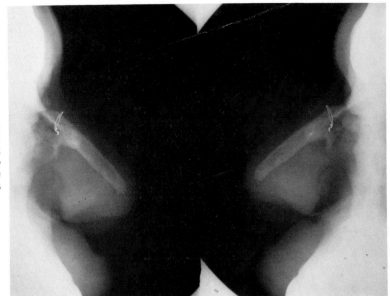

FIGURE 29-287. Cantilever bone graft for the support of the reconstructed nose. Roentgenograms taken five years after bone grafting show consolidation of the graft to the underlying framework of the nose. Wire fixation was provided, as illustrated in Figure 29-286.

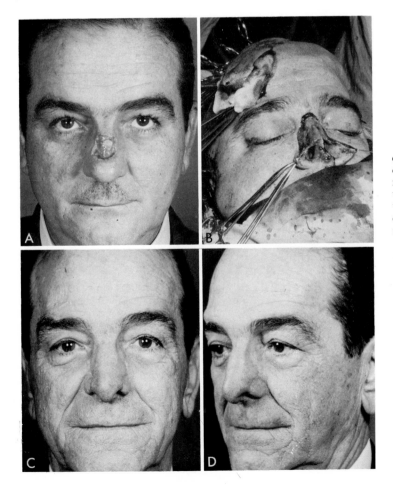

FIGURE 29-288. *A,* Ulcerated, recurrent, irradiated basal cell carcinoma of the nose. *B,* Appearance after the resection. An immediate reconstruction was done. Such a procedure is not advisable. Absolute certainty of the freedom of the margins of the defect from neoplastic involvement, whether by frozen section or routine sections, is an absolute prerequisite to repair. If doubt exists, the skin and mucosal edges should be sutured or the defect covered with a split-thickness graft until verification of freedom of involvement is obtained. *C, D,* Appearance 20 years after the scalping flap reconstruction of the nose and subsequent iliac bone grafting.

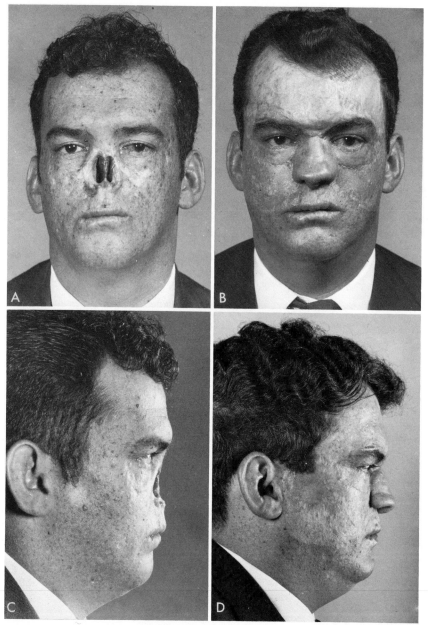

FIGURE 29–289. Total reconstruction of the nose by combined scalping flap and island flap techniques. *A,* Patient with xeroderma pigmentosum who had undergone total amputation of the nose for recurrent basal cell epithelioma. The patient was treated by dermabrasion and overgrafting, with split-thickness skin grafts covering the forehead and cheeks. Full-thickness retroauricular skin grafts replaced the skin of the lower eyelids. *B,* Reconstruction was achieved by a scalping flap for cutaneous coverage and an island flap for lining (see Fig. 29–275). *C,* Preoperative profile view, showing minimal residual nasal bones. *D,* After reconstruction and placement of a costal cartilage framework.

bones have been destroyed, as bone grafts require intimate contact with host bone for survival.

Total Reconstruction of the Nose

Total loss of the nasal pyramid is less frequent than subtotal loss. Patients with recurrent carcinoma may require total resection, and reconstruction can be considered only if control of the disease offers a reasonable chance that the risk of recurrence is not a contraindication to reconstructive surgery. Total loss of the nose resulting from trauma is rare. Various tropical diseases and amputation of the nose as a form of punishment are other causes of total nasal loss.

Total Reconstructive Rhinoplasty. The skin of the bony stump is not available when the entire nose (or nearly the entire nose) has been amputated. The patient shown in Figure 29–289 had undergone nasal amputation for recurrent basal cell carcinoma, and only a small amount of scarred tissue remained at the root of the nose and was poorly suited to furnish any portion of the nasal lining. The surrounding tissue could not be used for hinged turn-in flaps. He was afflicted with an unusual type of xeroderma pigmentosum which involved only his face. When he was first seen, a number of basal cell carcinomas were diagnosed and excised. Later he was treated by sequential dermabrasion and split-thickness skin grafting of the major portion of his face, including the entire forehead (Fig. 29–289, *A, C*). When local flaps are unavailable for lining, tissue must be found eslewhere. In this patient an island forehead flap (see Fig. 29–275) furnished the lining, and a scalping forehead flap provided cutaneous coverage (Fig. 29–289, *B, D*). A costal

FIGURE 29–290. Placing the fulcrum to support the new bony framework. *A*, Outline of incisions around the defect and a median forehead flap. *B*, Lining tissue is obtained from the mucous membrane of the nasal cavity. *C*, The flap covers the mucous membrane. *D*, Two months later, the covering flap was raised from above; a mortised fulcrum is wired to the edges of the bony defect. *E*, The skin flap is then replaced and sutured. *F*, Coronal section, illustrating the position of the fulcrum. (After Millard, 1966.)

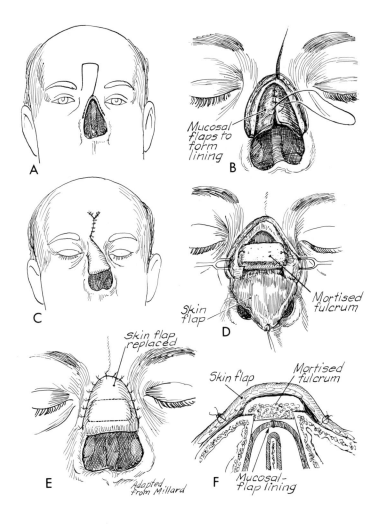

cartilage graft was inserted subsequently. The reconstruction was successful despite the prior skin overgrafting, the poorly vascularized recipient site, and the fact that the scalping flap was not delayed. Final surgical procedures were interrupted because the patient was obliged to return to his native country; he was, however, alive and well ten years after nasal reconstruction.

PRIMARY GRAFTING OF A SKELETAL FRAMEWORK IN SUBTOTAL AND TOTAL RHINOPLASTY. As a point of reference for total reconstruction when there is complete absence of a foundation in the form of any skeletal structure, placing a bone strut in the form of a cantilever bone graft fitted into a notch in the frontal bone and fixed to a bony platform wired to the maxilla (Millard, 1966) is a valuable asset. The danger of necrosis of the flap must be overcome by using a large flap and avoiding the infolding of the distal portion of the flap for the forming of the alae. Millard lined the portion of the forehead flap to serve as the future columella and alae with split-thickness grafts to avoid the infolding of the distal portion of the flap and the risk of necrosis as may occur in the procedure illustrated in Figure 29–265.

In a preliminary stage the cephalic portion of the defect is lined with mucous membrane dissected from within the nasal vault (Fig. 29–290, *A, B*) and is covered with a median forehead flap (Fig. 29–290, *C*). Two months later the cephalic portion of the flap is raised and a split rib graft, serving as a strut, is mortised and wired to the maxilla on each side (Fig. 29–290, *D*). The flap is sutured back into position (Fig. 29–290, *E, F*).

A large horizontal flap based on the vessels of the right supraorbital area is outlined. At its distal portion in the left temporal area, the future columella and alar rims are lined with thick split-thickness grafts (Fig. 29–291, *A*). Two months later the skin covering the fulcrum derived from the median forehead flap is raised and turned down as a hinge flap to furnish additional lining. The major portion of the rib graft taken previously and stored in the chest wall is shaped and fitted into a notch in the frontal bone in a position most suitable for the nasal profile when the graft is supported by the previously placed bony platform acting as fulcrum (Fig. 29–292). The cantilever graft is fixed to the frontal bone with a stainless steel wire and stabilized by means of guy sutures passing over the graft and through the bony platform on each side (Fig. 29–291, *B*).

The turned-down median flap is fitted to the undersurface of the cantilever bone graft by a suture looped around it and is joined by small turn-up flaps from the sides of the nasal cavity (Fig. 29–291, *C*). The forehead flap is draped over the bone graft. The alae and columella are sutured in position; the columella is reinforced by a labial mucosal flap brought through a buttonhole incision in the lip. The large secondary defect on the left side of the forehead is repaired by a flap transposed from the bald scalp, and the secondary defect is repaired by a split-thickness skin graft (Fig. 29–291, *D, E*). The result of the reconstruction is shown in Figure 29–293.

Complications of Forehead Flaps. The major complication is the loss of a portion of the flap resulting from inadequate vascularization. The usual causes are inadequate design of the flap, tension on the flap, hematoma formation, excessive thinning of the distal portion of the flap, and the presence of preexisting scars traversing the flap.

Inadequate design, an excessively narrow pedicle, and a short flap are usual causes of tension and ischemia after the flap is transferred to the nose; tension is the most frequent cause of ischemia. A hematoma within the tubed portion of a scalping flap, an unusual occurrence, causes circulatory embarrassment if it is not evacuated. Prudence must be exerted in thinning the distal portion of the flap and in excising subcutaneous tissue for the purpose of obtaining delicately modeled alae.

When the flap is not of adequate size and length, the complication of inadequate shaping of the new nose is inevitable. When the flap is too short, the tip of the new nose is retracted downward because of the short columella, a complication previously emphasized.

Stenosis of the reconstructed nares is another complication of the excessively short flap. Sufficient tissue must be available for adequate infolding of the flap. The infolded skin provides the lining of the new vestibules, ensures adequate airways, and prevents stenosis. Occasionally, a ringlike stenosis has been seen at the area of junction of the infolded scalping flap and the turned-down hinge flap from the dorsum of the nose. Relief by Z-plasty, inlay skin grafting, and long-term maintenance of the aperture by acrylic molds (see Fig. 29–280) may be required.

THE NECROTIC FLAP: SUBSEQUENT MANAGEMENT. When it becomes apparent that necrosis is inevitable, the flap should be detached and the sloughing area excised. The remainder

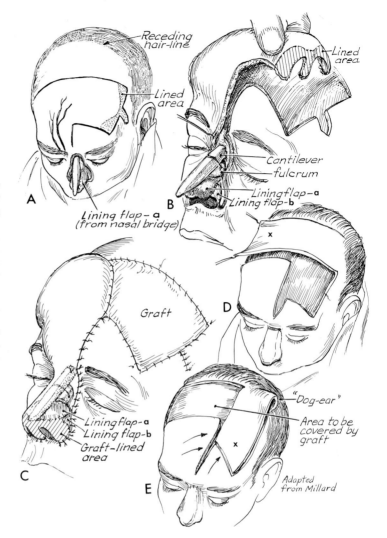

FIGURE 29–291. Transfer of flap for total nose reconstruction and repair of the forehead defect. *A,* Outline of flap. The dotted area at the distal end of the flap indicates the split-thickness skin graft lining placed in a preliminary stage. *B,* The skeletal framework (see Fig. 29–292) and the lining flaps are in place. *C,* The flap has been transferred and the forehead defect skin grafted. *D,* After severance of the pedicle, the unused portion of the forehead flap is returned to the forehead. Flap (*x*) is raised from the bald area over the calvarium. *E,* The flap (*x*) is transposed over the forehead defect, and the donor area is covered by a split-thickness skin graft. (After Millard.)

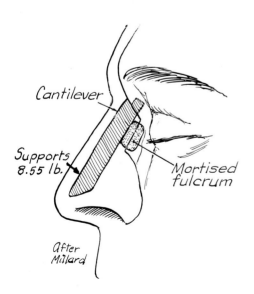

FIGURE 29–292. The cantilever rib graft has been shaped, inserted, and wired into the frontal bone, and, resting on the fulcrum, it is placed at a suitable nasal angle. (After Millard.)

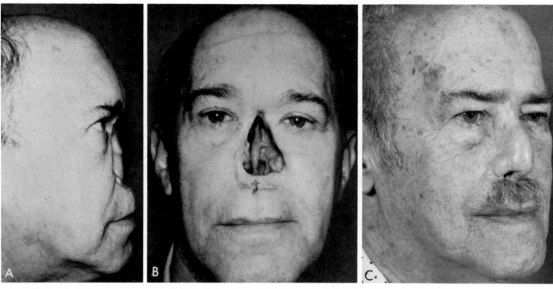

FIGURE 29–293. Total reconstruction of the nose. *A, B,* Photographs of patient after total resection of the nose. *C,* Result obtained by the techniques illustrated in Figures 29–290, 29–291, and 29–292. (From Millard, D. R., Jr: Total reconstructive rhinoplasty and a missing link. Plast. Reconstr. Surg., *37*:167, 1966. Copyright © 1966, The Williams & Wilkins Company, Baltimore.)

of the flap is returned to its donor bed, and the resulting defect on the forehead is skin-grafted.

Because the scalping flap utilizes the skin on the lateral aspect of the forehead, the remainder of the forehead is intact and may be utilized for a second nasal reconstruction. After a suitable time interval, the same scalping flap may be employed to transfer the forehead skin immediately medial to the sloughed area; preferably, another scalping flap is utilized to transfer skin from the opposite side of the forehead, one of the advantages of the scalping flap technique.

The scalping flap is remarkably sturdy. Not only is it capable of being used a second time to transplant skin from the contralateral side of the forehead, but also it has been used in reconstructing the nose in severely burned patients after the forehead donor site had been resurfaced by a split-thickness graft. In the latter procedure, an outline delay preceding transfer of the flap is advisable.

Reconstruction of the Nose by Methods Other than the Forehead Flap. The forehead flap is the method of choice in nasal reconstruction. In addition to the risks attending the transfer of a flap from a distant area and the discomfort endured by the patient, the results obtained in major nasal reconstruction using distant flaps have not been as satisfactory as those obtained using forehead flaps. The color and texture of

the transplanted skin are less satisfactory, and the flap is often too bulky.

According to Ortiz-Monasterio (1975), the forehead flap is contraindicated in patients with dark skin in whom a skin graft must be used to repair the secondary forehead defect, because the graft becomes darkly pigmented.

BRACHIAL FLAPS

The Tagliacotian technique. Tissue must be borrowed from another portion of the body when the forehead is unavailable as a donor site. The anteromedial aspect of the arm is hairless, and with the exception of its color, the skin is suitable for nasal covering. The technique described by Tagliacozzi (1597) employed a retrograde delayed flap from the arm. Because the Tagliacotian flap receives its blood supply from a distal base, the proximal base being detached for transplantation, a preliminary delay of the flap is necessary. Joseph (1931) designed an arm flap with a more laterally situated pedicle to improve the blood supply of the flap and to obviate the need for a preliminary delay procedure (Fig. 29–294). A tubed flap from the arm with a proximal or distal base may be employed for reconstruction of a defect of the nose (Fig. 29–295).

In the direct transfer of skin flaps from the arm to the nose, strict immobilization of the upper extremity to the head is necessary to ensure normal healing of the brachial flap and recipient site.

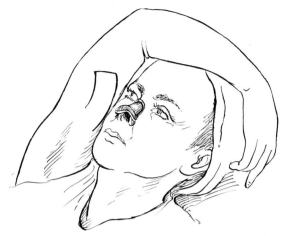

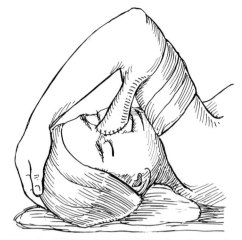

FIGURE 29–294. Brachial flap for nasal reconstruction. (After Joseph, 1931.)

FIGURE 29–295. Tube brachial flap for nasal reconstruction.

A number of methods have been employed to secure immobilization. Tagliacozzi used a leather harness. Malgaigne (1838) achieved fixation by an ingenious support which combined a cloth jacket and a harness. Another method of immobilization involves use of a plaster of Paris bandage head cap; an additional plaster bandage forms a splint around the arm and thus maintains the upper extremity and head in strict immobilization.

CERVICAL FLAPS. Tube flaps raised in the cervical area parallel to a line of minimal tension have been employed for reconstructing nasal defects (Young, 1946). In another technique, one end of the tube flap is detached and attached under the chin. The other end is then detached and extends to the nasal defect.

ACROMIOPECTORAL AND DELTOPECTORAL FLAPS. Other types of distant flaps have been employed. The acromiopectoral tube flap (Gillies, 1935) is usually detached at its medial

extremity and transferred to the nasal region, a satisfactory flap for resurfacing but a poor one for subtotal nasal reconstruction.

The unipedicle deltopectoral flap (see Chapter 63), which is an extended, nondelayed version of the Gillies acromiopectoral tubed flap, based on a medial pedicle, is available as an alternative method of immediate resurfacing of the nose (McGregor and Jackson, 1970; Song, Wise and Bromberg, 1973).

ABDOMINAL FLAPS. An abdominal tube flap is usually transferred to the nose by way of the upper extremity. A position of transfer for this flap is the "salute position" (Fig. 29–296) advocated by Kilner (1937). The upper end of an oblique abdominal tube flap is attached to the radial aspect of the wrist (Fig. 29–296, *A*). In a subsequent stage, the lower end of the tube flap is detached from the abdomen, and the flap is transferred to the face by way of the wrist, where it is opened and in-

FIGURE 29–296. Salute position (Kilner, 1937) for the transfer of an abdominal tube flap to the nose. *A*, Attachment of the abdominal tube flap to the radial aspect of the wrist. *B*, Salute position. The dorsal aspect of the wrist is applied against the forehead. The tube extends downward from the radial border.

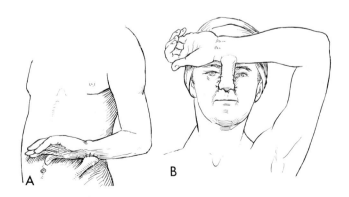

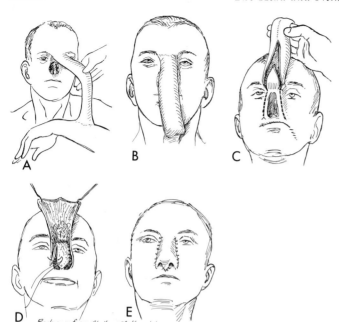

FIGURE 29–297.　　The abdominal tube flap in nose reconstruction. (After Chetrov, 1954, and Kavrakirov, 1961.) *A,* A long abdominal tube is transferred on the wrist to the glabellar region. *B,* In a later stage, the tube is detached from the wrist and attached to the submental area. *C,* Preparation of the lining flap from the undersurface of the tube. *D,* The lining flap is sutured to the edges of the nasal defect; the tube is defatted. *E,* Operation is completed.

Redrawn from Chetrov & Kavrakirov

serted over the nasal area. The dorsal aspect of the forearm is placed against the forehead and immobilized in the position illustrated in Figure 29–296, *B,* with the volar aspect of the forearm and hand facing forward.

The flap is severed from its connection with the arm 18 to 21 days after the flap transfer. Sufficient tissue must be left attached to the nose so that the alae and columella can be refined in a subsequent stage.

One of the difficulties in reconstructing the nose by means of an abdominal flap is the thickness of the reconstructed nose and the consequent difficulty of adequately shaping the alae, tip, and columella. Chetrov (1954) stripped the fat from the undersurface of the tube flap when using it for reconstruction of the nose. The removal of the fat permits more esthetic molding of the structures of the lower part of the nose.

Kavrakirov (1961) has employed Chetrov's method with good success. A long tube flap is raised on the abdomen and attached to the forearm; in a later stage, the flap is carried on the forearm and is inserted into the glabellar area. The length of the abdominal tube flap required for the reconstruction is at least 10 cm. When the flap on the abdomen is being designed, an excess in length and width of 1 to 2 cm should be allowed for shrinkage. The technique is illustrated in Figure 29–297. The upper part of the inner lining is provided by a tonguelike flap outlined on the undersurface of the base of the tube flap. The remainder of the lining is provided by infolding the distal end of the flap, which is stripped of its adipose tissue. A cartilaginous framework is later added to the reconstructed nose.

Ortiz-Monasterio (1975) has modified Chetrov's technique by transplanting the abdominal tube flap into a trapdoor flap in the scalp above the forehead instead of into the forehead itself.

DEFECTS OF THE COLUMELLA

Deformities of the columella vary from relatively minor deformities, such as retrusion or retraction of the structure, to major defects or total loss of the columella.

Minor defects of the columella include retrusion of the columella, loss of the columellar skin alone, shortness of the columella, and total absence of the columella combined with loss of the septum.

Retrusion of the Columella. Retrusion of the columella is observed in patients who have suffered septal trauma, fractures, or abscess in childhood, with subsequent loss of the caudal part of the septal framework. The techniques of repair are similar to those described earlier in the chapter (see p. 1095).

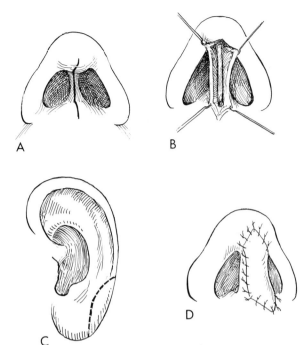

FIGURE 29-298. Composite skin-fat graft to repair a cicatricial columella. *A, B,* A vertical incision splits the columella. *C,* The composite graft consisting of skin and fat is removed from the outer border of the lobe of the ear. *D,* The composite graft is sutured to fill the defect in the columella.

In another type of deformity, the columella is deficient because of thin cicatricial skin. The deformity also causes a downward pull on the tip of the nose. The scar is excised in such cases; the skin on each side of the columella is freely undermined; and a retroauricular composite skin-fat graft from the outer border of the lobe of the ear or a composite skin-fat cartilage graft is transplanted into the defect (Fig. 29-298).

Reconstruction of the Columella. The columella is probably one of the most difficult structures to reconstruct, especially when it is totally destroyed either by trauma or by excision for malignant disease. Total absence of the columella is also occasionally found in patients with congenital anomalies.

The most frequent cause of congenital shortness of the columella is bilateral cleft lip. The various techniques for lengthening the columella in this type of deformity are discussed in Chapter 47.

Many techniques have been described for reconstruction following total loss of the columella. Paletta and Van Norman (1962) have reviewed the literature and have described seven categories of columellar reconstruction. Some of these techniques are illustrated in Figure 29-299.

Joseph (1912) published the earliest report of reconstruction in the modern literature; he utilized a composite graft from the ala. Gillies (1923, 1949), Ivy (1925), and Kazanjian (1937) advocated use of the forehead flap in their publications. The forehead flap was also used by Shaw and Fell (1948), Heanley (1955), Malbec and Beaux (1958), Cardoso (1958), and Paletta and Van Norman (1962). The columella was reconstructed using a flap from the arm by Malbec and Beaux (1958) and one from the hand by Blair and Byars (1946) and Young (1949).

RECONSTRUCTION OF THE COLUMELLA USING TISSUE FROM THE UPPER LIP. Dieffenbach (1833) preferred the upper lip as a source of columellar tissue. Lexer (1931) formed a tube of mucosa and brought it through an opening in the upper lip. This technique has been largely abandoned because of the persistence of the red coloration of the labial mucosa. The flap also tends to diminish in size. Millard (1963) stated that the technique is acceptable in dark-skinned individuals in whom the degree of pigmentation is sufficient to camouflage the mucosal color. The mucosal tube can also be resurfaced with a postauricular skin graft. Another technique suggested by Millard is to line a horizontal labial flap with a chondrocutaneous graft from the postauricular area. The technique provides adequate skin color for the anterior portion of the transplanted columella.

COMPOSITE GRAFTS. Composite grafts have been used with varying degrees of success in partial loss of the columella and in cleft lip deformities.

In a case of congenital retrusion of the tip of the nose caused by lack of development of the columella and alae of the nose, Millard (1971) has used three small composite auricular grafts consisting of wedges to increase the vertical dimension of the two alae (Fig. 29-300). The two grafts for the alar bases were taken from the junction of the helix and the lobe of each ear. The columellar defect was repaired using skin and subcutaneous tissue from the postauricular area. Five months later, cartilage removed from the septum was introduced into the columella to provide skeletal support.

THE CERVICAL FLAP. The columella may be reconstructed by means of a narrow cervical tube (see Fig. 29-299, *A, B*). In the female the tube is formed in the suprahyoid

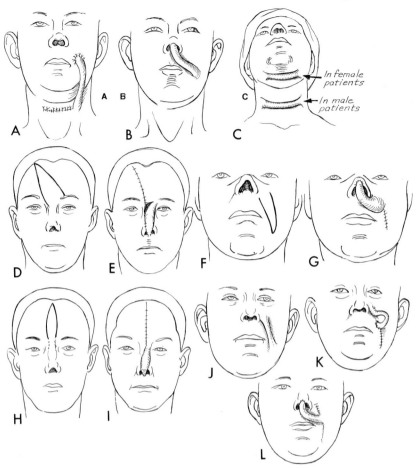

FIGURE 29–299. Various methods of reconstructing the columella. *A,* A horizontal cervical tube migrated to the nasolabial area. *B,* The tube is subsequently migrated to the tip of the nose. *C,* Cervical tube flaps for columella reconstruction. *D, E,* Oblique-median forehead flap. *F, G,* Nasolabial flap. *H, I,* Median forehead flap. *J, K, L,* Nasolabial tube flap.

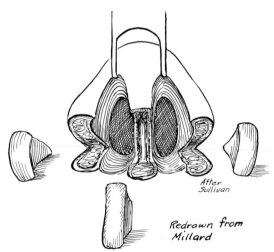

FIGURE 29–300. Millard's technique of using three composite grafts taken from the auricle to increase the projection of the tip of the nose. The two alar grafts were removed from the junction of the helical rim and the lobe; the columella graft consisted of skin and subcutaneous tissue from the retroauricular area.

region (see Fig. 29–299, *C*) and is transferred to the columella in two stages. In the male patient, the presence of hair follicles in the upper cervical skin makes it necessary for the cervical tube to be raised in the lower cervical region, entailing at least one more transfer procedure to enable the end of the tube to reach the defect.

THE FOREHEAD FLAP. A median forehead flap (Figs. 29–301 and 29–302) is the most expeditious and satisfactory method for use in cases of complete loss of the columella combined with loss of the caudal portion of the septum and a portion of the ala, a condition which is often associated with defects of the lip and adjacent tissues. It is evident that extensive repair of this type of deformity requires a greater amount of tissue. An oblique forehead flap (Fig. 29–299, *D, E*) or preferably a median forehead flap supplies sufficient tissue for the repair of such defects; the techniques are illus-

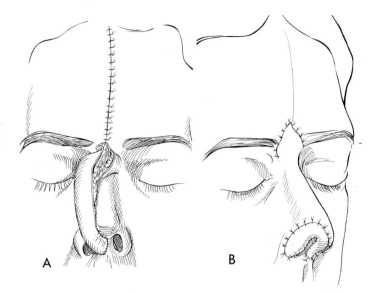

FIGURE 29–301. Technique of reconstruction of the columella and the ala by a median forehead flap. *A*, The median flap inserted into the columellar defect. *B*, Reconstructed columella and ala. (After Kazanjian.)

trated in Figure 29–299, *H* and *I*). In the patient with a low hairline, the median flap may be extended into the scalp, thus providing additional length to reach the base of the proposed columella. After completion of the reconstructive procedure and a suitable delay, the hair on the new columella is removed by progressively destroying the hair follicles through electrolysis or by removing the hair-bearing skin and replacing it with a full-thickness postauricular skin graft.

THE NASOLABIAL FLAP. Another technique for columella reconstruction feasible in older-patients is that of using a nasolabial flap based superiorly, partly tubed, and rotated to cover the defect, as depicted in Figure 29–299, *F, G*.

A variant of this technique is to prepare a tubed flap in the nasolabial area in a first stage, then advance the lower end of the tube to the upper lip, using the upper portion of the tube to reconstruct the columella (Fig. 29–299, *J, K, L*). In male patients the flap should be removed from the lower portion of the cervical area to avoid hair-bearing skin. An excellent technique is the modification of Da Silva (1964), which introduces a nasolabial flap through an incision temporarily detaching the ala, thus short-circuiting the distance between the donor and recipient areas. This technique, like all techniques that employ a nasolabial flap, is more applicable to defects in the older patient because of the looseness of aging tissues (see also Fig. 29–285).

THE FORESHORTENED NOSE

The problem of the patient with a short nose has been reserved for the last section of this chapter because lengthening may require many of the techniques previously described.

These deformities fall into a number of categories: (1) congenital deformities; (2) deformities resulting from naso-orbital fractures; (3) burn deformities; (4) deformities resulting from the treatment of malignancy by surgery, chemosurgery, or radiation; and (5) deformities resulting from overshortening of the nose during a corrective rhinoplasty (see Fig. 29–172, p. 1161).

Shortening of the nose results from one of four causes: (1) loss of nasal lining; (2) loss of the nasal framework; (3) destruction by trauma of the cutaneous covering of the nose; and (4) involvement of the three layers in injuries which include the full thickness of the nose.

The congenital short nose is seen in a variety of congenital anomalies. The treatment of nasomaxillary hypoplasia by the nasomaxillary skin graft inlay technique has been described (see p. 1201). The short nose deformity is also the sequela of trauma in infancy and childhood. The frequency of early injuries was noted in Chapter 26. The nose fails to develop in length, and frequently there is a nasomaxillary deformity. Traumatic foreshortening of the nose, the result of malunited naso-orbital fractures, has been discussed in Chapter 28.

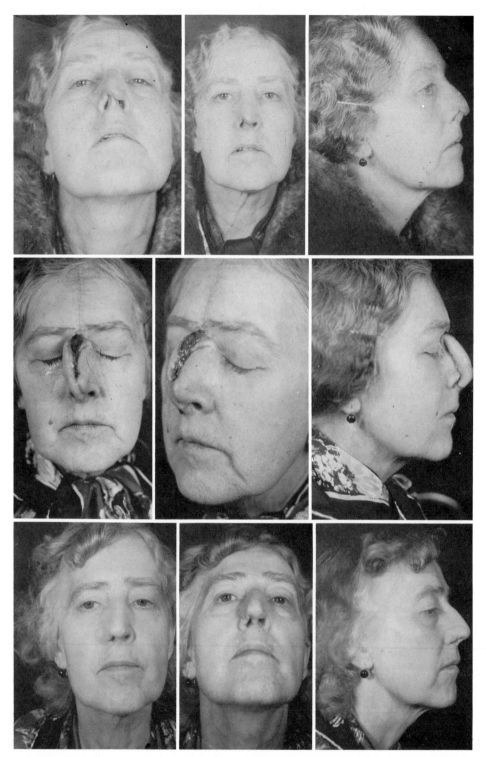

FIGURE 29–302.   Reconstruction of the columella by a median forehead flap. *Top,* Columellar and alar defect resulting from dog bite. *Middle,* The median flap secured to the columellar defect. *Bottom,* Result obtained by use of the median forehead flap illustrated in Figure 29–301. (After Kazanjian.)

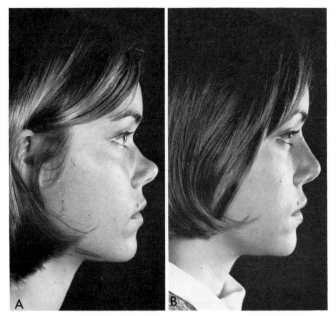

FIGURE 29-303. *A*, Foreshortened nose in a traumatic type of saddle-nose deformity. *B*, Result obtained after submucous resection of the septum, detelescoping of the cartilaginous structures as illustrated in Figure 29-307, and insertion of an iliac bone graft over the dorsum.

The deformity varies from a depression or saddle-nose deformity of the dorsum of the nose, with a slight amount of shortening and uptilt of the nasal tip, to the severely foreshort-ened nose (Fig. 29-303) and depressed glabellar portion of the frontal bone (Fig. 29-304) caused by full-thickness loss of the nasal tissue and frontal bone.

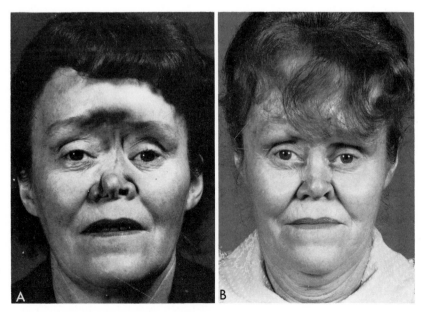

FIGURE 29-304. *A*, Deformity resulting from severe malunited and depressed naso-orbital fracture and fracture of the frontal bone. The patient had suffered brain damage which required neurosurgical care. *B*, Appearance after reconstruction of the frontal bone by an iliac bone graft and restoration of the contour of the nose with bilateral, consecutive, superimposed scalping flaps.

In many cases, foreshortening is the result of fracture and telescoping of the structures of the nasal framework without loss of cutaneous tissues; in others, additional skin or mucous membrane lining or full-thickness tissue replacement are required (see Chapter 28, Fig. 28–164, p. 1020).

The disruption of the bony nasal structures is not the only cause of nasal shortening following fractures. The lateral cartilages, which are firmly attached to the undersurface of the nasal bones, are displaced conjointly with the bones, or they may be detached and pushed under the bones by the traumatic force, together with the fractured septum to which they are attached. The fractured and shortened septum is a major cause of the shortened nose; the alar cartilages, because of the attachments of the nasal tip to the septum, may also be displaced in a cephalad direction over the lateral cartilages. Bony consolidation, hemorrhage, and fibrosis result in permanent deformity when early treatment is inadequate.

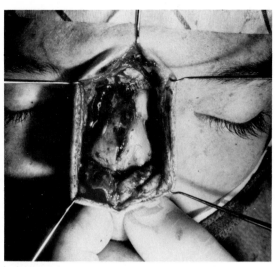

FIGURE 29–306. Photograph demonstrating the exposure of the nasal skeletal structures obtained by a vertical midline incision.

External Incisions. A transcutaneous approach is usually required in more severe deformities. These include bilateral incisions through the skin of the upper portion of the lateral wall of the nose on each side; a trapdoor incision, the transverse portion of which extends through the skin of the root of the nose and the lateral portions of which extend downward along the lateral wall of the nose (Fig. 29–305); and an inverted V-shaped incision extending into the glabellar region, which permits the gain of a certain amount of soft tissue covering by means of a V-Y advancement. Cutaneous scars resulting from the initial injury are an obvious route of approach to the nasal framework. A midline incision extending from the root of the nose to the supratip area leaves a scar which is relatively inconspicuous but limits its use to the more severe deformities (Fig. 29–305). It provides the ideal exposure of bones and cartilages for excision, detelescoping, narrowing, and remodeling procedures under direct vision (Fig. 29–306).

Lengthening the Cartilaginous Framework of the Nose. The shortened septum, which is the result of overlapping fractures of the cartilaginous and bony septal framework, will resist any attempts to lengthen the nasal pyramid. An extensive resection of the septal framework is usually an essential first step; the resection should include the dorsal portion of the septal cartilage in the severely foreshortened nose.

Additional lining, usually deficient in the foreshortened nose, may be gained by mobilizing the lateral cartilages and mucoperiosteum from the undersurface of the nasal bones (Fig. 29–307). This procedure was used by Kazanjian (1937) to obtain additional lining in unilateral defects of the nose and by Edgerton, Lewis and McKnelly (1967) to lengthen the short nose of a cleft lip-palate patient. A similar maneuver is employed (see Chapter 30, p. 1455) in the short nose of the nasomaxillary dish-face deformity (Converse, Horowitz, Valauri and

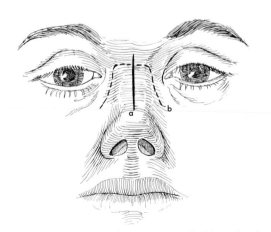

FIGURE 29–305. Various cutaneous incisions for the exposure of the nasal framework. A midline incision (*a*) provides the most complete exposure. Lateral incisions (*b*) over the frontal process of the maxilla may be joined across the midline by a transverse incision.

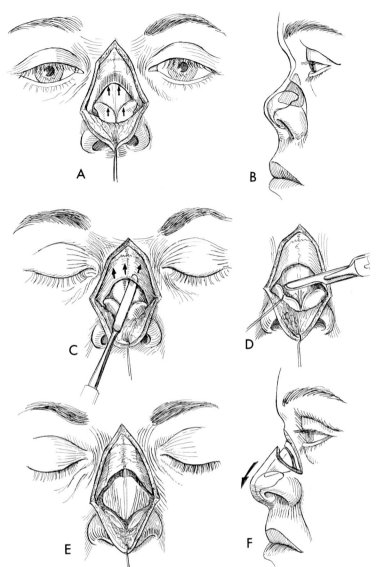

FIGURE 29–307.　Elongation of the cartilaginous framework. *A, B,* The arrows indicate the usual direction of the overlapping of the nasal bones and the alar cartilages over the lateral cartilages. *C,* Detaching the lateral cartilages and the mucoperiosteum from under the nasal bones. After the lining tissues have been severed transversely under the nasal bones, they can be drawn downward to elongate the lining of the nose. *D,* Further elongation is obtained by separating the alar from the lateral cartilages and sliding the alar cartilages caudad. *E, F,* Elongation obtained.

Montandon, 1970). The tissue binding the cartilages is incised and resected. The alar cartilage can then be drawn downward, releasing it from its retracted position over the lateral cartilage and thus allowing further lengthening of the nose. If the upper portion of the columella is seized between thumb and forefinger and downward traction is exerted, the nose does not resist lengthening.

When the shortened septum and nasal lining have been released and the detelescoping of the alar cartilages has been obtained, maintenance of contour and length is ensured by bone or cartilage grafts. When shortening is moderate, as seen in most traumatic saddle-nose deformities (see Fig. 29–303), an intranasal approach suffices. A periosteal elevator is introduced over the lateral cartilage to the undersurface of the nasal bone on each side. The lateral cartilage is separated from the undersurface of the nasal bone by the elevator, and the mucoperiosteum above this area is also raised

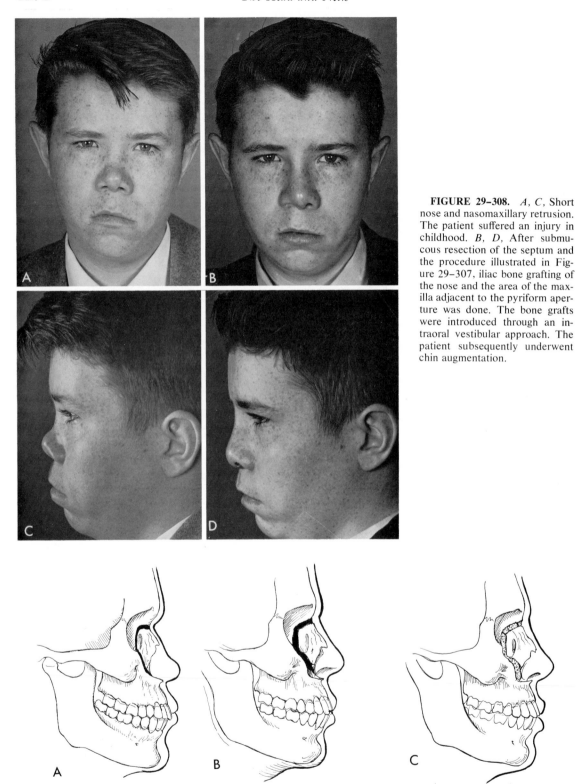

FIGURE 29–308. *A, C,* Short nose and nasomaxillary retrusion. The patient suffered an injury in childhood. *B, D,* After submucous resection of the septum and the procedure illustrated in Figure 29–307, iliac bone grafting of the nose and the area of the maxilla adjacent to the pyriform aperture was done. The bone grafts were introduced through an intraoral vestibular approach. The patient subsequently underwent chin augmentation.

FIGURE 29–309. The perinasal osteotomy. Further lengthening and increase in the projection of the nose is obtained by the perinasal osteotomy. *A,* Malunited naso-orbital fracture resulting in a foreshortened nose. *B,* The osteotomy begins at the nasofrontal junction, extends posteriorly to the lacrimal groove, descending along the medial orbital wall and rim and joining a line of osteotomy extending through the base of the frontal process of the maxilla. The nasal skeleton can then be lifted to increase its forward projection. *C,* Small iliac bone grafts are placed in the interstices left by the forward mobilization of the nasal structures.

as high as possible, at which point it is sectioned transversely. It is then possible to draw both lateral cartilages and the mucoperiosteum from the undersurface of the nasal bones in a caudal direction, thus providing an appreciable amount of additional lining and releasing the lateral cartilages from their telescoped position. In the patient with nasomaxillary hypoplasia shown in Figure 29–308, bone grafting was employed to provide nasal contour and lengthening, and onlay bone grafts were placed around the pyriform aperture through an oral vestibular incision.

An iliac bone graft is usually required to restore dorsal support and contour. The bone graft is introduced through a transcartilaginous incision near the caudal margin of the alar cartilage. The bone graft is placed under direct vision when a transcutaneous incision has been employed.

The periosteum is raised from the outer surface of the nasal bones, and an iliac bone graft restores dorsal support and adequate contour to the nose. A modification of the shape of the tip can be done at this stage, if necessary, and the distal end of the bone graft is placed between the domes of the alar cartilages. Fixation of the bone graft to the nasal bones by transosseous wiring is favored as an additional precaution to ensure stability (see Fig. 29–154).

Dingman and Walter (1969) have employed the following technique for the lengthening of a traumatic foreshortened nose. The nose is divided transversely across the dorsum below the nasal bones. The lining defect is repaired by a previously prepared median forehead flap which has been lined with a conchal composite graft; the composite graft furnishes the lining and the skeletal support, and the median forehead flap the outer skin cover. At the end of three weeks the pedicle of the median flap is severed, and the remainder of the flap is returned to the forehead. The skin is sutured over the transplanted composite graft.

Lengthening the Bony Framework of the Nose: The Perinasal Osteotomy. The perinasal osteotomy (Fig. 29–309) is required, in addition to the above procedures, to lengthen the cartilaginous and bony skeletal framework of the nose that has been shortened as a result of naso-orbital fracture.

Exposure is obtained through one of the external incisions previously described. The area of junction of the nasal bones with the frontal bone is exposed subperiosteally, and subperiosteal elevation is extended backward to the lacrimal groove, the lacrimal sac being raised from the groove. The lamina papyracea situated posterior to the posterior lacrimal crest is also exposed. The attachment of the medial canthal tendon is raised with the periosteum. The upper portion of the nasolacrimal duct is seen where it enters the nasolacrimal canal. The periosteum is then raised along the base of the lateral orbital wall. An incision made in the nasal vestibule immediately lateral to the base of the pyriform aperture allows the passage of a periosteal elevator, which raises the periosteum from the base of the lateral wall until the elevator rejoins the medial orbital area; exposure can also be obtained by an intraoral incision.

Exposure having been obtained, the perinasal osteotomy may now be performed. A transverse osteotomy is done at the junction of the nasal bone with the frontal bone. The bone is thick at this point, being reinforced by the nasal process of the frontal bone and thickened by overlapping fractured fragments. An air turbine–driven drill sections the bone in this area. The osteotomy is then extended backward horizontally above the lacrimal sac to an area situated posterior to the posterior lacrimal crest. The osteotomy then extends downward, posterior to the lacrimal sac through the medial portion of the orbital floor and rim and downward along the base of the lateral wall of the nose. This latter portion of the osteotomy can be done with a nasal saw or chisel. The separation of the nasal bones from the frontal bone can be completed with a small osteotome which is levered downward. The area of the root of the nose then opens up. If resistance to downward displacement of the bones is noted, scissors are introduced into the nasal cavity, and the posterior portion of the septum is divided. The cribriform plate, being situated sufficiently far posteriorly, is not involved in the osteotomy. Wedges of iliac bone are then placed between the frontal bone and the nasal bones, thus providing the desired lengthening of the bony portion of the nose. Thin plates of cancellous bone are placed over the areas of osteotomy along the medial wall of the orbit. Wedges of bone are placed between, and thin plates of bone over, the edges of the line of osteotomy in the lateral wall of the nose. The detelescoping procedures required to lengthen the cartilaginous nasal skeletal framework (see Fig. 29–307) are done when indicated. A bone graft placed along the dorsum of the nose is usually necessary to restore adequate contour and projection of the dorsum (Fig. 29–310).

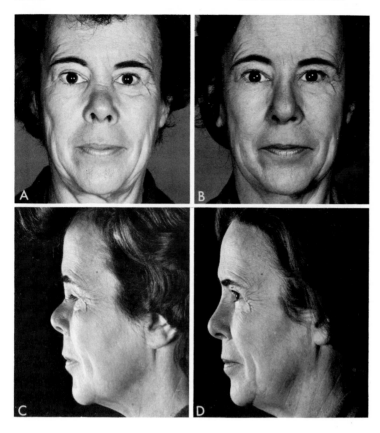

FIGURE 29–310. *A,* Foreshortened nose resulting from comminuted fracture of the nasal bones and telescoping of the cartilaginous structures. *B,* Elongation obtained by detelescoping of the cartilaginous structures (see Fig. 29–307), extensive submucous resection of the foreshortened septum, and perinasal osteotomy (see Fig. 29–309) through a midline incision. *C,* Extent of the nasal foreshortening. *D,* Extent of the nasal lengthening obtained by the procedures described. (Figs. 29–307 to 29–310 from Converse, J. M.: Surgical elongation of the traumatically foreshortened nose: The perinasal osteotomy. Plast. Reconstr. Surg., *47:*539, 1972. Copyright © 1971, The Williams & Wilkins Company, Baltimore.)

Lengthening the Nose after Loss of Nasal Tissue. The inordinately foreshortened nose following naso-orbital and nasofrontal fractures with full thickness loss of nasal tissue requires reconstructive procedures. A patient with this type of deformity was discussed in the preceding chapter (p. 1020).

In the older patient, nasolabial flaps may be utilized for the restoration of the defective nasal lining (see Figs. 29–211 and 29–212). Such flaps were employed in the patient shown in Figure 29–304. Reconstruction of the frontal bone defect was achieved by means of an iliac bone graft. Bilateral consecutive scalping flaps were superimposed in order to provide sufficient tissue. A first flap did not provide sufficient tissue bulk, and after it had been in place for a period of three months, it was dermabraded, and a second scalping flap taken from the contralateral side of the forehead was placed over the abraded initial flap.

Lengthening the Shortened Burned Nose. In the burned nose with contracture following healing of a full-thickness burn wound of the dorsum, the upward retraction of the tip and alae of the nose, combined with varying amounts of local tissue destruction, results in a severe deformity (Figs. 29–311, *A, B* and 29–312, *A, B*).

Skin grafts or flaps resurface the nose in favorable cases; an example of the use of a forehead flap is shown in Figure 29–312. The technique of elongation of the severely shortened burned nose follows.

In a first operation, the nasal tip and alae are replaced in their anatomical position by separating the lateral and alar cartilages from the septum using a transfixion incision similar to that employed in corrective nasal plastic operations (Fig. 29–311, *C, D*). A transverse incision through the dorsal skin and lateral cartilages (Fig. 29–311, *E*) releases the tip of the nose, and traction is exerted downward; a full thickness defect thus results (Figs. 29–311, *F, G* and Fig. 29–312, *B*). Recurrence of upward retraction is prevented by inserting into each lateral defect an acrylic mold, fabricated after an impression of the defect is taken.

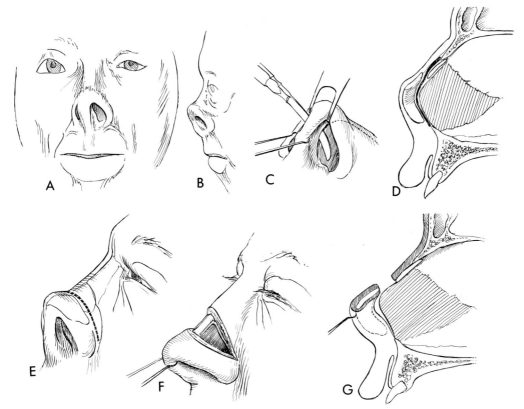

FIGURE 29–311. Elongation of the burned nose. *A, B,* Typical appearance of the nose following contracture of the covering soft tissues. *C, D,* Transfixion incision. *E,* Transverse incision through the soft tissues of the nose above the alar cartilages. *F, G,* The nasal tip is pulled down into an adequate position. The position is maintained by acrylic molds inserted into the defects; later an inner lining of the defect is provided by hinged turnover flaps or composite auricular grafts. The remainder of the scarred burned skin is resected, and a scalping forehead flap resurfaces the nose (see Fig. 29–312).

The mold is worn for at least two months or until the tendency for upward retraction has been arrested.

In a second operation, a scalping forehead flap (see Fig. 29–252) provides a new cutaneous covering; local hinged turnover flaps furnish the lining of the defects.

The upward retraction is less accentuated in most burn patients; the alar borders may be rolled downward, after being freed by a transverse incision through the skin, or reconstituted by hinged turnover flaps combined with a forehead flap.

Postoperative Shortening of the Nose. Postoperative shortening of the entire nose or unilateral or bilateral alar retraction is usually caused by overshortening of the septum and excessive resection of inner lining and cartilage during the corrective rhinoplasty. Dingman and Walter (1969) suggested the use of an auricular composite graft taken from either the scapha or the concha (Fig. 29–313).

Bilateral intercartilaginous incisions, as well as the transfixion incision, are employed. The skin of the nose is widely undermined to allow elongation of the nose. Downward traction is exerted on the tip of the nose and columella in order to lengthen the nose. A defect becomes apparent at the site of the intercartilaginous incisions, which are joined in the midline across the transfixion incision. A pattern made of the defect serves to indicate the amount of auricular skin and cartilage to be used as a composite graft. A long composite graft can be taken from the upper portion of the scapha. The excised tissue may be extended downward to the lower portion of the scapha.

The cartilage of the composite graft is incised, the incision extending through the carti-

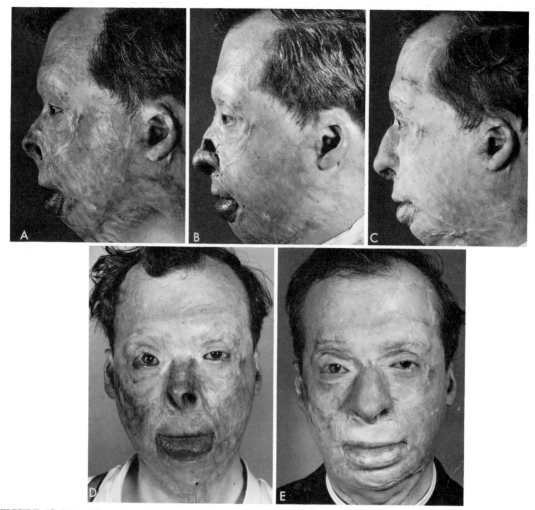

FIGURE 29–312.   Elongation of the burned nose. *A*, Burn contractures of the face following a chemical explosion and unsuccessful primary skin grafting. *B*, Lengthening of the nose obtained by the procedure illustrated in Figure 29–311. *C*, Final result. The nose has been resurfaced by a scalping flap. The inner lining of the full thickness defects was provided by hinged turnover local flaps. *D*, Preoperative appearance. Note the severe shortening of the nose. *E*, Postoperative appearance. Numerous skin grafting procedures were also required. (The treatment of severe burn ectropion of the eyelids is described in Chapter 33, p. 1631.)

lage only, sparing the skin. The graft can then be flexed into the curvature of the wings of a flying bird. The graft is placed over the transfixion incision after a small section of septal cartilage has been excised, and each wing fits into the defects produced by the intercartilaginous incisions on each side and is sutured to the adjacent nasal lining.

When the shortening of the nose affects the area of the nasal tip, a small amount of the dorsal border of the septal cartilage is resected, and a composite graft from the concha is placed across the septal dorsal border (Fig. 29–314). An incision is made through the skin of the composite graft so that the cartilage graft will be in contact with the septal cartilage. The skin of the composite graft is sutured to the inner lining of the nose after the graft is placed in the defect. The composite graft should be of sufficient length and width to furnish the missing tissue in the lateral walls of the nose, as well as the caudal portion of the septum. The graft is sutured in position between the lateral and alar cartilages on each side and between the columella and the caudal edge of the septum centrally.

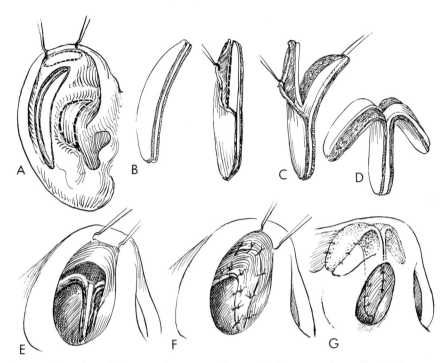

FIGURE 29–313. Elongation of the nose by means of an auricular composite graft. *A*, The composite graft is removed from various areas of the scapha. *B*, The graft is split longitudinally. *C*, A portion of the cartilage is removed, leaving an excess of skin on each side. *D*, The split portion of the graft is folded over, forming two wings. *E*, After the nasal framework has been exposed through intercartilaginous incisions and a transfixion incision. *F*, The graft is sutured in the resulting defect. *G*, Position of the graft in the nose. (After Dingman and Walter, 1969.)

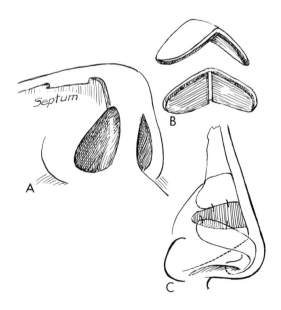

FIGURE 29–314. Elongation of the nose by means of an auricular composite graft. *A*, In this technique, a notch is prepared along the dorsal border of the septal cartilage for the reception of the composite graft. *B*, Technique of preparation of the composite graft. A narrow rectangle of cartilage is excised. This allows the downfolding of the two wings. *C*, The composite graft is fitted over the septal cartilage and into the intercartilaginous defects. (After Dingman and Walter, 1969.)

REFERENCES

Adams, W. S.: A bifurcating tubular dermoid of dorsum nasi. J. Laryngol., *79*:633, 1965.

Almast, S. C.: History and evolution of the Indian method of rhinoplasty. Trans. 4th Internatl. Congr. Plast. Reconstr. Surg., Rome, Oct., 1967. Amsterdam, Excerpta Medica Foundation, 1967, p. 19.

Ammon, F. A. von, and Baumgarten, M.: Die plastische Chirurgie nach ihren bisherigen Leistungen Kritisch dargestellt. Berlin, Reimer, 1842.

Anderson, J. R.: A new approach to rhinoplasty. Trans. Am. Acad. Ophthalmol. Otolaryngol., *70*:183, 1966.

Anderson, J. R., and Dykes, E. R.: Surgical treatment of rhinophyma. Plast. Reconstr. Surg., *30*:397, 1962.

Anderson, J. R., and Rubin, W.: Retrograde intramucosal hump removal in rhinoplasty. A. M. A. Arch. Otolaryngol., *68*:346, 1958.

Anglade, M., and Philip, W. C.: Le gliome des fosses nasales, Presse Med., *38*:464, 1920.

Antia, N. H.: The scope of plastic surgery in leprosy: A ten-year progress report. Clinics in Plastic Surgery, *1*:69, 1974.

Aufricht, G.: Combined nasal plastic and chin plastic; correction of microgenic by osteocartilaginous transplants from large hump nose. Am. J. Surg., *25*:292, 1934.

Aufricht, G.: A few hints and surgical details in rhinoplasty. Laryngoscope, *53*:317, 1943.

Aufricht, G.: Symposium on corrective rhinoplasty. Plast. Reconstr. Surg., *28*:241, 1961.

Ballantyne, D. L., and Converse, J. M.: Vascularization of composite auricular grafts transplanted to the chorioallantois of the chick embryo. Transplant. Bull., *5*:373, 1958.

Ballantyne, D. L., Uhlschmid, G. K., and Converse, J. M.: Massive rabbit skin zenografts in rats. Transplantation, *7*:274, 1969.

Baronio, G.: Degli Innesti Animali, Stamperia e Fonderia del Genio, Milan, 1804.

Barron, J. N.: Personal communication, 1959.

Barron, J. N., and Emmett, A. J. J.: Subcutaneous pedicle flaps. Br. J. Plast. Surg., *18*:51, 1965.

Becker, O. J.: Principles of Otolaryngologic Plastic Surgery. 2nd Ed. Rochester, Minn., American Academy of Ophthalmology and Otolaryngology, 1958.

Beinfield, H. H.: Congenital bilateral bony atresia of the posterior nares in a one-month premature infant who survived. J. Pediatr., *45*:679, 1954.

Beinfield, H. H.: Surgical management of complete and incomplete bony atresia of the posterior nares (choanal). Am. J. Surg., *89*:957, 1955.

Beinfield, H. H.: Surgical management of complete and incomplete bony atresia of the posterior nares. Trans. Am. Acad. Ophthalmol., Otolaryngol., *60*:778, 1956.

Beinfield, H. H.: Unsolved problems of infant suffocation. N.Y. J. Med., *57*:3160, 1957.

Beinfield, H. H.: Ways and means to reduce infant mortality due to suffocation. Importance of choanal atresia. J.A.M.A., *170*:647, 1959.

Bell, R. C.: Unsuccessful use of "Kiel" bone in nasal reconstruction. Br. J. Plast. Surg., *19*:271, 1966.

Berger, M., and Martin, C.: L'Arhinogenesie totale. (Absence congénitale du nez, et des fosses nasales.) A propos d'une observation exceptionnelle. Rev. Laryngol., *90*:300, 1969.

Berndorfer, A.: Quoted by Warkany (1971).

Black, B. K., and Smith, D. E.: Nasal glioma. Arch. Neurol. Psychiatr., *64*:614, 1950.

Blair, V. P.: Total and subtotal restoration of the nose. J.A.M.A., *85*:1931, 1925.

Blair, V. P.: Congenital atresia and obstruction of nasal air passage. Ann. Otol. Rhinol. Laryngol., *40*:1021, 1931.

Blair, V. P., and Brown, J. B.: Nasal abnormalities, fancied and real. Surg. Gynecol. Obstet., *53*:797, 1931.

Blair, V. P., and Byars, L.: Hits, strikes and outs in the use of pedicle flaps for nasal restoration. Surg. Gynecol. Obstet., *82*:367, 1946.

Blandin, P. F.: De l'autoplastie, ou restauration des parties du corps, qui ont été détruites, à la faveur d'une emprunt fait à d'autres parties plus ou mois éloignées. Thesis, Urtubie, Paris, 1836.

Blocksma, R., and Innis, C. O.: Reconstruction of the amputated nose. Plast. Reconstr. Surg., *15*:390, 1955.

Boo-Chai, K.: Augmentation of rhinoplasty in the orientals. Plast. Reconstr. Surg., *34*:81, 1964.

Boo-Chai, K.: The bifid nose. Plast. Reconstr. Surg., *36*:626, 1965.

Brown, J. B., and Cannon, B.: Composite free grafts of skin and cartilages from the ear. Surg. Gynecol. Obstet., *82*:253, 1946.

Brown, J. B., and McDowell, F.: Plastic Surgery of the Nose. St. Louis, Mo., C. V. Mosby Company, 1951.

Brown, J. B., and McDowell, F.: Plastic Surgery of the Nose. 3rd Ed. Springfield, Ill., Charles C Thomas, Publisher, 1965.

Brunk, A. A.: A new case of unilateral ossions occlusion: An operation through the palate. Z. Ohrenheilk., *59*:221, 1909.

Burian, F.: Proposta di una collaborazione internazionale per lo studio dei problemi inerenti alla labio-palatoschisi. Minerva Chir., *13*:931, 1958.

Calderini: Annali dell'Universita di Medicina, *194*:520, 1842.

Campbell, R. M.: Personal communication, 1957.

Cardoso, A. D.: Loss of columella after leishmaniasis; reconstruction with subcutaneous tissue pedicle flap. Plast. Reconstr. Surg., *21*:117, 1958.

Carpue, J. C.: An account of two successful operations for restoring a lost nose from the integuments of the forehead in the cases of two officers of His Majesty's Army. London, Longman, 1816.

Carter, C. H., Smith, G. F., and Schindeler, J.: Choanal atresia and bifid thumb associated with an abnormal D group chromosome. Mental Deficiency Research, *14*:221, 1970.

Cherry, J., and Bordley, J. E.: Surgical correction of choanal atresia. Ann. Otol. Rhinol. Laryngol., *75*:911, 1966.

Chetrov, F. M.: Plastic reconstruction of face and neck defects with Filatov's tubed flap. (Title translated from the Russian.) Moscow, Medgiz, 1954.

Conley, J. J.: Cancer of the skin of the nose. Arch. Otolaryngol., *84*:55, 1966.

Conley, J. J., and von Fraenkel, P. H.: The principle of cooling as applied to the composite graft in the nose. Plast. Reconstr. Surg., *17*:444, 1956.

Converse, J. M.: Corrective surgery of the nasal tip. Ann. Otol. Rhinol. Laryngol., *49*:895, 1940.

Converse, J. M.: New forehead flap for nasal reconstruction. Proc. R. Soc. Med., *35*:811, 1942.

Converse, J. M.: Reconstruction of the nasolabial area by a composite graft from the concha. Plast. Reconstr. Surg., *5*:247, 1950a.

Converse, J. M.: Corrective surgery of nasal deviations. Arch. Otolaryngol., *52*:671, 1950b.

Converse, J. M.: Technique of bone grafting for contour restoration of the face. Plast. Reconstr. Surg., *14*:332, 1954.

Converse, J. M.: The cartilaginous structures of the nose. Ann. Otol. Rhinol. Laryngol., *64*:220, 1955.

Converse, J. M.: Composite graft from the septum in nasal reconstruction. Trans. Lat. Am. Congr. Plast. Surg., 8:281, 1956.

Converse, J. M.: Corrective surgery of the nasal tip. Laryngoscope, 67:16, 1957.

Converse, J. M.: Reconstruction of the nose by the scalping flap technique. Surg. Clin. North Am., 39:335, 1959.

Converse, J. M.: Deformities of the Nose. *In* Converse, J. M. (Ed.): Reconstructive Plastic Surgery Vol. 2. Philadelphia, W. B. Saunders Company, 1964, p. 818.

Converse, J. M., Deformities of the nose (Fig. 21–60). *In* Converse, J. M. (Ed.): Reconstructive Plastic Surgery. Philadelphia, W. B. Saunders Company, 1964, p. 729.

Converse, J. M.: Clinical applications of the scalping flap in reconstruction of the nose. Plast. Reconstr. Surg., 43:247, 1969.

Converse, J. M.: The deformity termed "pug nose" and its correction by a simple operation. John O. Roe, Rochester, N.Y. (Reprinted from the Medical Record, June 4, 1887.) Plast. Reconstr. Surg., 45:78, 1970.

Converse, J. M.: Surgical elongation of the traumatically foreshortened nose: The perinasal osteotomy. Plast. Reconstr. Surg., 47:539, 1971.

Converse, J. M.: Unpublished technique, 1975.

Converse, J. M., and Brauer, R. O.: Transplantation of skin (Fig. 2–12). *In* Converse, J. M. (Ed.): Reconstructive Plastic Surgery. Philadelphia, W. B. Saunders Company, 1964a.

Converse, J. M., and Brauer, R. O.: Transplantation of skin (Figs. 2–15 and 2–16). *In* Converse, J. M. (Ed.): Reconstructive Plastic Surgery. Philadelphia, W. B. Saunders Company, 1964b.

Converse, J. M., and Casson, P. R.: Reconstructive surgery: An integral part of treatment of cancer of the nose. *In* Gaisford, J. C. (Ed.): Symposium on Cancer of the Head and Neck. Total treatment and reconstructive rehabilitation. Vol. 2. Proccedings of the Second Annual Symposium of the Educational Foundation of the American Society of Plastic and Reconstructive Surgeons Inc., held at Pittsburg, Pennsylvania, Dec. 2, 3, and 4, 1968. St. Louis, Mo., C. V. Mosby Company, 1969.

Converse, J. M., and Wood-Smith, D.: Experiences with the forehead island flap with a subcutaneous pedicle. Plast. Reconstr. Surg., 31:521, 1963.

Converse, J. M., Horowitz, S. L., Valauri, A. J., and Montandon, D.: The treatment of nasomaxillary hypoplasia. A new pyramidal naso-orbital maxillary osteotomy. Plast. Reconstr. Surg., 45:527, 1970.

Cottle, M. H.: Corrective surgery of the nasal septum and the external pyramid — Study notes and labortatory manual. Chicago, American Rhinologic Society, 1960.

Crockford, D. A., and Converse, J. M.: The ilium as a source of bone grafts in children. Plast. Reconstr. Surg., 50:270, 1972.

Da Silva, G.: Columella reconstruction with nasolabial flap. Plast. Reconstr. Surg., 34:63, 1964.

Davis, J. S.: Plastic Surgery — Its Principle and Practice. Philadelphia, P. Blakiston's and Son, 1919.

Davis, J. S.: The story of plastic surgery. Ann. Surg., 113:641, 1941.

DeKleine, E. H.: Nasal tip reconstruction through external incisions. Plast. Reconstr. Surg., 15:502, 1955.

Delpech, J. M.: Chirurgie Clinique de Montpellier, ou Observations et Réflexions Tirées des Travaux de Chirurgie de Cette École. Paris, Gabon et Cie, 1823–1828.

Demjén, S.: Personal communication, 1967.

Denonvilliers, M.: (States that he performed operation in 1854.) Bull. Gén. Thérap., 65:257, 1863.

de Quervain, F.: Ueber partielle seitliche Rhinoplastik. Zentralbl. Chir., 29:297, 1902.

Diamond, H. P.: Rhinoplasty technique. Surg. Clin. North Am., 51:317, 1971.

Diamond, H. P.: Personal communication, 1975.

Dieffenbach, J. F.: Chirurgische Erfahrungen, besonders ueber die Wiederherstellung Zerstoerter Theile des Menschlichen Koerpers nach neuen Methoden. Berlin, T. C. F. Enslin, 1829–1834.

Dieffenbach, J. F.: Surgical observations on restoration of the nose. Operative Chirurgie, 1:359, 1833.

Dieffenbach, J. F.: Die Nasenbehandlung in Operative Chirurgie. Leipzig, F. A. Brockhaus, 1845.

Dieffenbach, J. F.: Die Operative Chirurgie. Leipiz, F. A. Brockhaus, 1845–1848.

Dieffenbach, J. F.: Quoted by Erich, J. B.: Sebaceous, mucous, dermoid, and epidermoid cysts. Am. J. Surg., 50:672, 1940.

Dingman, R. O., and Walter, C.: Use of composite ear grafts in correction of short nose. Plast. Reconstr. Surg., 43:117, 1969.

Dupertuis, S. M.: Free ear lobe grafts of skin and fat; their value in reconstruction about nostrils. Plast. Reconstr. Surg., 1:135, 1946.

Durward, A., Lord, O. C., and Polson, C. J.: Congenital choanal atresia. J. Laryngol. Otol., 60:461, 1945.

Edgerton, M. T., Lewis, C. M., and McKnelly, L. O.: Lengthening of the short nasal columella by skin flaps from the nasal tip and dorsum. Plast. Reconstr. Surg., 40:343, 1967.

Emmert, C.: Cited by Luschka et al.: Bilateral Bony Atresia. Stuttgart, Lehrbuch d. Chir., 1853.

Ersner, M. S.: Operative and postoperative management of bilateral atresia of the choana. Arch. Otolaryngol., 58:96, 1953.

Esser, J. F. S.: Studies in plastic surgery of the face. Ann. Surg., 65:297, 1917.

Evans, J. N. G., and Maclachlan, R. F.: Choanal atresia. J. Laryngol. Otol., 85:903, 1971.

Falces, E., Wesser, D., and Gorney, M.: Cosmetic surgery of the non-caucasian nose. Plast. Reconstr. Surg., 45:317, 1970.

Fatin, M.: A rare case of congenital malformation. Total absence of half the nose. Egyptian Med. Assoc., 38:470, 1955.

Firmin, F., LePesteur, J., Mints, V., Peyronie, M., Quiliquini, J., Thon, A., Weshler, J., and Tessier, P.: The superficial musuloaponeurotic system — anatomical study. Presented at the French Society of the Plastic Surgery Meeting, October 1974.

Flowers, R. S., and Anderson, R.: Injury to the lacrimal apparatus during rhinoplasty. Plast. Reconstr. Surg., 42:577, 1968.

Fomon, S.: The Surgery of Injury and Plastic Repair. Baltimore, The Williams & Wilkins Company, 1939.

Fomon, S.: Cosmetic Surgery. Principles and Practice. Philadelphia, J. B. Lippincott Company, 1960.

Freeman, B. S.: Reconstructive rhinoplasty for rhinophyma. Plast. Reconstr. Surg., 46:265, 1970.

Freeman, R. G., Knox, J. M., and Heaton, C. L.: The treatment of skin cancer. Cancer, 17:353, 1964.

Freer, O.: Deflection of the nasal septum; a critical review of the methods of their correction, with a report of 116 operations. Ann. Otol. Rhinol. Laryngol., 15:213, 1902.

Friedrich, H. C.: Zur Therapie des Rhinophyma. Aesth. Med. (Berlin), 16:169, 1967.

Fry, J. H., and Robertson, W. B.: Interlocked stresses in human septal cartilage. Br. J. Plast. Surg., 19:392, 1967.

Furakawa, M.: Oriental rhinoplasty. Clinics in Plastic Surgery, 1:129, 1974.

Furnas, D. W.: Neonatal nasolabial gangrene. Plast. Reconstr. Surg., 41:381, 1968.

Gibson, T., and Davis, W. B.: The distortion of autogenous cartilage grafts: Its cause and prevention. Br. J. Plast. Surg., *10*:257, 1958.

Gibson, T., Curran, R. C., and Davis, W. B.: The survival of living homograft cartilages in man. Transplant. Bull., *4*:105, 1957.

Gifford, G. H., Swanson, L., and MacCollum, D. W.: Congenital absence of the nose and anterior nasopharynx. Plast. Reconstr. Surg., *50*:5, 1972.

Gillies, H. D.: Plastic Surgery of the Face. London, Oxford University Press, 1920, p. 274.

Gillies, H. D.: Deformities of the syphilitic nose. Br. Med. J., *29*:977, 1923.

Gillies, H. D.: Experiences with the tubed pedicle flaps. Surg. Gynecol. Obstet., *60*:291, 1935.

Gillies, H. D.: A new free graft applied to the reconstruction of the nostril. Br. J. Surg., *30*:305, 1943.

Gillies, H.: The columella. Br. J. Plast. Surg., *2*:192, 1949.

Gillies, H. D., and Kristensen, H. K.: Ox cartilage in plastic surgery. Br. J. Plast. Surg., *4*:63, 1951.

Gillies, H. D., and Millard, D. R., Jr.: Principles and Art of Plastic Surgery. Boston, Little, Brown and Company, 1957.

Gitlin, G., and Behar, A. J.: Meningeal angeomatosis, arhinencephaly; agenesis of the corpus callosum and large hamartome of the brain with neoplasia, in an infant having bilateral nasal proboscis. Acta Anat., *41*:56, 1960.

Gnudi, M. T., and Webster, J. P.: The Life and Times of Gaspare Tagliacozzi, Surgeon of Bologna, 1545–1599. New York, H. Reichner, 1950.

Graefe, C. F. von: Rhinoplastik, oder die Kunst den verlust der Nase organisch zu ersetzen in ihren früheren Verhältnissne erforscht und durch neue Verfahrungsweisen zur höheren Vollkommenheit gefördert. Berlin, Realschulbuchhandlung, 1818.

Grattan, J. F.: Rhinophyma. Surg. Gynecol. Obstet., *41*:99, 1925.

Gruenwald, L.: Quoted by Brunner and Harned (1942).

Haas, E.: Experience with "kiel bone graft" in the correction of saddle nose deformities. J. Laryngol. Rhinol. Otol., *42*:440, 1963.

Hadley, R. C.: Personal communication, 1975.

Heanley, C.: The subcutaneous tissue pedicle flap in columellar and other nasal reconstruction. Br. J. Plast. Surg., *8*:60, 1955.

Herceg, S. J., and Harding, R. L.: Gradenigo's syndrome following correction of a posterior choanal atresia. Plast. Reconstr. Surg., *48*:181, 1971.

Herrmann, I. F., and Klein, P. P.: Electrocoagulation in the treatment of choanal atresia in the newborn. J. Laryngol. Otol., *84*:1257, 1971.

Hilger, J. A.: The internal osteotomy in rhinoplasty. Arch. Otolaryngol., *88*:211, 1968.

Howarth, J. C., Medovy, H., and Lewis, A. J.: Cebocephaly with endocrine dysgenesis. Report of three cases. J. Pediatr., *59*:726, 1961.

Israel, J.: Zwei neue Methoden der Nasenplastik. Lagenbecks Arch. Klin. Chir., *53*:255, 1896.

Ivy, R. H.: Repair of acquired defects of the face. J.A.M.A., *84*:181, 1925.

Jobert, A. J.: Traité de Chirurgie Plastique. Paris, J. B. Baillière et fils, 1849.

Johnson, G. F., and Weisman, P. A.: Radiological features of dermoid cyst of nose. Radiology, *82*:1016, 1964.

Johnson, N. E.: Septal surgery and rhinoplasty. Trans. Am. Acad. Ophthalmol. Otolaryngol., *68*:869, 1964.

Joseph, J.: Handbuch d. Spezielle Chir., Kats, Preysing, Blumenfeld, 1912.

Joseph, J.: Nasenplastik und sontige Gesichtplastik (nebst einem Anhang uber Mammaplastik und einige weitere Operationen aus dem Gebiete ausserer Korperplastik;

ein Atlas und Lehrbuch). Leipzig, Kabitzsch, 1931, pp. 498–842.

Jost, G., and Mahé, E.: Le bec de corbin. Ann. Chir. Plast., *17*:5, 1972.

Jost, G., Vergnon, L., and Hadjean, E.: Les asymétries nasales postopératoires. Ann. Chir. Plast., *20*:123, 1973.

Kavrakirov, V.: On the problem of total rhinoplasty with a Filatov's flap stripped of fat. Acta Chir. Plast., *3*:241, 1961.

Kazanjian, V. H.: Plastic repair of deformities about the lower part of the nose resulting from loss of tissue. Trans. Am. Acad. Ophthalmol. Otolaryngol., *42*:338, 1937.

Kazanjian, V. H.: The treatment of congenital atresia. Ann. Otol. Rhinol. Laryngol., *51*:704, 1942.

Kazanjian, V. H.: The repair of nasal defects with the median forehead flap. Primary closure of the forehead wound. Surg. Gynecol. Obstet., *83*:37, 1946.

Kazanjian, V. H.: Nasal deformities of syphilitic origin. Plast. Reconstr. Surg., *3*:517, 1948.

Kazanjian, V. H., and Roopenian, A.: The surgical treatment of basal cell carcinoma of the external nose. Trans. Am. Acad. Ophthalmol. Otolaryngol., *67*:37, 1963.

Keegan, D. G.: Rhinoplastic Operations. London, Ballière, Tindall & Cox, 1900.

Kernahan, D. A., and Littlewood, A. H.: Experiences in use of arterial flaps about the face. Plast. Reconstr. Surg., *28*:207, 1961.

Killian, G.: Die submucose Fensterresektion der Nasenscheidewand. Arch. Laryngol. Rhinol. (Berl.), *16*:362, 1904.

Kilner, T. P.: Plastic surgery. *In* Maingot, R. (Ed.): Postgraduate Surgery. Vol. 3. New York, Appleton-Century-Crofts, 1937.

Kilner, T. P.: Unusual congenital malformation of the face. Rev. Chir. Structive, *8*:164, 1938.

Kirschner, J. A.: Traumatic nasal deformity in the newborn. A. M. A. Arch. Otolaryngol., *62*:139, 1955.

König, F.: Eine neue Methode der Aufrichtung eingesunkener Nasen durch Bildung des Nasenruckens aus einem Haut-Periost-Knochenlappen der Stirn. Verh. Dtsch. Ges. Chir. (Berl.), *15*:41, 1886.

König, F.: Eine neue Methode der Aufrichtung eingesunkener Nasen durch Bildung des Nasenruckens aus einem Haut-Periost-Knochenlappen der Stirn. Arch. Klin. Chir., *34*:165, 1887.

Kravits, H., Driessen, G., Gomberg, R., and Korach, A.: Accidental falls from elevated surfaces in infants from birth to one year of age. Pediatrics (Suppl), *44*:869, 1969.

Kubaček, V.: Transposition of flaps in the face on a subcutaneous pedicle. Acta Chir. Plast., *2*:108, 1960.

Labat, M.: De la rhinoplastie. Ann. Med. Physiol., *23*:319, 1833.

Labat, M.: De la rhinoplastie, art de restaurer ou de refaire complètement le nez. Thesis, Paris, 1834.

Lewin, M. L.: Total rhinoplasty in infants. Report of a case of Waterhouse-Friderichsen syndrome. Trans. 1st Internatl. Congr. Soc. Plast. Surg., Baltimore, The Williams & Wilkins Company, 1957.

Lewin, M. L.: Subtotal nasal reconstruction in infants and children for the correction of acquired defects. *In* Hueston, J. T. (Ed.): Transactions of the Fifth International Congress of Plastic and Reconstructive Surgery. Melbourne, Australia, Butterworths, 1971.

Lexer, E.: Die gesamte Wiederherstellurge-Chirurgie. Leipzig, Johann Ambrosius Barth, 1931.

Lipschutz, H.: A clinical evaluation of subdermal and subcutaneous silicone implants. Plast. Reconstr. Surg., *37*:249, 1966.

Lipschutz, H., and Abramson, B.: Complete bilateral bony choanal atresia: A new approach to its correction and report of a case. Plast. Reconstr. Surg., *39*:465, 1967.

Lipsett, E. M.: A new approach to surgery of the lower cartilaginous vault. Arch. Otolaryngol., *70*:42, 1959.

Lisfranc, J.: Rhinoplastie. Clin. Hôp. Paris, *2*:285, 1827.

Liston, R.: Practical Surgery. London, J. & A. Churchill, 1837.

Longacre, J. J., and DeStefano, G. A.: Reconstruction of extensive defects of the skull with split rib grafts. Plast. Reconstr. Surg., *19*:186, 1957.

Lössen, H.: Ueber Rhinoplastik mit Einfügen einer Prosthesis. Münch. Med. Wochenschr., *45*:1527, 1898.

McDonald, T. J., Devine, K. D., and Hayles, A. B.: Nasopharyngeal stenosis following tonsillectomy and adenoidectomy. Arch. Otolaryngol., *98*:38, 1973.

McDowell, F.: Personal observation, 1969.

McDowell, F., Valone, J. A., and Brown, J. B.: Bibliography and historical note on plastic surgery of nose. Plast. Reconstr. Surg., *10*:149, 1952.

McGovern, F. H.: The association of congenital choanal atresia and congenital heart disease. Ann. Otolaryngol. (Paris), *62*:894, 1953.

McGovern, F. H.: Bilateral choanal atresia in the newborn. A new method of medical management. Laryngoscope, *71*:480, 1961.

McGovern, F. H., and Fitzhugh, G. S.: Surgical management of congenital choanal atresia. Arch. Otolaryngol., *73*:627, 1961.

McGregor, I. A., and Jackson, I. T.: The extended role of the deltopectoral flap. Br. J. Plast. Surg., *23*:173, 1970.

McLaughlin, C. R.: Composite ear grafts and their blood supply. Br. J. Plast. Surg., *7*:274, 1954.

Malbec, E. F., and Beaux, A. R.: Reconstruction of columella. Br. J. Plast. Surg., *11*:142, 1958.

Malgaigne, J. F.: Traité d'Anatomie Chirurgicale et Chirurgie Expérimentale. Paris, G. Ballière, 1838.

Maliniac, J. W.: Rhinophyma, Compte Rendu. Acad. Sci. (Paris), 1930, pp. 250–257.

Mangold, F. von: Ueber die Einpflanzung von Rippenknorpel in den Kehlkopf zur Heilung Schwerer Stenosen und Defecte. Arch. Klin. Chir., *59*:926, 1899.

Marks, B.: Pathogenesis of rosacea. Br. J. Dermatol., *80*:170, 1968.

Matton, G., Pickrell, K., Hugher, W., and Pound, E.: The surgical treatment of rhinophyma. Plast. Reconstr. Surg., *30*:403, 1962.

Medawar, P. D.: Notes on problems of skin homografts. Bull. War Med., *4*:1, 1942.

Meyer, R.: Nasal-septal perforation and nostril stenosis. *In* Goldwyn, R. M. (Ed.): The Unfavorable Result in Plastic Surgery. Boston, Little, Brown and Company, 1972.

Millard, D. R., Jr.: The triad of columella deformities. Plast. Reconstr. Surg., *31*:370, 1963.

Millard, D. R., Jr.: Total reconstructive rhinoplasty and a missing link. Plast. Reconstr. Surg., *37*:167, 1966.

Millard, D. R., Jr.: Hemirhinoplasty. Plast. Reconstr. Surg., *40*:440, 1967a.

Millard, D. R., Jr.: Alar margin sculpturing. Plast. Reconstr. Surg., *40*:337, 1967b.

Millard, D. R., Jr.: Secondary corrective rhinoplasty. Plast. Reconstr. Surg., *44*:545, 1969.

Millard, D. R., Jr.: Congenital nasal tip retrusion and three little composite ear grafts. Plast. Reconstr. Surg., *48*:501, 1971.

Millard, D. R., Jr.: Reconstructive rhinoplasty for the lower half of a nose. Plast. Reconstr. Surg., *53*:133, 1974.

Mink, P. J.: Physiologie der oberen Luftwege. Leipzig, Vogel, 1920.

Mohs, F. E.: Chemosurgery in Cancer. Springfield, Ill., Charles C Thomas, Publisher, 1956a.

Mohs, F. E.: The chemosurgical method for the microscopically controlled excision of cancer of the skin. N.Y. State J. Med., *56*:3481, 1956b.

Monks, G. H.: The restoration of a lower eyelid by new method. Boston Med. Surg., *139*:385, 1898.

Monvalliu, G.: Basal cell carcinomata of the head and neck. Br. J. Plast. Surg., *21*:200, 1968.

Mosher, H. P.: The direct method of correcting lateral deformity of the nasal bones. Laryngoscope, *16*:28, 1906.

Mowlem, R.: The use and behavior of iliac bone grafts in the restoration of nasal contour. Clinical and radiographic observations. Rev. Chir. Structive, *8*:23, 1938.

Murray, J. E., and Cannon, B.: Basal cell cancer in children and young adults. New Engl. J. Med., *262*:440, 1960.

Natvig, P.: Personal communication, 1975.

Natvig, P., Sether, L. A., Gingrass, R. P., and Gardner, W. D.: Anatomical details of the osseous-cartilaginous framework of the nose. Plast. Reconstr. Surg., *48*:528, 1971.

Nélaton, C.: Discussion sur la rhinoplastie. Bull. Mém. Soc. Chir. Paris, *28*:458, 1902.

Nélaton, C., and Ombrédanne, L.: La Rhinoplastie. Paris, G. Steinheil, 1904.

New, G. B.: Sickle flap for nasal reconstruction. Surg. Gynecol. Obstet., *80*:597, 1945.

New, G. B., and Erich, J. B.: Dermoid cyst of the head and neck. Surg. Gynecol. Obstet., *65*:48, 1937.

New, G. B., and Erich, J. B.: A method to prevent fresh costal cartilage grafts from warping. Am. J. Surg., *54*:435, 1941.

O'Connor, G. B., and McGregor, M. W.: Secondary rhinoplasties; their cause and prevention. Plast. Reconstr. Surg., *15*:404, 1955.

Odou, B. L., and Odou, E. R.: Rhinophyma. Am. J. Surg., *102*:3, 1961.

Ohmori, S., Tange, I., Fukada, O., Soeda, S., and Ito, M.: Median cleft nose: A report of two cases. Jap. J. Plast. Reconstr. Surg., *5*:199, 1962.

Ollier, L.: Application de l'ostéoplastie à la réstauration du nez; transplantation du périoste frontal. Bull. Gén. Thérapeut., *61*:510, 1861.

Orentreich, N.: Personal communication, 1976.

Orticochea, M.: A new method for total reconstruction of the nose: The ears as donor areas. Br. J. Plast. Surg., *24*:225, 1971.

Ortiz-Monasterio, F.: Personal communication, 1975.

Owens, H.: Observations in treating twenty-five cases of choanal atresia by the transpalatine approach. Laryngoscope, *75*:84, 1965.

Paletta, F. X., and Van Norman, R. T.: Total reconstruction of the columella. Plast. Reconstr. Surg., *30*:322, 1962.

Paré, A.: Les oeuvres de M. Ambroise Paré, conseiller et premier chirurgien du roy. Avec les figures et portraits tan de l'anatomie que des instruments de chirurgie, et de plusieurs monstres. Le tout divisé en vingt-six livres, comme il est contenu en la page suyvente. Paris, G. Buone, 1575.

Parkes, M. L., and Brennan, H. G.: High septal transfixion to shorten the nose. Plast. Reconstr. Surg., *45*:487, 1970.

Parkes, M. L., and Brennan, H. G.: Familial choanal atresia in a rhinoplasty candidate—A case report. Eye, Ear, Nose and Throat Monthly, *52*:46, 1973.

Peet, E. W., and Patterson, T. J.: The Essentials of Plastic Surgery. Oxford, Blackwell Scientific Publications, 1964.

Penn, J.: The reconstruction of the nose. Br. J. Plast. Surg., 20:369, 1967.

Pollet, J., and Baudelot, S.: Séquelles de la chirurgie esthétique de la base du nez. An.. Chir. Plast., 12:185, 1967.

Pratt, L. W.: Acquired nasopharyngeal stenosis. Laryngoscope, 84:707, 1974.

Rees, T. D.: Nasal plastic surgery in the Negro. Plast. Reconstr. Surg., 43:13, 1969.

Rees, T. D.: An aid in the reduction of the supratip swelling after rhinoplasty. Laryngoscope, 81:308, 1971.

Rees, T. D., Wood-Smith, D.: Cosmetic Facial Surgery. Philadelphia, W. B. Saunders Company, 1972.

Rees, T. D., Wood-Smith, D., Converse, J. M., and Guy, C. L.: Composite grafts. Third International Congress of Plastic Surgery, Excerpta Medica Foundation, Washington, D.C., 1963.

Rees, T. D., Krupp, S., and Wood-Smith, D.: Secondary rhinoplasty. Plast. Reconstr. Surg., 46:332, 1970.

Reid: Ueber angeboren Hirbruche in der Stirn und Nasenegend. Illus. Med. Ztg., 1:133, 1852.

Rethi, A.: Raccourcissement du nez trop long. Rev. Chir. Plast., 2:85, 1934.

Ribbert, V. A.: Ueber Bau, Wachstum und Genese der Angiome, nebst Bemerkungen ueber Ceptenbildung. Virchows Arch. Pathol. Anat., 151:381, 1898.

Robin, J. L.: Réduction extra-muqueuse contrôlée de l'arête nasale. Proceedings of the Ninth International Congress of Otolaryngology, Mexico. Amsterdam, Excerpta Medica International Series No. 206, 711, 1969.

Robin, J. L.: Rhinoplastie extra-muqueuse controlée avec measure pré-opératoire de la modification du profil. Ann. Chir. Plast., 18:119, 1973.

Robins, P.: Personal communication, 1975.

Roe, J. O.: See Converse (1970).

Rogers, B. O.: The importance of "delay" in timing secondary and tertiary correction of post-rhinoplastic deformities. Transactions of the Fourth International Congress of Plastic Reconstructive Surgery, 1967. Amsterdam, Excerpta Medica Foundation, 1969.

Rogers, B. O.: Rhinoplasty. *In* Goldwyn, R. M. (Ed.): The Unfavorable Result in Plastic Surgery. Boston, Little, Brown and Company, 1972.

Rogers, B. O.: The role of physical anthropology in plastic surgery today. Clinics in Plastic Surgery, 1:439, 1974.

Rogers, B. O., and Converse, J. M.: Bovine embryo skin zoografts as temporary biologic dressings for burns and other skin defects. Plast. Reconstr. Surg., 22:471, 1958.

Ronaldson, T. R.: Bilateral membranous atresia. Edinburgh Med. J., 26:1035, 1880–1881.

Roopenian, A., and Stemmer, A. L.: Congenital posterior choanal atresia. Am. J. Surg., 96:802, 1958.

Rose, D. E.: Nasal glioma. Laryngoscope, 76:1602, 1966.

Safian, J.: Corrective Rhinoplastic Surgery. New York, Paul B. Hoeber, 1934.

Schimmelbusch, C.: Ein veues Verfahren der Rhinoplastik und Operation der sattelnase. Verh. Dtsch. Ges. Chir., 28:342, 1895.

Schmid, E.: Ueber neue Wege in der plastischen Chirurgie der Nase. Beitr. Klin. Chir., 184:385, 1952.

Schmidt, M. D.: Ueber seltene Spaltbildungen in Bereiche des mittleren Stirnfortsatzes. Virchows Arch. Pathol. Anat., 162:340, 1900.

Sebenkoff: Quoted by Warkany (1971).

Sédillot, C.: Nouveau procédé et observation de rhinoplastie. Gaz. Med. Strasb., 16:269, 1856.

Serre, M.: Traité sur l'art de réstaurer les difformités de la face, selon la méthode par déplacement ou méthode française. Montpellier, L. Castel, 1842.

Shaw, M. H., and Fell, S. R.: Columella reconstruction. Br. J. Plast. Surg., 1:111, 1948.

Sheehan, J. E.: Plastic Surgery of the Nose. London, Oxford University Press, 1937.

Sheen, J. H.: Achieving more nasal tip projection by the use of a small autogenous vomer or septal cartilage graft. Plast. Reconstr. Surg., 56:35, 1975a.

Sheen, J. H.: Secondary rhinoplasty. Plast. Reconstr. Surg., 56:137, 1975b.

Sheen, J.: Personal communication, 1976.

Sheftel, M. P.: Operativnoe ustranenie Vrozhdennogo sradinnogo rasshschepleniia Naruzhnogo Nosa. Vestn. Otorinolaring., 20:21, 1958.

Singleton, G. T., and Hardcastle, B.: Congenital choanal atresia. Arch. Otolaryngol., 87:74, 1968.

Skoog, T.: A method of hump reduction in rhinoplasty. Arch. Otolaryngol., 83:115, 1966.

Skoog, T.: Plastic Surgery—New Methods and Refinements. Philadelphia, W. B. Saunders Company, 1974.

Smithdeal, C. D.: Personal communication, 1975.

Song, I. C., Wise, A. J., and Bromberg, B. E.: Total nasal reconstruction. Br. J. Plast. Surg., 26:414, 1973.

Spina, V.: Nariz negroide-technica personal. Presented at the Third Latin American Plastic Surgery Congress, Lima, Peru, Oct., 1966.

Steiss, C. F.: Errors in rhinoplasty and their prevention. Plast. Reconstr. Surg., 28:276, 1951.

Stoll, H. L., Milgrom, H., and Traenkle, H. L.: Results of roentgen therapy of carcinoma of the nose. Arch. Dermatol., 90:577, 1964.

Straatsma, B. R., and Straatsma, C. R.: The anatomical relationship of the lateral nasal cartilage to the nasal bone and the cartilaginous nasal septum. Plast. Reconstr. Surg., 8:443, 1951.

Stupkaw, W.: Quoted by Warkany (1971).

Sussenguth, L.: Ueber Nasegliome. Virchows Arch. Pathol. Anat., 195:537, 1909.

Szymanowski, J. von: Handbuch der Operativen Chirurgie. Braunschweig, F. Vieweg. u. Sohn, 1870.

Tagliacozzi, G.: De Curtorum Chirurgia per Institionem. Venetiis, B. Bindonus, 1597.

Testut, L., and Jacob, O.: Traité d'Anatomie Topographique avec Applications Médico-chirurgicales. Paris, Octave Doin & Cie, 1929.

Thiersch, C.: Ueber eine rhinoplastische Modification. Verh. Dtsch. Ges. Chir., 8:67, 1879.

Thomas, L.: Observation de fissure congénitale du nez. Bull. Soc. Chir. Paris, 2:162, 1873.

Thomson, S. C.: Disease of the Nose. *In* Thomson, S. C., and Negus, V. E.: Disease of the Nose and Throat. 4th Ed. New York, D. Appleton, 1937.

Uchida, J.: The Practice of Plastic Surgery. Tokyo, Kinbara, 1958.

Van Dishoek, H. A. E.: Elektograms der Nasenflugelmuskein und Nasenwiderstandskurve. Acta Otolaryngol., 25:285, 1937.

Velpeau, A. A. L. M.: Nouveaux Eléments de Médecine Opératoire. Paris, J. B. Balliére, 1839.

Vergnon, L., and Jost, G.: A propos du bec de corbin physio-pathogènia et prévention. Ann. Chir. Plast., 20:69, 1975.

Verneuil, A.: Mémoires de Chirurgie. Paris, B. Masson, 1877–1888.

Volkmann, A. W.: Technique described in Gesellschft. für Chir., 3:20, 1874.

Voltaire, F. M. D. de: Oeuvres Complètes. Imprimerie de la Societé littéraire-typographique. Paris, 1785.

Wahby, B.: Abnormal nasal bones. J. Anat. Physiol., 38:49, 1903.

Walker, D. G.: Malformation of the Face. Edinburgh, E. & S. Livingston, 1961, p. 31.

Walsh, T. S., and Tompkins, V. N.: Some observations on the strawberry nevus of infancy. Cancer, *9*:869, 1956.

Ward, N.: A case of rhinoplastic operation. Med. Times Gaz., London, *12*:285, 1856.

Warkany, J.: Congenital Malformation. Chicago, Year Book Medical Publishers, 1971.

Warren, J. M.: Rhinoplastic operation. Boston Med. Surg. J., *16*:69, 1837.

Washio, H.: Retroauricular temporal flap. Plast. Reconstr. Surg., *43*:162, 1969.

Washio, H.: Further experiences with the retroauricular temporal flap. Plast. Reconstr. Surg., *50*:160, 1972.

Weaver, D. F., and Billings, D. H.: Bifid nose with midline cleft of the upper lip. Arch. Otolaryngol., *44*:480, 1946.

Webster, J. P., and Deming, E. G.: Surgical treatment of bifid nose. Plast. Reconstr. Surg., *6*:1, 1950.

Weir, R. R.: On restoring sunken noses without scarring the face. N.Y. Med. J., *56*:499, 1892.

Wen, I. C.: Ontogeny and phylogeny of the nasal cartilages. Contributions to Embryology, Carnegie Institution, *414*:109, 1921.

Wilke, J.: Beitrag zum Problem der Nasendoppelbildungen. Z. Laryngol., *37*:770, 1958.

Williams, H.: Posterior choanal atresia. Am. J. Roentgenol. Radium Ther. Nucl. Med., *112*:1, 1971.

Young, F.: The repair of nasal losses. Surgery, *20*:670, 1946.

Young, F.: The surgical repair of nasal deformities. Plast. Reconstr. Surg., *4*:59, 1949.

Zeis, E.: Handbuch der plastischen Chirurgie (nebst einer Vorrede von J. F. Dieffenbach). Berlin, Reiner, 1838.

Zukerhandl, E.: Normal u. Pathol. Anat. der Nasenhohlen. Wien, Braumuller, 1892.

INDEX

i

Apertognathism. See *Open bite.*
Apert's syndrome, *31, 33,* 832, 2321–2327, 2407, 2465, 2466
  anatomical pathology in, 2468–2472
  calvarium in, 2468, 2469, *2469*
  coronal synostosis in, 2495
  cranial fossa and orbits in, 2469–2471
  etiopathogenesis of, 2321, 2322
  extremity and skeletal deformities in, 2322–2326, *2326,* 2327, 2472, *2472*
  facial deformities in, 2324, 2472
  history of, 2321
  Le Fort III osteotomy in, 2477, 2480
  maxilla in, 2471, 2472
  neurosurgery in, 2324, 2325
  ocular deformities in, 2322, *2323,* 2471
  orbital hypertelorism in, 2437, *2439, 2443*
  physical characteristics of, 2322–2324
  preoperative cephalometric planning in, 2482, *2484*
  ptosis of upper eyelid in, 2472, 2485
  reconstructive surgery in, 2325–2327
  skull deformities in, 2322, *2326*
  syndactyly in, 3311, 3313–3319
  treatment of, 2324–2327
Apical ectodermal ridge (AER), and hand and limb deformities, 3308, 3309, *3309,* 3310
Aplasia cutis congenita, 827, 828
Apocrine sweat glands, *153,* 155
Arch and band appliances, in maxillofacial prosthetics, 2920, *2920,* 2921
Arch bar fixation, 649–651, *651–653*
  in jaw deformities, 1300, *1301*
  in mandibular fractures, 669, *669,* 670
  in maxillary fractures, 700–702
Arch bars, prefabricated, in mandibular fractures, 665, 667, *667*
Arch wires, banded dental, in mandibular fractures, 667, *668,* 669
  cable, in fixation of facial bone fractures in children, 800, *801*
  in mandibular fractures, 667, *668*
Areola, simulation of by tattooing, *3722,* 3723
Areola-nipple complex, reconstruction of after radical mastectomy, *3716–3719,* 3720–3723
Arhinencephaly, 2128
  orbital hypotelorism in, 2462, *2462,* 2463, *2463, 2464*
  with median cleft lip, *1180,* 1181
Aries-Pitanguy technique of breast reduction, 3667, *3668, 3669*
Arm. See also *Extremity, upper.*
  thoracobrachial flap in repair of, 215, *215*
Arm flap technique, of nose repair, 5, 6
Arrector pili muscle, 154, 155
  in dermis graft, *249*
Arsenical keratoses, 2858, 3456
Arterial flaps, 194, *194,* 217
Arterial occlusion, in microvascular replants, 371
Arterial repair, microvascular, 358, *358–362*
Arteriovenous aneurysm, of jaws, 2567, *2567, 2568*
Arteriovenous fistula, of hand, *3483*
Artery(arteries)
  auricular, 1521
  direct cutaneous, 193, *193*
  epigastric, 3041, *3042*
  facial, transverse, 1779
  lingual, distribution of, 2701, *2701*
  microvascular repair patency rates for, 353, 353t, 354
  musculocutaneous, 193, *193*

Artery(arteries) *(Continued)*
  occipital, 1779
  of abdominal wall, 3729
  radial, 2976
  stylomastoid, 1779
  superficial temporal, 1779
    and forehead flap, 217, *217*
  ulnar, 2976
Artery island flap, 959, *961, 962*
Arthritis, of hand, 3507–3518
  correction of early ulnar drift in, 3514, 3515, *3515*
  degenerative, 3507–3511
  digital joints in, 3515–3517
  gouty, 3511, *3511*
  intrinsic muscle release in, 3514, *3514*
  muscles in, 3513–3515
  rheumatoid, 3511–3518
  surgical treatment of, 3512–3518
  synovectomy for, 3512, 3513
  tendons and tendon sheaths in, 3512, 3513
  thumb in, 3517, 3518
Arthrodesis, small joint, in arthritic hand, 3510, 3511, *3511*
Arthroplasty, in arthritic hand, 3508, 3516
Arthrosis, temporomandibular, 1529, *1529*
Articular disc, 1521, 1522, *1522*
Asche forceps, for reduction of nasal fractures, 727, *727,* 728, *785*
Asche metal, in splinting of nose, 1087, *1087, 1088*
Ascites, chylous, 3586, *3587*
Ascorbic acid depletion, and wound healing, 92, 93
Ashley operation, in repair of lower lip defect, 1567, 1568, *1568*
Ashley prosthesis, for mammary augmentation, 3697, 3698
L-Asparaginase, and immunosuppression, 138
Asphyxia neonatorum, 1165
Aspirin, and craniofacial clefts, 2123
  in microvascular surgery, 367
Atheroma, 2784–2786
Atriodigital dysplasia, 3334
Atropine absorption test, of flap circulation, 195
Auditory canal, external, stenosis of, 1735, *1735,* 1736
Auditory meatus, external, 2309
Aufricht retractor, 1070, *1070*
Auricle. See also *Ear.*
  amputated, replantation of, 1725–1732
    as composite graft, 1728, 1731, 1732, *1734*
    dermabrasion and, 1727, 1728, *1731*
    microsurgery and, 1732
    upon removal of medial auricular skin and fenestration of cartilage, 1728, *1732*
    with auricular cartilage, 1727, *1729, 1730*
    with auricular tissue as composite graft, 1727, *1728*
    with auricular tissue attached by narrow pedicle, *1726,* 1727, *1727*
  anatomy of, 1672, *1672, 1673*
  avulsion of, *1747*
  deformities of, 1671–1773
    acquired, 1724–1768
      amputation, 1725–1732
      full-thickness, 1744–1768
        following trauma, 1744–1750
        partial, 1750–1761
      with loss of auricular tissue, 1736–1743
      without loss of auricular tissue, 1732–1736
    burn, 1636